renal ex

11, 12, 5, 6

(1, 2, 3, 4) combining
forms

The Language
of Medicine

resp
card.   86%.
8 J

michele 5693552
jola - 846 33 26
6e NINA - 918 1069

Davi-Ellen Chabner, BA, MAT

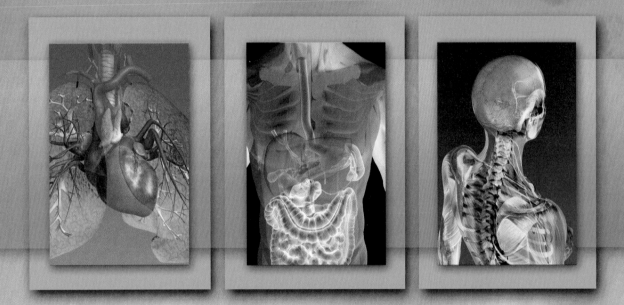

The Language of Medicine

Eighth Edition

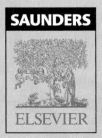

SAUNDERS

ELSEVIER

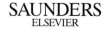

SAUNDERS
ELSEVIER

11830 Westline Industrial Drive
St. Louis, Missouri 63146

THE LANGUAGE OF MEDICINE, EIGHTH EDITION

ISBN 13: 978-1-4160-3492-6
ISBN 10: 1-4160-3492-7

ISBN 13: 978-1-4160-3492-6
ISBN 10: 1-4160-3492-7

Executive Editor: Jeanne Wilke
Senior Developmental Editor: Becky Swisher
Publishing Services Manager: Patricia Tannian
Project Manager: John Casey
Senior Designer: Ellen Zanolle

Illustrations by Jim Perkins

Printed in United States of America

Last digit is the print number: 9   8   7   6   5   4   3   2   1

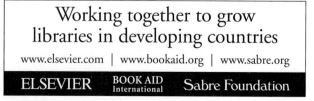

*To my students, past and present, who are my devoted
classroom partners. Your enthusiasm and excitement for learning
are my inspiration.*

and

*To my fellow instructors of medical terminology who
share my passion for teaching. Your insights, communication,
and encouragement are vital to my writing.*

Preface

Welcome to the 8th edition of *The Language of Medicine*. The focus of this new edition is **illumination** . . . the act of brightening and enlightening to enhance understanding. From the brilliant cover design with dynamic anatomic images to the colorfully crafted new interior, the book attracts and draws today's student into the exciting world of medical concepts and terms!*

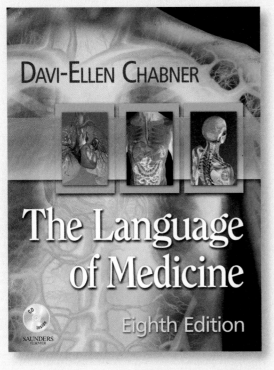

While the year 2007 marks the 31st anniversary of the 1st edition, *The Language of Medicine* continues to speak to students of all backgrounds and levels by presenting an engaging and accessible pathway to learning. Students interact on practically every page of this workbook text through writing and reviewing terms, labeling diagrams, and answering questions. As in all past editions, my primary objective is to explain terminology in its proper context, which is the structure and function of the human body in health and disease.

The Language of Medicine is written in simple, non-technical language so that ideas and terminology are easy to understand. Throughout this revision, I have listened to scores of students and instructors and incorporated their valuable suggestions and comments. Expert medical reviewers have once again provided insight and advice about relevant and cutting edge clinical medical terminology. New information and illustrations reflect the impact of each reviewer.

My continued goal in writing *The Language of Medicine* is to help students learn and to help instructors teach. Using an interactive, logical, interesting, and easy-to-follow method, you will find that medical terminology comes "alive" and stays with you. Undeniably, the study of this language requires commitment and hard work, but the benefits are great. The knowledge that you gain will jump-start your career in the medical workplace and help you for years to come!

---

*Continuing in this edition is the omission of the possessive form of all eponyms (e.g., Down syndrome, Tourette syndrome, Alzheimer disease). While the possessive form remains acceptable, this text is responding to a growing trend in promoting consistency and clarity. This decision is supported by The American Association for Medical Transcription in their *Manual of Style* (2002) and the American Medical Association in their *Manual of Style,* 10th edition (Williams & Wilkins), as well as by major medical dictionaries. Note: When eponyms appear without a noun (such as disease or syndrome), it is recommended that the possessive be retained (e.g., The patient is seen for Alzheimer's).

NEW TO THE 8TH EDITION

While the essential elements of *The Language of Medicine* remain in place, the 8th edition is more visually dynamic and engaging than ever before.

The exciting body system images on each two-page chapter opener actively introduce each chapter and invite you to explore. You can navigate the book easily with this new visual approach, and instructors can more effectively use and teach medical terminology.

Each illustration is realistic and three dimensional. New images have been added to enhance your understanding of anatomy, physiology, and pathology.

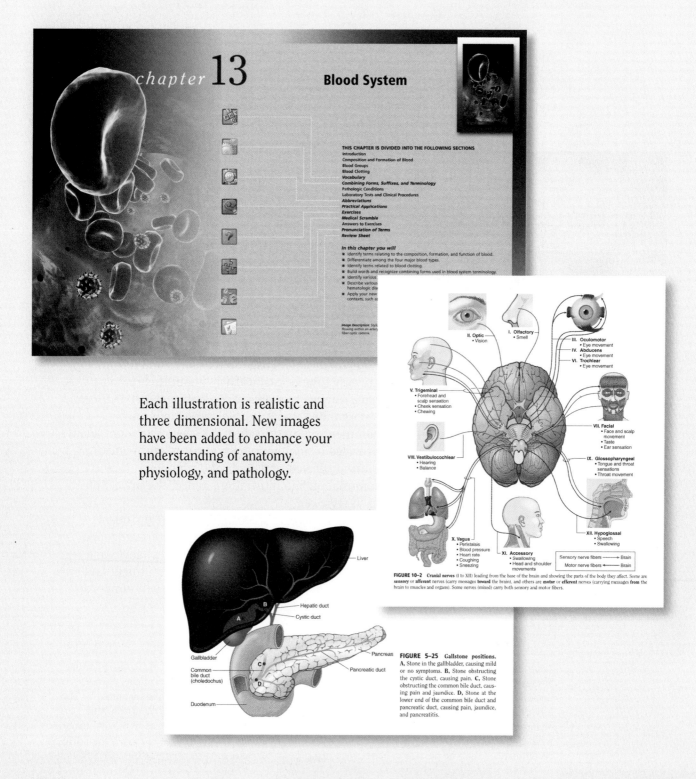

FIGURE 10-2 Cranial nerves (I to XII) leading from the base of the brain and showing the parts of the body they affect. Some are *sensory* or **afferent** nerves (carry messages **toward** the brain), and others are *motor* or **efferent** nerves (carrying messages **from** the brain to muscles and organs). Some nerves (mixed) carry both sensory and motor fibers.

FIGURE 5-25 Gallstone positions. **A,** Stone in the gallbladder, causing mild or no symptoms. **B,** Stone obstructing the cystic duct, causing pain. **C,** Stone obstructing the common bile duct, causing pain and jaundice. **D,** Stone at the lower end of the common bile duct and pancreatic duct, causing pain, jaundice, and pancreatitis.

New photographs of conditions and medical procedures have been added as well. This helps you see terminology in action.

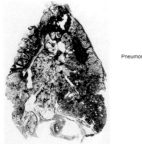
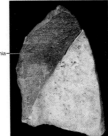

FIGURE 12–11   A. Anthracosis or black lung disease. Notice the dark black deposits of coal dust throughout the lung. **B. Lobar pneumonia** (at autopsy). Notice that the condition affects a lobe of the lung. The patient's signs and symptoms included fever, chills, cough, dark sputum, rapid shallow breathing, and cyanosis. If diagnosis is made early, antibiotic therapy is successful.

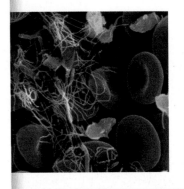
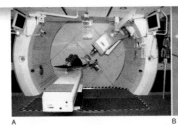

FIGURE 19–11   A. Proton therapy machine. Proton beam radiation therapy is useful in treating a variety of cancers including head and neck, brain, sarcomas, eye tumors, prostate, chest, and GI tumors. **B. Proton stereotactic radiosurgery.** A model poses to show how a proton beam device is brought near a patient in preparation for stereotactic radiosurgery. (Courtesy of Dr. Jay Loeffler, Massachusetts General Hospital Radiation Oncology Department, Boston.)

SPOTLIGHTS

Chapters include a new feature called Spotlights. The purpose of these Spotlights is to give you extra information, or in many cases, alert you to commonly confused medical terms.

Shift to the Left
The phrase "shift to the left" derives from the early practice of reporting percentages of each WBC type across the top of a page, starting with blasts (immature cells) on the left and more mature cell on the right. An increase in immature neutrophils (as seen with severe infection) would be noted on a "shift to the left" indicates an infection and the body's effort to fight it b

MEDICAL SCRAMBLE

Each chapter now includes a new feature called Medical Scramble to reinforce spelling and comprehension of terms.

MEDICAL SCRAMBLE

Unscramble the letters to form urinary system terms from the clues. Use the letters in squares to complete the bonus term. Answers are found on page 243.

1. *Clue:* Pus in the urine

   _ _ _ _ _ _   RAPIYU

2. *Clue:* Blood in the urine

   _ _ _ _ _ _ _ _   TAMIHUERA

3. *Clue:* Sugar in the urine

   _ _ _ _ _ _ _ _ _   CILASGUYRO

4. *Clue:* Protein in the urine

   _ _ _ _ _ _ _ _ _   NLIBAIMURAU

5. *Clue:* An electrolyte

   _ _ _ _ _ _   MIDOSU

BONUS TERM: *Clue:* Examination of urine to determine its contents.

How to Use the Book

One of the most important aspects of *The Language of Medicine* is that it makes learning **easy**. The book **guides** and **coaches** you step by step through the learning experience. Don't get overwhelmed! Approach it systematically, step by step. I've helped you study each chapter by organizing the information in small pieces. These new icons will help you navigate the sections of the text.

After basic material in the chapter is introduced, the key terms you need to learn are presented in vocabulary lists. These lists help you study and stay focused.

Vocabulary

arteriole	Small artery.
Bowman capsule	Enclosing structure surrounding each glomerulus.
calyx *or* **calix** (*plural:* **calyces** *or* **calices**)	Cup-like collecting region of the renal pelvis.
catheter	Tube for injecting or removing fluids.
cortex	Outer region; the renal cortex is the outer region of the kidney (**cortical** means pertaining to the cortex).
creatinine	Waste product of muscle metabolism; nitrogenous waste urine. Creatinine clearance is a measure of the efficiency in removing creatinine from the blood.
electrolyte	A chemical element that carries an electrical charge when water. Examples are potassium (K^+) and sodium (Na^+), ea positive charge. The most important negatively charged el bicarbonate (HCO_3^-) and chloride (Cl^-). Electrolytes are e cellular function and transmission of impulses in nerve ar

You cannot get lost using *The Language of Medicine*. You learn and engage in small incremental steps. The book imparts the most important concepts, allowing you to concentrate on things that are essential.

Combining Forms and Terminology

Write the meanings of the medical terms in the spaces provided.

Combining Form	Meaning	Terminology	Meaning
andr/o	male	androgen *Testosterone is an androgen. The testes in males and the adrenal glands in both men and women produce androgens.*	
balan/o	glans penis (Greek *balanos*, acorn)	balanitis *Caused by overgrowth of organisms (bacteria and yeast) under the foreskin. See Figure 9–5, A.*	
cry/o	cold	cryogenic surgery *New techniques for prostate cancer treatment use cryosurgery to freeze and kill cells that radical prostatectomy cannot reach.*	
crypt/o	hidden	cryptorchism *In this congenital condition, one or both testicles do not descend, by the time of birth, into the scrotal sac from the abdominal cavity. See Figure 9–5, B.*	
epididym/o	epididymis	epididymitis *Symptoms are fever, chills, pain in the groin, tender, swollen epididymis*	
gon/o	seed (Greek *gone*, seed)	gonorrhea *See page •••.*	
hydr/o	water, fluid	hydrocele *See page •••.*	

Practical Applications

Medical terminology is connected to real life by the incorporation of scenarios, medical cases, and vignettes throughout the text and on the companion CD.

Answers to the questions about the case report and the urinalysis findings are on page 243.

UROLOGIC CASE REPORT

The patient, a 50-year-old woman, presented herself at the clinic complaining of dysuria. This symptom was followed by sudden onset of hematuria and clots. There had been no history of urolithiasis, pyuria, or previous hematuria. Nocturia had been present about 5 years earlier. Panendoscopy revealed a carcinoma located about 2 cm from the left ureteral orifice. A partial cystectomy was carried out and the lesion cleared. No ileal conduit was necessary. A metastatic workup was negative. Bilateral pelvic lymphadenectomy revealed no positive nodes.

Questions about the Case Report

1. Urologic refers to which system of the body?
   a. Digestive
   b. Reproductive
   c. Excretory
2. What was the patient's reason for appearing at the clinic?
   a. Scanty urination
   b. Inability to urinate
   c. Painful urination
3. What acute symptom followed?
   a. Blood in the feces
   b. Blood in the urine
   c. Excessive urea in the blood

As you study with *The Language of Medicine,* you are engaged in each step of the learning process. On nearly every page you are actively involved in labeling diagrams, dividing words into component parts, writing meanings to terms, testing, reviewing, and evaluating exactly what you have learned.

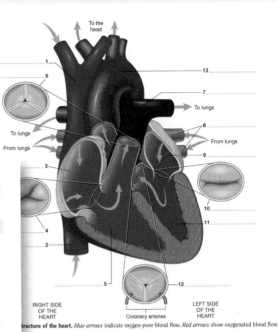

To the head

To lungs

To lungs

From lungs

From lungs

RIGHT SIDE OF THE HEART   Coronary arteries   LEFT SIDE OF THE HEART

Structure of the heart. *Blue arrows* indicate oxygen-poor blood flow. *Red arrows* show oxygenated blood flow.

EXERCISES

Remember to check your answers carefully with those given in the Answers to Exercises.

A. Match the following cells with their meanings as given below.

basophil   hematopoietic stem cell   neutrophil
eosinophil   lymphocyte   platelet
erythrocyte   monocyte

1. mononuclear white blood cell (agranulocyte) formed in lymph tissue; it is a phagocyte and the

   precursor of a macrophage _____

2. thrombocyte or cell that helps blood clot _____

3. cell in the bone marrow that gives rise to different types of blood cells _____

4. mononuclear leukocyte formed in lymph tissue; produces antibodies _____

5. leukocyte with dense, reddish granules having an affinity for red acidic dye; associated with allergic

   reactions _____

6. red blood

7. leukocyte

   granules

8. leukocyte

heparin

ABBREVIATIONS

ABMT	autologous bone marrow transplantation—patient serves as his or her own donor for stem cells	**diff.**	differential count (of white blood cells)
ABO	four main blood types—A, B, AB, and O	**EBV**	Epstein-Barr virus, the cause of mononucleosis
ALL	acute lymphocytic leukemia	**eos**	eosinophils
AML	acute myelogenous leukemia	**EPO**	erythropoietin
ASCT	autologous stem cell transplantation	**ESR**	erythrocyte sedimentation rate
baso	basophils	**G-CSF**	granulocyte colony-stimulating factor
BMT	bone marrow transplantation	**GM-CSF**	granulocyte-macrophage colony-stimulating factor
CBC	complete blood count	**g/dL**	
CLL	chronic lymphocytic leukemia	**GVHD**	
CML	chronic myelogenous leukemia		
DIC	disseminated intravascular		

Abbreviations are listed and explained in each body systems chapter.

A review sheet at the end of each chapter helps you organize and test yourself on what you have learned!

REVIEW SHEET

Write the meanings of the combining forms in the spaces provided and test yourself. Check your answers with the information in the text or in the glossary (Medical Terms—English) at the back of the book.

COMBINING FORMS

Combining Form	Meaning	Combining Form	Meaning
fluor/o	_____	roentgen/o	_____
ion/o	_____	son/o	_____
is/o	_____	therapeut/o	_____
myel/o	_____	vitr/o	_____
pharmaceut/o	_____	viv/o	_____
radi/o	_____		

SUFFIXES

Suffix	Meaning	Suffix	Meaning
-gram	_____	-lucent	_____
-graphy	_____	-opaque	_____

PREFIXES

Prefix	Meaning	Prefix	Meaning
cine-	_____	ultra-	_____
echo-	_____		

The Pronunciation of Terms section shows you how to pronounce each new term in the chapter and gives you the chance to practice writing its meaning. You can also hear these terms pronounced on the companion CD. The answers to the Pronunciation of Terms sections are found on the CD as well.

PRONUNCIATION OF TERMS

PRONUNCIATION GUIDE

ā as in āpe	ă as in ăpple
ē as in ēven	ĕ as in ĕvery
ī as in īce	ĭ as in ĭnterest
ō as in ōpen	ŏ as in pŏt
ū as in ūnit	ŭ as in ŭnder

To test your understanding of the terminology in this chapter, write the meaning of each term in the space provided. In addition, you may wish to cover the terms and write them by looking at your definitions. Make sure your spelling is correct.

The page number after each term indicates where it is defined or used in the book, so you can easily check your responses. You will find complete definitions for all of these terms and their audio-pronunciations on the CD.

VOCABULARY AND TERMINOLOGY

Term	Pronunciation	Meaning
albumin (___)	ăl-BŪ-mĭn	_____
anisocytosis (___)	ăn-ī-sō-sī-TŌ-sĭs	_____
antibody (___)	ĂN-tĭ-bŏd-ē	_____
anticoagulant (___)	ăn-tĭ-cō-ĂG-ū-lănt	_____
antigen (___)	ĂN-tĭ-jĕn	_____
basophil (___)	BĀ-sō-fĭl	_____
bilirubin (___)	bĭl-ĭ-ROO-bĭn	_____
coagulation (___)	kō-ăg-ū-LĀ-shŭn	_____
coagulopathy (___)	kō-ăg-ū-LŎP-ă-thē	_____
colony-stimulating factor (___)	KŎL-ō-nē STĬM-ū-lā-tĭng FĂK-tŏr	_____
cytology (___)	sī-TŎL-ō-jē	_____
differentiation (___)	dĭf-ĕr-ĕn-shē-Ā-shŭn	_____

ALSO AVAILABLE

STUDENT CD (included in this text)

The CD included with this new edition is packed with additional information, images, and video clips to expand your understanding and with activities to test your knowledge. Chapter by chapter you will find case studies, examples of medical records, and a wealth of images to illustrate terminology. Additionally, on the CD, you can hear me pronounce the terms corresponding to the Pronunciation of Terms section in each chapter (more than 3000 terms in all).

NEW to the student CD for the 8th edition

- Answers to the Pronunciations of Terms sections in the text. Terms are clearly and simply defined.
- More animations of human anatomy and illustrations of actual clinical procedures.
- Fun games test your knowledge of medical terms.

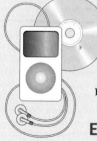

NEW! AUDIO STUDY COMPANION (for sale separately)

The new audio study guide provides pronunciation and comprehension practice in a portable format. The audio companion is available for download and as a set of audio CDs. Included are definitions, coaching notes, and mini review quizzes.

EVOLVE LEARNING RESOURCES

Go online to this companion website to access study tips, a new glossary of Greek and Latin word parts, new electronic flashcards, games, and more at http://evolve.elsevier.com/Chabner/language.

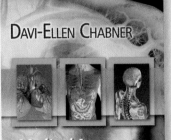

MEDICAL LANGUAGE INSTANT TRANSLATOR
(for sale separately)

The Medical Language Instant Translator is a uniquely useful resource for all allied health professionals and students of medical terminology. It is a pocket-sized medical terminology reference with convenient information at your fingertips!

- NEW Illustrated Guide to Surgical Instruments
- NEW Specialized Terms Used in Medical Records
- NEW Complementary and Alternative Medicine Terms

INSTRUCTOR'S RESOURCE MANUAL

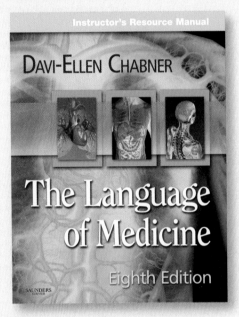

The Language of Medicine Instructor's Resource Manual (includes an instructor's manual and a CD with test bank and Power Point image collection) is available with even more new quizzes, teaching suggestions, crossword puzzles, medical reports, and reference material. The image collection contains all figures and photos from the 8th edition. The instructor materials can also be accessed online at http://evolve.elsevier.com/Chabner/language.

The fundamental features you have come to trust in learning and teaching medical terminology remain strong in this new edition. These are:

- Simple, nontechnical explanations of medical terms.
- Workbook format with ample space to write answers.
- Explanations of clinical procedures, laboratory tests, and abbreviations related to each body system.
- Pronunciations of Terms sections with phonetic spellings and spaces to write meanings of terms.
- Practical Applications sections with case reports, operative and diagnostic tests, and laboratory and x-ray reports.
- Exercises that test your understanding of terminology as you work through the text step by step (answers are included).
- Review Sheets that pull together terminology to help you study.
- Comprehensive glossaries and appendices for reference in class and on the job.

Each student and teacher who selects *The Language of Medicine* becomes my partner in the exciting adventure of learning medical terms. Continuity is crucial. Continue to communicate with me through email (Meddavi@aol.com) with your suggestions and comments so that future printings and editions may benefit. A website connected to *The Language of Medicine* and dedicated to helping students and teachers is located at http://evolve.elsevier.com/Chabner/language. I hope you will tell me about additional resources you would like to see on that website so that we can make it an even more useful part of the learning process. You should know that I still experience the thrill and joy of teaching new students. I love being in a classroom and feel privileged to continue to write this text. I hope that my enthusiasm and passion for the medical language are transmitted to you through these pages.

Work hard, but have fun with
The Language of Medicine!

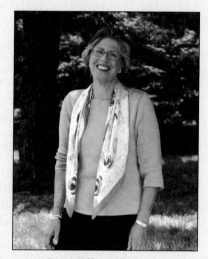

Davi-Ellen Chabner

Acknowledgments

Writing *The Language of Medicine* and its ancillaries is not possible as a solitary effort any longer. I need all the help that I can get! First and foremost, I am supremely grateful to my loyal and energetic editor, Maureen Pfeifer. Armed with an amazingly positive attitude, she provided the essential support and brilliant counsel that brought this eighth edition to completion. She tackled any and all projects with extraordinary intelligence, insight, and good judgment. I continue to count on her as a vital partner in my work, every step of the way. Thank you, Maureen!

Ellen Zanolle, Senior Book Designer, Art/Design, deserves great credit for masterminding the new look to *The Language of Medicine*. She spent countless hours selecting images for the cover and two-page chapter openers and created a dynamic, new interior design to make it easier for students to navigate the text. She skillfully supervised the complicated layout and composition of the book as well. Ellen's long association with *The Language of Medicine* is a valuable asset to the book. I am also grateful to Bill Donnelly, page layout designer, who, in association with Ellen, expertly crafted each chapter's layout.

Jim Perkins, Assistant Professor of Medical Illustration, Rochester Institute of Technology, redrew the artwork so that it is more realistic and three dimensional. I continue to appreciate his excellent work highlighted by detail, clarity, and accuracy in each image.

Elizabeth Galbraith copyedited the manuscript of the text and other ancillaries to the book. Her methodical and careful attention to grammar and consistency has made this edition even easier to read and study. I am grateful to Cathy Ward for her comprehensive review and organization of a glossary of Latin and Greek derivations for combining forms, suffixes, and prefixes, which is included on the companion Evolve website. This will be a valuable reference for both students and instructors.

Two devoted family members, as well as physicians, never hesitated to advise and provide help on any aspect of the project. My husband, Bruce A. Chabner, MD, and my daughter, Elizabeth Chabner Thompson, MD, MPH, have made essential contributions in editing and bringing new ideas to this edition. In addition, Elizabeth expertly reviewed and recorded the terms and definitions on the new audio Study Companion and is currently teaching medical terminology at Lehman College, Bronx, New York. As an enthusiastic classroom instructor, she contributed valuable insights and suggestions. I am grateful to Ann Sacher, MD, who also teaches medical terminology at Lehman College. She shared creative and effective materials for the instructor's resource manual.

During the last 2 years, my assistant, Joelle Reidy, accepted me as an after-hours project, and the edition benefited greatly from her talents. She energetically organized my office and my life and spent countless hours typing manuscript, finding new and exciting images for the book, and solving problems. Thank you, Joelle!

I especially appreciated the medical reviewers (listed on a page xvii), who took time away from busy schedules to provide expert advise on specific chapters of the text. Their outstanding guidance makes this edition current, accurate, and up-to-date.

Selected classroom instructors (listed on page xviii) extensively reviewed the text and provided their experienced and helpful feedback. I have made every effort to incorporate their comments in this edition. Many instructors personally communicated with me via email and gave valuable suggestions for this edition. Special thank you to Jeanne Amato, Judy Aronow, Charlotte Bowers, Jim Dresbach, Karla Duran, Bob Fischer, Delores Jevsnik, Rich Lehrer, Diane Malcolm, Nancy Marks, Jolene K. Miller, Linda Murtagh, Joyce Nakano, Alice Noblin, Martha Payne, David Petersen, Sharon Rahilly, Alan Rosenberg, Will Russell, Janet Stiles, Kathy Trawick, Gloria Vachino, Patricia Valleau, Rosemary Van Vranken, Jane Van't Hof, Susan Webb, and Linda Wilson.

I am always happy to hear from my current and past students and all others who take the time to comment on the book. They bring practical and insightful suggestions. Special thank you to Lisa Aune, Nadine Baxter, Sharon Glassman, Ronald Gaudette, Carol TeRondo, Eqerem Mete, Virginia Snowden, Joe Santora, Al Speetles, Isla Nortrud, Leah Ames, Shannon Hargis, Sharon Florano, Cheryl Hussey, Janet McClintic, Mark Schnell, Pat Dickerson, Sara Dodd, Catherine Matson, Irina Abramova, and Muhammed Khalid.

The excellent staff at Elsevier Health Sciences worked very hard on this edition. Jeanne Wilke, Executive Editor, Health Professions II, directed the entire project in a calm and skillful manner. Thank you, Jeanne, for all that you do for the book. Becky Swisher, Senior Developmental Editor, Health Professions II, was crucial to coordinating and managing the many details of the text and its ancillaries. I continue to rely on her excellent work, encouragement, and enthusiastic support. Thank you, Becky! Luke Held, Editorial Assistant, Health Professions II, was always available and helpful for any and all projects.

John Casey, Senior Project Manager, did a great job of keeping the manuscript rolling and selecting the best people to work on the book. He was superb in coordinating a complicated production effort.

I am grateful to Sally Schrefer, Executive Vice President, Nursing and Health Professions, and Andrew Allen, Publishing Director, Health Professions II, for their continuing support and confidence in my work. Thanks to Peggy Fagen, Director of US Health Sciences Book Production, Linda McKinley, Product Manager, and Trish Tannian, Publishing Services Manager, for their ongoing production efforts. I am grateful for the enthusiastic and hard-working Marketing and Creative Services staff, and in particular, Kim Hamby, Market Segment Manager, Sharon Korn, Director of Creative Services, Chris O'Brien, Senior Copywriter, and Connie Boone, Graphic Designer. Thanks to Tyson Sturgeon, Multimedia Manager, and Jeanne Crook, Executive Producer, Multimedia, for their talent and help.

My family and friends are always a haven of comfort. Besides my two wonderful children, Brandon and Elizabeth, five precious grandchildren, Bebe, Solomon, Ben, Gus, and Louisa, help me relax with countless hours of fun and play. Juliana Do Carmo faithfully and consistently puts my house and life in order so that I can work more effectively. My husband, Bruce, patiently provides answers to countless medical queries, and even more important, nourishes and calms my spirit. For 43 years now, he continues to be my essential source of strength.

Reviewers

The following persons reviewed the text and/or the ancillaries:

MEDICAL REVIEWERS

Elizabeth Chabner Thompson, MD, MPH
Scarsdale, New York

Bruce A. Chabner, MD
Clinical Director
Massachusetts General Hospital Cancer Center
Professor of Medicine
Harvard Medical School
Boston, Massachusetts

Giuliana Arcovio, BS, CNMT, RT(N)
Nuclear Medicine
Massachusetts General Hospital
Boston, Massachusetts

Ronald Arellano, MD
Assistant Radiologist
Massachusetts General Hospital
Instructor in Radiology
Harvard Medical School
Boston, Massachusetts

Richard Bender, MD, FACP
Medical Director
Hematology/Oncology
Quest Diagnostics Inc.
San Juan Capistrano, California

Christine Bethune, RN
Cardiac Nurse Manager
Electrophysiology and Pacemaker Laboratory
Massachusetts General Hospital
Boston, Massachusetts

Thomas N. Byrne, MD
Department of Brain and Cognitive Sciences
Massachusetts Institute of Technology
Cambridge, Massachusetts

Richard N. Channick, MD
Professor of Medicine
Pulmonary and Critical Care Division
University of California, San Diego
La Jolla, California

Carlos Jamis Dow, MD
Department of Radiology
Georgetown University Hospital
Washington, DC

Keith B. Isaacson, MD
Medical Director, Minimally Invasive GYN
    Surgery Center
Newton-Wellesley Hospital
Newton, Massachusetts

Jennifer E. Lawrence, MD, FACE
Director
Diabetes Management Center
Chief of Endocrinology
South Georgia Medical Center
Valdosta, Georgia

Jay Loeffler, MD
Chief of Radiation Oncology
Massachusetts General Hospital Cancer Center
Boston, Massachusetts

Fredric J. Mintz, MD
Digestive Center of Huntington NY
Huntington, New York

Diane J. Orlinsky, MD
Simmons-O'Brien & Orlinsky LLC
Towson, Maryland

Henry E. Schniewind, MD
Instructor in Psychiatry
Harvard Medical School
Boston, Massachusetts

Marcy L. Schwartz, MD
Department of Cardiology
Children's Hospital
Boston, Massachusetts

Amy R. Simon, MD
Associate Professor of Medicine
Tufts University School of Medicine
Pulmonary Critical Care Division
Boston, Massachusetts

Daniel I. Simon, MD
Chief
Division of Cardiovascular Medicine
Director
Heart and Vascular Institute
Case Medical Center
University Hospital of Cleveland
Herman K. Hellerstein Professor of
    Cardiovascular Research
Case Western Reserve University
School of Medicine
Cleveland, Ohio

Norman M. Simon, MD
Evanston Northwestern Healthcare
Professor of Medicine
Northwestern University
Feinberg School of Medicine
Chicago, Illinois

Jill Smith, MD
Associate Chief of Ophthalmology
Newton-Wellesley Hospital
Newton, Massachusetts

Julie E. Wilbur, MD
Clinical Fellow
Massachusetts General Hospital
Boston, Massachusetts

INSTRUCTOR REVIEWERS

Victoria Agyekum, MSN, RN
Department Head/Instructor
Savannah Technical College
Savannah, Georgia

Mercedes N. Alafriz-Gordon
Associate Vice President of Education
High Tech Institute, Inc.
Phoenix, Arizona

LaBera Ard, BA, MA, CPC
Professor
Bluegrass Community and Technical College
Lexington, Kentucky

Lori A. Artler-Vargo, BS, PE
MedStart Academy Lead
Marana High School
Pima Community College, Northwest Medical
    Center
Tucson, Arizona

**Susan Balman, BA (Elem. Educ.),
MA (Adult Educ.)**
Instructor
Butler Community College
El Dorado, Kansas

Victoria L. Bastecki-Perez, EdD
Dean, Health and Physical Education
Montgomery County Community College
Blue Bell, Pennsylvania

Caren Burford-Henry, CMA
National Registered Certified Medical Assistant
Certified Medical Assistant
Remington College
Dallas, Texas

Shawnmarie Carpenter, BS, MEd,
Certified Teacher, Certified Spiritual Director
Professor
University of Alaska South East
Ketchikan High School
Ketchikan, Alaska

Cathleen Currie, RN, BS
Program Manager—Allied Health and Health
  Sciences
College of Southern Idaho
Twin Falls, Idaho

James R. Dickerson, NR-CMA, NRC-EKG
Associate Program Chair
NAHP, Remington College
Gardner, Kansas

Karla Knaussman Duran, AS, BS, MLS
Instructor
Butler Community College
Andover, Kansas

Susan K. England, MSN, RN
HSTE Instructor
HCISD
Buda, Texas

Deborah Fazio, CMAS, RMA
Medical Billing and Coding Program Director
Sanford Brown Institute
Middleburg Heights, Ohio

Geri Lynn Finn, NRCMA, EMT-B, LYN
Medical Assisting Instructor
Remington College–Dallas Campus
Garland, Texas

Anita Hazelwood, MLS, RHIS, FAHIMA
Professor
University of Louisiana at Lafayette
Lafayette, Louisiana

Lisa Johnson, RD/LD, MBA, MEd
Advanced Health Occupations Specialist
Twin Falls High School
Twin Falls, Idaho

Cathy Kelley-Arney, CMA, MLTC, BSHS
Institutional Director of Health Care
  Education
National College
Bluefield, Virginia

Judith T. Land, EdS, MEd, BA, CMT, FAAMT
Instructor
Medical Transcription Training School (M-TEC)
Cincinnati, Ohio

Kathy Magorian, RN, MSN
Assistant Professor, Division of Nursing
Mt. Marty College
Yankton, South Dakota

Michelle Moy, M.Ad.Ed., MT (ACSP) SC
Instructor/Supervisor
Rush University Medical Center—College of
  Health Sciences
Chicago, Illinois

Alice Noblin, MBA, RHIA
Visiting Instructor, HIM Program
University of Central Florida
Orlando, Florida

Lynda Norris-Donathan, MS, RT(R)(M)(CT)
Assistant Professor of Imaging Sciences
Morehead State University
Morehead, Kentucky

Nancy L. Olrech, MSHP, BSN, RN
Adjunct Faculty, Allied Health Science
Austin Community College
Austin, Texas

Stella J. Olson, CMT, FAAMT
Consultant–Educator
AAMT
Modesto, California

Sue E. Ouellette, PhD, LCPC, LMFT, CRC, NCC
Professor and Chair, Department of
  Communicative Disorders
Northern Illinois University
Dekalb, Illinois

Angela Parmley, BS
MBC Program Director/Clinical Coordinator
American-International University
Hoffman Estates, Illinois

David B. Peterson, PhD, CRC, NCC,
Licensed Clinical Psychologist
Associate Professor
Illinois Institute of Technology
Chicago, Illinois

Terry Powell, RPh
Instructor
Edmonds Community College
Everett, Washington

Lara Denise Skaggs, MA, ATC
State Program Manager, Health Careers
    Education
Oklahoma Department of Career and
    Technology Education
Stillwater, Oklahoma

Leesa Gray Whicker, BA, CMA
Program Chair
Central Piedmont Community College
Charlotte, North Carolina

Contents

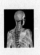

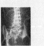

xxi

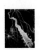

chapter 22
Psychiatry 893

Glossary

appendix I
Plurals 953

appendix II
Abbreviations, Acronyms, and Symbols 955

appendix III
Normal Hematologic Reference Values and Implications of Abnormal Results 965

appendix IV
Drugs 969

appendix V
Complementary and Alternative Medicine Terms 973

The Language of Medicine

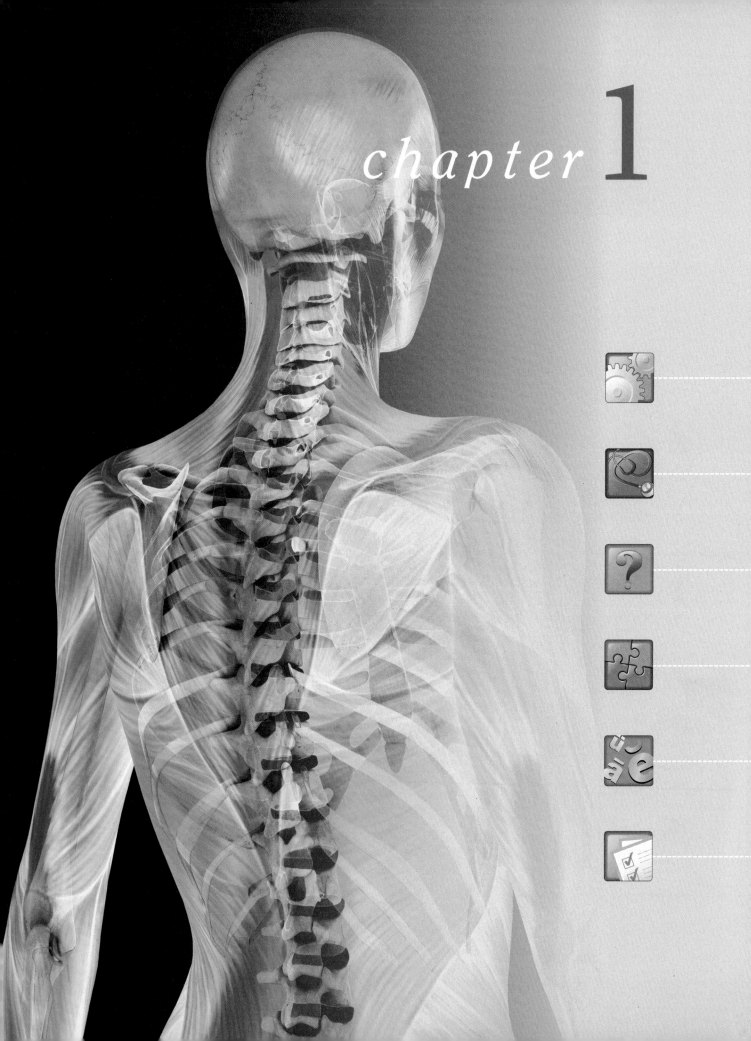

chapter 1

Basic Word Structure

In this chapter you will

- Identify basic objectives to guide your study of the medical language.
- Divide medical words into their component parts.
- Learn the meanings of basic combining forms, suffixes, and prefixes of the medical language.
- Use these combining forms, suffixes, and prefixes to build medical words.

Image Description: Posterior stylized view, angled to the right side, of the female musculoskeletal system.

3

OBJECTIVES IN STUDYING THE MEDICAL LANGUAGE

There are three objectives to keep in mind as you study medical terminology:

1. **Analyze words by dividing them into component parts.** Your goal is to learn the *tools* of word analysis that will make understanding complex terminology easier. Do not simply memorize terms; think about dividing terms into component parts. This book will show you how to separate both complicated and simple terms into understandable word elements. Medical terms are much like individual jigsaw puzzles in that they are constructed of small pieces that make each word unique, with one major difference: The pieces can be shuffled up and used in lots of combinations to make other words as well. As you become familiar with word parts and learn what each means, you will be able to recognize those word parts in totally new combinations in other terms.

2. **Relate the medical terms to the structure and function of the human body.** Memorization of terms, although essential to retention of the language, should not become the primary objective of your study. A major focus of this book is to *explain* terms in the context of how the body works in health and disease. Medical terms explained in their proper context also will be easier to remember. Thus, the term **hepatitis,** meaning inflammation **(-itis)** of the liver **(hepat),** is better understood when you know where the liver is and how it functions. No previous knowledge of biology, anatomy, or physiology is needed for this study. Explanations in this book are straightforward and basic.

3. **Be aware of spelling and pronunciation problems.** Some medical terms are pronounced alike but are spelled differently, which accounts for their different meanings. For example, **ilium** and **ileum** have identical pronunciations, but the first term, **ilium,** means a part of the hip bone, whereas the second term, **ileum,** refers to a part of the small intestine. Even when terms are spelled correctly, they can be misunderstood because of incorrect pronunciation. For example, the **urethra** (ū-RĒ-thrăh) is the tube leading from the urinary bladder to the outside of the body, whereas a **ureter** (ŪR-ĕ-tĕr) is one of two tubes each leading from a single kidney and inserting into the urinary bladder. Figure 1–1 illustrates the difference between the urethra and the ureters.

WORD ANALYSIS

Studying medical terminology is very similar to learning a new language. At first, the words sound strange and complicated, although they may stand for commonly known English terms. For example, the word **otalgia** means "earache," and an **ophthalmologist** is an "eye doctor."

Your first job in learning the language of medicine is to understand how to divide words into their component parts. Logically, most terms, whether complex or simple, can be broken down into basic parts and then understood. For example, consider the following term:

HEMATOLOGY   HEMAT/O/LOGY

root | suffix

combining vowel

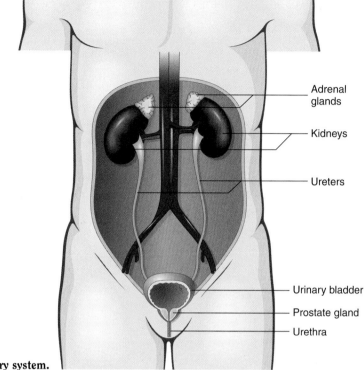

FIGURE 1–1   Urinary system.

The **root** is the *foundation of the word*. All medical terms have one or more roots. For example, the root **hemat** means **blood**.

The **suffix** is the *word ending*. All medical terms have a suffix. The suffix **-logy** means **process of study**.

The **combining vowel**—usually **o**, as in this term—*links the root to the suffix or the root to another root*. A combining vowel has no meaning of its own; it joins one word part to another.

It is useful to read the meaning of medical terms *starting from the suffix and then going back to the beginning of the term*. Thus, the term **hematology** means **process of study of blood**.

Here is another familiar medical term:

ELECTROCARDIOGRAM   ELECTR/O/CARDI/O/GRAM
                         root   root   suffix

                         combining vowel

The root **electr** means **electricity**.
The root **cardi** means **heart**.
The suffix **-gram** means **record**.
The entire word (reading from the suffix back to the beginning of the term) means **record of the electricity in the heart**.

Notice that there are two combining vowels—both **o**—in this term. The first o links the two roots **electr** and **cardi**; the second o links the root **cardi** and the suffix **-gram**.

Try another term:

GASTRITIS   GASTR/ITIS
           ↓   ↓
       root   suffix

The root **gastr** means **stomach.**
The suffix **-itis** means **inflammation.**
The entire word, reading from the end of the term (suffix) to the beginning, means **inflammation of the stomach.**

Notice that the combining vowel, o, is missing in this term. This is because the suffix, **-itis,** begins with a vowel. The combining vowel is dropped before a suffix that begins with a vowel. It is retained, however, between two roots, even if the second root begins with a vowel. Consider the following term:

GASTROENTEROLOGY   GASTR/O/ENTER/O/LOGY
      ↓   ↓   ↓
    root   root   suffix

combining vowel

The root **gastr** means **stomach.**
The root **enter** means **intestines.**
The suffix **-logy** means **process of study.**
The entire term means **process of study of the stomach and intestines.**

Notice that the combining vowel is used between **gastr** and **enter,** even though the second root, **enter,** begins with a vowel. When a term contains two or more roots related to parts of the body, anatomic position often determines which root goes before the other. For example, the stomach receives food first, before the small intestine—so the word is formed as **gastroenterology,** not "enterogastrology."

> In summary, remember three general rules:
> 1. Read the meaning of medical terms from the suffix back to the beginning of the term and across.
> 2. Drop the combining vowel (usually o) before a suffix beginning with a vowel: **gastritis,** *not* "gastroitis."
> 3. Keep the combining vowel between two roots: **gastroenterology,** *not* "gastrenterology."

In addition to the root, suffix, and combining vowel, two other word parts are commonly found in medical terms. These are the **combining form** and the **prefix.** The combining form is simply the root plus the combining vowel. For example, you already are familiar with the following combining forms and their meanings:

HEMAT/O   means   **blood**

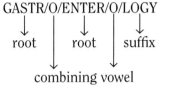

Root + combining vowel = COMBINING FORM

GASTR/O   means   **stomach**

Root + combining vowel = COMBINING FORM

CARDI/O   means   **heart**

Root + combining vowel = COMBINING FORM

Combining forms are used with many different suffixes. Remembering the meaning of a combining form will help you understand different medical terms.

The **prefix** is a small part that is attached to the *beginning of a term*. Not all medical terms contain prefixes, but the prefix can have an important influence on the meaning. Consider the following examples:

SUB/GASTR/IC   means   **pertaining to <u>under</u> the stomach**

prefix   root   suffix
(under) (stomach) (pertaining to)

EPI/GASTR/IC   means   **pertaining to <u>above</u> the stomach**

prefix   root   suffix
(above) (stomach) (pertaining to)

In summary, the important elements of medical terms are the following:
1. **Root:** foundation of the term
2. **Suffix:** word ending
3. **Prefix:** word beginning
4. **Combining vowel:** vowel (usually o) that links the root to the suffix or the root to another root
5. **Combining form:** combination of the root and the combining vowel

COMBINING FORMS, SUFFIXES, AND PREFIXES

In previous examples you have been introduced to the combining forms **gastr/o** (stomach), **hemat/o** (blood), and **cardi/o** (heart). This section of the chapter presents a list of additional combining forms, suffixes, and prefixes, with examples of medical words using those word parts. (Similar lists are included for each chapter in the book.) Write the *meaning* of the medical term in the space provided. Then check the correct pronunciation for each term with the Pronunciation of Terms list on page 26. Your CD contains audio-pronunciations of terms from this list.

Most medical terms are derived from Greek and Latin roots. Although it is not necessary to memorize these Greek and Latin derivations, they are presented (for Chapters 1 to 4) on the Evolve website.

CHAPTER STUDY GUIDE

1. **Use slashes to divide each term** into component parts *(aden/oma)*, and **write its meaning** *(tumor of a gland)* in the space provided. Although most medical terms are divided easily into component parts and understood, others defy simple explanation. Information in *italics* under a medical term helps you define and understand the term. See the CD (Combining Forms, Suffixes, and Prefixes List) to check your meanings.
2. **Complete the Exercises,** pages 16 to 23, and **check your answers against those provided on** pages 24 to 26.
3. **Write meanings for terms on the Pronunciation of Terms list,** pages 26 to 29. Definitions are on the CD.
4. **Complete the Review Sheet,** pages 30 and 31. Check your answers with the Glossary, page 931. Finally, **test yourself** by writing Review Sheet terms and meanings on a separate sheet of paper.

Notice that you are actively engaging in the learning process by **WRITING** terms and their meanings and **TESTING** yourself repeatedly. I guarantee success if you follow these simple steps. This is a proven method—it really works!

COMBINING FORMS

Combining Form	Meaning	Terminology	Meaning
aden/o	gland	adenoma *tumor of a gland*	
		The suffix -oma means tumor or mass.	
		adenitis *inflamation of the gland*	
		The suffix -itis means inflammation.	
arthr/o	joint	arthritis *inflamation join*	
bi/o	life	biology *study of life*	
		The suffix -logy is composed of the root log (study) and the final suffix -y (process or condition).	
		biopsy *viewing of living tissue*	
		The suffix -opsy means process of viewing. Living tissue is removed from the body and viewed under a microscope.	
carcin/o	cancerous, cancer	carcinoma *CANCEROUS TUMOR*	
		A carcinoma is a cancerous tumor. Carcinomas grow from epithelial (surface or skin) cells that cover the outside of the body and line organs, cavities, and tubes within the body.	
cardi/o	heart	cardiology *study of the heart*	
cephal/o	head	cephalic *pertaining to head*	
		(sĕ-FAL-ĭk) The suffix -ic means pertaining to. If an infant is born with the head delivered first, it is a cephalic presentation.	

1

Combining Form	Meaning	Terminology	Meaning
cerebr/o	cerebrum (largest part of the brain)	cerebral _pertaining to the brain_	
		The suffix -al means pertaining to. A cerebrovascular accident (CVA) occurs when damage to blood vessels (vascul/o means blood vessels) in the cerebrum causes injury to nerve cells of the brain. This condition also is called a stroke.	
cis/o	to cut	incision _process to cut IN_	
		The prefix in- means into, and the suffix -ion means process.	
		excision _process to cut out_	
		The prefix ex- means out.	
crin/o	to secrete (to form and give off)	endocrine glands _secrete with them_	
		The prefix endo- means within; endocrine glands (e.g., thyroid, pituitary, and adrenal glands) secrete hormones directly within (into) the bloodstream. Other glands, called exocrine glands, secrete chemicals (e.g., saliva, sweat, tears) through tubes (ducts) to the outside of the body.	
cyst/o	urinary bladder; a sac or a cyst (sac containing fluid)	cystoscopy _vie bladder_	
		(sĭs-TŎS-kō-pē) The suffix -scopy means process (y) of visual examination (scop).	
cyt/o	cell	cytology _study of cell_	
derm/o dermat/o	skin	dermatitis _inflamation skin_	
		hypodermic _Low_	
		The prefix hypo- means under, below. _Record of the_	
electr/o	electricity	electrocardiogram _electricity in the heart_	
		The suffix -gram means record. Abbreviated ECG (or sometimes EKG).	
encephal/o	brain	electroencephalogram _Record of electricity of the brain_	
		Abbreviated EEG.	
enter/o	intestines (usually the small intestine)	enteritis _INFLAMATION OF INTESTINE_	
		The small intestine is narrower but much longer than the large intestine (colon)	
erythr/o	red	erythrocyte _red blood cell_	
		The suffix -cyte means cell. Erythrocytes carry oxygen in the blood.	
gastr/o	stomach	gastrectomy _excision of the stomach_	
		The suffix -ectomy means excision or removal. All or, more commonly, part of the stomach is removed.	
		gastrotomy _INCISION of the stomach_	
		The suffix -tomy means incision or process (y) of cutting (tom).	

Combining Form	Meaning	Terminology	Meaning
gnos/o	knowledge	diagnosis	*State OF complete Knowlege.*

The prefix dia- means complete. The suffix -sis means state or condition of. A diagnosis is made after sufficient information has been obtained about the patient's condition. Literally, it is a "state of complete knowledge."

		prognosis	*Knowlege before.*

The prefix pro- means before. Literally "knowledge before," a prognosis is a prediction about the outcome of an illness, but it is always given after the diagnosis has been determined.

Combining Form	Meaning	Terminology	Meaning
gynec/o	woman, female	gynecology	*"Study of female reproduct sw*
hemat/o	blood	hematology	*study OF the blood*
hem/o		hematoma	*mass collection of blood*

In this term, -oma means a mass or collection of blood, rather than a growth of cells (tumor). A hematoma forms when blood escapes from blood vessels and collects as a clot in a cavity, organ, or under the skin.

		hemoglobin	*protein of the blood*

The suffix -globin means protein. Hemoglobin carries oxygen in red blood cells.

Combining Form	Meaning	Terminology	Meaning
hepat/o	liver	hepatitis	*inflamation of the liver*
iatr/o	treatment, physician	iatrogenic	*pertaining*

The suffix -genic means pertaining to producing, produced by, or produced in. Iatrogenic conditions are adverse side effects that result from treatment or intervention by a physician.

Combining Form	Meaning	Terminology	Meaning
leuk/o	white	leukocyte	*white blood cell*

This blood cell helps the body fight disease.

Combining Form	Meaning	Terminology	Meaning
nephr/o	kidney	nephritis	*inflamation of the kidney*
		nephrology	*study of the kidney*
neur/o	nerve	neurology	*study of the nerve*
onc/o	tumor	oncology	*study of the tumor*
		oncologist	*study of the tumor*

The suffix -ist means one who specializes in a field of medicine (or other profession).

Combining Form	Meaning	Terminology	Meaning
ophthalm/o	eye	ophthalmoscope	*instrument of the eye.*

(ŏf-THĂL-mō-skōp) The suffix -scope means an instrument for visual examination. (To help with spelling, notice that just as there are two eyes, there are two "h"s in this term.)

1

Combining Form	Meaning	Terminology	Meaning
oste/o	bone	osteitis	_INFLAMATION of the bones_
		osteoarthritis	_infla. join and bones_

This condition is actually a degeneration of bones and joints that occurs with aging. It often is accompanied by inflammation.

| path/o | disease | pathology | _study of disease_ |
| | | pathologist | |

A pathologist examines biopsy samples microscopically and examines a dead body to determine the cause of death.

| ped/o | child | pediatric | _pert. to children_ |

Notice that ped/o is also in the term ortho**ped**ist. Orthopedists once were doctors who straightened (orth/o means straight) children's bones and corrected deformities. Nowadays, orthopedists specialize in disorders of bones and muscles in people of all ages.

psych/o	mind	psychology	_study of the mind_
		psychiatrist	
radi/o	x-rays	radiology	_study of XRAYS_

Low-energy x-rays are used for diagnostic imaging.

| ren/o | kidney | renal | _pertaining to the KIDNEY_ |

Ren/o (Latin) and nephr/o (Greek) both mean kidney. Ren/o is used with -al (Latin) to describe the kidney, whereas nephr/o is used with other suffixes such as -osis, -itis, and -ectomy (Greek) to describe abnormal conditions and operative procedures.

| rhin/o | nose | rhinitis | _INFLAMATION NOSe_ |
| sarc/o | flesh | sarcoma | |

This is a cancerous (malignant) tumor. A sarcoma grows from cells of "fleshy" connective tissue such as muscle, bone, and fat, whereas a carcinoma (another type of cancerous tumor) grows from epithelial cells that line the outside of the body or the inside of organs in the body.

| sect/o | to cut | resection | _PROCESS TO CUT OUT_ |

The prefix re- means back. A resection is a cutting back in the sense of cutting out or removal (excision). A gastric resection is a gastrectomy, or excision of the stomach.

| thromb/o | clot, clotting | thrombocyte | _CONDITION OF clot formation_ |

Also known as **platelets**, these cells help clot blood. A **thrombus** is the actual clot that forms, and **thrombosis** (-osis means condition) is the condition of clot formation.

| ur/o | urinary tract, urine | urology | _study of the urinary tract_ |

A urologist is a surgeon who operates on the organs of the urinary tract and the organs of the male reproductive system.

SUFFIXES

Suffix	Meaning	Terminology	Meaning
-ac	pertaining to	cardiac	*pertaining to the heart*
-al	pertaining to	neural	*'' '' to the nerve*
-algia	pain	arthralgia	*pain of the join*
		neuralgia	*pain of the nerv.*
-cyte	cell	erythrocyte	*Red cell*
-ectomy	excision, removal	nephrectomy	*Remove of the kidney*
-emia	blood condition	leukemia	*condition of the white cell*

Literally, this term means "a blood condition of white (blood cells)." Actually, it is a condition of blood in which cancerous white blood cells proliferate (increase in number).

Suffix	Meaning	Terminology	Meaning
-genic	pertaining to producing, produced by, or produced in	carcinogenic	*pert of cancer*

Cigarette smoke is carcinogenic.

pathogenic _____ *pert to produce disease*

A virus or a bacterium is a pathogenic organism.

iatrogenic _____

In this term, -genic means produced by.

Suffix	Meaning	Terminology	Meaning
-globin	protein	hemoglobin	*blood protein*
-gram	record	electroencephalogram	
-ic, -ical	pertaining to	gastric	*pertaining to the stomach*
		neurologic	*study of the nerve*

Log/o means study of.

Suffix	Meaning	Terminology	Meaning
-ion	process	excision	*process to cut out*
-ist	specialist	gynecologist	*specialist of female Reprod syste*
-itis	inflammation	cystitis	*INFLAMATION OF URINARY bladder*
-logy	process of study	endocrinology	
-oma	tumor, mass, swelling	hepatoma	*tumor of the liver*

A hepatoma (hepatocellular carcinoma) is a malignant tumor of the liver.

Suffix	Meaning	Terminology	Meaning
-opsy	process of viewing	biopsy	

Biopsy specimens are viewed under a microscope.

1

Suffix	Meaning	Terminology	Meaning
-osis	condition, usually abnormal (slight increase in numbers when used with blood cells)	nephrosis _abnormal cond. of the kidney_	
		leukocytosis _____	
		This condition, a slight increase in normal white blood cells, occurs as white blood cells multiply to fight an infection. Don't confuse leukocytosis with leukemia, which is a cancerous (malignant) condition marked by high levels of abnormal, immature white blood cells.	
-pathy	disease condition	enteropathy _____ (ĕn-tĕ-RŎP-ă-thē)	
		adenopathy _____ (ă-dĕ-NŎP-ă-thē)	
-scope	instrument to visually examine	endoscope _____ _End- means within. A cystoscope is an endoscope._	
-scopy	process of visually examining with an endoscope	endoscopy _____ (ĕn-DŎS-kō-pē)	
-sis	state of; condition	prognosis _____	
-tomy	process of cutting, incision	osteotomy _INCISION to the bone_ (ŏs-tē-ŎT-tō-mē)	
-y	process, condition	gastroenterology _process to the stomach_	

PREFIXES

Prefix	Meaning	Terminology	Meaning
a-, an-	no, not, without	anemia _NO blood_ _Anemia is a decreased number of erythrocytes or an abnormality of the hemoglobin (a chemical) within the red blood cells. This results in decreased delivery of oxygen to cells of the body. Anemic patients look so pale that early physicians thought they were literally "without blood."_	
aut-, auto-	self, own	autopsy _PROCESS OF VIEWING by oneself_ _This term literally means "process of viewing by oneself." Hence, an autopsy is the examination of a dead body with one's own eyes to determine the cause of death and nature of disease._	
dia-	through, complete	diagnosis _____	
end-, endo-	within	endoscopy _process_	
		endocrinologist _especialist_	

1

Prefix	Meaning	Terminology	Meaning
epi-	above, upon	epigastric	*per to above the stomach*
		epidermis	*per to above the skin*
			This outermost layer of skin lies above the middle layer of skin, known as the dermis.
ex-	out	excision	*process to take out*
exo-	outside of, outward	exocrine glands	
hyper-	excessive, above, more than normal	hyperglycemia	
			The combining form glyc/o means sugar.
		hyperthyroidism	*condition*
			The suffix -ism means process or condition.
hypo-	deficient, below, under, less than normal	hypogastric	
			When hypo- is used with a part of the body, it means below.
		hypoglycemia	
			In this term, hypo- means deficient.
in-	into, in	incision	*process*
peri-	surrounding, around	pericardium	*structure surrounds heart*
			The suffix -um means a structure. The pericardium is the membrane that surrounds the heart.
pro-	before, forward	prostate gland	
			This exocrine gland "stands" (-state) before or in front of the urinary bladder (see Figure 1-1). It produces semen, which contains fluid and sperm cells.

Hyperglycemia and Diabetes
Hyperglycemia (high blood sugar) most frequently is associated with **diabetes.** People with diabetes have high blood sugar levels because they lack **insulin** (in **type 1 diabetes**) or have ineffective insulin (in **type 2 diabetes**). Insulin is the hormone normally released by the pancreas (an endocrine gland near the stomach) to "escort" sugar from the bloodstream into cells.

The term **diabetes** comes from the Greek word *diabainein*, meaning "to pass through." Thus, one symptom of diabetes is **polyuria** (frequent urination). Another symptom is **glycosuria** (sugar in the urine), as high blood sugar causes the kidneys to release sugar into the urine.

Long-term complications of diabetes mellitus (DM) include **neuropathy** (nerve damage) and **nephropathy** (kidney disease), as well as **ophthalmic** conditions leading to blindness.

Understanding Hyperthyroidism
In **hyperthyroidism,** a hyperactive **thyroid gland** (an endocrine gland in the neck) secretes a greater than normal amount of **thyroxine** (thyroid hormone, or T_4). Because thyroxine causes cells to burn fuel and release energy, signs and symptoms of hyperthyroidism are increased energy level and nervousness, **tachycardia** (increased heart rate), weight loss, and **exophthalmos** (bulging eyeballs).

Treatment includes **antithyroid** (anti- means against) drugs, surgery **(thyroidectomy),** and radioactive iodine therapy for severe cases. Untreated hyperthyroidism may lead to death from **cardiac** failure.

Prefix	Meaning	Terminology	Meaning
re-	back, backward, again	resection _____ *This is an operation in which tissue is "cut back" or removed. The Latin "resectio" means a trimming or pruning.*	
retro-	behind	retrocardiac _____	
sub-	below, under	subhepatic ___ *perl*	
trans-	across, through	transhepatic ___ *pert. across the liver*	

PRACTICAL APPLICATIONS

This section provides an opportunity for you to use your skill in understanding medical terms and to increase your knowledge of new terms. Be sure to check your answers with the Answers to Practical Applications on page 26. You should find helpful explanations there.

SPECIALISTS

Match the **abnormal condition** in Column I with the **physician (specialist) who treats** it in Column II. Write the letter of the correct specialist in the space provided.

Column I

1. heart attack — D
2. ovarian cysts — F
3. bipolar (manic-depressive) disorder — J
4. breast adenocarcinoma — E
5. iron deficiency anemia — B
6. retinopathy — H
7. cerebrovascular accident — I
8. renal failure — G C
9. inflammatory bowel disease — A
10. cystitis — G

Column II

A. gastroenterologist
B. hematologist
C. nephrologist
D. cardiologist
E. oncologist
F. gynecologist
G. urologist
H. ophthalmologist
I. neurologist
J. psychiatrist

EXERCISES

1

The exercises that follow are designed to help you learn the terms presented in the chapter. Writing terms over and over again is a good way to study this new language. You will find the answers to these exercises starting on p. 24. This makes it easy to check your work. As you check each answer, you not only will reinforce your understanding of a term but often will gain additional information from the answer. Each exercise is designed not as a test, but rather as an opportunity for you to learn the material.

A. Complete the following sentences.

1. Word beginnings are called ___prefix___.

2. Word endings are called ___suffix___.

3. The foundation of a word is known as the ___root___.

4. A letter linking a suffix and a root, or linking two roots, in a term is the ___combining vowel___.

5. The combination of a root and a combining vowel is known as the ___combining form___.

B. Give the meanings of the following combining forms.

1. cardi/o ___heart___

2. aden/o ___gland___

3. bi/o ___life___

4. cerebr/o ___cerebrum (large part of the brain)___

5. cephal/o ___head___

6. arthr/o ___joint___

7. carcin/o ___cancerous, cancer___

8. cyst/o ___urinary bladder, sac___

9. cyt/o ___cell___

10. derm/o or dermat/o ___skin___

11. encephal/o ___brain___

12. electr/o ___electricity___

C. Give the meanings of the following suffixes.

1. -oma ___tumor, mass, swelling___

2. -al ___pertaining to___

3. -itis ___inflammation___

4. -logy ___process of study___

5. -scopy ___process of visually exam. with endoscope___

6. -ic ___pertaining to___

7. -gram ___record___

8. -opsy ___process of viewing___

D. Using slashes, divide the following terms into parts, and give the meaning of the entire term.

cerebr/al 1. cerebral ___pertaining to the cerebrum (largest part of the brain)___

bi/opsy 2. biopsy ___process of viewing life under a microscope___

aden/itis 3. adenitis ___inflammation of the gland___

cephal/ic 4. cephalic _pertaining to head_

5. carcinoma _cancerous tumor - carcin/oma_

cyst/o/scopy 6. cystoscopy _process of visually examining the urinary bladder._

7. electrocardiogram _electr/o/cardiogram -electricity of the heart. record_

8. cardiology _cardi/o/logy - study of the heart_

9. electroencephalogram _electro/encephal/e/gram - record of electricity in the brain_

10. dermatitis _derm/it/itis - inflammation of the skin_

11. arthroscopy _arthr/o/scopy - process of visual examination of a joint._

12. cytology _cyt/o/logy - study of the cell._

E. Give the meanings of the following combining forms.

1. erythr/o _Red_ 7. nephr/o _kidney_

2. enter/o _intestine_ 8. leuk/o _White_

3. gastr/o _stomach_ 9. iatr/o _treatment_

4. gnos/o _Knowledge_ 10. hepat/o _liver_

5. hemat/o _blood_ 11. neur/o _NERVE_

6. cis/o _to cut_ 12. gynec/o _woman / female_

F. Complete the medical term, based on its meaning as provided.

1. white blood cell: _leuko_ cyte

2. inflammation of the stomach: gastr _itis_

3. pertaining to being produced by treatment: _iatro_ genic

4. study of kidneys: _nephro_ logy -

5. red blood cell: _erythro_ cyte

6. mass of blood: _hemat_ oma

7. process of viewing living tissue (using a microscope): bi _opsy_

8. pain of nerves: neur _neuralgia_

9. process of visual examining of the eye: _ophthalmo_ scopy

10. inflammation of the small intestine: _enter_ itis

G. Match the English term in Column I with its combining form in Column II. Write the correct combining form in the space provided.

Column I
English Term

Column II
Combining Form

1. kidney _____ren/o_____
2. disease _____path/o_____
3. eye _____ophthalm/o_____
4. to cut _____sect/o_____
5. nose _____rhin/o_____
6. flesh _____sarc/o_____
7. mind _____psych/o_____
8. urinary tract _____ur/o_____
9. bone _____oste/o_____
10. x-rays _____radi/o_____
11. clotting _____thromb/o_____
12. tumor _____onc/o_____

onc/o
ophthalm/o
oste/o
path/o
psych/o
radi/o
ren/o
rhin/o
sarc/o
sect/o
thromb/o
ur/o

H. Underline the suffix in each term and then give the meaning of the term.

1. ophthalmo_scopy_ __process of visual examination of the eyes__
2. ophthalmo_scope_ __instrument to visually examine the eye__
3. onco_logy_ __study of tumors__
4. oste_itis_ __inflammation of the bone__
5. psych_osis_ __abnormal condition of the mind__
6. thrombo_cyte_ __clotting cell (platelet)__
7. ren_al_ __pertaining to the kidney__
8. nephr_ectomy_ __removal of the kidney (excision or resection)__
9. osteo_tomy_ __incision of a bone (process of cutting into)__
10. re_section_ __process of cutting back (cutting out or remove)__
11. carcino_genic_ __pertaining to producing cancer__
12. sarc_oma_ __tumor of flesh (cancerous tumor of flesh tissue__

I. Match the suffix in Column I with its meaning in Column II. Write the correct meaning in the space provided.

Column I
Suffix

Column II
Meaning

1. -algia ___pain___

2. -ion ___process___

3. -emia ___blood condition___

4. -gram ___record___

5. -scope ___instrument___

6. -osis ___abnormal condition___

7. -ectomy ___Removal, excision___

8. -genic ___pertaining to producing...___

9. -pathy ___disease condition___

10. -tomy ___incision/process of cutting___

11. -itis ___inflammation___

12. -cyte ___cell___

abnormal condition
blood condition
cell
disease condition
incision, process of cutting into
inflammation
instrument to visually examine
pain
pertaining to producing, produced by, or produced in
process
record
removal, excision, resection

J. Select from the listed terms to complete the following sentences.

arthralgia
carcinogenic
cystitis
endocrine
enteropathy

exocrine
hematoma
hepatoma (hepatocellular carcinoma)

iatrogenic
leukemia
leukocytosis
neuralgia

1. When Paul smoked cigarettes, he inhaled a ___carcinogenic___ substance with each puff.

2. Sally's sore throat, fever, and chills made her doctor order a white blood cell count. The results, indicating infection, showed a slight increase in normal cells, a condition called ___Leukocytosis___.

3. Mr. Smith's liver enlarged, giving him abdominal pain. His radiologic tests and biopsy revealed a malignant tumor, or ___hepatoma___.

4. Mrs. Rose complained of pain in her hip joints, knees, and shoulders each morning. She was told that she had painful joints, or ___Arthralgia___.

5. Dr. Black was trained to treat disorders of the pancreas, thyroid gland, adrenal glands, and pituitary gland. Thus, he was an expert in the ___endocrine___ glands.

1

6. Ms. Walsh told her doctor she had pain when urinating. After tests, the doctor's diagnosis was

inflammation of the urinary bladder, or ___cystitis___.

7. Elizabeth's overhead tennis shot hit David in the thigh, producing a large ___hematoma___. His skin looked bruised and was tender.

8. Mr. Bell's white blood cell count is 10 times higher than normal. Examination of his blood shows

cancerous white blood cells. His diagnosis is ___leukemia___.

9. Mr. Kay was resuscitated (revived from potential or apparent death) in the emergency room after experiencing a heart attack. Unfortunately, he suffered a broken rib as a result of the physician's

chest compressions. This is an example of a (an) ___iatrogenic___ fracture.

10. After coming back from a trip during which he had eaten strange foods, Mr. Cameron had a disease

of his intestines called ___enteropathy___.

K. Give the meanings of the following prefixes.

1. dia- ___complete___

2. pro- ___before / forward___

3. aut-, auto- ___self / own___

4. a-, an- ___one / not / without___

5. hyper- ___excessive / above___

6. hypo- ___deficient / below / less than around___

7. epi- ___above / upon___

8. end-, endo- ___within___

9. retro- ___behind___

10. trans- ___across, through___

11. peri- ___surrounding / around___

12. ex-, exo- ___out___

13. sub- ___below / under___

14. re- ___back / backward / again___

L. Underline the prefix in the following terms and give the meaning of the entire term.

1. <u>dia</u>gnosis complete /knowledge ; decision about patient's condition after test.

2. <u>pro</u>gnosis before/ knowledge ; a prediction about

3. <u>sub</u>hepatic under/ pertaining to below the liver.

4. <u>peri</u>cardium surrounding /the membrane surrounding the heart

5. <u>hyper</u>glycemia excessive/ sugar in the blood.

6. <u>hypo</u>dermic deficient/ pertaining to under the skin

7. <u>epi</u>gastric above/ pertaining to above the stomach.

8. <u>re</u>section again/ process of cutting back

9. <u>hypo</u>glycemia below/ condition of deficient/low sugar in the blood

10. <u>an</u>emia one/ without/ condition of low nº of erythrocytes or deficient of hemoglobin in these cells.

M. Complete the following terms (describing areas of medicine), based on their meanings as given.

1. study of the urinary tract: _____urology_____ logy

2. study of women and women's diseases: _____gynecology_____ logy

3. study of blood: _____hematology_____ logy

4. study of tumors: _____oncology_____ logy

5. study of the kidneys: _____nephrology_____ logy

6. study of nerves: _____neurology_____ logy

7. treatment of children: _____Pediatrics_____ iatrics

8. study of x-rays in diagnostic imaging: _____Radiology_____ logy

9. study of the eyes: _____ophthalmology_____ logy

10. study of the stomach and intestines: _____gastroenterology_____ logy

11. study of glands that secrete hormones: _____endocrinology_____ logy

12. treatment of the mind: _____Psychiatry_____ iatry

13. study of disease: _____pathology_____ logy

14. study of the heart: _____cardiology_____ logy

N. Give the meaning of the underlined word part and then define the term.

1. cerebro vascular accident _____cerebrum/is damage to the blood vessels of the cerebrum_____

2. encephalitis _____brain/ is inflammation of the brain_____

3. cystoscope _____urinary bladder/is an instrument used to visually examine the urine bladder_____

4. transhepatic _____across/through-means pertaining to across the liver_____

5. iatrogenic _____treatment- means pertaining to an adverse side effect produced by treatment._____

6. hypogastric _____under/deficient- pertaining to below the stomach._____

7. endocrine glands _____within- Endocrine glands secret hormones within the body_____

8. nephrectomy _____excision- resection/ is the removal of a kidney_____

9. exocrine glands _____outside-secrete chemicals to the outside of the body. (Sweet tear-_____

10. neuralgia _____-pain - is nerve pain_____

1

O. Select from the listed terms to complete the following sentences.

anemia
biopsy
diagnosis
leukemia
nephrologist
neuropathy

oncogenic
oncologist
osteoarthritis
pathogenic
prognosis

psychiatrist
psychologist
thrombocyte
thrombosis
urologist

1. Seventy-two-year-old Ms. Crick suffers from a degenerative joint disease that is caused by the wearing away of tissue around her joints. This disease, which literally means "inflammation of bones and joints," is _____osteoarthritis_____.

2. The ___biopsy___ sample was removed during surgery and sent to a pathologist to be examined under a microscope for a proper diagnosis.

3. A (an) ___urologist___ performed surgery to remove Mr. Simon's cancerous kidney.

4. Ms. Rose has suffered from diabetes with hyperglycemia for many years. This condition can lead to long-term complications, such as the disease of nerves called diabetic ___neuropathy___.

5. A virus or a bacterium produces disease and is therefore a (an) ___pathogenic___ organism.

6. Jordan has a disease caused by abnormal hemoglobin in his erythrocytes. The erythrocytes change shape, collapsing to form sickle-shaped cells that can become clots and stop the flow of blood. His condition is called sickle cell ___anemia___.

7. Dr. Max Shelby is a physician who treats carcinomas and sarcomas. He is a (an) ___oncologist___.

8. Bill had difficulty stopping the bleeding from a cut on his face while shaving. He knew his medication caused him to have decreased platelets, or a low ___thrombocyte___ count, and that probably was the reason his blood was not clotting very well.

9. Dr. Susan Parker told Paul that his condition would improve with treatment in a few weeks. She said his ___prognosis___ is excellent and he can expect total recovery.

10. After fleeing the World Trade Center on September 11, 2001, Mrs. Jones had many problems with her job, her husband, and her family relationships. She went to see a ___psychiatrist___, who prescribed drugs to treat her depression.

P. Circle the correct term to complete each sentence.

1. Ms. Brody had a cough and fever. Her doctor instructed her to go to the (pathology, radiology, hematology) department for a chest x-ray examination.

2. After delivery of her third child, Ms. Thompson had problems holding her urine (a condition known as urinary incontinence). She made an appointment with a (gastroenterologist, pathologist, urologist) to evaluate her condition.

3. Dr. Monroe told a new mother she had lost much blood during delivery of her child. She had **(anemia, leukocytosis, adenitis)** and needed a blood transfusion immediately.

4. Mr. Preston was having chest pain during his morning walks. He made an appointment to discuss his new symptom with a **(nephrologist, neurologist, cardiologist)**.

5. After my skiing accident, Dr. Curtin suggested **(cystoscopy, biopsy, arthroscopy)** to visually examine my swollen, painful knee.

MEDICAL SCRAMBLE

Unscramble the letters to form medical terms from the clues. Use the letters in squares to complete the bonus term. Answers are found on page 26.

1. *Clue:* Complete knowledge of a patient's condition

   D I A G N O S I S   SIGOADSNI

2. *Clue:* Outermost layer of skin

   E P I D E R M E S   SREMEIDPI

3. *Clue:* Collection of blood below the skin

   H E M A T O M A   MATEHOAM

4. *Clue:* Pertaining to treatment of the mind

   P S Y C H I A T R I C   ICAITSHYRPC

5. *Clue:* Study of malignant tumors

   O N C O L O G Y   OCLOYGNO

BONUS TERM: *Clue:* A condition marked by deficiency of hemoglobin or decreased erythrocytes.

   A N E M I A

ANSWERS TO EXERCISES

A

1. prefixes
2. suffixes
3. root
4. combining vowel
5. combining form

B

1. heart
2. gland
3. life
4. cerebrum, largest part of the brain
5. head
6. joint
7. cancer, cancerous
8. urinary bladder
9. cell
10. skin
11. brain
12. electricity

C

1. tumor, mass, swelling
2. pertaining to
3. inflammation
4. process of study
5. process of visual examination
6. pertaining to
7. record
8. process of viewing

D

1. cerebr/al—pertaining to the cerebrum or largest part of the brain
2. bi/opsy—process of viewing life (removal of living tissue and viewing it under the microscope)
3. aden/itis—inflammation of a gland
4. cephal/ic—pertaining to the head
5. carcin/oma—tumor that is cancerous (cancerous tumor)
6. cyst/o/scopy—process of visually examining the urinary bladder
7. electr/o/cardi/o/gram—record of the electricity in the heart
8. cardi/o/logy—process of study of the heart
9. electr/o/encephal/o/gram—record of the electricity in the brain
10. dermat/itis—inflammation of the skin
11. arthr/o/scopy—process of visual examination of a joint
12. cyt/o/logy—process of study of cells

E

1. red
2. intestines (usually small intestine)
3. stomach
4. knowledge
5. blood
6. to cut
7. kidney
8. white
9. treatment, physician
10. liver
11. nerve
12. woman, female

F

1. leukocyte
2. gastritis
3. iatrogenic
4. nephrology
5. erythrocyte
6. hematoma
7. biopsy
8. neuralgia
9. ophthalmoscopy
10. enteritis

G

1. ren/o
2. path/o
3. ophthalm/o
4. sect/o
5. rhin/o
6. sarc/o
7. psych/o
8. ur/o
9. oste/o
10. radi/o
11. thromb/o
12. onc/o

H

1. ophthalmoscopy—process of visual examination of the eye
2. ophthalmoscope—instrument to visually examine the eye
3. oncology—study of tumors
4. osteitis—inflammation of bone
5. psychosis—abnormal condition of the mind
6. thrombocyte—clotting cell (platelet)
7. renal—pertaining to the kidney
8. nephrectomy—removal (excision or resection) of the kidney
9. osteotomy—incision of (process of cutting into) a bone
10. resection—process of cutting back (in the sense of "cutting out" or removal)
11. carcinogenic—pertaining to producing cancer
12. sarcoma—tumor of flesh (cancerous tumor of flesh tissue, such as bone, fat, and muscle)

I

1. pain
2. process
3. blood condition
4. record
5. instrument to visually examine
6. abnormal condition
7. removal, excision, resection
8. pertaining to producing, produced by, or produced in
9. disease condition
10. incision, process of cutting into
11. inflammation
12. cell

J

1. carcinogenic
2. leukocytosis
3. hepatoma (hepatocellular carcinoma)
4. arthralgia
5. endocrine
6. cystitis
7. hematoma
8. leukemia
9. iatrogenic
10. enteropathy

K

1. complete, through
2. before
3. self, own
4. no, not, without
5. excessive, above, more than normal
6. deficient, below, less than normal
7. above, upon
8. within
9. behind
10. across, through
11. surrounding
12. out
13. below, under
14. back

L

1. diagnosis—complete knowledge; a decision about the nature of the patient's condition after the appropriate tests are done
2. prognosis—before knowledge; a prediction about the outcome of treatment, given after the diagnosis
3. subhepatic—pertaining to below the liver. A combining vowel is not needed between the prefix and the root.
4. pericardium—the membrane surrounding the heart
5. hyperglycemia—condition of excessive sugar in the blood
6. hypodermic—pertaining to under the skin
7. epigastric—pertaining to above the stomach
8. resection—process of cutting back (in the sense of cutting out)
9. hypoglycemia—condition of deficient (low) sugar in the blood
10. anemia—condition of low numbers of erythrocytes (red blood cells) or deficient hemoglobin in these cells. Notice that the root in this term is *em*, which is shortened from *hem*, meaning blood.

M

1. urology
2. gynecology
3. hematology
4. oncology
5. nephrology
6. neurology
7. pediatrics (combining vowel *o* has been dropped between ped and iatr)
8. radiology
9. ophthalmology
10. gastroenterology
11. endocrinology
12. psychiatry
13. pathology
14. cardiology

N

1. cerebrum (largest part of the brain). A cerebrovascular accident is damage to the blood vessels of the cerebrum, leading to death of brain cells; also called a stroke.
2. brain. Encephalitis is inflammation of the brain.
3. urinary bladder. A cystoscope is an instrument used to visually examine the urinary bladder. The cystoscope is placed through the urethra into the urinary bladder.
4. across, through. Transhepatic means pertaining to across or through the liver.
5. treatment. Iatrogenic means pertaining to an adverse side effect produced by treatment.
6. under, below, deficient. Hypogastric means pertaining to below the stomach.
7. within. Endocrine glands secrete hormones within the body.
8. excision or resection. Nephrectomy is the removal of a kidney.
9. outside. Exocrine glands secrete chemicals to the outside of the body (sweat, lacrimal or tear-producing, prostate, and salivary glands).
10. pain. Neuralgia is nerve pain.

Examples of these are the pituitary, thyroid, and adrenal glands.

O

1. osteoarthritis
2. biopsy
3. urologist (a nephrologist is a medical doctor who treats kidney disorders but does not operate on patients)
4. neuropathy
5. pathogenic
6. anemia
7. oncologist
8. thrombocyte
9. prognosis
10. psychiatrist (a psychologist can treat mentally ill patients but is not a medical doctor and cannot prescribe medications)

P

1. radiology
2. urologist
3. anemia
4. cardiologist
5. arthroscopy

ANSWERS TO PRACTICAL APPLICATIONS

1. **D** A **cardiologist** is an internal medicine specialist who takes additional (fellowship) training in the diagnosis and treatment of heart disease.
2. **F** A **gynecologist** trains in both surgery and internal medicine in order to diagnose and treat disorders of the female reproductive system. Ovarian cysts are sacs of fluid that form on and in the ovaries (female organs that produce eggs and hormones).
3. **J** A **psychiatrist** is a specialist in diagnosing and treating mental illness. In bipolar disorder (manic-depressive illness), the mood switches periodically from excessive mania (excitability) to deep depression (sadness, despair, and discouragement).
4. **E** An **oncologist** is an internal medicine specialist who takes fellowship training in the diagnosis and medical (drug) treatment of cancer.
5. **B** A **hematologist** is an internal medicine specialist who takes fellowship training in the diagnosis and treatment of blood disorders such as anemia and clotting diseases.
6. **H** An **ophthalmologist** trains in both surgery and internal medicine to diagnose and treat disorders of the eye. The retina is a sensitive layer of light receptor cells in the back of the eye. Retinopathy can occur as a secondary complication of chronic diabetes (from hyperglycemia).
7. **I** A **neurologist** is an internal medicine specialist who takes fellowship training in the diagnosis and treatment of disorders of nervous tissue (brain, spinal cord, and nerves). A CVA causes damage to areas of the brain, resulting in loss of function.
8. **C** A **nephrologist** is an internal medicine specialist who takes fellowship training in the diagnosis and medical treatment of kidney disease. A nephrologist does not perform surgery on the urinary tract, but treats kidney disease with drugs.
9. **A** A **gastroenterologist** is an internal medicine specialist who takes fellowship training in the diagnosis and treatment of disorders of the gastrointestinal tract. Examples of inflammatory bowel disease are ulcerative colitis (inflammation of the large intestine) and Crohn's disease (inflammation of the last part of the small intestine).
10. **G** A **urologist** is a surgical specialist who treats and operates on organs of the urinary tract (such as the urinary bladder) and the male reproductive system.

ANSWERS TO MEDICAL SCRAMBLE

1. DIAGNOSIS 2. EPIDERMIS 3. HEMATOMA 4. PSYCHIATRIC 5. ONCOLOGY

BONUS TERM: ANEMIA

PRONUNCIATION OF TERMS

PRONUNCIATION GUIDE

ā as in āpe	ă as in ăpple
ē as in ēven	ĕ as in ĕvery
ī as in īce	ĭ as in ĭnterest
ō as in ōpen	ŏ as in pŏt
ū as in ūnit	ŭ as in ŭnder

The markings ¯ and ˘ above the vowels—a, e, i, o, and u—indicate the proper sounds of the vowels in a term. When ¯ is above a vowel, its sound is long—that is, exactly like its name. The ˘ marking indicates a short vowel sound.

To test your understanding of the terminology in this chapter, write the meaning of each term in the space provided. In addition, you may wish to cover the terms and write them by looking at your definitions. Make sure your spelling is correct. The page number after each term indicates where it is defined or used in the book, so you can easily check your responses. You will find complete definitions for all of these terms and their audio pronunciations on the CD.

VOCABULARY AND TERMINOLOGY

Term	Pronunciation	Meaning
adenitis (8)	ăd-ĕ-NĪ-tĭs	______________
adenoma (8)	ăd-ĕ-NŌ-mă	______________

Term	Pronunciation	Meaning
adenopathy (13)	ăd-ĕ-NŎP-ă-thē	_____
anemia (13)	ă-NĒ-mē-ă	_____
arthralgia (12)	ăr-THRĂL-jă	_____
arthritis (8)	ăr-THRĪ-tĭs	_____
autopsy (13)	ĂW-tŏp-sē	_____
biology (8)	bī-ŎL-ō-jē	_____
biopsy (12)	BĪ-ŏp-sē	_____
carcinogenic (12)	kăr-sĭ-nō-JĔN-ĭk	_____
carcinoma (8)	kăr-sĭ-NŌ-mă	_____
cardiac (12)	KĂR-dē-ăk	_____
cardiology (8)	kăr-dē-ŎL-ō-jē	_____
cephalic (8)	sĕ-FĂL-ĭk	_____
cerebral (9)	sĕ-RĒ-brăl or SĔR-ĕ-brăl	_____
cystitis (12)	sĭs-TĪ-tĭs	_____
cystoscopy (9)	sĭs-TŎS-kō-pē	_____
cytology (9)	sī-TŎL-ō-jē	_____
dermatitis (9)	dĕr-mă-TĪ-tĭs	_____
dermatology (9)	dĕr-mă-TŎL-ō-jē	_____
diagnosis (10)	dī-ăg-NŌ-sĭs	_____
electrocardiogram (5)	ē-lĕk-trō-KĂR-dē-ō-grăm	_____
electroencephalogram (9)	ē-lĕk-trō-ĕn-SĔF-ă-lō-grăm	_____
endocrine glands (9)	ĔN-dō-krĭn glăndz	_____
endocrinologist (13)	ĕn-dō-krĭ-NŎL-ō-jĭst	_____
endocrinology (12)	ĕn-dō-krĭ-NŎL-ō-jē	_____
endoscope (13)	ĔN-dō-skōp	_____
endoscopy (13)	ĕn-DŎS-kō-pē	_____
enteritis (9)	ĕn-tĕ-RĪ-tĭs	_____
enteropathy (13)	ĕn-tĕ-RŎP-ă-thē	_____
epidermis (14)	ĕp-ĭ-DĔR-mĭs	_____
epigastric (14)	ĕp-ĭ-GĂS-trĭk	_____
erythrocyte (9)	ĕ-RĬTH-rō-sīt	_____
excision (9)	ĕk-SĬ-zhŭn	_____
exocrine glands (14)	ĔK-sō-krĭn glăndz	_____

Term	Pronunciation	Meaning
gastrectomy (9)	găs-TRĔK-tō-mē	_____
gastric (12)	GĂS-trĭk	_____
gastroenterology (13)	găs-trō-ĕn-tĕr-ŎL-ō-jē	_____
gastrotomy (9)	găs-TRŎT-ō-mē	_____
gynecologist (12)	gī-nĕ-KŎL-ō-jĭst	_____
gynecology (10)	gī-nĕ-KŎL-ō-jē	_____
hematology (10)	hē-mă-TŎL-ō-jē	_____
hematoma (10)	hē-mă-TŌ-mă	_____
hemoglobin (10)	HĒ-mō-glō-bĭn	_____
hepatitis (10)	hĕp-ă-TĪ-tĭs	_____
hepatoma (12)	hĕp-ă-TŌ-mă	_____
hyperglycemia (14)	hī-pĕr-glī-SĒ-mē-ă	_____
hyperthyroidism (14)	hī-pĕr-THĪ-rŏyd-ĭsm	_____
hypodermic (9)	hī-pō-DĔR-mĭk	_____
hypogastric (14)	hī-pō-GĂS-trĭk	_____
hypoglycemia (14)	hī-pō-glī-SĒ-mē-ă	_____
iatrogenic (10)	ī-ăt-rō-JĔN-ĭk	_____
incision (9)	ĭn-SĬ-zhŭn	_____
leukemia (12)	lū-KĒ-mē-ă	_____
leukocyte (10)	LŪ-kō-sīt	_____
leukocytosis (13)	lū-kō-sī-TŌ-sĭs	_____
nephrectomy (12)	nĕ-FRĔK-tō-mē	_____
nephritis (10)	nĕ-FRĪ-tĭs	_____
nephrology (10)	nĕ-FRŎL-ō-jē	_____
nephrosis (13)	nĕ-FRŌ-sĭs	_____
neural (12)	NŪ-răl	_____
neuralgia (12)	nū-RĂL-jă	_____
neurologic (12)	nū-rō-LŎJ-ĭk	_____
neurology (10)	nū-RŎL-ō-jē	_____
oncologist (10)	ŏn-KŎL-ō-jĭst	_____
oncology (10)	ŏn-KŎL-ō-jē	_____

Term	Pronunciation	Meaning
ophthalmologist (26)	ŏf-thăl-MŎL-ō-jĭst	_____
ophthalmoscope (10)	ŏf-THĂL-mō-skōp	_____
osteitis (11)	ŏs-tē-Ī-tĭs	_____
osteoarthritis (11)	ŏs-tē-ō-ăr-THRĪ-tĭs	_____
osteotomy (13)	ŏs-tē-ŎT-ō-mē	_____
pathogenic (12)	păth-ō-JĔN-ĭk	_____
pathologist (11)	pă-THŎL-ŏ-jĭst	_____
pathology (11)	pă-THŎL-ō-jē	_____
pediatric (11)	pē-dē-ĂT-rĭk	_____
pericardium (14)	pĕr-ĭ-KĂR-dē-ŭm	_____
prognosis (13)	prŏg-NŌ-sĭs	_____
prostate gland (14)	PRŎS-tāt gland	_____
psychiatrist (11)	sī-KĪ-ă-trĭst	_____
psychiatry (26)	sī-KĪ-ă-trē	_____
psychology (11)	sī-KŎL-ō-jē	_____
radiology (11)	rā-dē-ŎL-ō-jē	_____
renal (11)	RĒ-năl	_____
resection (15)	rē-SĔK-shŭn	_____
retrocardiac (15)	rĕ-trō-KĂR-dē-ăc	_____
rhinitis (11)	rī-NĪ-tĭs	_____
sarcoma (11)	săr-KŌ-mă	_____
subhepatic (15)	sŭb-hĕ-PĂT-ĭk	_____
thrombocyte (11)	THRŎM-bō-sīt	_____
transhepatic (15)	trănz-hĕ-PĂT-ĭk	_____
urology (11)	ū-RŎL-ō-jē	_____

REVIEW SHEET

This Review Sheet and the others that follow each chapter are complete lists of the word elements contained in that chapter. The Review Sheets are designed to pull together the terminology and to reinforce your learning by giving you the opportunity to write the meanings of each word part in the spaces provided and to test yourself. Check your answers with the information in the chapter or in the Glossary (Medical Word Parts—English) at the end of the book.

COMBINING FORMS

Combining Form	Meaning	Combining Form	Meaning
aden/o		hem/o, hemat/o	
arthr/o		hepat/o	
bi/o		iatr/o	
carcin/o		leuk/o	
cardi/o		log/o	
cephal/o		nephr/o	
cerebr/o		neur/o	
cis/o		onc/o	
crin/o		ophthalm/o	
cyst/o		oste/o	
cyt/o		path/o	
derm/o, dermat/o		ped/o	
electr/o		psych/o	
encephal/o		radi/o	
enter/o		ren/o	
erythr/o		rhin/o	
gastr/o		sarc/o	
glyc/o		sect/o	
gnos/o		thromb/o	
gynec/o		ur/o	

SUFFIXES

Suffix	Meaning	Suffix	Meaning
-ac		-ectomy	
-al		-emia	
-algia		-genic	
-cyte		-globin	

SUFFIXES—cont'd

Suffix	Meaning	Suffix	Meaning
-gram	_____	-osis	_____
-ic, -ical	_____	-pathy	_____
-ion	_____	-scope	_____
-ist	_____	-scopy	_____
-itis	_____	-sis	_____
-logy	_____	-tomy	_____
-oma	_____	-y	_____
-opsy	_____		

PREFIXES

Prefix	Meaning	Prefix	Meaning
a-, an-	_____	in-	_____
aut-, auto-	_____	peri-	_____
dia-	_____	pro-	_____
end-, endo-	_____	re-	_____
epi-	_____	retro-	_____
ex-, exo-	_____	sub-	_____
hyper-	_____	trans-	_____
hypo-	_____		

 Please refer to the enclosed CD for additional exercises and images related to this chapter.

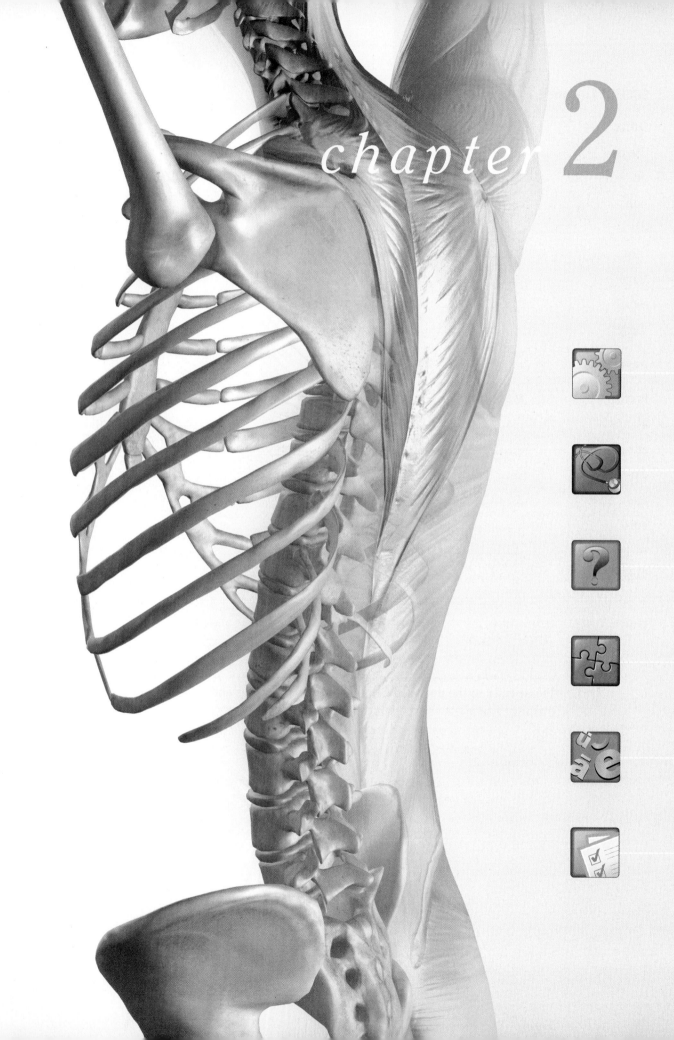

chapter 2

Terms Pertaining to the Body as a Whole

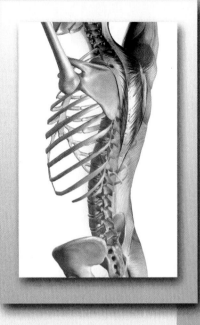

THIS CHAPTER IS DIVIDED INTO THE FOLLOWING SECTIONS

In this chapter you will

- Define terms that apply to the structural organization of the body.
- Identify the body cavities and recognize the organs contained within those cavities.
- Locate and identify the anatomic and clinical divisions of the abdomen.
- Locate and name the anatomic divisions of the back.
- Become acquainted with terms that describe positions, directions, and planes of the body.
- Identify the meanings for new word elements and use them to understand new medical terms.

Image Description: Posterior angled view of a male body with musculature highlighted.

STRUCTURAL ORGANIZATION OF THE BODY

This chapter provides you with an orientation to the body as a whole—cells, tissues, organs, systems, and terminology describing positions and directions within the body. We begin with the smallest living unit, the **cell,** and build to an understanding of complex body systems. In order to know how organs function in both health and disease, it is important to appreciate the workings of their individual cellular units.

Cells

The cell is the fundamental unit of all living things (animal or plant). Cells are everywhere in the human body—every tissue, every organ is made up of these individual units.

Similarity in Cells. All cells are similar in that they contain a gelatinous substance composed of water, protein, sugar, acids, fats, and various minerals. Several parts of a cell, described next, are pictured in Figure 2–1 as they might look when photographed with an electron microscope. *Label* the structures on Figure 2–1. Throughout the book, numbers in *brackets* indicate that the boldface term preceding it is to be used in labeling.

The **cell membrane** [1] not only surrounds and protects the cell but also regulates what passes into and out of the cell.

The **nucleus** [2] controls the operations of the cell. It directs cell division and determines the structure and function of the cell.

Chromosomes [3] are rod-like structures within the nucleus. All human body cells—except for the sex cells the egg and the sperm (short for spermatozoon)—contain 23 pairs of chromosomes. Each sperm and each egg cell have only 23 unpaired chromosomes. After an egg and a sperm cell unite to form the embryo, each cell of the embryo then has 46 chromosomes (23 pairs) (Fig. 2–2).

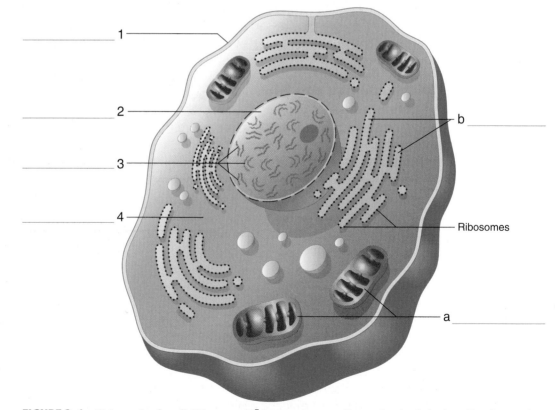

FIGURE 2–1   **Major parts of a cell.** Ribosomes (RĪ-bō-sōmz) are small granules that help the cell make proteins.

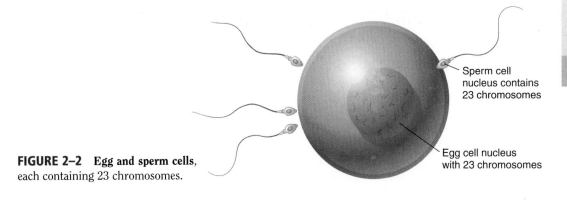

FIGURE 2–2 **Egg and sperm cells,** each containing 23 chromosomes.

Sperm cell nucleus contains 23 chromosomes

Egg cell nucleus with 23 chromosomes

Chromosomes contain regions called **genes.** There are several thousand genes, in an orderly sequence, on every chromosome. Each gene is composed of a chemical called **DNA** (deoxyribonucleic acid). DNA regulates the activities of the cell by its sequence (arrangement into genes) on each chromosome. The DNA sequence resembles a series of recipes in code. The code, when passed out of the nucleus to the rest of the cell, directs the activities of the cell, such as cell division and synthesis of proteins.

Chromosomes within the nucleus are analyzed in terms of their size, arrangement, and number by determining a **karyotype.** Karyotyping of chromosomes determines whether the chromosomes are normal in number and structure. For example, obstetricians often recommend an amniocentesis (puncture of the sac around the fetus for removal of fluid and cells) for a pregnant woman so that the karyotype of the baby can be examined. Figure 2–3 shows a karyotype, or chromosomal map, for a normal male. The chromosomes have been treated with chemicals so that bands (light and dark areas) can be seen.

If a baby is born with an abnormal number of chromosomes, serious problems can result. In Down syndrome, the karyotype shows 47 chromosomes instead of the normal number of 46. The extra number 21 chromosome results in the development of a child with Down syndrome (also called trisomy 21 syndrome). Its incidence is about 1 in every 750 live births, but as the mother's age increases, the presence of the chromosomal (genetic) abnormality increases. A typical Down syndrome infant is born with physical malformations that may include a small, flattened skull; a short, flat-bridged nose; wide-set, slanted eyes; and short, broad hands and feet with a wide gap between the first and second toes. Reproductive organs often are underdeveloped, congenital heart defects are not uncommon, and some degree of mental retardation is evident (Fig. 2–4).

Continue labeling Figure 2–1.

The **cytoplasm** [4] (cyt/o = cell, -plasm = formation) includes all the material outside the nucleus and enclosed by the cell membrane. It carries on the work of the cell (e.g., in a muscle cell, it does the contracting; in a nerve cell, it transmits impulses). The cytoplasm contains specialized apparatus to supply the chemical needs of the cell:

Mitochondria [a] are small, sausage-shaped bodies that, like miniature power plants, produce energy by burning food in the presence of oxygen. During this chemical process, called **catabolism** (cata = down, bol = to cast, -ism = process), complex foods (sugar and fat) are broken down into simpler substances. The catabolism of sugar and fat releases needed energy to do the work of the cell.

The **endoplasmic reticulum** [b] is a network (reticulum) of canals within the cell. These canals (containing small structures called ribosomes) are a cellular tunnel system in which proteins are manufactured for use in the cell. This process of building up complex materials, such as proteins, from simpler parts is called **anabolism** (ana = up, bol = to cast, -ism = process). During anabolism, small pieces of protein (called amino acids) are fitted together like links in a chain to make larger proteins.

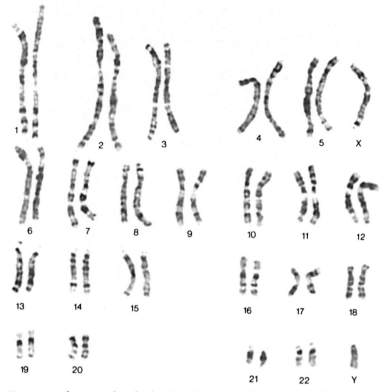

FIGURE 2–3 **Karyotype of a normal male** showing 23 pairs of chromosomes. The 23rd pair is the XY pair. In a normal female karyotype, the 23rd pair is XX. (X chromosome is near number 5 pair and Y chromosome is near number 22 pair.) (From Behrman RE, Kliegman RM, Jensen HB [eds]: Nelson Textbook of Pediatrics, 16th ed. Philadelphia, WB Saunders, 2000, p 326.)

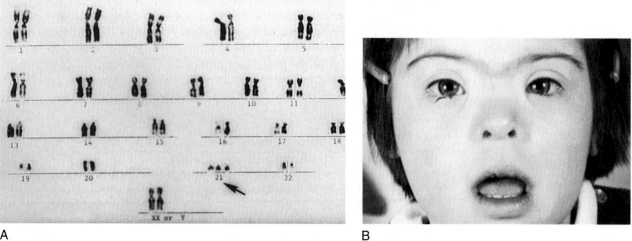

A   B

FIGURE 2–4 **A, Karyotype of a female patient with Down syndrome, showing trisomy 21. B, Photograph of a 3½-year-old girl with the typical facial appearance that occurs in Down syndrome.** Features include a flat nasal bridge, an upward slant of the eyes, and a protruding tongue. Other characteristics of Down syndrome patients are mental deficiency and heart defects. (**A** courtesy of Urvashi Surti, PhD, Pittsburgh Cytogenetics Laboratory. From Zitelli BJ, Davis HW: Atlas of Pediatric Physical Diagnosis, 4th ed. St. Louis, Mosby, 2002, p. 11. **B** From Baralos M, Baramki TA: Medical Cytogenics, Baltimore, Lippincott Williams and Wilkins, 1967.)

Together, these two processes—anabolism and catabolism—are known as **metabolism** (meta = change, bol = to cast, -ism = process). Metabolism is the total of the chemical processes occurring in a cell. If a person has a "fast metabolism," then foods such as sugar and fat are thought to be used up very quickly, and energy is released. If a person has a "slow metabolism," foods are thought to be burned slowly, and fat accumulates in cells.

STUDY SECTION 1

Practice spelling each term, and know its meaning.

anabolism	Process of building up complex materials (proteins) from simple materials.
catabolism	Process of breaking down complex materials (foods) to form simpler substances and release energy.
cell membrane	Structure surrounding and protecting the cell. It determines what enters and leaves the cell.
chromosomes	Rod-shaped structures in the nucleus that contain regions of DNA called genes. There are 46 chromosomes (23 pairs) in every cell except for the egg and sperm cells, which contain only 23 individual, unpaired chromosomes.
cytoplasm	All the material that is outside the nucleus and yet contained within the cell membrane.
DNA	Chemical found within each chromosome. Arranged like a sequence of recipes in code, it directs the activities of the cell.
endoplasmic reticulum	Structure (canals) within the cytoplasm. Site in which large proteins are made from smaller protein pieces. **Ribosomes** are found on the endoplasmic reticulum (see Figure 2–1).
genes	Regions of DNA within each chromosome.
karyotype	Picture of chromosomes in the nucleus of a cell. The chromosomes are arranged in numerical order to determine their number and structure.
metabolism	The total of the chemical processes in a cell. It includes both catabolism and anabolism.
mitochondria	Structures in the cytoplasm in which foods are burned to release energy.
nucleus	Control center of the cell. It contains chromosomes and directs the activities of the cell.

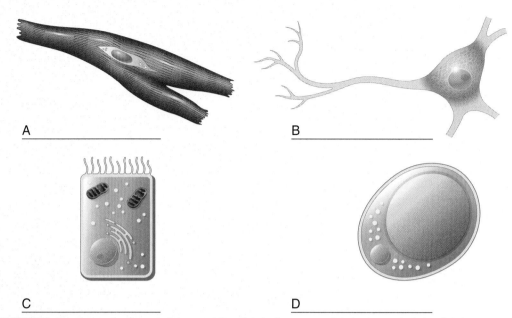

A _____   B _____

C _____   D _____

FIGURE 2–5   **Types of cells.** Label the **muscle cell (A)**, the **nerve cell (B)**, the **epithelial cell (C)**, and the **fat cell (D)**.

Differences in Cells. Cells are different, or specialized, throughout the body to carry out their individual functions. For example, a **muscle cell** is long and slender and contains fibers that aid in contracting and relaxing; an **epithelial cell** (a lining and skin cell) may be square and flat to provide protection; a **nerve cell** may be long and have various fibrous extensions that aid in its job of carrying impulses; a **fat cell** contains large, empty spaces for fat storage. These are only a few of the many types of cells in the body. Figure 2–5 illustrates the different sizes and shapes of muscle, nerve, fat, and epithelial cells.

Tissues

A tissue is a group of similar cells working together to do a specific job. A **histologist** (hist/o = tissue) is a scientist who specializes in the study of tissues. Several different types of tissue are recognized. Tissues of the same type may be located in various regions of the body.

Epithelial Tissue. Epithelial tissue, located all over the body, forms the linings of internal organs, and the outer surface of the skin covering the body. It also lines exocrine and endocrine glands. The term **epithelial** originally referred to the tissue above (epi-) the breast nipple (thel/o). Now it describes all tissue that covers the outside of the body and lines the inner surface of internal organs.

Muscle Tissue. Voluntary muscle found in arms and legs and parts of the body where movement is under conscious control. Involuntary muscle, found in the heart and digestive system, as well as other organs, allows movement that is not under conscious control. Cardiac muscle is a specialized type of muscle found only in the heart. Contractions of this muscle type can be seen as a beating heart in an ultrasound scan of a 6-week-old fetus.

Connective Tissue. Examples are **adipose** (fat) tissue, **cartilage** (elastic, fibrous tissue attached to bones), bone, and blood.

Nerve Tissue. Nerve tissue conducts impulses all over the body.

Organs

Organs are structures composed of several types of tissue. For example, an organ such as the stomach is composed of muscle tissue, nerve tissue, and glandular epithelial tissue. The medical term for internal organs is **viscera** (singular: **viscus**). Examples of abdominal viscera (organs located in the abdomen) are the liver, stomach, intestines, pancreas, spleen, and gallbladder.

Systems

Systems are groups of organs working together to perform complex functions. For example, the mouth, esophagus, stomach, and small and large intestines are organs that do the work of the digestive system to digest food and absorb it into the bloodstream.

The body systems with their individual organs are listed next. Learn to spell and identify the organs in **boldface.**

System	Organs
Digestive	Mouth, **pharynx** (throat), esophagus, stomach, intestines (small and large), liver, gallbladder, pancreas.
Urinary or excretory	Kidneys, **ureters** (tubes from the kidneys to the urinary bladder), urinary bladder, **urethra** (tube from the bladder to the outside of the body).
Respiratory	Nose, pharynx, **larynx** (voice box), **trachea** (windpipe), bronchial tubes, lungs (where the exchange of gases takes place).
Reproductive	*Female*: Ovaries, fallopian tubes, **uterus** (womb), vagina, mammary glands.
	Male: Testes and associated tubes, urethra, penis, prostate gland.
Endocrine	**Thyroid gland** (in the neck), **pituitary gland** (at the base of the brain), sex glands (ovaries and testes), adrenal glands, pancreas (islets of Langerhans), parathyroid glands.
Nervous	Brain, spinal cord, nerves, and collections of nerves.
Circulatory	Heart, blood vessels (arteries, veins, and capillaries), lymphatic vessels and nodes, spleen, thymus gland.
Musculoskeletal	Muscles, bones, and joints.
Skin and sense organs	Skin, hair, nails, sweat glands, and sebaceous (oil) glands; eye, ear, nose, and tongue.

2

STUDY SECTION 2

Practice spelling each term, and know its meaning.

adipose tissue	Collection of fat cells.
cartilage	Flexible connective tissue attached to bones at joints. For example, it surrounds the trachea and forms part of the external ear and nose.
epithelial cells	Skin cells that cover the external body surface and line the internal surfaces of organs.
histologist	Specialist in the study of tissues.
larynx (LĂR-ĭnks)	"Voice box"; located at the upper part of the trachea.
pharynx (FĂR-ĭnks)	Throat. The pharynx serves as the common passageway for both food (from the mouth going to the esophagus) and air (from the nose to the trachea).
pituitary gland	Endocrine gland at the base of the brain.
thyroid gland	Endocrine gland that surrounds the trachea in the neck.
trachea	"Windpipe" (tube leading from the throat to the bronchial tubes).
ureter	One of two tubes, each leading from a single kidney to the urinary bladder. *Spelling clue*: Ureter has two e's, and there are two ureters.
urethra	Tube from the urinary bladder to the outside of the body. *Spelling clue*: Urethra has one e, and there is only one urethra.
uterus	The womb. The organ that holds the embryo/fetus as it develops.
viscera	Internal organs.

BODY CAVITIES

A body cavity is a space within the body that contains internal organs (viscera). Label Figure 2–6 as you learn the names of the body cavities. Some of the important viscera contained within those cavities are listed as well.

Cavity	Organs
Cranial [1]	Brain, pituitary gland.
Thoracic [2]	Lungs, heart, esophagus, trachea, bronchial tubes, thymus gland, aorta (large artery).
	The thoracic cavity is divided into two smaller cavities (Fig. 2–7): a. **Pleural cavity**—space surrounding each lung. A double-folded membrane, or **pleura**, lines the pleural cavity. If the pleura becomes inflamed (as in pleuritis or pleurisy), the pleural cavity can fill with fluid. b. **Mediastinum**—centrally located area outside of and between the lungs. It contains the heart, aorta, trachea, esophagus, thymus gland, bronchial tubes, and many lymph nodes.

Abdominal [3]   Stomach, small and large intestines, spleen, pancreas, liver, and gallbladder. The diaphragm (a muscular wall), divides the abdominal and thoracic cavities (see Figure 2–6).

The **peritoneum** is the double-folded membrane surrounding the abdominal cavity (Fig. 2–8). The kidneys are two bean-shaped organs situated behind (retroperitoneal area) the abdominal cavity on either side of the backbone (see Figs. 2–8 and 2–10).

Pelvic [4]   Portions of the small and large intestines, rectum, urinary bladder, urethra, and ureters; uterus and vagina in the female.

Spinal [5]   Nerves of the spinal cord.

The cranial and spinal cavities are the **dorsal** body cavities because of their location on the back (posterior) portion of the body. The thoracic, abdominal, and pelvic cavities are **ventral** body cavities because they are on the front (anterior) portion of the body. See Figure 2–6.

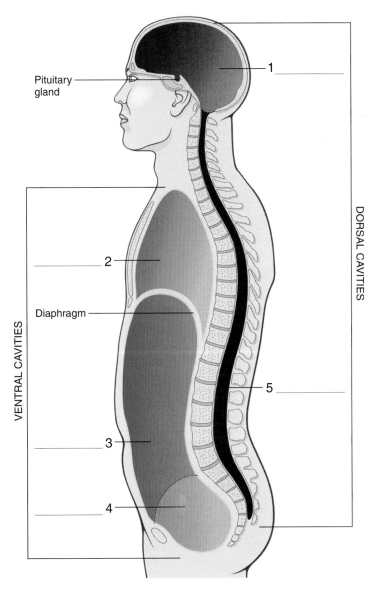

FIGURE 2–6 **Body cavities.** Ventral (anterior) cavities are in the front of the body. Dorsal (posterior) cavities are in the back.

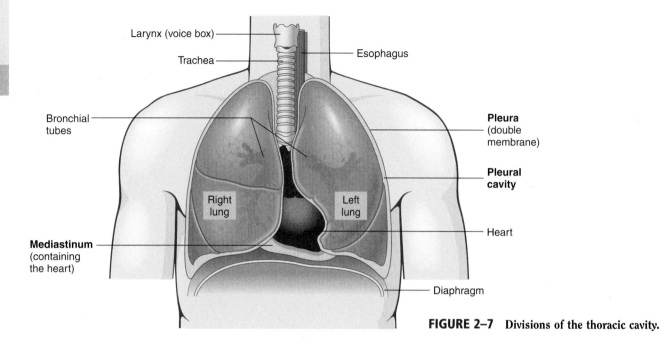

FIGURE 2–7   Divisions of the thoracic cavity.

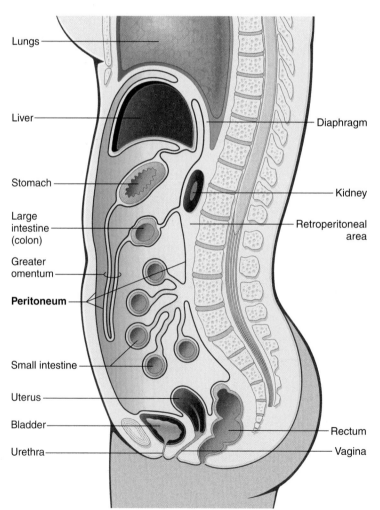

FIGURE 2–8 **Abdominal cavity** *(side view and in light blue).* Notice the **peritoneum** *(in dark red),* which is a membrane surrounding the organs in the abdominal cavity. The **retroperitoneal area** is behind the peritoneum. The **greater omentum** is a part of the peritoneum in the front of the abdomen. It contains fat and hangs down loosely like an apron over the intestines to keep them warm.

The thoracic and abdominal cavities are separated by a muscular wall called a diaphragm. Since the abdominal and pelvic cavities are not separated by a diaphragm, they are frequently referred together as the **abdominopelvic cavity.** Figures 2–9 and 2–10 show the abdominal and thoracic viscera from anterior (ventral) and posterior (dorsal) views.

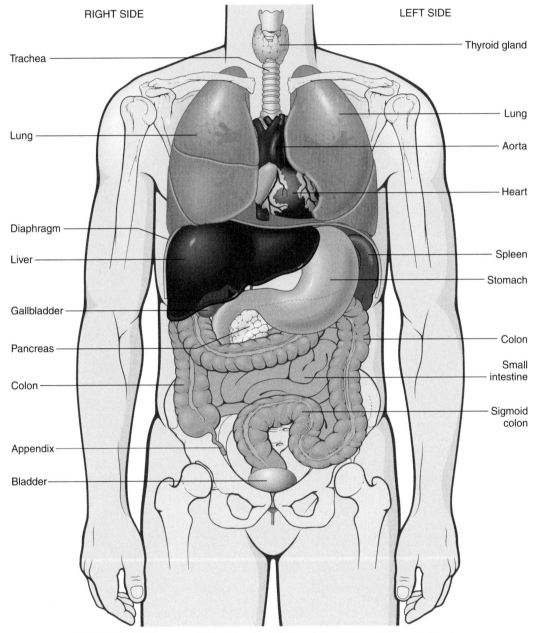

RIGHT SIDE

LEFT SIDE

Trachea

Thyroid gland

Lung

Lung

Aorta

Heart

Diaphragm

Spleen

Liver

Stomach

Gallbladder

Colon

Pancreas

Small intestine

Colon

Sigmoid colon

Appendix

Bladder

FIGURE 2–9   **Organs of the abdominopelvic and thoracic cavities,** anterior view.

2

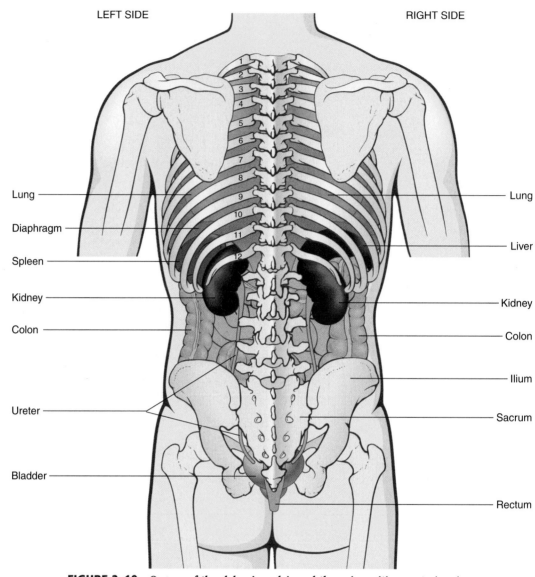

LEFT SIDE   RIGHT SIDE

Lung

Diaphragm

Spleen

Kidney

Colon

Ureter

Bladder

Lung

Liver

Kidney

Colon

Ilium

Sacrum

Rectum

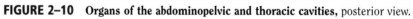

FIGURE 2–10 **Organs of the abdominopelvic and thoracic cavities,** posterior view.

2

STUDY SECTION 3

Practice spelling each term, and know its meaning.

abdominal cavity	Space below the chest containing organs such as the liver, stomach, gallbladder, and intestines; also called the **abdomen.**
cranial cavity	Space in the head containing the brain and surrounded by the skull. **Cranial** means **pertaining to the skull.**
diaphragm	Muscle separating the abdominal and thoracic cavities.
dorsal (posterior)	Pertaining to the back.
mediastinum	Centrally located space between the lungs.
pelvic cavity	Space below the abdomen containing portions of the intestines, rectum, urinary bladder, and reproductive organs. **Pelvic** means **pertaining to the pelvis,** composed of the hip bones surrounding the pelvic cavity.
peritoneum	Double-layered membrane surrounding the abdominal organs.
pleura	Double-layered membrane surrounding each lung.
pleural cavity	Space between the pleural membranes and surrounding each lung.
spinal cavity	Space within the spinal column (backbones) and containing the spinal cord. Also called the **spinal canal.**
thoracic cavity	Space in the chest containing the heart, lungs, bronchial tubes, trachea, esophagus, and other organs.
ventral (anterior)	Pertaining to the front.

Pleural/Plural

Don't confuse *pleural,* which relates to the membranes surrounding the lungs, with *plural,* which means more than one.

ABDOMINOPELVIC REGIONS AND QUADRANTS

REGIONS

Doctors divide the abdominopelvic area into nine regions. Label these regions in Figure 2–11.

Hypochondriac region [1]: upper right and left region below (hypo-) the cartilage (chondr/o) of the ribs that extend over the abdomen.

Epigastric region [2]: region above the stomach.

Lumbar region [3]: middle right and left region near the waist.

Umbilical region [4]: region of the navel or umbilicus.

Inguinal region [5]: lower right and left region near the groin (inguin/o = groin), which is the area where the legs join the trunk of the body. This region, on right and left, is also known as the **iliac** region because it is near the ilium, which is the upper portion of the hip bone.

Hypogastric region [6]: lower middle region below the umbilical region.

QUADRANTS

The abdominopelvic area can be divided into four quadrants by two imaginary lines—one horizontal and one vertical—that cross at the midsection of the body. Figure 2–12 shows

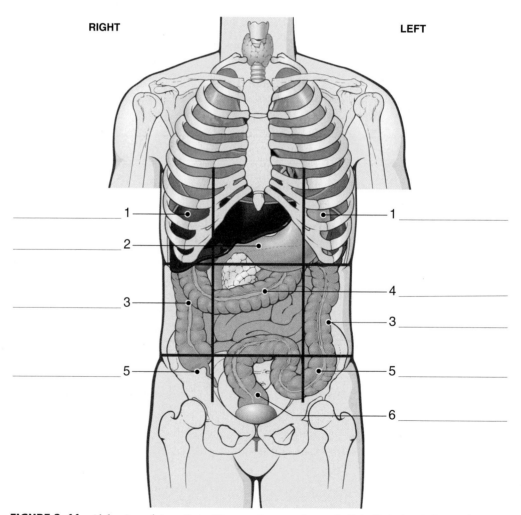

FIGURE 2–11   Abdominopelvic regions. These regions can be used clinically to locate internal organs.

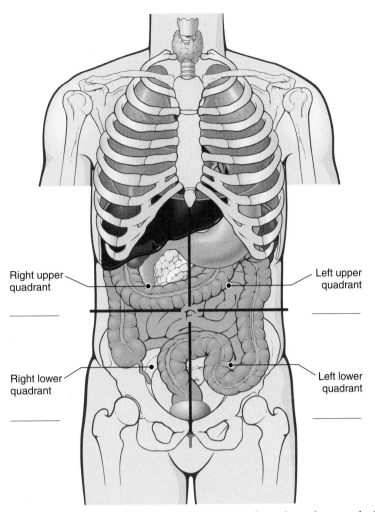

Right upper quadrant

Left upper quadrant

Right lower quadrant

Left lower quadrant

FIGURE 2–12 **Abdominopelvic quadrants.** Give the abbreviation for each quadrant on the line provided.

the four abdominopelvic quadrants; add the proper abbreviation on the line under each label on the diagram.

Right upper quadrant (RUQ)—contains the liver (right lobe), gallbladder, part of the pancreas, parts of the small and large intestines

Left upper quadrant (LUQ)—contains the liver (left lobe), stomach, spleen, part of the pancreas, parts of the small and large intestines

Right lower quadrant (RLQ)—contains parts of the small and large intestines, right ovary, right fallopian tube, appendix, right ureter

Left lower quadrant (LLQ)—contains parts of the small and large intestines, left ovary, left fallopian tube, left ureter

DIVISIONS OF THE BACK (SPINAL COLUMN)

The spinal column is composed of a series of bones that extend from the neck to the tailbone. Each bone is a **vertebra** (plural: **vertebrae**).

Label the divisions of the back on Figure 2–13 as you study the following:

Division of the Back	Abbreviation	Location
Cervical [1]	C	Neck region. There are seven cervical vertebrae (C1 to C7).
Thoracic [2]	T	Chest region. There are 12 thoracic vertebrae (T1 to T12). Each bone is joined to a rib.
Lumbar [3]	L	Loin (waist) or flank region (between the ribs and the hipbone). There are five lumbar vertebrae (L1 to L5).
Sacral [4]	S	Five bones (S1 to S5) are fused to form one bone, the **sacrum.**
Coccygeal [5]		The **coccyx** (tailbone) is a small bone composed of four fused pieces.

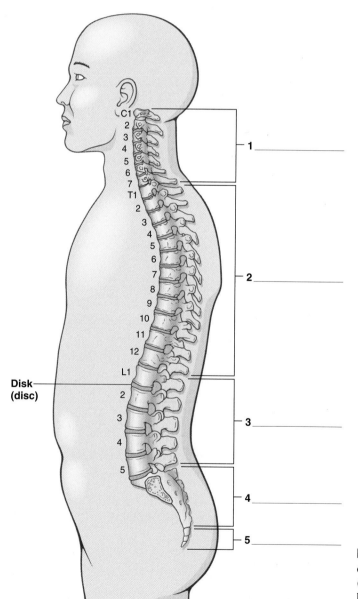

C1
2
3
4
5
6
7
T1
2
3
4
5
6
7
8
9
10
11
12
L1
2
3
4
5

Disk (disc)

1 _____
2 _____
3 _____
4 _____
5 _____

FIGURE 2–13 **Anatomic divisions of the back (spinal column).** A disk (disc) is a small pad of cartilage between each backbone.

Do not confuse the **spinal column** (back bones or vertebrae) and the **spinal cord** (nerves surrounded by the column). The column is bone tissue, whereas the cord is nervous tissue.

The spaces between the vertebrae (intervertebral spaces) are identified according to the two vertebrae between which they occur—for example, the L5–S1 space is between the fifth lumbar vertebra and the first sacral vertebra; T2–3 is between the second and third thoracic vertebrae. Within the space and between vertebrae is a small pad called a **disk,** or **disc.** The disk, composed of water and cartilage, is a shock absorber. Occasionally, a disk may move out of place (rupture) and put pressure on a nerve. This is a **slipped disk,** which causes back pain.

STUDY SECTION 4

Practice spelling each term, and know its meaning.

ABDOMINOPELVIC REGIONS

hypochondriac	Upper right and left regions beneath the ribs.
epigastric	Upper middle region above the stomach.
lumbar	Middle right and left regions near the waist.
umbilical	Central region near the navel.
inguinal	Lower right and left regions near the groin. Also called **iliac regions.**
hypogastric	Lower middle region below the umbilical region.

ABDOMINOPELVIC QUADRANTS

RUQ	Right upper quadrant.
LUQ	Left upper quadrant.
RLQ	Right lower quadrant.
LLQ	Left lower quadrant.

DIVISIONS OF THE BACK

cervical	Neck region (C1 to C7).
thoracic	Chest region (T1 to T12).
lumbar	Loin (waist) region (L1 to L5).
sacral	Region of the sacrum (S1 to S5).
coccygeal	Region of the coccyx (tailbone).

RELATED TERMS

vertebra	A single backbone.
vertebrae	Backbones.
spinal column	Bone tissue surrounding the spinal cavity.
spinal cord	Nervous tissue within the spinal cavity.
disk (disc)	A pad of cartilage between vertebrae.

POSITIONAL AND DIRECTIONAL TERMS

Label Figure 2–14, *A* and *B,* to identify the following positional and directional terms.

Location	Relationship
Anterior (ventral) [1]	Front surface of the body. *Example*: The forehead is on the **anterior** side of the body.
Posterior (dorsal) [2]	The back side of the body. *Example*: The back of the head is **posterior (dorsal)** to the face.
Deep [3]	Away from the surface. *Example*: The stab wound penetrated **deep** into the abdomen.
Superficial [4]	On the surface. *Example*: **Superficial** veins can be viewed through the skin.
Proximal [5]	Near the point of attachment to the trunk or near the beginning of a structure. *Example*: The **proximal** end of the upper armbone (humerus) joins with the shoulder bone.

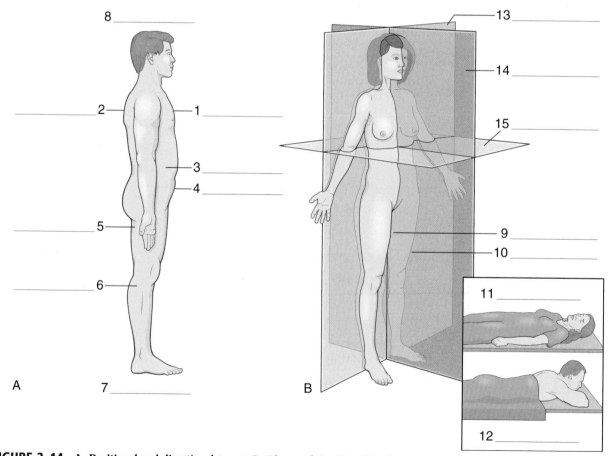

FIGURE 2–14   A, Positional and directional terms. B, Planes of the body. The figure is standing in the **anatomic position,** with the palms of the hands facing outward and the fifth (little) finger in a medial position (closer to the center of the body).

Distal [6]	Far from the point of attachment to the trunk or far from the beginning of a structure. *Example*: At its **distal** end, the humerus joins with the lower armbones at the elbow.
Inferior [7]	Below another structure. *Example*: The feet are at the **inferior** part of the body. They are inferior to the knees. The term **caudal** (pertaining to the tail, or to the lower portion of the body) also means away from the head or below another structure.
Superior [8]	Above another structure. *Example*: The head is **superior** to the neck. **Cephalic** (pertaining to the head) also means above another structure.
Medial [9]	Pertaining to the middle or nearer the medial plane of the body. *Example*: The inner thigh is **medial** in relation to the body.
Lateral [10]	Pertaining to the side. *Example*: The outer thigh is **lateral** in relation to the body.
Supine [11]	Lying on the back. *Example*: The patient lies **supine** during an examination of the abdomen. (The face is **up** in the **sup**ine position.)
Prone [12]	Lying on the belly. *Example*: The backbones are examined with the patient in a **prone** position. (The patient lies **on** his or her stomach in the **pro**ne position.)

PLANES OF THE BODY

A plane is an imaginary flat surface. Label Figure 2–14, *B*, to identify the following planes of the body:

Plane	Location
Frontal (coronal) plane [13]	Vertical plane dividing the body or structure into anterior and posterior portions. A common chest x-ray view is a PA (posteroanterior—viewed from back to front) view, which is in the **frontal (coronal)** plane.
Sagittal (lateral) plane [14]	Lengthwise vertical plane dividing the body or structure into right and left sides. The **midsagittal** plane divides the body into right and left halves. A **lateral** (side-to-side) chest x-ray film is taken in the **sagittal** plane.
Transverse plane [15] (cross-sectional or axial)	Horizontal plane running across the body parallel to the ground. This **cross-sectional** plane divides the body or structure into upper and lower portions. A CT (computed tomography) scan is one of a series of x-ray pictures taken in the transverse (axial or cross-sectional) plane.

STUDY SECTION 5

Practice spelling each term, and know its meaning.

anterior (ventral)	Front surface of the body.
deep	Away from the surface.
distal	Far from the point of attachment to the trunk or far from the beginning of a structure.
frontal (coronal) plane	Vertical plane dividing the body or structure into anterior and posterior portions.
inferior (caudal)	Below another structure; pertaining to the tail or lower portion of the body.
lateral	Pertaining to the side.
medial	Pertaining to the middle or near the medial plane of the body.
posterior (dorsal)	Back surface of the body.
prone	Lying on the belly (face down, palms down).
proximal	Near the point of attachment to the trunk or near the beginning of a structure.
sagittal (lateral) plane	Lengthwise, vertical plane dividing the body or structure into right and left sides. From the Latin *sagitta*, meaning arrow. As an arrow is shot from a bow it enters the body in the sagittal plane, dividing right from left. The **midsagittal** plane divides the body into right and left halves.
superficial	On the surface.
superior (cephalic)	Above another structure; pertaining to the head.
supine	Lying on the back (face up, palms up).
transverse (cross-sectional or axial) plane	Horizontal plane dividing the body into upper and lower portions.

COMBINING FORMS, PREFIXES, AND SUFFIXES

Divide each term into its component parts, and write its meaning in the space provided.

COMBINING FORMS

Combining Form	Meaning	Terminology	Meaning
abdomin/o	abdomen	abdominal _____ *The abdomen is the region below the chest containing internal organs (such as the liver, intestines, stomach, and gallbladder).*	
adip/o	fat	adipose _____ *The suffix -ose means pertaining to or full of.*	
anter/o	front	anterior _____ *The suffix -ior means pertaining to.*	

Combining Form	Meaning	Terminology	Meaning
bol/o	to cast (throw)	anabolism _____ *The prefix ana- means up. The suffix -ism means process. In this cellular process, proteins are built up (protein synthesis).*	
cervic/o	neck (of the body or of the uterus)	cervical _____ *The cervix is the neck of the uterus. The term cervical can mean pertaining to the neck of the body or the neck (lower part) of the uterus.*	
chondr/o	cartilage (type of connective tissue)	chondroma _____ *This is a benign tumor.* chondrosarcoma _____ *This is a malignant tumor. The term sarc indicates that the malignant tumor arises from a type of flesh or connective tissue.*	
chrom/o	color	chromosomes _____ *These nuclear structures absorb the color of dyes used to stain the cell. The suffix -somes means bodies. Literally, this term means "bodies of color," because this is how they appeared to researchers who first saw them under the microscope.*	
coccyg/o	coccyx (tailbone)	coccygeal _____	
crani/o	skull	craniotomy _____	
cyt/o	cell	cytoplasm _____ *The suffix -plasm means formation.*	
dist/o	far, distant	distal _____	
dors/o	back portion of the body	dorsal _____ *The dorsal fin of a fish is on its back.*	
hist/o	tissue	histology _____	
ili/o	ilium (part of the pelvic bone)	iliac _____ *See Figure 2–10 for a picture of the ilium.*	
inguin/o	groin	inguinal _____	
kary/o	nucleus	karyotype _____ *The suffix -type means classification or picture.*	
later/o	side	lateral _____	
lumb/o	lower back (side and back between the ribs and the pelvis)	lumbosacral _____	
medi/o	middle	medial _____	

Combining Form	Meaning	Terminology	Meaning
nucle/o	nucleus	nucleic _____	
pelv/i	pelvis	pelvic _____	
		The pelvis includes all the bones that surround the pelvic cavity (Fig. 2–15).	
poster/o	back, behind	posterior _____	
proxim/o	nearest	proximal _____	
sacr/o	sacrum	sacral _____	
sarc/o	flesh	sarcoma _____	
spin/o	spine, backbone	spinal _____	
thel/o	nipple	epithelial cell _____	
		This cell, originally identified in the skin of the nipples, lies on body surfaces, externally (outside the body) and internally (lining cavities and organs).	
thorac/o	chest	thoracic _____	
		thoracotomy _____	
trache/o	trachea, windpipe	tracheal _____	

Pelvis: Comparison of Female and Male

The female pelvis is wider and more massive than the male pelvis. The female pelvis is a larger, rounded, oval shape, whereas the male pelvis is deep, narrow, and funnel- or heart-shaped. Thus, the female pelvis can accommodate the fetus during pregnancy and its downward passage through the pelvic cavity in childbirth.

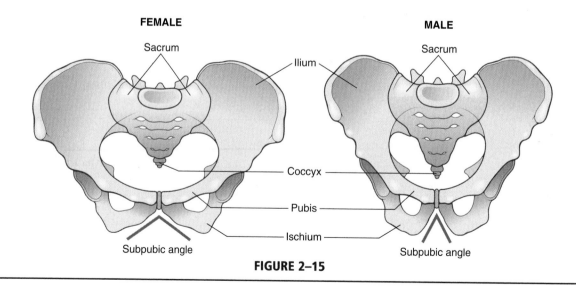

FIGURE 2–15

Combining Form	Meaning	Terminology	Meaning
umbilic/o	navel, umbilicus	umbilical _____	
ventr/o	belly side of the body	ventral _____ *The ventral fin of a fish is on its belly.*	
vertebr/o	vertebra(e), backbone(s)	vertebral _____	
viscer/o	internal organs	visceral _____	

PREFIXES

Prefix	Meaning	Terminology	Meaning
ana-	up	anabolic _____	
cata-	down	catabolism _____ *The cellular process of breaking down foods to release energy.*	
epi-	above	epigastric _____	
hypo-	below	hypochondriac region _____ *The Greeks thought that organs (liver and spleen) in the hypochondriac region of the abdomen were the origin of imaginary illnesses—hence the term hypochondriac, a person with unusual anxiety about his or her health and with symptoms not attributable to any disease process.*	
inter-	between	intervertebral _____ *A disk (disc) is an intervertebral structure.*	
meta-	change	metabolism _____ *Literally, to cast (bol/o) a change (meta-), meaning the chemical changes (processes) that occur in a cell.*	

SUFFIXES

The following are some new suffixes introduced in this chapter. See the Glossary, page 930, for additional suffixes meaning "pertaining to."

Suffix	Meaning	Suffix	Meaning
-eal	pertaining to	**-ose**	pertaining to, full of
-iac	pertaining to	**-plasm**	formation
-ior	pertaining to	**-somes**	bodies
-ism	process, condition	**-type**	picture, classification

PRACTICAL APPLICATIONS

Be sure to check your answers with the Answers to Practical Applications on page 65.

SURGICAL PROCEDURES

Match the **surgical procedure** in Column I with a *reason for performing* it in Column II. Note: You are not looking for the exact meaning of each surgical procedure, but rather why it would be performed.

Column I	*Column II*
1. Craniotomy _____	A. Emergency effort to remove foreign material from the windpipe
2. Thoracotomy _____	B. Inspection and repair of torn cartilage in the knee
3. Diskectomy _____	C. Removal of a diseased or injured portion of the brain
4. Mediastinoscopy _____	D. Inspection of lymph nodes* in the region between the lungs
5. Tracheotomy _____	E. Removal of a squamous cell† carcinoma in the voicebox
6. Laryngectomy _____	F. Open heart surgery, or removal of lung tissue
7. Arthroscopy _____	G. Inspection of abdominal organs and removal of diseased tissue
8. Peritoneoscopy _____	H. Relief of symptoms from a bulging intervertebral disk

*Lymph nodes are collections of tissue containing white blood cells called lymphocytes.
†A squamous cell is a type of epithelial cell.

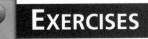 **EXERCISES**

Remember to check your answers carefully with Answers to Exercises, page 64.

A. The listed terms are parts of a cell. Match each term with its correct meaning.

cell membrane   DNA   mitochondria
chromosomes   endoplasmic reticulum   nucleus
cytoplasm   genes

1. material of the cell located outside the nucleus and yet enclosed by the cell membrane

   _____

2. regions of DNA within each chromosome _____

3. small, sausage-shaped structures; the place where food is burned to release energy

   _____

4. canal-like structure in the cytoplasm; the site of protein synthesis_____

5. structure that surrounds and protects the cell _____

6. control center of the cell, containing chromosomes _____

7. chemical found within each chromosome_____

8. rod-shaped structures in the nucleus that contain regions called genes_____

B. Use medical terms or numbers to complete the following sentences.

1. A picture of chromosomes in the nucleus of a cell is a (an) _____.

2. The number of chromosomes in a normal male's muscle cell is _____.

3. The number of chromosomes in a female's egg cell is _____.

4. The process of building up proteins in a cell is _____.

5. The process of chemically burning or breaking down foods to release energy in cells is

   _____.

6. The total of the chemical processes in a cell is _____.

7. A scientist who studies tissues is a (an) _____.

8. The medical term for internal organs is _____.

2

C. Match each of the listed body parts or tissues with its correct description below.

adipose tissue	pharynx	trachea
cartilage	pituitary gland	ureter
epithelial tissue	pleura	urethra
larynx	thyroid gland	uterus

1. voice box _____

2. membrane surrounding the lungs _____

3. throat _____

4. tube from the kidney to the urinary bladder _____

5. collection of fat cells _____

6. endocrine organ located at the base of the brain _____

7. windpipe_____

8. flexible connective tissue attached to bones at joints _____

9. surface cells covering the outside of the body and lining internal organs_____

10. endocrine gland surrounding the windpipe in the neck_____

11. womb _____

12. tube leading from the urinary bladder to the outside of the body _____

D. Name the five cavities of the body.

1. cavity surrounded by the skull _____

2. cavity in the chest surrounded by the ribs _____

3. cavity below the chest containing the stomach, liver, and gallbladder _____

4. cavity surrounded by the hip bones _____

5. cavity surrounded by the bones of the back _____

E. Select from the following definitions to complete the sentences below.

space surrounding each lung
space between the lungs
muscle separating the abdominal and thoracic cavities
membrane surrounding the abdominal organs
area below the umbilicus (as well as below the stomach)
area above the stomach
area of the navel
areas near the groin
nervous tissue within the spinal cavity
bone tissue surrounding the spinal cavity
pad of cartilage between each vertebra

1. The hypogastric region is the _____.

2. The mediastinum is the _____.

3. The spinal cord is _____.

4. The diaphragm is a (an) _____.

5. An intervertebral disk is_____.

6. The pleural cavity is _____.

7. The spinal column is _____.

8. Inguinal areas are the _____.

9. The peritoneum is the _____.

10. The umbilical region is the _____.

11. The epigastric region is the _____.

F. Name the five divisions of the back.

1. region of the neck_____

2. region of the chest _____

3. region of the waist_____

4. region of the sacrum_____

5. region of the tailbone _____

2

G. Give the meanings of the following abbreviations.

1. LLQ _____

2. L5–S1 _____

3. RUQ _____

4. C3–C4 _____

5. RLQ _____

H. Give the opposites of the following terms.

1. deep _____   4. medial _____

2. proximal _____   5. dorsal _____

3. supine _____   6. superior _____

I. Select from the following medical terms to complete the sentences below.

distal   midsagittal   transverse (cross-sectional)
frontal (coronal)   proximal   vertebra
inferior (caudal)   superior (cephalic)   vertebrae
lateral

1. The kidney lies _____ to the spinal cord. (*Hint:* to the side of.)

2. The _____ end of the thigh bone (femur) joins with the knee cap (patella).

3. The _____ plane divides the body into an anterior and a posterior portion.

4. Each backbone is a (an) _____.

5. Several backbones are _____.

6. The diaphragm lies _____ to the organs in the thoracic cavity.

7. The _____ plane divides the body into right and left halves.

8. The _____ end of the upper armbone (humerus) is at the shoulder.

9. The _____ plane divides the body into upper and lower portions.

10. The pharynx is located _____ to the esophagus.

J. Use slashes to divide the following terms into component parts, and give meanings for each.

1. craniotomy _____

2. cervical _____

3. chondroma _____

4. chondrosarcoma _____

5. nucleic _____

K. Give the medical term for the following definitions. Pay attention to spelling!

1. space below the chest containing the liver, stomach, gallbladder, and intestines:

   _____

2. flexible connective tissue attached to bones at joints: _____

3. rod-shaped structures in the cell nucleus, containing regions of DNA:_____

4. muscle separating the abdominal and thoracic cavities:_____

5. voice box: _____

6. vertical plane dividing the body into right and left sides:_____

7. pertaining to the neck: _____

8. tumor (benign) of cartilage: _____

9. control center of the cell; directs the activities of the cell:_____

10. pertaining to the windpipe:_____

L. Complete each term based on the meaning provided.

1. pertaining to internal organs: _____al

2. tumor of flesh tissue (malignant): _____oma

3. pertaining to the chest: _____ic

4. picture of the chromosomes in the cell nucleus: _____type

5. sausage-shaped cellular structures in which catabolism takes place: mito_____

6. space between the lungs: media_____

7. endocrine gland at the base of the brain: _____ary gland

8. pertaining to skin (surface) cells: epi_____

9. pertaining to far from the beginning of a structure: _____al

10. on the surface of the body: super_____

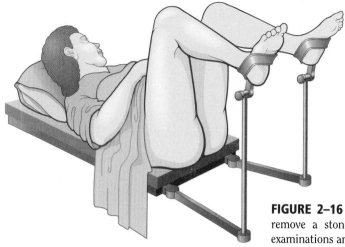

FIGURE 2–16   Dorsal lithotomy position. Lithotomy means incision to remove a stone (lith/o = stone). This position is used for gynecologic examinations and for removal of stones from the urinary tract.

M. Circle the correct term to complete each sentence.

1. Dr. Curnen said the **(inguinal, superior, superficial)** wound barely scratched the surface.

2. Because the liver and spleen are on opposite sides of the body, the liver is in the **(RUQ, LUQ, LLQ)** of the abdominopelvic cavity and the spleen is in the **(RUQ, LUQ, RLQ)**.

3. When a gynecologist performs a pelvic examination, the patient lies on her back in the **(ventral, dorsal, medial)** lithotomy position. See Figure 2–16.

4. Sally complained of pain in the area surrounding her navel. The doctor described the pain as **(periumbilical, epigastric, hypogastric)**.

5. After sampling the fluid surrounding her 16-week-old fetus and reviewing the chromosomal picture, the doctor explained to Mrs. Jones that the fetus had trisomy 21. The diagnosis was made by analysis of an abnormal **(urine sample, x-ray film, karyotype)**.

6. The **(spinal, sagittal, abdominal)** cavity contains digestive organs.

7. The emergency department physician suspected appendicitis when Brandon was admitted with sharp **(LLQ, RLQ, RUQ)** pain.

8. Susan had hiccups after rapidly eating spicy Indian food. Her physician explained that the hiccups were involuntary contractions or spasms of the **(umbilicus, diaphragm, mediastinum)** resulting in uncontrolled breathing in of air.

9. Everyone in the society pages was noticeably slimmer this year. Could the popularity of liposuction surgery to remove unwanted **(cartilage, epithelial tissue, adipose tissue)** have something to do with this phenomenon?

10. Maria's coughing and sneezing were a result of an allergy to animal dander that affected her **(respiratory, cardiovascular, urinary)** system.

11. While ice skating, Natalie fell and landed on her buttocks. She had persistent **(cervical, thoracic, coccygeal)** pain for a few weeks but no broken bones on x-ray examination.

MEDICAL SCRAMBLE

Unscramble the letters to form medical terms from the clues. Use the letters in the squares to complete the bonus term. Answers are found on page 65.

1. *Clue:* Endocrine gland in the neck

   ___ ___ ☐ ___ ___ ☐ ___   R Y D I H O T

2. *Clue:* Control center of a cell

   ___ ___ ___ ___ ___ ☐ ___   L U S N E C U

3. *Clue:* Internal organs

   ___ ☐ ___ ___ ___ ___ ___   A C S R V E I

4. *Clue:* Windpipe

   ☐ ___ ___ ___ ___ ___ ☐   A H C R A T E

5. *Clue:* Tube connecting the kidneys and urinary bladder

   ___ ___ ___ ☐ ___ ___   T R U E R E

6. *Clue:* The double-layered membrane surrounding the lung

   ☐ ___ ___ ___ ☐ ___   A U P E L R

BONUS TERM: *Clue:* The gland at the base of the brain that secretes growth hormone, thyroid-stimulating hormone, and hormones that affect the ovaries and testes.

☐ ☐ ☐ ☐ ☐ ☐ ☐ ☐ ☐

ANSWERS TO EXERCISES

A

1. cytoplasm
2. genes
3. mitochondria
4. endoplasmic reticulum
5. cell membrane
6. nucleus
7. DNA
8. chromosomes

B

1. karyotype
2. 46 (23 pairs)
3. 23
4. anabolism
5. catabolism
6. metabolism
7. histologist
8. viscera

C

1. larynx
2. pleura
3. pharynx
4. ureter
5. adipose tissue
6. pituitary gland
7. trachea
8. cartilage
9. epithelial tissue
10. thyroid gland
11. uterus
12. urethra

D

1. cranial
2. thoracic
3. abdominal
4. pelvic
5. spinal

E

1. area below the umbilicus
2. space between the lungs
3. nervous tissue within the spinal cavity
4. muscle separating the abdominal and thoracic cavities
5. pad of cartilage between two adjoining vertebrae
6. space surrounding each lung
7. bone tissue surrounding the spinal cavity
8. areas near the groin
9. membrane surrounding the abdominal organs
10. area of the navel
11. area above the stomach

F

1. cervical
2. thoracic
3. lumbar
4. sacral
5. coccygeal

G

1. left lower quadrant (of the abdominopelvic cavity)
2. between the fifth lumbar vertebra and the first sacral vertebra (a common place for a slipped disk)
3. right upper quadrant (of the abdominopelvic cavity)
4. between the third and fourth cervical vertebrae
5. right lower quadrant (of the abdominopelvic cavity)

H

1. superficial
2. distal
3. prone
4. lateral
5. ventral (anterior)
6. inferior (caudal)

I

1. lateral
2. distal
3. frontal (coronal)
4. vertebra
5. vertebrae
6. inferior (caudal)
7. midsagittal
8. proximal
9. transverse
10. superior (cephalic)

J

1. crani/o/tomy—incision of the skull
2. cervic/al—pertaining to the neck (of the body or the cervix of the uterus)
3. chondr/oma—tumor of cartilage (benign or noncancerous tumor)
4. chondr/o/sarc/oma—flesh tumor of cartilage (cancerous, malignant tumor)
5. nucle/ic—pertaining to the nucleus

K

1. abdomen or abdominal cavity	5. larynx	9. nucleus
2. cartilage	6. sagittal—note spelling with two t's	10. tracheal
3. chromosomes	7. cervical	
4. diaphragm	8. chondroma	

L

1. visceral	5. mitochondria—*memory tip:* **cat**abolism and **m**itochondria, **cat** and **m**ouse!	7. pituitary gland
2. sarcoma		8. epithelial
3. thoracic		9. distal
4. karyotype	6. mediastinum	10. superficial

M

1. superficial	4. periumbilical	8. diaphragm
2. RUQ; LUQ	5. karyotype	9. adipose tissue
3. dorsal; often called the dorsolithotomy position	6. abdominal	10. respiratory
	7. RLQ	11. coccygeal

ANSWERS TO PRACTICAL APPLICATIONS

1. **C** A trephine is a type of circular saw used for craniotomy.
2. **F**
3. **H** Endoscopic diskectomy is performed through a small incision on the back, lateral to the spine. All or a portion of the disk is removed.

4. **D** A small incision is made above the breastbone and an endoscope is inserted to inspect the lymph nodes around the trachea.
5. **A**
6. **E**
7. **B**

8. **G** A small incision is made near the navel, and a laparoscope is inserted. The procedure, also called laparoscopy (lapar/o means abdomen) or minimally invasive surgery, is used to examine organs and perform less complex surgical operations, such as removal of the gallbladder or appendix or tying off of the fallopian tubes.

ANSWERS TO MEDICAL SCRAMBLE

1. THYROID   2. NUCLEUS   3. VISCERA   4. TRACHEA   5. URETER   6. PLEURA

BONUS TERM: PITUITARY

PRONUNCIATION OF TERMS

PRONUNCIATION GUIDE

ā as in āpe	ă as in ăpple
ē as in ēven	ĕ as in ĕvery
ī as in īce	ĭ as in ĭnterest
ō as in ōpen	ŏ as in pŏt
ū as in ūnit	ŭ as in ŭnder

To test your understanding of the terminology in this chapter, write the meaning of each term in the space provided. In addition, you may wish to cover the terms and write them by looking at your definitions. Make sure your spelling is correct. The page number after each term indicates where it is defined or used in the book, so you can easily check your responses. You will find complete definitions for all of these terms and their audio pronunciations on the CD.

Term	Pronunciation	Meaning
abdomen (45)	ĂB-dō-mĕn	_____
abdominal cavity (45)	ăb-DŎM-ĭ-năl KĂ-vĭ-tē	_____
adipose (52)	ĂD-ĭ-pōs	_____
anabolism (37)	ă-NĂB-ō-lĭzm	_____
anterior (45)	an-TĒ-rē-ŏr	_____
cartilage (40)	KĂR-t-lĭj	_____

2

Term	Pronunciation	Meaning
catabolism (37)	kă-TĂB-ō-lĭzm	_____
caudal (52)	KĂW-dăl	_____
cell membrane (37)	sĕl MĔM-brān	_____
cephalic (52)	SEF-ă-lĭk	_____
cervical (53)	SĔR-vĭ-kăl	_____
chondroma (53)	kŏn-DRŌ-mă	_____
chondrosarcoma (53)	kŏn-drō-săr-KŌ-mă	_____
chromosome (37)	KRŌ-mō-sōm	_____
coccygeal (49)	kŏk-sĭ-JĒ-ăl	_____
coccyx (48)	KŎK-sĭks	_____
cranial cavity (45)	KRĀ-nē-ăl KĂ-vĭ-tē	_____
craniotomy (53)	krā-nē-ŎT-ō-mē	_____
cytoplasm (37)	SĪ-tō-plăzm	_____
deep (52)	dēp	_____
diaphragm (45)	DĪ-ă-frăm	_____
disk (disc) (49)	dĭsk	_____
distal (52)	DĬS-tăl	_____
dorsal (45)	DŎR-săl	_____
endoplasmic reticulum (37)	ĕn-dō-PLĂZ-mĭk rē-TĬK-ū-lŭm	_____
epigastric region (49)	ĕp-ĭ-GĂS-trĭk RĒ-jŭn	_____
epithelial cells (40)	ĕp-ĭ-THĒ-lē-ăl sĕlz	_____
frontal plane (52)	FRŬN-tăl plān	_____
genes (37)	jēnz	_____
histology (53)	hĭs-TŎL-ō-jē	_____
hypochondriac region (49)	hī-pō-KŎN-drē-ăk RĒ-jŭn	_____
hypogastric region (49)	hĭ-pō-GĂS-trĭk RĒ-jŭn	_____
iliac (53)	ĬL-ē-ăk	_____
inguinal region (49)	ĬNG-gwĭ-năl RĒ-jŭn	_____
intervertebral (55)	ĭn-tĕr-VĔR-tĕ-brăl or ĭn-tĕr-vĕr-TĒ-brăl	_____
karyotype (37)	KĂR-ē-ō-tīp	_____
larynx (40)	LĂR-ĭnks	_____
lateral (52)	LĂT-ĕr-al	_____

Term	Pronunciation	Meaning
lumbar region (49)	LŬM-băr RĒ-jŭn	_____
lumbosacral (53)	lŭm-bō-SĀ-krăl	_____
medial (52)	MĒ-dē-ăl	_____
mediastinum (45)	mē-dē-ă-STĪ-nŭm	_____
metabolism (37)	mĕ-TĂB-ō-lĭzm	_____
mitochondria (37)	mī-tō-KŎN-drē-ă	_____
nucleic (54)	nū-KLĒ-ĭk	_____
nucleus (37)	NŪ-klē-ŭs	_____
pelvic cavity (45)	PĔL-vĭk KĂ-vĭ-tē	_____
peritoneum (45)	pĕ-rĭ-tō-NĒ-um	_____
pharynx (40)	FĂR-ĭnks	_____
pituitary gland (40)	pĭ-TŪ-ĭ-tăr-ē glănd	_____
pleura (45)	PLOO-ră	_____
pleural cavity (45)	PLOOR-ăl KĂ-vĭ-tē	_____
posterior (45)	pōs-TĒR-ē-ŏr	_____
prone (52)	prōn	_____
proximal (52)	PRŎKS-ĭ-măl	_____
sacral (49)	SĀ-krăl	_____
sacrum (48)	SĀ-krŭm	_____
sagittal plane (52)	SĂJ-ĭ-tăl plān	_____
sarcoma (54)	săr-KŌ-mă	_____
spinal cavity (45)	SPĪ-năl KĂ-vĭ-tē	_____
spinal column (49)	SPĪ-năl KŎL-ŭm	_____
spinal cord (49)	SPĪ-năl kŏrd	_____
superficial (52)	sū-pĕr-FĬSH-ăl	_____
supine (52)	SŪ-pīn	_____
thoracic cavity (45)	thō-RĂS-ĭk KĂ-vĭ-tē	_____
thoracotomy (54)	thō-ră-KŎT-ō-mē	_____
thyroid gland (39)	THĪ-royd glănd	_____
trachea (39)	TRĀ-kē-ă	_____
tracheal (54)	TRĀ-kē-ăl	_____
transverse plane (52)	trănz-VĔRS plān	_____
umbilical region (49)	ŭm-BĬL-ĭ-kăl RĒ-jŭn	_____

Term	Pronunciation	Meaning
ureter (40)	Ū-rĕ-tĕr *or* ū-RĒ-tĕr	_____
urethra (40)	ū-RĒ-thră	_____
uterus (40)	Ū-tĕ-rŭs	_____
ventral (45)	VĔN-trăl	_____
vertebra (49)	VĔR-tĕ-bră	_____
vertebrae (49)	VĔR-tĕ-brā	_____
vertebral (55)	VĔR-tĕ-brăl *or* vĕr-TĒ-brăl	_____
viscera (40)	VĬS-ĕr-ă	_____
visceral (55)	VĬS-ĕr-ăl	_____

REVIEW SHEET

Write the meaning of each combining form in the space provided and test yourself. Check your answers with the information in the chapter or in the Glossary (Medical Word Parts—English) at the end of the book.

COMBINING FORMS

Combining Form	Meaning	Combining Form	Meaning
abdomin/o	_____	lumb/o	_____
adip/o	_____	medi/o	_____
anter/o	_____	nucle/o	_____
bol/o	_____	pelv/i	_____
cervic/o	_____	poster/o	_____
chondr/o	_____	proxim/o	_____
chrom/o	_____	sacr/o	_____
coccyg/o	_____	sarc/o	_____
crani/o	_____	spin/o	_____
cyt/o	_____	thel/o	_____
dist/o	_____	thorac/o	_____
dors/o	_____	trache/o	_____
hist/o	_____	umbilic/o	_____
ili/o	_____	ventr/o	_____
inguin/o	_____	vertebr/o	_____
kary/o	_____	viscer/o	_____
later/o	_____		

PREFIXES

Prefix	Meaning	Prefix	Meaning
ana-	_____	hypo-	_____
cata-	_____	inter-	_____
epi-	_____	meta-	_____

SUFFIXES

Suffix	Meaning	Prefix	Meaning
-eal	_____	-ose	_____
-ectomy	_____	-plasm	_____
-iac	_____	-somes	_____
-ior	_____	-tomy	_____
-ism	_____	-type	_____
-oma	_____		

Label the regions and quadrants of the abdominopelvic cavity.

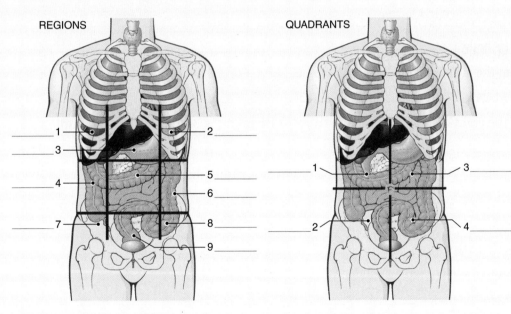

Name the divisions of the spinal column.

neck region (C1 to C7) _____

chest region (T1 to T12) _____

lower back (loin) region (L1 to L5) _____

region of the sacrum (S1 to S5) _____

tailbone region _____

Name the planes of the head as pictured below:

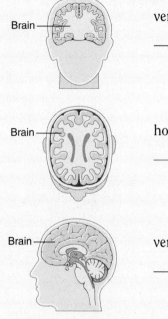

vertical plane that divides the body into anterior and posterior portions

_____

horizontal plane that divides the body into upper and lower portions

_____

vertical plane that divides the body into right and left portions

_____

Name the positional and directional terms.

front of the body _____

back of the body _____

away from the surface of the body _____

on the surface of the body _____

far from the point of attachment to the trunk or far from the beginning of a structure

_____

near the point of attachment to the trunk or near the beginning of a structure

_____

below another structure _____

above another structure _____

pertaining to the side _____

pertaining to the middle _____

lying on the belly _____

lying on the back _____

Give the meanings of the following terms that pertain to the cell.

chromosomes _____

mitochondria _____

nucleus _____

DNA _____

endoplasmic reticulum _____

cell membrane _____

catabolism _____

anabolism _____

metabolism _____

Give the term that suits the meaning provided.

membrane surrounding the lungs _____

membrane surrounding the abdominal viscera _____

muscular wall separating the thoracic and abdominal cavities _____

space between the lungs, containing the heart, windpipe, aorta _____

a backbone _____

a pad of cartilage between each backbone and the next _____

 Please refer to the enclosed CD for additional exercises and images related to this chapter.

chapter 3

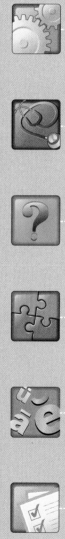

Suffixes

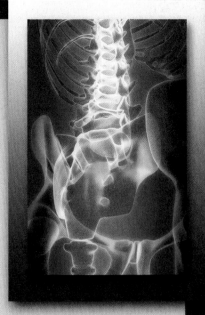

THIS CHAPTER IS DIVIDED INTO THE FOLLOWING SECTIONS

In this chapter you will

- Define new suffixes and review those presented in previous chapters.
- Gain practice in word analysis by using these suffixes with combining forms to build and understand terms.
- Identify the functions of the different types of blood cells in the body.

Image Description: Posterior x-ray view, angled to the right side and below, of the pelvic region.

INTRODUCTION

This chapter has three purposes. The first purpose is to teach many of the most common suffixes in the medical language. As you work through the entire book, these suffixes will appear often. An additional group of suffixes is presented in Chapter 6.

The second goal is to master additional combining forms and then use them to make words with suffixes. Your analysis of the words in the section on Suffixes and Terminology will increase your medical language vocabulary.

The third goal is to expand your understanding of terminology beyond basic word analysis. The appendices contain images and give more detailed explanations of new terms.

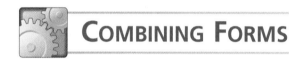

COMBINING FORMS

Read the following list, and underline those combining forms that are unfamiliar.

COMBINING FORMS

Combining Form	Meaning	Combining Form	Meaning
abdomin/o	abdomen	carcin/o	cancer
acr/o	extremities, top, extreme point	cardi/o	heart
		chem/o	drug, chemical
acu/o	sharp, severe, sudden	chondr/o	cartilage
aden/o	gland	chron/o	time
adip/o	fat	col/o	colon (large intestine)
amni/o	amnion (sac surrounding the embryo in the uterus)	cyst/o	urinary bladder
angi/o	vessel	encephal/o	brain
arteri/o	artery	erythr/o	red
arthr/o	joint	hem/o	blood
axill/o	armpit	hepat/o	liver
bi/o	life	hydr/o	water, fluid
blephar/o	eyelid	inguin/o	groin
bronch/o	bronchial tubes (two tubes, one right and one left, that branch from the trachea to enter the lungs)	isch/o	to hold back
		lapar/o	abdomen, abdominal wall
		laryng/o	larynx (voice box)

Combining Form	Meaning	Combining Form	Meaning
leuk/o	white	peritone/o	peritoneum
lymph/o	lymph	phag/o	to eat, swallow
	Lymph, a clear fluid that bathes tissue spaces, is contained in special lymph vessels and nodes throughout the body.	phleb/o	vein
		plas/o	formation, development
		pleur/o	pleura (membrane surrounding lungs and adjacent to chest wall)
mamm/o	breast		
mast/o	breast	pneumon/o	lungs
morph/o	shape, form	pulmon/o	lungs
muc/o	mucus	radi/o	x-rays
my/o	muscle	rect/o	rectum
myel/o	spinal cord, bone marrow	ren/o	kidney
	Context of usage indicates the meaning intended.	rhin/o	nose
		sarc/o	flesh
necr/o	death (of cells or whole body)	splen/o	spleen
		staphyl/o	clusters
nephr/o	kidney	strept/o	twisted chains
neur/o	nerve	thorac/o	chest
neutr/o	neutrophil (a white blood cell)	thromb/o	clot
		tonsill/o	tonsils
nucle/o	nucleus	trache/o	trachea (windpipe)
ophthalm/o	eye	ven/o	vein
oste/o	bone		
ot/o	ear		
path/o	disease		

SUFFIXES AND TERMINOLOGY

3

NOUN SUFFIXES

The following list includes common noun suffixes. After the meaning of each suffix, terminology illustrates the use of the suffix in various words. Remember the basic rule for building a medical term: Use a combining vowel, such as o, to connect the root to the suffix. However, drop the combining vowel if the suffix begins with a vowel—for example, **gastr/itis,** *not* "gastr/o/itis."

The numbered footnotes keyed to some terms refer you to the Appendices (beginning on page 82). These Appendices are provided to help you gain a fuller understanding of the terminology. Remember, your CD contains definitions for all terms presented here.

Suffix	Meaning	Terminology	Meaning
-algia	pain	arthralgia _____	
		otalgia _____	
		neuralgia _____	
		myalgia _____	
-cele	hernia[1]	rectocele _____	
		cystocele _____	
-centesis	surgical puncture to remove fluid	thoracentesis _____	
		Notice that this term is shortened from thoracocentesis.	
		amniocentesis[2] _____	
		abdominocentesis _____	
		This procedure is more commonly known as abdominal paracentesis (para- means beside or near). A tube is placed through an incision in the abdomen and fluid is removed from the peritoneal cavity (beside the abdominal organs).	
-coccus (plural: **-cocci**)[3]	berry-shaped bacterium (plural: bacteria)	streptococcus[4] _____	
		staphylococci _____	
-cyte	cell	erythrocyte[5] _____	
		leukocyte _____	
		thrombocyte _____	
-dynia	pain	pleurodynia _____	
		Pain in the chest wall muscles that is aggravated by breathing.	

[1]See Appendix A, page 82.
[2]See Appendix B, page 82.
[3]See Appendix C, page 82.
[4]See Appendix D, page 83.
[5]See Appendix E, page 84.

3

Suffix	Meaning	Terminology	Meaning
-ectomy	excision, removal, resection	laryngectomy[6] _____	
		mastectomy _____	
-emia	blood condition	anemia[7] _____	
		ischemia[8] _____	
-genesis	condition of producing, forming	carcinogenesis _____	
		pathogenesis _____	
		angiogenesis _____	
-gram	record	electroencephalogram _____	
		myelogram _____	
		Myel/o means spinal cord in this term. This is an x-ray record taken after injection of contrast material into membranes (meninges) surrounding the spinal cord.	
		mammogram _____	
-graph	instrument for recording	electroencephalograph _____	
-graphy	process of recording	electroencephalography _____	
		angiography _____	
-itis	inflammation	bronchitis _____	
		tonsillitis[9] _____	
		thrombophlebitis _____ *Also called phlebitis.*	
-logy	study of	ophthalmology _____	
		morphology _____	
-lysis	breakdown, destruction, separation	hemolysis _____ *Breakdown of red blood cells with release of hemoglobin.*	
-malacia	softening	osteomalacia _____	
		chondromalacia _____	

---

[6]See Appendix F, page 85.
[7]See Appendix G, page 85.
[8]See Appendix H, page 85.
[9]See Appendix I, page 85.

3

Suffix	Meaning	Terminology	Meaning
-megaly	enlargement	acromegaly[10] _____	
		splenomegaly[11] _____	
-oma	tumor, mass, collection of fluid	myoma _____ *A benign tumor.*	
		myosarcoma _____ *A malignant tumor. Muscle is a type of flesh (sarc/o) tissue.*	
		multiple myeloma _____ *Myel/o means bone marrow in this term. This malignant tumor occurs in bone marrow tissue throughout the body.*	
		hematoma _____	
-opsy	to view	biopsy _____	
		necropsy _____ *This is an autopsy or postmortem examination.*	
-osis	condition, usually abnormal	necrosis _____	
		hydronephrosis _____	
		leukocytosis _____	
-pathy	disease condition	cardiomyopathy _____ *Primary disease of the heart muscle in the absence of a known underlying etiology (cause).*	
-penia	deficiency	erythropenia _____	
		neutropenia _____ *In this term, neutr/o indicates neutrophil (a type of white blood cell).*	
		thrombocytopenia _____	
-phobia	fear	acrophobia _____ *Fear of heights. Acr/o means extremities, in the sense of extreme or far points.*	
		agoraphobia _____ *An anxiety disorder marked by fear of venturing out into a crowded place. Agora means marketplace.*	
-plasia	development, formation, growth	achondroplasia[12] _____	

[10]See Appendix J, page 86.
[11]See Appendix K, page 86.
[12]See Appendix L, page 86.

3

Suffix	Meaning	Terminology	Meaning
-plasty	surgical repair	angio<u>plasty</u> _____	
		An interventional cardiologist opens a narrowed blood vessel (artery) using a balloon that is inflated after insertion into the vessel. Stents, or slotted tubes, are then put in place to keep the artery open.	
-ptosis[13]	drooping, sagging, prolapse	blepharo<u>ptosis</u> _____	
		*Physicians use **ptosis** (TŌ-sĭs) alone to indicate drooping of the upper eyelids or the breasts.*	
-sclerosis	hardening	arterio<u>sclerosis</u> _____	
		In atherosclerosis (a form of arteriosclerosis), deposits of fat (ather/o means fatty material) collect in an artery.	
-scope	instrument for visual examination	laparo<u>scope</u> _____	
-scopy	process of visual examination (with an endoscope)	laparo<u>scopy</u>[14] _____	
-stasis	stopping, controlling	meta<u>stasis</u> _____	
		Meta- means beyond. A metastasis is the spread of a malignant tumor beyond its original site to a secondary organ or location.	
		hemo<u>stasis</u> _____	
		*Blood flow is stopped naturally by clotting or artificially by compression or suturing of a wound. A surgical clamp is a **hemostat**.*	
-stomy	opening to form a mouth (stoma)	colo<u>stomy</u> _____	
		tracheo<u>stomy</u> _____	
-therapy	treatment	hydro<u>therapy</u> _____	
		chemo<u>therapy</u> _____	
		radio<u>therapy</u> _____	
		High-energy radiation is used to treat, not diagnose, illness.	
-tomy	incision, cutting into	laparo<u>tomy</u> _____	
		Also referred to as a "lap," this procedure is creation of a large incision into the peritoneal cavity, often performed on an exploratory basis.	
		phlebo<u>tomy</u> _____	
		tracheo<u>tomy</u>[15] _____	

---

[13]See Appendix M, page 86.
[14]See Appendix N, page 87.
[15]See Appendix O, page 88.

3

Suffix	Meaning	Terminology	Meaning
-trophy	development, nourishment	hypertrophy _____ *Cells increase in size, not number. Muscles of weight lifters often hypertrophy (hī-PĔR-trō-fē).* atrophy _____ *Cells decrease in size. Muscles atrophy when immobilized in a cast and not in use.*	

The following are shorter noun suffixes that usually are attached to roots in words.

Suffix	Meaning	Terminology	Meaning
-er	one who	radiographer _____ *A technologist who assists in the making of diagnostic x-ray pictures.*	
-ia	condition	leukemia _____ pneumonia _____	
-ist	specialist	nephrologist _____	
-ole	little, small	arteriole[16] _____	
-ule	little, small	venule	
-um, -ium	structure, tissue	pericardium _____ *This membrane surrounds the heart.*	
-us	structure, substance	mucus _____ esophagus _____ *Eso- means within or inward.*	
-y	condition, process	nephropathy _____	

ADJECTIVE SUFFIXES

The following are adjective suffixes. No simple rule will explain which suffix meaning "pertaining to" is used with a specific combining form. Concentrate on identifying the suffix in each term; then write the meaning of the term.

Suffix	Meaning	Terminology	Meaning
-ac, -iac	pertaining to	cardiac _____	
-al	pertaining to	peritoneal _____ inguinal _____ pleural _____	

---

[16]See Appendix P, page 88.

Suffix	Meaning	Terminology	Meaning
-ar	pertaining to	tonsillar _____	
-ary	pertaining to	pulmonary _____	
		axillary _____	
-eal	pertaining to	laryngeal _____	
-genic	pertaining to producing, produced by, or in	carcinogenic _____	
		osteogenic _____	
		An osteogenic sarcoma is a malignant tumor produced in bone.	
-ic, -ical	pertaining to	chronic _____	
		Acute *is the opposite of chronic. It describes a disease that is of rapid onset and has severe symptoms and brief duration.*	
		pathologic _____	
-oid	resembling	adenoids[17] _____	
		mucoid _____	
-ose	pertaining to, full of	adipose _____	
-ous	pertaining to	mucous membrane _____	
		*Mucous membranes produce the sticky secretion called **mucus** (a noun).*	
-tic	pertaining to	necrotic _____	

_____

[17]See Appendix Q, page 88.

APPENDICES

APPENDIX A: HERNIA

A **hernia** is protrusion of an organ or the muscular wall of an organ through the cavity that normally contains it. A **hiatal hernia** occurs when the stomach protrudes upward into the mediastinum through the esophageal opening in the diaphragm (see Fig. 5–19, page 160), and an **inguinal hernia** occurs when part of the intestine protrudes downward into the groin region and commonly into the scrotal sac in the male (see Fig. 5–19, page 160). A **rectocele** is the protrusion of a portion of the rectum toward the vagina through a weak part of the vaginal wall muscles. An **omphalocele** (omphal/o = umbilicus, navel) is a herniation of the intestines through the navel occurring in infants at birth. A **cystocele** occurs when part of the urinary bladder herniates through the vaginal wall as a result of weakness of the pelvic muscles (Fig. 3–1).

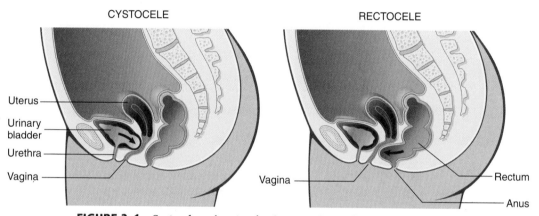

FIGURE 3–1 **Cystocele** and **rectocele.** *Arrows* point to the areas of herniation.

APPENDIX B: AMNIOCENTESIS

The amnion is the sac (membrane) that surrounds the embryo (called the fetus after the 8th week) in the uterus. Fluid accumulates within the sac and can be withdrawn (by **amniocentesis**) for analysis between the 12th and 18th weeks of pregnancy. The fetus sheds cells into the fluid, and these cells are grown (cultured) for microscopic analysis. A karyotype is made to analyze chromosomes, and the fluid is examined for high levels of chemicals indicating defects in the developing spinal cord and spinal column of the fetus (Fig. 3–2).

APPENDIX C: PLURALS

Words ending in **-us** commonly form their plural by dropping the **-us** and adding **-i.** Thus, nucleus becomes nuclei and coccus becomes cocci (KŎK-sī). Here are two other examples of plural formations: For words ending in **-is** drop the **-is** and add **-es**: diagnosis becomes diagnoses. For words ending in **-um** drop the **-um** and add **-a**: bacterium becomes bacteria.

For additional information on formation of plurals, refer to Appendix I, page 953.

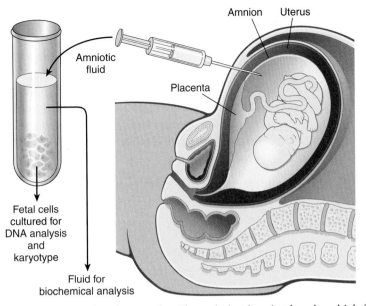

FIGURE 3–2 **Amniocentesis.** Under ultrasound guidance (using imaging based on high-frequency sound waves), the physician inserts a needle through the uterus wall and amnion (the membrane surrounding the fetus) into the amniotic cavity. Amniotic fluid, containing fetal cells, is withdrawn for analysis. The physician uses continuous ultrasound pictures to locate the fetus and other structures within the uterus, and to ensure the proper placement of the needle.

APPENDIX D: STREPTOCOCCUS

Streptococcus, a berry-shaped bacterium, grows in twisted chains. One group of streptococci causes such conditions as "strep throat," tonsillitis, rheumatic fever, and certain kidney ailments, whereas another group causes infections in teeth, in the sinuses (cavities) of the nose and face, and in the valves of the heart.

Staphylococci, other berry-shaped bacteria, grow in small clusters, like grapes. Staphylococcal lesions may be external (skin abscesses, boils, styes) or internal (abscesses in bone and kidney). An **abscess** is a collection of pus, white blood cells, and protein that is present at the site of infection.

Examples of **diplococci** (berry-shaped bacteria organized in pairs; dipl/o = two) are **pneumococci** (pneum/o = lungs) and **gonococci** (gon/o = seed). Pneumococci cause bacterial pneumonia, and gonococci invade the reproductive organs, causing gonorrhea. Figure 3–3 illustrates the different growth patterns of streptococci, staphylococci, and diplococci.

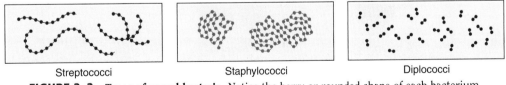

| Streptococci | Staphylococci | Diplococci |

FIGURE 3–3 **Types of coccal bacteria.** Notice the berry or rounded shape of each bacterium.

3

APPENDIX E: BLOOD CELLS

Study Figure 3–4 as you read the following to note the differences among the three different types of cells in the blood. **Erythrocytes**, or red blood cells, are the first type. These cells are made in the bone marrow (soft tissue in the center of certain bones). They carry oxygen from the lungs through the blood to all body cells. Body cells use oxygen to burn food and release energy (catabolism). **Hemoglobin** (globin = protein), an important protein in erythrocytes, carries the oxygen through the bloodstream.

Leukocytes, or white blood cells, are the second type. There are five different kinds of leukocytes: three granulocytes, or polymorphonuclear cells, and two mononuclear cells.

- **Granulocytes**, or polymorphonuclear cells, contain dark-staining granules in their cytoplasm and have a multilobed nucleus. They are formed in the bone marrow, and there are three types:
    1. **Eosinophils** (granules stain red [eosin/o = rosy] with acidic stain) are active and increased in number in allergic conditions such as asthma. About 3 percent of leukocytes are eosinophils.
    2. **Basophils** (granules stain blue with basic [bas/o = basic] stain). The function of basophils is not clear, but the number of these cells increases in the healing phase of inflammation. Less than 1 percent of leukocytes are basophils.

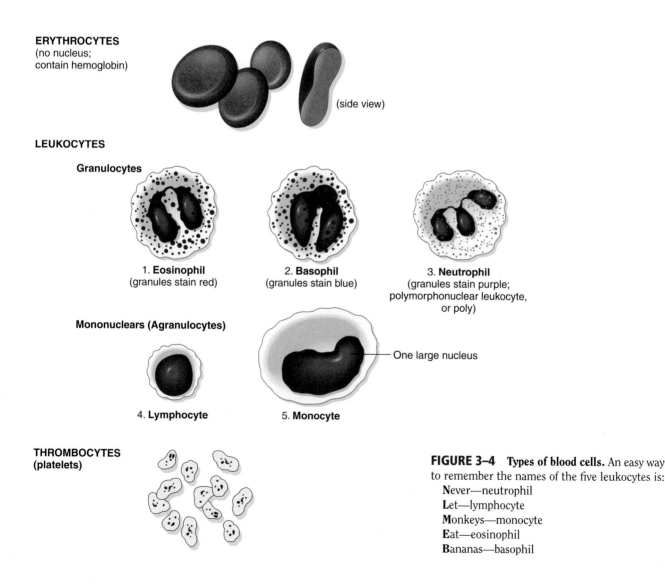

ERYTHROCYTES
(no nucleus;
contain hemoglobin)

(side view)

LEUKOCYTES

Granulocytes

1. **Eosinophil**
(granules stain red)

2. **Basophil**
(granules stain blue)

3. **Neutrophil**
(granules stain purple;
polymorphonuclear leukocyte,
or poly)

Mononuclears (Agranulocytes)

One large nucleus

4. **Lymphocyte**

5. **Monocyte**

THROMBOCYTES
(platelets)

FIGURE 3–4   Types of blood cells. An easy way to remember the names of the five leukocytes is:

Never—neutrophil
Let—lymphocyte
Monkeys—monocyte
Eat—eosinophil
Bananas—basophil

3. **Neutrophils** (granules stain blue and red [purple] with neutral stain) are important disease-fighting cells. They are **phagocytes** (phag/o = eating, swallowing)—they engulf and digest bacteria. They are the most numerous disease-fighting "soldiers" (50 to 60 percent of leukocytes are neutrophils) and are referred to as "polys" or **polymorphonuclear leukocytes** (poly = many, morph/o = shape) because of their multilobed nucleus.

• **Mononuclear leukocytes (agranulocytes)** have one large nucleus and only a few granules in their cytoplasm. They are produced in bone marrow as well as lymph nodes and spleen. There are two types of mononuclear leukocytes (see Fig. 3–4):

4. **Lymphocytes** (lymph cells) fight disease by producing antibodies, thereby destroying foreign cells. They also may attach directly to foreign cells and destroy them. Two types of lymphocytes are T cells and B cells. About 32 percent of leukocytes are lymphocytes.

5. **Monocytes** (cells with one [mon/o = one] very large nucleus) engulf and destroy cellular debris after neutrophils have attacked foreign cells. Monocytes leave the bloodstream and enter tissues (such as lung and liver) to become **macrophages,** which are large phagocytes. Monocytes make up about 4 percent of all leukocytes.

Thrombocytes or **platelets** (clotting cells) are the third type of blood cell. These are actually tiny fragments of cells formed in the bone marrow and necessary for blood clotting.

APPENDIX F: PRONUNCIATION CLUE

The letters **g** and **c** are soft (as in ginger and cent) when followed by an **i** or **e,** and are hard (as in good and can) when followed by an **o** or **a.** This is true even with words based on the same combining form—for example:

laryngitis (lăr-ĭn-JĪ-tĭs)
laryngotomy (lă-rĭn-GŎT-ō-mē)

APPENDIX G: ANEMIA

Anemia literally means no blood. However, in medical language and usage, anemia is a condition of *reduction* in the number of erythrocytes or in the amount of hemoglobin in the circulating blood. Anemias are classified according to the different problems that arise with red blood cells. **Aplastic** (a- = no, plas/o = formation) **anemia,** a severe type, occurs when bone marrow fails to produce not only erythrocytes but leukocytes and thrombocytes as well.

APPENDIX H: ISCHEMIA

Ischemia literally means to hold back (isch/o) blood (-emia) from a part of the body. Tissue that becomes **ischemic** loses its normal flow of blood and becomes deprived of oxygen. The ischemia can be caused by mechanical injury to a blood vessel, by blood clots lodging in a vessel, or by the closing off (occlusion) of a vessel caused by collection of fatty material.

APPENDIX I: TONSILLITIS

The tonsils (notice the spelling with one letter l, whereas the combining form has a double letter l) are lymphatic tissue in back of the throat. They contain white blood cells (lymphocytes), which filter and fight bacteria. However, tonsils also can become infected and inflamed. Streptococcal infection of the throat causes **tonsillitis,** which may require **tonsillectomy.**

APPENDIX J: ACROMEGALY

Acromegaly is an endocrine disorder. It occurs when the **pituitary gland,** attached to the base of the brain, produces an excessive amount of growth hormone *after* the completion of puberty. The excess growth hormone most often results from a benign tumor of the pituitary gland. A person with acromegaly typically is of normal height because the long bones have stopped growth after puberty, but bones and soft tissue in the hands, feet, and face grow abnormally. High levels of growth hormone *before* completion of puberty produce excessive growth of long bones (gigantism), as well as acromegaly.

APPENDIX K: SPLENOMEGALY

The spleen is an organ in the left upper quadrant (LUQ) of the abdomen (below the diaphragm and to the side of the stomach). Composed of lymph tissue and blood vessels, it disposes of dying red blood cells and manufactures white blood cells (lymphocytes) to fight disease. Splenomegaly occurs with development of high blood pressure in hepatic veins (portal hypertension) and hemolytic blood diseases (anemias involving excessive destruction or lysis of red blood cells). If the spleen is removed (splenectomy), other organs carry out these functions.

APPENDIX L: ACHONDROPLASIA

Achondroplasia is an inherited disorder in which the bones of the arms and legs fail to grow to normal size because of a defect in both cartilage and bone. It results in a type of dwarfism characterized by short limbs, a normal-size head and body, and normal intelligence (Fig. 3–5).

APPENDIX M: -PTOSIS

The suffix **-ptosis** is pronounced TŌ-sĭs. When two consonants begin a word, the first is silent. If the two consonants are found in the middle of a word, both are pronounced—for example, blepharoptosis (blĕf-ăr-ŏp-TŌ-sĭs). This condition occurs when eyelid muscles weaken; the affected person then has difficulty keeping the eye open (Fig. 3–6).

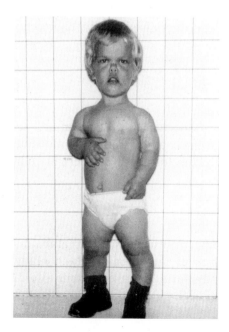

FIGURE 3–5 A boy with achondroplasia. His abnormalities include short stature with normal length of the trunk, short limbs and fingers, bowed legs, a relatively large head, a prominent forehead, and a depressed nasal bridge. (Courtesy of Dr. A. E. Chudley, Professor of Pediatrics and Child Health, Children's Hospital and University of Manitoba, Winnipeg, Manitoba, Canada.)

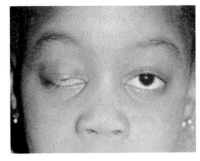

FIGURE 3–6 **Ptosis of the upper eyelid (blepharoptosis).** This condition may be congenital (appear at birth), can occur with aging, or may be associated with cerebrovascular accidents, cranial nerve damage, and other neurologic disorders. The eyelid droops because of muscle weakness. (From Seidel HM, Ball D, Dains J, Benedict GW: Mosby's Guide to Physical Examination, 5th ed. St. Louis, Mosby, 2003, p. 286.)

APPENDIX N: LAPAROSCOPY

Laparoscopy, or peritoneoscopy (a **minimally invasive surgery**), is visual examination of the abdominal (peritoneal) cavity using a laparoscope. The laparoscope, a lighted telescopic instrument, is inserted through an incision in the abdomen near the navel, and gas (carbon dioxide) is infused into the peritoneal cavity, to prevent injury to abdominal structures during surgery. Surgeons use laparoscopy to examine abdominal viscera for evidence of disease (performing biopsies) or for procedures such as removal of the appendix, gallbladder, adrenal gland, spleen, or ovary, colon resection, and repair of hernias. It also is used to clip and collapse the fallopian tubes (tubal ligation), which prevents sperm cells from reaching eggs that leave the ovary (Fig. 3–7).

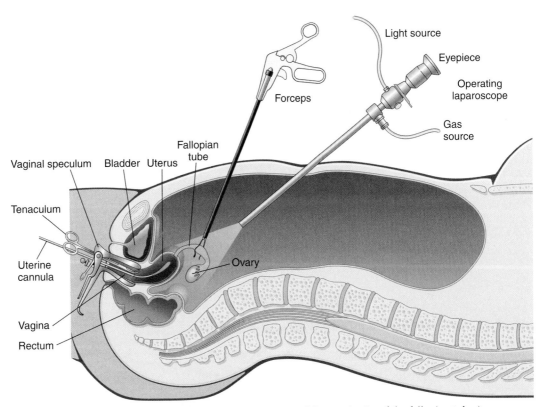

FIGURE 3–7 **Laparoscopy for tubal ligation** (interruption of the continuity of the fallopian tubes) as a means of preventing future pregnancy. The **tenaculum** grasps the cervix. The **vaginal speculum** keeps the vaginal cavity open. The **uterine cannula** is a tube placed into the uterus to manipulate the uterus during the procedure. **Forceps,** placed through the laparoscope, grasp or move tissue.

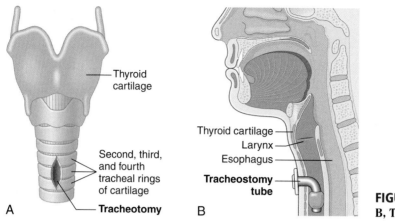

FIGURE 3–8 A, Tracheotomy. B, Tracheostomy.

APPENDIX O: TRACHEOTOMY

A tracheo**tomy** is an **incision** into the trachea to open it below a blockage. Tracheotomy may be performed to remove a foreign body or to obtain a biopsy specimen. See Figure 3–8, *A*.

A tracheo**stomy** is an **opening** into the trachea through which an indwelling tube is inserted. The tube is required to allow air to flow into the lungs or to help remove secretions (mucus) from the bronchial tubes. See Figure 3–8, *B*.

APPENDIX P: ARTERIOLE

Notice the relationship among an artery, **arterioles,** capillaries (the tiniest of blood vessels), **venules** (small veins), and a vein as illustrated in Figure 3–9.

APPENDIX Q: ADENOIDS

The **adenoids** are small masses of lymphatic tissue in the part of the pharynx (throat) near the nose and nasal passages. The literal meaning, "resembling glands," is appropriate because they are neither endocrine nor exocrine glands. Enlargement of adenoids may cause blockage of the airway from the nose to the pharynx, and adenoidectomy may be advised. The tonsils also are lymphatic tissue, and their location as well as that of the adenoids is indicated in Figure 3–10.

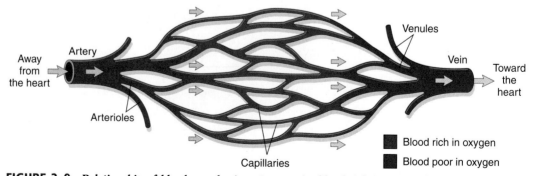

FIGURE 3–9 **Relationship of blood vessels.** An **artery** carries blood rich in oxygen from the heart to the organs of the body. In the organs, the artery narrows to form **arterioles** (small arteries), which branch into **capillaries** (the smallest blood vessels). Through the thin walls of capillaries, oxygen leaves the blood and enters cells. Thus, the capillaries branching into **venules** (small veins) carry blood poor in oxygen. Venules lead to a **vein,** which brings oxygen-poor blood back to the heart.

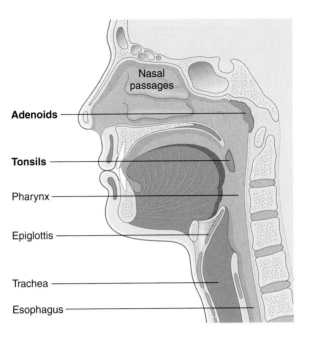

Nasal passages

Adenoids

Tonsils

Pharynx

Epiglottis

Trachea

Esophagus

FIGURE 3–10 Adenoids and tonsils.

PRACTICAL APPLICATIONS

Check your answers with the Answers to Practical Applications on page 99.

PROCEDURES

Choose the correct diagnostic or treatment procedure for each of the numbered definitions.

amniocentesis   colostomy   mastectomy   tonsillectomy
angiography   laparoscopy   paracentesis
angioplasty   laparotomy   thoracentesis

1. removal of abdominal fluid from the peritoneal space _____
2. large abdominal incision to remove an ovarian adenocarcinoma _____
3. removal of an adenocarcinoma of the breast _____
4. a method used to determine the karyotype of a fetus _____
5. surgical procedure to remove pharyngeal lymphatic tissue _____
6. surgical procedure to open clogged coronary arteries _____
7. method of removing fluid from the chest (pleural effusion) _____
8. procedure to drain feces from the body after bowel resection _____
9. x-ray procedure used to examine blood vessels before surgery _____
10. minimally invasive surgery within the abdomen _____

? EXERCISES

3

Remember to check your answers carefully with those given in the Answers to Exercises, page 98.

A. Give the meanings for the following suffixes.

1. -cele _____

2. -emia _____

3. -coccus _____

4. -gram _____

5. -cyte _____

6. -algia _____

7. -ectomy _____

8. -centesis _____

9. -genesis _____

10. -graph _____

11. -itis _____

12. -graphy _____

B. Using the combining forms below and your knowledge of suffixes, build the following medical terms.

amni/o	isch/o	ot/o
angi/o	laryng/o	rect/o
arthr/o	mast/o	staphyl/o
bronch/o	my/o	strept/o
carcin/o	myel/o	thorac/o
cyst/o		

1. hernia of the urinary bladder _____

2. pain of muscle _____

3. process of producing cancer _____

4. record (x-ray) of the spinal cord _____

5. berry-shaped bacteria in twisted chains _____

6. surgical puncture to remove fluid from the chest _____

7. removal of the breast _____

8. inflammation of the tubes leading from the windpipe to the lungs _____

9. to hold back blood from cells _____

10. process of recording (x-ray) blood vessels _____

11. visual examination of joints _____

12. berry-shaped bacteria in clusters _____

13. resection of the voice box _____

14. surgical procedure to remove fluid from the sac around the fetus _____

C. Match the following terms, which describe blood cells, with their meanings below.

basophil   lymphocyte   neutrophil
eosinophil   monocyte   thrombocyte
erythrocyte

1. granulocytic white blood cell (granules stain purple) that destroys foreign cells by engulfing and

   digesting them; also called a polymorphonuclear leukocyte _____

2. mononuclear white blood cell that destroys foreign cells by making antibodies

   _____

3. clotting cell; also called a platelet _____

4. leukocyte with reddish-staining granules and numbers elevated in allergic reactions

   _____

5. red blood cell _____

6. mononuclear white blood cell that engulfs and digests cellular debris; contains one large nucleus

   _____

7. granulocytic white blood cell that increases during the healing phase of inflammation

   _____

D. Give the meanings of the following suffixes.

1. -logy _____   8. -megaly _____

2. -lysis _____   9. -oma _____

3. -pathy _____   10. -opsy _____

4. -penia _____   11. -plasia _____

5. -malacia _____   12. -plasty _____

6. -osis _____   13. -sclerosis _____

7. -phobia _____   14. -stasis _____

E. **Using the combining forms below and your knowledge of suffixes, build the following medical terms.**

acr/o	hem/o	phleb/o
arteri/o	hydr/o	rhin/o
bi/o	morph/o	sarc/o
blephar/o	my/o	splen/o
cardi/o	myel/o	
chondr/o	nephr/o	

1. enlargement of the spleen_____

2. study of the shape (of cells) _____

3. softening of cartilage_____

4. abnormal condition of water (fluid) in the kidney _____

5. disease condition of heart muscle _____

6. hardening of arteries_____

7. tumor (benign) of muscle_____

8. flesh tumor (malignant) of muscle_____

9. surgical repair of the nose _____

10. tumor of bone marrow _____

11. fear of heights _____

12. view of living tissue under the microscope _____

13. stoppage of the flow of blood (by mechanical or natural means) _____

14. inflammation of the eyelid _____

15. incision of a vein _____

F. **Match the following terms with their meanings below.**

achondroplasia	colostomy	laparoscopy
acromegaly	hydrotherapy	metastasis
atrophy	hypertrophy	necrosis
chemotherapy	laparoscope	osteomalacia

1. treatment using drugs_____

2. condition of death (of cells) _____

3. softening of bone_____

4. opening of the large intestine to the outside of the body _____

5. no development; shrinkage of cells _____

6. beyond control; spread of a cancerous tumor to another organ _____

7. instrument to visually examine the abdomen _____

8. enlargement of extremities; an endocrine disorder that causes excess growth hormone to be

   produced by the pituitary gland after puberty _____

9. condition of improper formation of cartilage in the embryo that leads to short bones and

   dwarfism _____

10. process of viewing the peritoneal (abdominal) cavity _____

11. treatment using water_____

12. excessive development of cells (increase in size of individual cells)_____

G. Give the meanings of the following suffixes.

1. -ia _____

2. -trophy _____

3. -stasis _____

4. -stomy_____

5. -tomy _____

6. -ole _____

7. -um _____

8. -ule _____

9. -y _____

10. -oid _____

11. -genic_____

12. -ptosis _____

H. Using the list of combining forms and suffixes below, build the following medical terms.

Combining Forms

arteri/o	pleur/o
lapar/o	pneumon/o
mamm/o	radi/o
nephr/o	ven/o

Suffixes

-dynia	-ole	-therapy
-ectomy	-pathy	-tomy
-gram	-plasty	-ule
-ia	-scopy	

1. incision of the abdomen _____

2. process of visual examination of the abdomen _____

3. a small artery_____

4. condition of the lungs_____

5. treatment using x-rays _____

6. record (x-ray film) of the breast _____

7. pain of the chest wall and the membranes surrounding the lungs _____

8. a small vein _____

9. disease condition of the kidney_____

10. surgical repair of the breast _____

I. Underline the suffix in the following terms, and give the meaning of the entire term.

1. laryngeal _____

2. inguinal _____

3. chronic _____

4. pulmonary _____

5. adipose _____

6. peritoneal _____

7. axillary _____

8. necrotic _____

9. mucoid _____

10. mucous _____

11. agoraphobia _____

12. esophagus _____

J. Select from the following terms relating to blood and blood vessels to complete the sentences below.

anemia	hemolysis	leukocytosis
angioplasty	hemostasis	multiple myeloma
arterioles	ischemia	thrombocytopenia
hematoma	leukemia	venules

1. Billy was diagnosed with excessively high numbers of cancerous white blood cells, or

   _____. His doctor prescribed chemotherapy and expected an excellent
   prognosis.

2. Mr. Clark's angiogram showed that he had serious atherosclerosis of one of the arteries supplying

   blood to his heart. His doctor recommended that _____ would be helpful
   to open up his clogged artery by threading a catheter (tube) through his artery and opening a
   balloon at the end of the catheter to widen the artery.

3. Mrs. Jackson's blood count showed a reduced number of red blood cells, indicating

   _____. Her erythrocytes were being destroyed by _____.

4. Doctors refused to operate on Joe because of his low platelet count, a condition called

   _____.

5. Blockage of an artery leading to Mr. Stein's brain led to the holding back of blood flow to nerve

   tissue in his brain. This condition, called _____, could lead to necrosis of
   tissue and a cerebrovascular accident.

6. Small arteries, or _____, were broken under Ms. Bein's scalp when she was struck on the head with a rock. She soon developed a mass of blood, a (an)

   _____, under the skin in that region of her head.

7. Sarah Jones had a staphylococcal infection causing elevation of her white blood cell count. She

   was treated with antibiotics and the _____ returned to normal.

8. Within the body, the bone marrow (soft tissue within bones) is the "factory" for making blood cells.

   Mr. Scott developed _____, a malignant condition of the bone marrow cells in his hip, upper arm, and thigh bones.

9. During operations, surgeons use clamps to close off blood vessels and prevent blood loss. Thus,

   they maintain _____ and avoid blood transfusions.

10. Small vessels that carry blood toward the heart from capillaries and tissues are

    _____.

K. Complete the medical term for the following definitions.

Definition	*Medical Term*
1. the membrane surrounding the heart	peri_____
2. hardening of arteries	arterio _____
3. enlargement of the liver	hepato _____
4. new opening of the windpipe to the outside of the body	tracheo_____
5. inflammation of the tonsils	_____itis
6. surgical puncture to remove fluid from the abdomen	abdomino_____
7. muscle pain	my _____
8. pertaining to the membranes surrounding the lungs	_____al
9. study of the eye	_____logy
10. berry-shaped (spheroidal) bacteria in clusters	_____cocci
11. beyond control (spread of a cancerous tumor)	meta_____
12. pertaining to the voice box	_____eal

3

L. Circle the correct term to complete the following sentences.

1. Ms. Daley, who has nine children, visited her general practitioner because she was experiencing problems with urination. After examining her, the doctor found that her bladder was protruding into her vagina and told her she had a (**rectocele, cystocele, hiatal hernia**).

2. Susan coughed constantly for a week. Her physician told her that her chest x-ray examination showed evidence of pneumonia. Her sputum (material coughed up from the bronchial tubes) was found to contain (**ischemic, pleuritic, pneumococcal**) bacteria.

3. Mr. Manion went to see his family doctor because he couldn't keep his left upper eyelid from sagging. His doctor told him that he had a neurologic problem called Horner syndrome, characterized by (**necrosis, hydronephrosis, ptosis**) of his eyelid.

4. Jill broke her left arm in a fall while mountain biking. After 6 weeks in a cast to treat the fracture, her left arm was noticeably smaller and weaker than her right arm—the muscles had (**atrophied, hypertrophied, metastasized**). Her physician recommended physical therapy to strengthen the affected arm.

5. Ms. Brody was diagnosed with breast cancer. The first phase of her treatment included a (**nephrectomy, mastectomy, pulmonary resection**) to remove her breast and the tumor. After the surgery, her doctors recommended (**chemotherapy, radiotherapy, hydrotherapy**) using drugs such as doxorubicin (Adriamycin) and paclitaxel (Taxol).

6. At age 29, Kevin's facial features became coarser and his hands and tongue enlarged. After a head CT (computed tomography) scan, doctors diagnosed the cause of these changes as (**hyperglycemia, hyperthyroidism, acromegaly**), a slowly progressive endocrine condition involving the pituitary gland.

7. Each winter during "cold and flu season," Daisy developed (**chondromalacia, bronchitis, cardiomyopathy**). Her doctor prescribed antibiotics and respiratory therapy to help her recover.

8. After (**arthroscopy, laparotomy, radiotherapy**) on his knee, Alan had swelling and inflammation near the small incisions. Dr. Nicholas assured him that this was a common side effect of the procedure that would resolve spontaneously.

9. Under the microscope, Dr. Vance could see grape-like clusters of bacteria called (**eosinophils, streptococci, staphylococci**). She made the diagnosis of (**staphylococcemia, eosinophilia, streptococcemia**), and the patient was started on antibiotic therapy.

10. David enjoyed weight lifting, but he recently noticed a bulge in his right groin region. He visited his doctor, who made the diagnosis of (**hiatal hernia, rectocele, inguinal hernia**) and recommended surgical repair.

MEDICAL SCRAMBLE

Unscramble the letters to form suffixes from the clues. Use the letters in squares to complete the bonus term. Answers are found on page 99.

1. *Clue:* Surgical puncture to remove fluid

   - ☐ ___ ☐ ___ ___ ___ ___ ___   ESTICESN

2. *Clue:* Hardening ⁻ ___ ___ ___ ___ ___ ☐ ___ ___ ___   LSOSSECRI

3. *Clue:* Treatment ⁻ ___ ___ ☐ ☐ ___ ___ ___   RHPEYAT

4. *Clue:* Softening ⁻ ☐ ___ ___ ___ ___ ☐ ___   ACLAMAI

5. *Clue:* Surgical repair ⁻ ☐ ___ ___ ___ ☐ ___   YSLTAP

6. *Clue:* Development ⁻ ___ ___ ☐ ___ ___ ___   HYPTOR

7. *Clue:* Enlargement ⁻ ___ ___ ___ ___ ___ ☐   AGYMLE

8. *Clue:* Excision ⁻ ___ ___ ☐ ☐ ___ ___   MCYOET

9. *Clue:* Pain ⁻ ___ ___ ___ ___ ☐   IGLAA

10. *Clue:* Fear ⁻ ___ ☐ ___ ☐ ___ ___   AIBHPO

BONUS TERM: *Clue:* Deficiency of platelets

☐ ☐ ☐ ☐ ☐ ☐ ☐ ☐ ☐ ☐ ☐ ☐ ☐ ☐ ☐ ☐

ANSWERS TO EXERCISES

A

1. hernia
2. blood condition
3. berry-shaped bacterium
4. record
5. cell
6. pain
7. removal, excision, resection
8. surgical puncture to remove fluid
9. process of producing, forming
10. instrument to record
11. inflammation
12. process of recording

B

1. cystocele
2. myalgia ("myodynia" is not used)
3. carcinogenesis
4. myelogram
5. streptococci (*bacteria* is a plural term)
6. thoracocentesis or thoracentesis
7. mastectomy
8. bronchitis
9. ischemia
10. angiography
11. arthroscopy
12. staphylococci
13. laryngectomy
14. amniocentesis

C

1. neutrophil
2. lymphocyte
3. thrombocyte
4. eosinophil
5. erythrocyte
6. monocyte
7. basophil

D

1. process of study
2. breakdown, separation, destruction
3. process of disease
4. deficiency, less than normal
5. softening
6. condition, abnormal condition
7. fear of
8. enlargement
9. tumor, mass
10. process of viewing
11. condition of formation, growth
12. surgical repair
13. hardening, to harden
14. to stop, control

E

1. splenomegaly
2. morphology
3. chondromalacia
4. hydronephrosis
5. cardiomyopathy
6. arteriosclerosis
7. myoma
8. myosarcoma
9. rhinoplasty
10. myeloma (called multiple myeloma)
11. acrophobia
12. biopsy
13. hemostasis
14. blepharitis
15. phlebotomy

F

1. chemotherapy
2. necrosis
3. osteomalacia
4. colostomy
5. atrophy
6. metastasis
7. laparoscope
8. acromegaly
9. achondroplasia
10. laparoscopy
11. hydrotherapy
12. hypertrophy

G

1. condition
2. development, nourishment
3. to stop, control
4. new opening
5. incision, cut into
6. small, little
7. structure
8. small, little
9. condition, process
10. resembling
11. pertaining to producing, produced by or in
12. prolapse, drooping, sagging

H

1. laparotomy
2. laparoscopy
3. arteriole
4. pneumonia (this condition is actually *pneumonitis*)
5. radiotherapy
6. mammogram
7. pleurodynia
8. venule
9. nephropathy
10. mammoplasty

3

I

1. laryngeal—pertaining to the voice box
2. inguinal—pertaining to the groin
3. chronic—pertaining to time (over a long period of time)
4. pulmonary—pertaining to the lung
5. adipose—pertaining to (or full of) fat
6. peritoneal—pertaining to the peritoneum (membrane around the abdominal organs)
7. axillary—pertaining to the armpit, under arm
8. necrotic—pertaining to death
9. mucoid—resembling mucus
10. mucous—pertaining to mucus
11. agoraphobia—fear of open spaces (agora means marketplace)
12. esophagus—tube leading from the throat to the stomach

J

1. leukemia
2. angioplasty
3. anemia; hemolysis
4. thrombocytopenia
5. ischemia
6. arterioles; hematoma
7. leukocytosis
8. multiple myeloma
9. hemostasis
10. venules

K

1. pericardium
2. arteriosclerosis
3. hepatomegaly
4. tracheostomy
5. tonsillitis
6. abdominocentesis (this procedure also is known as paracentesis)
7. myalgia
8. pleural
9. ophthalmology
10. staphylococci
11. metastasis
12. laryngeal

L

1. cystocele
2. pneumococcal
3. ptosis
4. atrophied
5. mastectomy; chemotherapy
6. acromegaly
7. bronchitis
8. arthroscopy
9. staphylococci; staphylococcemia
10. inguinal hernia

ANSWERS TO PRACTICAL APPLICATIONS

1. paracentesis
2. laparotomy
3. mastectomy
4. amniocentesis
5. tonsillectomy
6. angioplasty
7. thoracentesis
8. colostomy
9. angiography
10. laparoscopy

ANSWERS TO MEDICAL SCRAMBLE

1. -CENTESIS   2. -SCLEROSIS   3. -THERAPY   4. -MALACIA   5. -PLASTY   6. -TROPHY   7. -MEGALY   8. -ECTOMY
9. -ALGIA   10. -PHOBIA
BONUS TERM: THROMBOCYTOPENIA

PRONUNCIATION OF TERMS

PRONUNCIATION GUIDE

ā as in āpe   ă as in ăpple
ē as in ēven   ĕ as in ĕvery
ī as in īce   ĭ as in ĭnterest
ō as in ōpen   ŏ as in pŏt
ū as in ūnit   ŭ as in ŭnder

To test your understanding of the terminology in this chapter, write the meaning of each term in the space provided. In addition, you may wish to cover the terms and write them by looking at your definitions. Make sure your spelling is correct. The page number after each term indicates where it is defined or used in the text, so you can check your responses. You will find complete definitions for all of these terms and their audio pronunciations on the CD.

Term	Pronunciation	Meaning
abdominocentesis (76)	ăb-dŏm-ĭ-nō-sĕn-TĒ-sĭs	_____
achondroplasia (78)	ā-kŏn-drō-PLĀ-zē-ă	_____
acromegaly (77)	ăk-rō-MĔG-ă-lē	_____

3

Term	Pronunciation	Meaning
acrophobia (78)	ăk-rō-FŌ-bē-ă	
acute (81)	ă-KŪT	
adenoids (81)	ĂD-ĕ-noydz	
adipose (81)	Ă-dĭ-pōs	
agoraphobia (78)	ă-gŏr-ă-FŌ-bē-ă	
amniocentesis (76)	ăm-nē-ō-sĕn-TĒ-sĭs	
anemia (77)	ă-NĒ-mē-ă	
angiogenesis (77)	ăn-jē-ō-JĔN-ĕ-sĭs	
angiography (77)	ăn-jē-ŎG-ră-fē	
angioplasty (78)	ăn-jē-ō-PLĂS-tē	
arteriole (80)	ăr-TĒR-ē-ōl	
arteriosclerosis (79)	ăr-tē-rē-ō-sklĕ-RŌ-sĭs	
arthralgia (76)	ăr-THRĂL-jă	
atrophy (80)	ĂT-rō-fē	
axillary (81)	ĂK-sĭ-lār-ē	
basophil (84)	BĀ-sō-fĭl	
biopsy (78)	BĪ-ŏp-sē	
blepharoptosis (79)	blĕf-ă-rŏp-TŌ-sĭs	
bronchitis (77)	brŏng-KĪ-tĭs	
carcinogenesis (77)	kăr-sĭ-nō-JĔN-ĕ-sĭs	
carcinogenic (81)	kăr-sĭ-nō-JĔN-ik	
cardiomyopathy (78)	kăr-dē-ō-mī-ŎP-ă-thē	
chemotherapy (79)	kē-mō-THĔR-ĕ-pē	
chondromalacia (77)	kŏn-drō-mă-LĀ-shă	
chronic (81)	KRŎN-ĭk	
colostomy (79)	kō-LŎS-tō-mē	
cystocele (76)	SĬS-tō-sēl	
electroencephalogram (77)	ē-lĕk-trō-ĕn-SĔF-ă-lō-grăm	
electroencephalograph (77)	ē-lĕk-trō-ĕn-SĔF-ă-lō-grăf	
electroencephalography (77)	ē-lĕk-trō-ĕn-sĕf-ă-LŎG-ră-fē	
eosinophil (84)	ē-ō-SĬN-ō-fĭl	
erythrocyte (76)	ĕ-RĬTH-rō-sīt	
erythropenia (78)	ĕ-rĭth-rō-PĒ-nē-ă	

Term	Pronunciation	Meaning
esophagus (80)	ĕ-SŎF-ă-gus	_____
hematoma (78)	hē-mă-TŌ-mă	_____
hemolysis (77)	hē-MŎL-ĭ-sĭs	_____
hemostasis (79)	hē-mō-STĀ-sĭs	_____
hydronephrosis (78)	hī-drō-nĕ-FRŌ-sĭs	_____
hydrotherapy (79)	hī-drō-THĔR-ă-pē	_____
hypertrophy (80)	hī-PĔR-trō-fē	_____
inguinal (80)	ĬNG-wĭ-năl	_____
ischemia (77)	ĭs-KĒ-mē-ă	_____
laparoscope (79)	LĂP-ă-rō-skōp	_____
laparoscopy (79)	lă-pă-RŎS-kō-pē	_____
laparotomy (79)	lăp-ă-RŎT-ō-mē	_____
laryngeal (81)	lă-RĬN-jē-ăl _or_ lăr-ĭn-JĒ-ăl	_____
laryngectomy (77)	lăr-ĭn-JĔK-tō-mē	_____
leukemia (80)	lū-KĒ-mē-ă	_____
leukocytosis (78)	lū-kō-sī-TŌ-sĭs	_____
lymphocyte (85)	LĬM-fō-sīt	_____
mammogram (77)	MĂM-mō-grăm	_____
mastectomy (77)	măs-TĔK-tō-mē	_____
metastasis (79)	mĕ-TĂS-tă-sĭs	_____
monocyte (85)	MŎN-ō-sīt	_____
morphology (77)	mŏr-FŎL-ō-jē	_____
mucoid (81)	MŪ-koyd	_____
mucous membrane (81)	MŪ-kŭs MĔM-brān	_____
mucus (81)	MŪ-kŭs	_____
myalgia (76)	mī-ĂL-jă	_____
myelogram (77)	MĪ-ĕ-lō-grăm	_____
myeloma (78)	mī-ĕ-LŌ-mă	_____
myoma (78)	mī-Ō-mă	_____
myosarcoma (78)	mī-ō-săr-KŌ-mă	_____
necropsy (78)	NĔ-krŏp-sē	_____
necrosis (78)	nĕ-KRŌ-sĭs	_____
necrotic (81)	nĕ-KRŎT-ĭk	_____
nephrologist (80)	nĕ-FRŎL-ō-jĭst	_____

Term	Pronunciation	Meaning
nephropathy (80)	nĕ-FRŎP-ă-thē	
neuralgia (76)	nū-RĂL-jă	
neutropenia (78)	nū-trō-PĒ-nē-ă	
neutrophil (87)	NŪ-trō-fĭl	
ophthalmology (77)	ŏf-thăl-MŎL-ō-jē	
osteogenic (81)	ŏs-tē-ō-JĔN-ĭk	
osteomalacia (77)	ŏs-tē-ō-mă-LĀ-shă	
otalgia (76)	ō-TĂL-jă	
paracentesis (76)	pă-ră-cĕn-TĒ-sĭs	
pathogenesis (77)	păth-ŏ-JĔN-ĕ-sĭs	
pathologic (81)	păth-ō-LŎJ-ĭk	
pericardium (80)	pĕr-ē-KĂR-dē-ŭm	
peritoneal (80)	pĕr-ĭ-tō-NĒ-ăl	
peritoneoscopy (88)	pĕr-ĭ-tō-nē-ŎS-kō-pē	
phlebotomy (79)	flĕ-BŎT-ō-mē	
platelet (85)	PLĀT-lĕt	
pleurodynia (76)	plūr-ō-DĬN-ē-ă	
pneumonia (80)	nū-MŌN-yă	
polymorphonuclear leukocyte (85)	pŏl-ē-mŏr-fō-NŪ-klē-ăr LŪ-kō-sīt	
ptosis (79)	TŌ-sĭs	
pulmonary (81)	PŪL-mō-nā-rē	
radiographer (80)	rā-dē-ŎG-ră-fĕr	
radiotherapy (79)	rā-dē-ō-THĔR-ă-pē	
rectocele (76)	RĔK-tō-sēl	
splenomegaly (77)	splē-nō-MĔG-ă-lē	
staphylococci (76)	stăf-ĭ-lō-KŎK-sī	
streptococcus (76)	strĕp-tō-KŎK-ŭs	
thoracentesis (76)	thō-ră-sĕn-TĒ-sĭs	
thrombocytopenia (78)	thrŏm-bō-sī-tō-PĒ-nē-ă	
thrombophlebitis (77)	thrŏm-bō-flĕ-BĪ-tĭs	
tonsillitis (77)	tŏn-sĭ-LĪ-tĭs	
tracheostomy (79)	trā-kē-ŎS-tō-mē	
venule (80)	VĔN-ūl	

3

REVIEW SHEET

Write the meanings of each word part in the space provided and test yourself. Check your answers with the information in the chapter or in the Glossary (Medical Word Parts—English) at the end of the book.

NOUN SUFFIXES

Suffix	Meaning	Suffix	Meaning
-algia	_____	-oma	_____
-cele	_____	-opsy	_____
-centesis	_____	-osis	_____
-coccus (-cocci)	_____	-pathy	_____
-cyte	_____	-penia	_____
-dynia	_____	-phobia	_____
-ectomy	_____	-plasia	_____
-emia	_____	-plasty	_____
-er	_____	-ptosis	_____
-genesis	_____	-sclerosis	_____
-gram	_____	-scope	_____
-graph	_____	-scopy	_____
-graphy	_____	-stasis	_____
-ia	_____	-stomy	_____
-ist	_____	-therapy	_____
-itis	_____	-tomy	_____
-logy	_____	-trophy	_____
-lysis	_____	-ule	_____
-malacia	_____	-um, -ium	_____
-megaly	_____	-us	_____
-ole	_____	-y	_____

ADJECTIVE SUFFIXES

Suffix	Meaning	Suffix	Meaning
-ac, -iac	_____	-ic, -ical	_____
-al	_____	-oid	_____
-ar	_____	-ose	_____
-ary	_____	-ous	_____
-eal	_____	-tic	_____
-genic	_____		

COMBINING FORMS

Combining Form	Meaning	Combining Form	Meaning
abdomin/o	_____	inguin/o	_____
acr/o	_____	isch/o	_____
acu/o	_____	lapar/o	_____
aden/o	_____	laryng/o	_____
adip/o	_____	leuk/o	_____
amni/o	_____	lymph/o	_____
angi/o	_____	mamm/o	_____
arteri/o	_____	mast/o	_____
arthr/o	_____	morph/o	_____
axill/o	_____	muc/o	_____
bi/o	_____	my/o	_____
blephar/o	_____	myel/o	_____
bronch/o	_____	necr/o	_____
carcin/o	_____	nephr/o	_____
cardi/o	_____	neur/o	_____
chem/o	_____	neutr/o	_____
chondr/o	_____	nucle/o	_____
chron/o	_____	ophthalm/o	_____
col/o	_____	oste/o	_____
cyst/o	_____	ot/o	_____
encephal/o	_____	path/o	_____
erythr/o	_____	peritone/o	_____
hem/o	_____	phag/o	_____
hepat/o	_____	phleb/o	_____
hydr/o	_____	plas/o	_____

3

Combining Form	Meaning	Combining Form	Meaning
pleur/o	_____	splen/o	_____
pneumon/o	_____	staphyl/o	_____
pulmon/o	_____	strept/o	_____
radi/o	_____	thorac/o	_____
rect/o	_____	thromb/o	_____
ren/o	_____	tonsill/o	_____
rhin/o	_____	trache/o	_____
sarc/o	_____	ven/o	_____

Give the medical term for the following blood cells:

    red blood cell _____

    clotting cell _____

    white blood cell _____

Name 5 different types of white blood cells (the first letter is given):

    e_____

    b_____

    n_____

    l_____

    m_____

 Please refer to the enclosed CD for additional exercises and images related to this chapter.

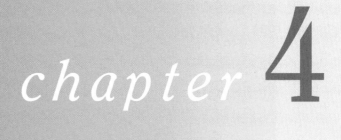

chapter 4

Prefixes

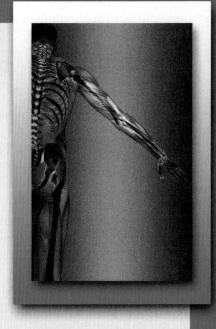

In this chapter you will

- Define basic prefixes used in the medical language.
- Analyze medical terms that combine prefixes and other word elements.
- Learn about the Rh condition as an example of an antigen-antibody reaction.

Image Description: Posterior angled view of a male body with skeleton and musculature.

INTRODUCTION

This chapter on prefixes, like the preceding chapter on suffixes, gives you practice in word analysis and provides a foundation for the study of the terminology of body systems that follows.

The list of combining forms, suffixes, and meanings helps you analyze terminology in the rest of the chapter. The appendices are included to provide more complete understanding of the terms and to explain the words with reference to the anatomy, physiology, and pathology of the body.

 # COMBINING FORMS AND SUFFIXES

COMBINING FORMS

Combining Form	Meaning	Combining Form	Meaning
carp/o	wrist bones	norm/o	rule, order
cib/o	meals	ox/o	oxygen
cis/o	to cut	pub/o	pubis (pubic bone); anterior portion of the pelvic or hipbone
cost/o	rib		
cutane/o	skin	seps/o	infection
dactyl/o	fingers, toes	somn/o	sleep
duct/o	to lead, carry	son/o	sound
flex/o	to bend	the/o	to put, place
furc/o	forking, branching	thel/o	nipple
gloss/o	tongue	thyr/o	thyroid gland; shield (the shape of the thyroid gland resembled (-oid) a shield to those who named it)
glyc/o	sugar		
immun/o	protection		
morph/o	shape, form	top/o	place, position, location
mort/o	death	tox/o	poison
nat/i	birth	trache/o	windpipe, trachea
nect/o	to bind, tie, connect	urethr/o	urethra

SUFFIXES

Suffix	Meaning	Suffix	Meaning
-blast	embryonic, immature	-partum	birth, labor
-crine	to secrete	-phoria	to bear, carry; feeling (mental state)
-cyesis	pregnancy	-physis	to grow
-drome	to run	-plasia	development, formation
-fusion	coming together; to pour	-plasm	structure or formation
-gen	substance that produces	-pnea	breathing
-lapse	to side, fall, sag	-ptosis	droop, sag, prolapse
-lysis	breakdown, separation, loosening	-rrhea	flow, discharge
-meter	to measure	-stasis	stop, control
-mission	to send	-trophy	nourishment, development
-or	one who		

PREFIXES AND TERMINOLOGY

Write the meaning of the medical term in the space provided. Remember, your CD contains definitions for all terms.

Prefix	Meaning	Terminology	Meaning
a-, an-	no, not, without	apnea _____	
		anoxia _____	
ab-	away from (notice that the b faces away from the a)	abnormal _____	
		abductor _____ *A muscle that draws a limb away from the body.*	
ad-	toward (notice that the d faces toward the a)	adductor _____ *A muscle that draws a limb toward the body.*	
		adrenal glands[1] _____ *These glands actually lie on top of each kidney.*	

[1]See Appendix A, page 115.

Abduction/Adduction
Abduction means moving away from (often dictated as "A-B-duction"), while *adduction* means moving toward (often dictated as "A-D-duction").

Prefix	Meaning	Terminology	Meaning
ana-	up, apart	anabolism _____	
		analysis _____	
		Urinalysis (urin/o + [an]/alysis) is a laboratory examination of urine that aids in the diagnosis of many medical conditions.	
ante-	before, forward	ante cibum _____	
		The notation a.c., seen on prescription orders, means before meals.	
		anteflexion _____	
		antepartum _____	
anti-	against	antisepsis _____	
		An antiseptic (-sis changes to -tic to form an adjective) substance fights infection. Anti- is pronounced an-tĭ.	
		antibiotic[2] _____	
		antigen[3] _____	
		In this term, anti- is short for antibody. An antigen (bacterium or virus) is a substance that produces (-gen) an antibody.	
		antibody _____	
		Protein produced against an antigen (foreign body).	
		antitoxin _____	
		This is an antibody, often from an animal (such as a horse), that acts against a toxin. An example is tetanus antitoxin.	
auto-	self, own	autoimmune disease[4] _____	
		Autoimmune means producing antibodies against one's own normal cells.	
bi-	two	bifurcation _____	
		Normal splitting into two branches, such as bifurcation of the trachea to form the bronchi.	
		bilateral _____	
brady-	slow	bradycardia _____	
		Usually, a pulse of less than 60; a slow heart rate.	
cata-	down	catabolism _____	
con-	with, together	congenital anomaly[5] _____	
		connective _____	
		Connective tissue supports and binds other body tissue and parts. Bone, cartilage, and fibrous tissue are connective tissues.	

[2]See Appendix B, page 115.
[3]See Appendix C, page 115.
[4]See Appendix D, page 116.
[5]See Appendix E, page 117.

Prefix	Meaning	Terminology	Meaning
contra-	against, opposite	contraindication _____ *Contra- means against in this term.*	
		contralateral[6] _____ *Contra- means opposite in this term.*	
de-	down, lack of	dehydration _____	
dia-	through, complete	diameter _____	
		diarrhea _____	
		dialysis[7] _____	
dys-	bad, painful, difficult, abnormal	dyspnea _____ *Often caused by respiratory or cardiac conditions, strenuous exercise, or anxiety*	
		dysplasia _____	
ec-, ecto-	out, outside	ectopic pregnancy[8] _____ *Ectopic means pertaining to out of place and modifies the noun "pregnancy."*	
en-, endo-	in, within	endocardium _____	
		endoscope _____	
		endotracheal _____ *An endotracheal tube, placed through the mouth into the trachea, is used for giving oxygen and in general anesthesia procedures.*	
epi-	upon, on, above	epithelium _____	
eu-	good, normal	euphoria _____ *Exaggerated feeling of well-being.*	
		euthyroid _____ *Normal thyroid function.*	
ex-	out, away from	exophthalmos _____ *Protrusion of the eyeball associated with enlargement and overactivity of the thyroid gland; also called proptosis (pro = forward, -ptosis = prolapse)*	
hemi-	half	hemiglossectomy _____	

[6]See Appendix F, page 117.
[7]See Appendix G, page 118.
[8]See Appendix H, page 118.

4

Prefix	Meaning	Terminology	Meaning
hyper-	excessive, above	hyperglycemia _____ *This is diabetes mellitus. Lack of insulin (type 1 diabetes) or ineffective insulin (type 2 diabetes) causes high levels of sugar in the blood.*	
		hyperplasia _____ *Increase in cell numbers. Hyperplasia is a characteristic of tumor growth.*	
		hypertrophy _____ *Increase in size of individual cells. Muscle, cardiac, and renal cells exhibit hypertrophy when workload is increased.*	
hypo-	deficient, under	hypodermic injection _____	
		hypoglycemia _____	
in-	not	insomniac _____	
in-	into, within	incision _____	
infra-	beneath	infracostal _____	
inter-	between	intercostal _____ *Intercostal muscles lie between adjacent ribs.*	
intra-	into, within	intravenous _____	
macro-	large	macrocephaly _____ *This is a congenital anomaly.*	
mal-	bad	malignant _____ *From the Latin ignis, meaning fire.* **Benign** *(ben- = good) means noncancerous, whereas* **malignant** *means cancerous.*	
		malaise _____ *Originally a French word meaning a vague feeling of bodily discomfort.*	
meta-	beyond, change	metacarpal bones _____ *The five hand bones lie beyond the wrist bones but before the finger bones (phalanges).*	
		metamorphosis _____ *Meta- means change in this term. The change in development from the larval (caterpillar) stage to the adult (butterfly) is a form of metamorphosis. Embryonic (immature)* **stem cells** *spontaneously change (undergo metamorphosis) to form many different types of mature cells.*	
		metastasis _____ *Meta = beyond and -stasis = control, or meta = change and -stasis = place. A metastasis is a cancerous tumor that has spread to a secondary location.*	

Inter-, infra-, intra-
Be careful not to confuse these prefixes: *inter-* means between; *infra-* means below or beneath; *intra-* means within.

4

Prefix	Meaning	Terminology	Meaning
micro-	small	microscope _____	
neo-	new	neonatal _____	
		The neonatal period is the interval from birth to 28 days.	
		neoplasm _____	
		A neoplasm may be benign or malignant.	
pan-	all	pancytopenia _____	
		Deficiency of erythrocytes, leukocytes, and thrombocytes.	
para-	abnormal, beside, near	paralysis _____	
		Abnormal disruption of the connection between nerve and muscle. Originally from the Greek paralusis, *meaning to separate, loosen on one side, describing the loss of movement on one side of the body (occurring in stroke patients).*	
		parathyroid glands[9] _____	
		Para- means beside. There are four parathyroid glands behind the thyroid gland.	
per-	through	percutaneous _____	
peri-	surrounding	pericardium _____	
		periosteum _____	
poly-	many, much	polymorphonuclear _____	
		polyneuritis _____	
post-	after, behind	postmortem _____	
		postpartum _____	
pre-	before, in front of	precancerous _____	
		prenatal _____	
pro-	before, forward	prodrome _____	
		Prodromal symptoms (rash, fever) appear before the actual illness and signal its onset.	
		prolapse[10] _____	
pseudo-	false	pseudocyesis _____	
		Development of signs of pregnancy but without the presence of an embryo. The origin of this condition may be psychogenic, or caused by tumor and endocrine dysfunction.	

---

[9]See Appendix I, page 118.
[10]See Appendix J, page 118.

4

Prefix	Meaning	Terminology	Meaning
re-	back, again	relapse _____	
		A disease or its symptoms return after an apparent recovery.	
		remission _____	
		Symptoms lessen and the patient feels better. Remission may be spontaneous or the result of treatment. In some cases the remission is permanent and the disease is cured.	
		recombinant DNA[11] _____	
		Genetic engineering uses recombinant DNA techniques.	
retro-	behind, backward	retroperitoneal _____	
		retroflexion _____	
		An abnormal position of an organ, such as the uterus, bent or tilted backward.	
sub-	under	subcutaneous _____	
supra-	above, upper	suprapubic _____	
		The pubis is one of a pair of pubic bones that forms the anterior part of the pelvic (hip) bone.	
syn-, sym-	together, with	syndactyly _____	
		Webbed fingers or toes.	
		synthesis _____	
		In protein synthesis, complex proteins are built up from simpler amino acids.	
		syndrome[12] _____	
		Before the letters b, m, and p, syn becomes sym.	
		symbiosis[13] _____	
		symmetry _____	
		Equality of parts on opposite sides of the body. What is asymmetry?	
		symphysis[14] _____	
tachy-	fast	tachypnea _____	
		(tă-KĬP-nē-ă)	

---

[11]See Appendix K, page 118.
[12]See Appendix L, page 119.
[13]See Appendix M, page 119.
[14]See Appendix N, page 120.

Prefix	Meaning	Terminology	Meaning
trans-	across, through	transfusion _____	
		Transfer of blood or blood parts from one person to another.	
		transurethral[15] _____	
		Trans- = through in this term.	
ultra-	beyond, excess	ultrasonography[16] _____	
uni-	one	unilateral _____	

[15]See Appendix O, page 120.
[16]See Appendix P, page 120.

APPENDICES

APPENDIX A: ADRENAL GLANDS

The **adrenal glands** (Fig. 4–1) are endocrine glands located above each kidney. They secrete chemicals (hormones) that affect the body's functioning. One of these hormones is adrenaline (epinephrine). It causes the bronchial tubes to widen, the heart to beat more rapidly, and blood pressure to rise.

APPENDIX B: ANTIBIOTIC

An **antibiotic** destroys or inhibits the growth of microorganisms (small living things) such as bacteria. Penicillin, the first antibiotic, was cultured from immature plants (molds) and found to inhibit bacterial growth.

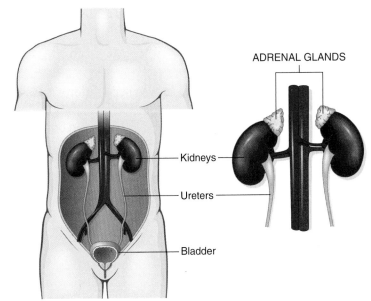

FIGURE 4–1 Adrenal glands.

4

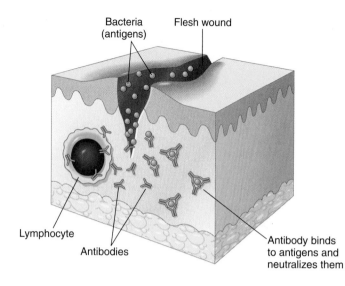

Bacteria
(antigens)   Flesh wound

Lymphocyte

Antibodies

Antibody binds
to antigens and
neutralizes them

FIGURE 4–2 **Antigens, antibodies, and the immune response.** When you receive a **vaccine**, it contains dead or weakened antigens that stimulate lymphocytes to make antibodies, which remain in your blood to protect against those specific antigens when encountered later on.

APPENDIX C: ANTIGENS AND ANTIBODIES; THE Rh CONDITION

An **antigen** is a substance, usually foreign to the body (such as a poison, virus, or bacterium), that stimulates the production of **antibodies.** Antibodies are protein substances made by white blood cells in response to the presence of foreign antigens. For example, the flu virus (antigen) enters the body, causing the production of antibodies in the bloodstream. These antibodies then attach to and destroy the antigens (viruses) that produced them. The reaction between an antigen and an antibody is an **immune response** (immun/o means protection) (Fig. 4–2).

Another example of an antigen-antibody is the **Rh condition.** A person who is Rh positive (Rh$^+$) has a protein coating (antigen) on his or her red blood cells (RBCs). This specific antigen factor is something that the person is born with and is normal. People who are Rh negative (Rh$^-$) have normal RBCs as well, but their red cells lack the Rh factor antigen.

If an Rh$^-$ woman and an Rh$^+$ man conceive an embryo, the embryo may be Rh$^-$ or Rh$^+$. A dangerous condition arises only when the embryo is Rh$^+$ (because this is different from the Rh$^-$ mother). During delivery of the first Rh$^+$ baby, some of the baby's blood cells containing Rh$^+$ antigens can escape into the mother's bloodstream. This sensitizes the mother so that she produces a low level of antibodies to the Rh$^+$ antigen. Because this occurs at delivery, the first baby is generally not affected and is normal at birth. Sensitization can also occur after a miscarriage, abortion, or blood transfusions (with Rh$^+$ blood).

Difficulties arise with the second Rh$^+$ pregnancy. If this embryo also is Rh$^+$, during pregnancy the mother's acquired antibodies (from the first pregnancy) enter the embryo's bloodstream. These antibodies attack and destroy the embryo's Rh$^+$ RBCs. The embryo attempts to compensate for this loss by making many new, but immature RBCs (erythroblasts). The infant is born with **hemolytic disease of the newborn (HDN)** or **erythroblastosis fetalis.** HDN can occur in the first pregnancy if a mother has had an Rh$^+$ blood transfusion.

One of the clinical signs of HDN is **jaundice** (yellow skin pigmentation). Jaundice results from excessive destruction of RBCs. When RBCs break down (hemolysis), the hemoglobin within the cells produces **bilirubin** (a chemical pigment). High levels of bilirubin in the bloodstream (hyperbilirubinemia) cause jaundice. To prevent bilirubin from affecting the brain cells of the infant, newborns are treated with exposure to bright lights (phototherapy). The light decomposes the bilirubin, which is excreted from the infant's body.

Physicians administer Rh immune globulin to an Rh⁺ woman within 72 hours after each Rh⁺ delivery, abortion, or miscarriage. The globulin binds to Rh⁺ cells that escape into the mother's circulation and prevents formation of Rh⁺ antibodies. This protects future babies from developing HDN. Figure 4–3 reviews the Rh antigen-antibody reaction.

APPENDIX D: AUTOIMMUNE DISEASE

Part of the normal immune reaction (protecting the body against foreign invaders) involves making antibodies to fight against viruses and bacteria. In an **autoimmune** disease, however, the body makes antibodies against its own good cells and tissues, causing inflammation and injury. Examples of autoimmune disorders are rheumatoid arthritis, affecting joints; systemic lupus erythematosus (SLE), affecting connective tissues, skin, and internal organs; and Graves disease, causing hyperthyroidism.

APPENDIX E: CONGENITAL ANOMALY

An anomaly is an irregularity in a structure or organ. Examples of **congenital anomalies** (those that an infant is born with) include webbed fingers or toes (syndactyly) and heart defects. Some congenital anomalies are hereditary (passed to the infant through chromosomes from the father or mother, or both), whereas others are produced by factors present during pregnancy. For example, cocaine addiction in the pregnant mother produces addiction and subsequent brain damage in the infant at birth.

APPENDIX F: CONTRALATERAL

After a stroke involving the motor (movement) area of the brain, the **contralateral** side of the body often demonstrates a deficit. This means that if brain damage is on the right side of the brain, the patient will have paralysis on the left side of the body. Muscles on one side of the body are controlled by nerves on the opposite (contralateral) side of the brain. **Ipsilateral** (**ipsi-** means same) means the same side.

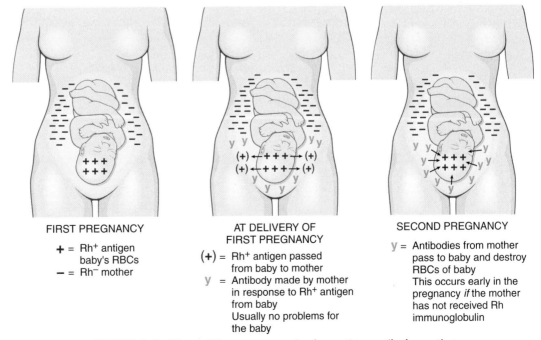

FIGURE 4–3 **Rh condition** as an example of an antigen-antibody reaction.

APPENDIX G: DIALYSIS

Dialysis literally means complete separation. In hemodialysis, waste materials from the blood are removed via a machine (artificial kidney) when the kidneys no longer function.

APPENDIX H: ECTOPIC PREGNANCY

In a normal pregnancy, the embryo develops within the uterus. In an **ectopic pregnancy**, the zygote (early stage embryo), develops outside the uterus—most often in a fallopian tube (Fig. 4–4).

APPENDIX I: PARATHYROID GLANDS

There are four **parathyroid glands** located on the dorsal side of the thyroid gland. They are endocrine glands that produce a hormone and function entirely separately from the thyroid gland. **Parathyroid hormone** increases blood calcium and maintains it at a normal level.

APPENDIX J: PROLAPSE

The suffix **-lapse** means to slide, sag, or fall. If an organ or tissue **prolapses**, it slides forward or downward. For example, if the muscles that hold the uterus in place become weak, the uterus may slide downward, or prolapse, toward the vagina (Fig. 4–5).

APPENDIX K: RECOMBINANT DNA

Recombinant DNA technology is the process of taking a gene (a region of DNA) from one organism and inserting it (recombining it) into the DNA of another organism. For example, recombinant techniques are used to manufacture insulin outside the body. The gene that

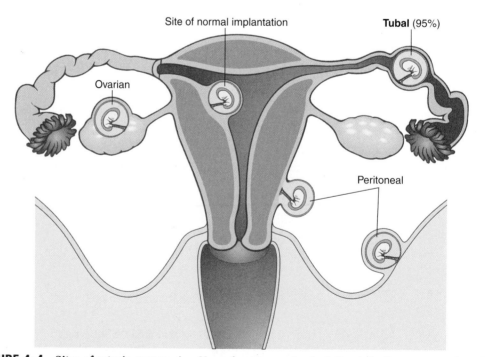

FIGURE 4–4 **Sites of ectopic pregnancies.** Normal pregnancy implantation is in the upper portion of the uterus. Ectopic pregnancy occurs most commonly in the fallopian tube (i.e., tubal pregnancy) and infrequently in the ovary or peritoneal (abdominal) cavity. (Modified from Damjanov I: Pathology for the Health-Related Professions, 3rd ed. Philadelphia, WB Saunders, 2006, p. 376.)

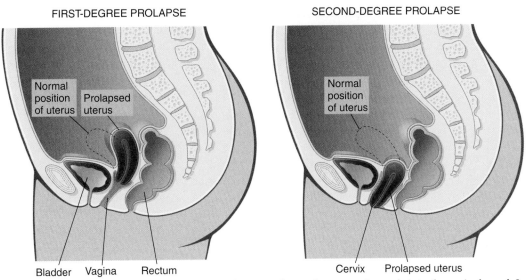

FIRST-DEGREE PROLAPSE   SECOND-DEGREE PROLAPSE

Normal position of uterus | Prolapsed uterus

Normal position of uterus

Bladder   Vagina   Rectum   Cervix   Prolapsed uterus

FIGURE 4–5 **Prolapse of the uterus.** In **first-degree** prolapse, the uterus descends into the vaginal canal. In **second-degree** prolapse, the body of the uterus is still within the vagina, but the cervix protrudes from the vaginal orifice (opening). In **third-degree** prolapse (not pictured), the entire uterus projects permanently outside the orifice. As treatment, the uterus may be held in position by a plastic pessary (oval supporting object) that is inserted into the vagina. Some affected women may require hysterectomy (removal of the uterus).

codes for insulin (i.e., contains the recipe for making insulin) is cut out of a human chromosome (using special enzymes) and transferred into a bacterium, such as *Escherichia coli.* The bacterium then contains the gene for making human insulin and, because it multiplies very rapidly, can produce insulin in large quantities. Diabetic patients, unable to make their own insulin, can use this synthetic product. Scientists also have developed the technique of **polymerase chain reaction (PCR),** a method of producing multiple copies of a single gene, which is an important tool in recombinant DNA technology.

APPENDIX L: SYNDROME

A **syndrome** (from the Greek *dromes,* meaning a course for running) is a group of signs or symptoms that appear together and present a clinical picture of a disease or inherited abnormality. For example, **Reye syndrome** is characterized by vomiting, swelling of the brain, increased intracranial pressure, hypoglycemia, and dysfunction of the liver. It may occur in children after a viral infection that has been treated with aspirin.

Fetal alcohol syndrome affects infants whose mothers consumed excessive amounts of alcohol during pregnancy. This syndrome is characterized by prenatal and postnatal growth deficiency, craniofacial anomalies such as microcephaly, and limb and heart defects.

Marfan syndrome is an inherited connective tissue disorder marked by a tall, thin body type with long, "spidery" fingers and toes (arachnodactyly), elongated head, and heart, blood vessel, and ophthalmic abnormalities. It is generally considered that President Abraham Lincoln had Marfan syndrome.

APPENDIX M: SYMBIOSIS

Symbiosis refers to two organisms living together in close association, either for mutual benefit or not. The bacteria that normally live in the digestive tract of humans live in symbiosis with the cells lining the intestine. **Parasitism,** another example of symbiosis, occurs when one organism benefits and the other does not.

In psychiatry, symbiosis is a relationship between two persons who are emotionally dependent on each other.

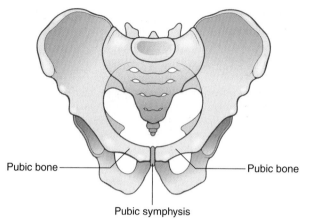

Pubic bone

Pubic bone

Pubic symphysis

FIGURE 4–6 Pubic symphysis.

APPENDIX N: SYMPHYSIS

A **symphysis** is a joint in which the bony surfaces are firmly united by a layer of fibrocartilage. The **pubic symphysis** is the area in which the pubic bones of the pelvis have grown together. The two halves of the lower jaw bone (mandible) unite before birth and form a symphysis. See Figure 4–6.

APPENDIX O: TRANSURETHRAL

In **transurethral** resection of the prostate gland (TURP), a portion of the prostate gland is removed with an instrument (resectoscope) passed through **(trans-)** the urethra. The procedure is indicated when prostatic tissue increases and interferes with urination. Figure 4–7 shows the location of the prostate gland at the base of the urinary bladder.

APPENDIX P: ULTRASONOGRAPHY

Ultrasonography is a diagnostic technique using ultrasound waves (inaudible sound waves) to produce an image or photograph of an organ or tissue. A machine records ultrasonic echoes as they pass through different types of tissue. **Echocardiograms** are ultrasound images of the heart. Figure 4–8 shows a fetal ultrasound image **(sonogram).**

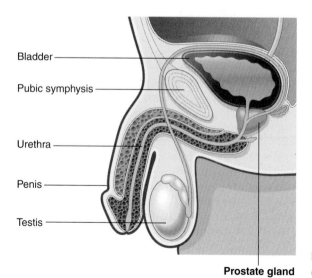

Bladder

Pubic symphysis

Urethra

Penis

Testis

Prostate gland

FIGURE 4–7 Location of the prostate gland *(side view).*

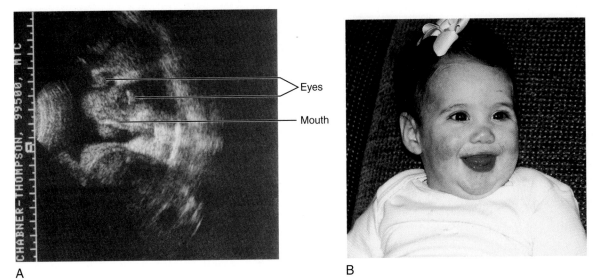

A   B

FIGURE 4–8 Ultrasonography. A, Notice the facial features of this beautiful 30-week-old fetus, in a (very) early "baby picture" of my granddaughter, Beatrix Bess Thompson! **B,** Bebe smiling at 3 months of age. (Courtesy of Dr. Elizabeth Chabner Thompson.)

PRACTICAL APPLICATIONS

Check your answers with the Answers to Practical Applications on page 130. You should find helpful explanations there.

PROCEDURES

Match the **procedure** or **treatment** in Column I with the best **reason for using it** in Column II. Write the letter of the answer in the space provided.

Column I		Column II
1. Ultrasonography	_____	A. Diagnose hepatopathy
2. Hemiglossectomy	_____	B. Treat renal failure
3. Percutaneous liver biopsy	_____	C. Obtain prenatal images
4. Transfusion of blood cells	_____	D. Determine the postmortem status of organs
5. Gastric endoscopy	_____	E. Treat carcinoma of the tongue
6. Autopsy	_____	F. Treat benign prostatic hypertrophy
7. Endotracheal intubation	_____	G. Diagnose disease in the stomach
8. Dialysis	_____	H. Establish an airway during surgery
9. Antibiotics	_____	I. Treat pancytopenia
10. Transurethral resection	_____	J. Treat staphylococcemia

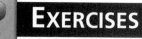

EXERCISES

4

Remember to check your answers carefully with those given in the Answers to Exercises, page 128.

A. Give the meanings of the following prefixes.

1. ante- _____

2. ab-_____

3. ana-_____

4. anti- _____

5. a-, an- _____

6. ad-_____

7. auto- _____

8. cata-_____

9. brady- _____

10. contra- _____

11. bi- _____

12. con- _____

B. Match the following terms with their meanings below.

adductor   anteflexion   bilateral
adrenal   antepartum   bradycardia
analysis   antisepsis   congenital anomaly
anoxia   apnea   contralateral

1. bending forward _____

2. muscle that carries the limb toward the body _____

3. before birth _____

4. slow heartbeat _____

5. gland located near (above) each kidney _____

6. not breathing_____

7. pertaining to the opposite side _____

8. against infection _____

9. to separate apart _____

10. pertaining to two (both) sides_____

11. condition of no oxygen in tissues_____

12. irregularity present at birth _____

C. Select from the following terms to match the descriptions below.

anabolism   antigen   catabolism
antibiotic   antitoxin   congenital anomaly
antibody   autoimmune disease   contraindication

1. chemical substance, such as erythromycin (-mycin = mold), made from molds and used against

   bacterial life _____

2. process of burning food (breaking it down) and releasing the energy stored in the food

   _____

3. reason that a doctor would advise against taking a specific medication _____

4. disorder in which the body's own leukocytes make antibodies that damage its own good tissue

   _____

5. a foreign agent (virus or bacterium) that causes production of antibodies_____

6. an antibody that acts against poisons that enter the body _____

7. process of building up proteins in cells by putting together small pieces of proteins, called amino

   acids _____

8. protein made by lymphocytes in response to the presence in the blood of a specific antigen is a (an)

   _____

D. Give the meanings of the following prefixes.

1. ec- _____   9. en- _____

2. dys- _____   10. eu- _____

3. de- _____   11. in- _____

4. dia- _____   12. inter- _____

5. hemi- _____   13. intra- _____

6. hypo- _____   14. infra- _____

7. epi- _____   15. macro- _____

8. hyper- _____

4

E. Complete the following terms, based on their meanings as given.

1. normal thyroid function: _____thyroid

2. painful breathing: _____pnea

3. pregnancy that is out of place (outside the uterus): _____topic

4. instrument to visually examine within the body: endo_____

5. removal of half of the tongue: _____glossectomy

6. good (exaggerated) feeling (of well-being): _____phoria

7. pertaining to within the windpipe: endo_____

8. blood condition of less than normal sugar: _____glycemia

9. condition (congenital anomaly) of large head: _____cephaly

10. pertaining to between the ribs: _____costal

11. pertaining to within a vein: intra_____

12. condition of bad (abnormal) formation (of cells): dys_____

13. condition of excessive formation (numbers of cells): _____plasia

14. structure (membrane) that forms the inner lining of the heart: endo_____

15. pertaining to below the ribs: infra_____

16. blood condition of excessive amount of sugar: hyper_____

F. Match the following terms with their meanings below.

dehydration   incision   metamorphosis
dialysis   insomnia   metastasis
diarrhea   malaise   microscope
exophthalmos   malignant   pancytopenia

1. vague feeling of bodily discomfort _____

2. inability to sleep _____

3. lack of water_____

4. spread of a cancerous tumor to a secondary organ or tissue _____

5. instrument used to see small objects_____

6. to cut into an organ or tissue_____

7. outward bulging of the eyeballs (proptosis)_____

8. condition of change in shape or form _____

9. watery discharge of wastes from the colon _____

10. deficiency of all (blood) cells _____

11. separation of wastes from the blood by using a machine that does the job of the kidney

_____

12. harmful, cancerous _____

G. Give the meanings of the following prefixes.

1. mal- _____	11. sub- _____
2. pan- _____	12. supra- _____
3. per- _____	13. re- _____
4. meta- _____	14. retro- _____
5. para- _____	15. tachy- _____
6. peri- _____	16. syn- _____
7. poly- _____	17. uni- _____
8. post- _____	18. trans- _____
9. pro- _____	19. neo- _____
10. pre- _____	20. epi- _____

H. Underline the prefix in the following terms, and give the meaning of the entire term.

1. periosteum _____

2. percutaneous _____

3. retroperitoneal _____

4. suprapubic _____

5. polyneuritis _____

6. retroflexion _____

7. transurethral _____

8. subcutaneous _____

9. tachypnea _____

10. unilateral _____

11. pseudocyesis _____

I. Match the following terms with their meanings below.

adrenal	parathyroid	recombinant DNA	syndactyly
neoplasm	prodrome	relapse	syndrome
paralysis	prolapse	remission	ultrasonography

1. return of a disease or its symptoms _____

2. loss of movement in muscles _____

3. congenital anomaly in which fingers or toes are webbed (formed together)_____

4. four endocrine glands that are located near (behind) another endocrine gland in the neck

   _____

5. glands that are located above the kidneys _____

6. symptoms that come before the actual illness_____

7. technique of transferring genetic material from one organism into another _____

8. sliding, sagging downward or forward _____

9. new growth or tumor _____

10. process of using sound waves to create an image of organs and structures in the body

    _____

11. group of symptoms that occur together and indicate a particular disorder _____

12. symptoms lessen and a patient feels better _____

J. Complete the following terms, based on their meanings as given.

1. pertaining to new birth: neo_____

2. after death: post_____

3. spread of a cancerous tumor: meta_____

4. branching into two: bi_____

5. increase in development (size of cells): hyper_____

6. pertaining to a chemical that works against bacterial life: _____biotic

7. hand bones (beyond the wrist): _____carpals

8. protein produced by leukocytes to fight foreign organisms: anti_____

9. group of symptoms that occur together: _____drome

10. surface or skin tissue of the body: _____thelium

K. Circle the correct term to complete the following sentences.

1. Dr. Tate felt that Mrs. Snow's condition of thrombocytopenia was a clear **(analysis, contraindication, synthesis)** to performing elective surgery.

2. Medical science was revolutionized by the introduction of **(antigens, antibiotics, antibodies)** in the 1940s. Now some infections can be treated with only one dose.

3. Robert's 82-year-old grandfather complained of **(malaise, dialysis, insomnia)** despite taking the sleeping medication that his doctor prescribed.

4. During her pregnancy, Ms. Payne described pressure on her **(pituitary gland, parathyroid gland, pubic symphysis),** making it difficult for her to find a comfortable position, even when seated.

5. Many times, people with diabetes accidentally take too much insulin. This results in lowering their blood sugar so much that they may be admitted to the emergency department with **(hyperplasia, hypoglycemia, hyperglycemia).**

6. Before his migraine headaches began, John noticed changes in his eyesight, such as bright spots, zigzag lines, and double vision. His physician told him that these were **(symbiotic, exophthalmal, prodromal)** symptoms.

7. After hiking in the Grand Canyon without an adequate water supply, Julie experienced **(hyperglycemia, dehydration, hypothyroidism).**

8. At 65 years of age, Paul Smith often felt fullness in his urinary bladder but had difficulty urinating. He visited his **(cardiologist, nephrologist, urologist),** who examined his prostate gland and diagnosed **(hypertrophy, atrophy, ischemia).** The doctor advised **(intracostal, transurethral, peritoneal)** resection of Paul's prostate.

9. After running the Boston Marathon, Elizabeth felt nauseated and dizzy. She realized that she was experiencing **(malaise, euphoria, hypoglycemia)** and drank a sports drink containing sugar, which made her feel better.

10. While she was taking an antibiotic that reacted with sunlight, Ruth's physician advised her that sunbathing was **(unilateral, contraindicated, contralateral)** and might cause a serious sunburn.

MEDICAL SCRAMBLE

Unscramble the letters to form a medical term from the clues. Use the letters in squares to complete the bonus term. Answers are found on page 130.

4

1. *Clue:* Bodily discomfort

   ☐ __ __ __ __ ☐ __   I S A M E L A

2. *Clue:* Well-being

   ☐ __ __ __ ☐ __ __ __   R H U A E P O I

3. *Clue:* Difficult breathing

   ☐ ☐ __ __ ☐ __ __   N A Y D E P S

4. *Clue:* Loss of movement

   __ __ ☐ __ __ __ ☐ __ __   Y S A L S A I P R

BONUS TERM: *Clue:* Examples are carpal tunnel, Down, Reye, and toxic shock.

   ☐ ☐ ☐ ☐ ☐ ☐ ☐ ☐ ☐

ANSWERS TO EXERCISES

A

1. before, forward
2. away from
3. up, apart
4. against

5. no, not, without
6. toward
7. self, own
8. down

9. slow
10. against, opposite
11. two
12. together, with

B

1. anteflexion
2. adductor
3. antepartum
4. bradycardia

5. adrenal
6. apnea
7. contralateral
8. antisepsis

9. analysis
10. bilateral
11. anoxia
12. congenital anomaly

C

1. antibiotic
2. catabolism
3. contraindication

4. autoimmune disease
5. antigen
6. antitoxin

7. anabolism
8. antibody

D

1. out, outside
2. bad, painful, difficult
3. down, lack of
4. through, complete
5. half
6. deficient, under
7. upon, on, above
8. excessive, above, beyond
9. in, within
10. good, well
11. in, not
12. between
13. within
14. below, inferior
15. large

E

1. euthyroid
2. dyspnea
3. ectopic
4. endoscope
5. hemiglossectomy
6. —
7. endotracheal
8. hypoglycemia
9. macrocephaly
10. intercostals
11. intravenous
12. dysplasia
13. hyperplasia
14. endocardium
15. infracostal
16. hyperglycemia

F

1. malaise
2. insomnia
3. dehydration
4. metastasis
5. microscope
6. incision
7. exophthalmos (proptosis)
8. metamorphosis
9. diarrhea
10. pancytopenia
11. dialysis
12. malignant

G

1. bad
2. all
3. through
4. change, beyond
5. near, beside, abnormal
6. surrounding
7. many, much
8. after, behind
9. before, forward
10. before, in front of
11. under
12. above
13. back, again
14. behind, backward
15. fast
16. together, with
17. one
18. across, through
19. new
20. above, upon, on

H

1. periosteum—membrane (structure) surrounding bone
2. percutaneous—pertaining to through the skin
3. retroperitoneal—pertaining to behind the peritoneum
4. suprapubic—above the pubic bone
5. polyneuritis—inflammation of many nerves
6. retroflexion—bending backward
7. transurethral—pertaining to through the urethra
8. subcutaneous—pertaining to below the skin
9. tachypnea—rapid, fast breathing
10. unilateral—pertaining to one side
11. pseudocyesis—false pregnancy (no pregnancy actually exists)

I

1. relapse
2. paralysis
3. syndactyly
4. parathyroid
5. adrenal
6. prodrome
7. recombinant DNA
8. prolapse
9. neoplasm
10. ultrasonography
11. syndrome
12. remission

J

1. neonatal
2. postmortem
3. metastasis
4. bifurcation
5. hypertrophy
6. antibiotic
7. metacarpals
8. antibody
9. syndrome
10. epithelium

K

1. contraindication
2. antibiotics
3. insomnia
4. pubic symphysis
5. hypoglycemia
6. prodromal
7. dehydration
8. urologist; hypertrophy; transurethral
9. hypoglycemia
10. contraindicated

ANSWERS TO PRACTICAL APPLICATIONS

1. **C** Ultrasonography is especially useful to detect fetal structures because no x-rays are used.
2. **E** Malignancies of the oral (mouth) cavity often are treated with surgery to remove the cancerous growth.
3. **A** Diseases such as hepatitis or hepatoma are diagnosed by performing a liver biopsy.
4. **I** Transfusion of leukocytes, erythrocytes, and platelets will increase numbers of these cells in the bloodstream.
5. **G** Placement of an endoscope through the mouth and esophagus and into the stomach is used to diagnose gastric (stomach) disease.
6. **D** A veterinarian performs a postmortem examination of an animal, which is called a necropsy.
7. **H** Endotracheal intubation is necessary during surgery in which general anesthesia is used.
8. **B** Patients experiencing loss of kidney function need dialysis to remove waste materials from the blood.
9. **J** Examples of antibiotics are penicillin, erythromycin, and amoxicillin.
10. **F** A TURP is a transurethral resection of the prostate gland.

ANSWERS TO MEDICAL SCRAMBLE

1. MALAISE   2. EUPHORIA   3. DYSPNEA   4. PARALYSIS
BONUS TERM: SYNDROMES

PRONUNCIATION OF TERMS

PRONUNCIATION GUIDE

ā as in āpe	ă as in ăpple
ē as in ēven	ĕ as in ĕvery
ī as in īce	ĭ as in ĭnterest
ō as in ōpen	ŏ as in pŏt
ū as in ūnit	ŭ as in ŭnder

To test your understanding of the terminology in this chapter, write the meaning of each term in the space provided. In addition, you may wish to cover the terms and write them by looking at your definitions. Make sure your spelling is correct. The page number after each term indicates where it is defined or used in the text so you can easily check your responses. You will find complete definitions for all of these terms and their audio pronunciations on the CD.

Term	Pronunciation	Meaning
abductor (109)	ăb-DŬK-tŏr	_____
adductor (109)	ă-DŬK-tŏr	_____
adrenal glands (109)	ă-DRĒ-năl glăndz	_____
anabolism (110)	ă-NĂ-bō-lĭzm	_____
analysis (110)	ă-NĂL-ĭ-sĭs	_____
anoxia (109)	ă-NŎK-sē-ă	_____
ante cibum (110)	ĂN-tē SĒ-bŭm	_____
anteflexion (110)	ăn-tē-FLĔK-shŭn	_____
antepartum (110)	ăn-tē-PĂR-tŭm	_____
antibiotic (110)	ăn-tĭ-bī-ŎT-ĭk	_____
antibody (110)	ĂN-tĭ-bŏd-ē	_____
antigen (110)	ĂN-tĭ-jĕn	_____
antisepsis (110)	ăn-tĭ-SĔP-sĭs	_____
antitoxin (110)	ăn-tĭ-TŎK-sĭn	_____
apnea (109)	ĂP-nē-ă *or* ăp-NĒ-ă	_____
autoimmune disease (110)	ăw-tō-ĭ-MŪN dĭ-ZĒZ	_____
benign (112)	bē-NĪN	_____

Term	Pronunciation	Meaning
bifurcation (110)	bī-fŭr-KĀ-shŭn	_____
bilateral (110)	bī-LĂT-ĕr-ăl	_____
bradycardia (110)	brăd-ē-KĂR-dē-ă	_____
congenital anomaly (110)	kŏn-JĔN-ĭ-tăl ă-NŎM-ă-lē	_____
connective tissue (110)	kŏn-NĔK-tĭv TĬ-shū	_____
contraindication (111)	kŏn-tră-ĭn-dĭ-KĀ-shŭn	_____
contralateral (111)	kŏn-tră-LĂT-ĕr-ăl	_____
dehydration (111)	dē-hī-DRĀ-shŭn	_____
dialysis (111)	dī-ĂL-ĭ-sĭs	_____
diameter (111)	dī-ĂM-ĭ-tĕr	_____
diarrhea (111)	dī-ă-RĒ-ă	_____
dysplasia (111)	dĭs-PLĀ-zē-ă	_____
dyspnea (111)	DĬSP-nē-ă _or_ dĭsp-NĒ-ă	_____
ectopic pregnancy (111)	ĕk-TŎP-ĭk PRĔG-năn-sē	_____
endocardium (111)	ĕn-dō-KĂR-dē-ŭm	_____
endoscope (111)	ĔN-dō-skōp	_____
endotracheal (111)	ĕn-dō-TRĀ-kē-ăl	_____
epithelium (111)	ĕp-ĭ-THĒ-lē-ŭm	_____
euphoria (111)	ū-FŎR-ē-ă	_____
euthyroid (111)	ū-THĪ-royd	_____
exophthalmos (111)	ĕk-sŏf-THĂL-mŏs	_____
hemiglossectomy (111)	hĕm-ē-glŏs-SĔK-tō-mē	_____
hyperglycemia (112)	hī-pĕr-glī-SĒ-mē-ă	_____
hyperplasia (112)	hī-pĕr-PLĀ-zē-ă	_____
hypertrophy (112)	hī-PĔR-trō-fē	_____
hypodermic injection (112)	hī-pō-DĔR-mĭk ĭn-JĔK-shŭn	_____
hypoglycemia (112)	hī-pō-glī-SĒ-mē-ă	_____
infracostal (112)	ĭn-fră-KŎS-tăl	_____
insomniac (112)	ĭn-SŎM-nē-ăk	_____
intercostal (112)	ĭn-tĕr-KŎS-tăl	_____
intravenous (112)	ĭn-tră-VĒ-nŭs	_____
macrocephaly (112)	măk-rō-SĔF-ă-lē	_____
malaise (112)	măl-ĀZ	_____
malignant (112)	mă-LĬG-nănt	_____
metacarpal bones (112)	mĕ-tă-KĂR-păl bōnz	_____

Term	Pronunciation	Meaning
metamorphosis (112)	mĕt-ă-MŎR-fŏ-sĭs	
metastasis (112)	mĕ-TĂS-tă-sĭs	
microscope (113)	MĪ-krō-skōp	
neonatal (113)	nē-ō-NĀ-tăl	
neoplasm (113)	NĒ-ō-plăzm	
pancytopenia (113)	păn-sī-tō-PĒ-nē-ă	
paralysis (113)	pă-RĂL-ĭ-sĭs	
parathyroid glands (113)	păr-ă-THĪ-royd glănz	
percutaneous (113)	pĕr-kū-TĀ-nē-ŭs	
periosteum (113)	pĕr-ē-ŎS-tē-ŭm	
polymorphonuclear (113)	pŏl-ĕ-mŏr-fō-NŪ-klē-ăr	
polyneuritis (113)	pŏl-ē-nū-RĪ-tĭs	
postmortem (113)	pōst-MŎR-tĕm	
postpartum (113)	pōst-PĂR-tŭm	
precancerous (113)	prē-KĂN-sĕr-ŭs	
prenatal (113)	prē-NĀ-tăl	
prodrome (113)	PRŌ-drōm	
prolapse (113)	PRŌ-lăps	
pseudocyesis (113)	sū-dō-sī-Ē-sĭs	
recombinant DNA (114)	rē-KŎM-bĭ-nănt DNA	
relapse (114)	RĒ-lăps	
remission (114)	rē-MĬ-shŭn	
retroflexion (114)	rĕt-rō-FLĔK-shŭn	
retroperitoneal (114)	rĕt-rō-pĕr-ĭ-tō-NĒ-ăl	
subcutaneous (114)	sŭb-kū-TĀ-nē-ŭs	
suprapubic (114)	sū-pră-PŪ-bĭk	
symbiosis (114)	sĭm-bē-Ō-sĭs	
symmetry (114)	SĬM-mĕ-trē	
symphysis (114)	SĬM-fĭ-sĭs	
syndactyly (114)	sĭn-DĂK-tĭ-lē	
syndrome (114)	SĬN-drōm	
synthesis (114)	SĬN-thĕ-sĭs	
tachypnea (114)	tă-KĬP-nē-ă *or* tăk-ĭp-NĒ-ă	
transfusion (115)	trăns-FŪ-zhŭn	
transurethral (115)	trăns-ū-RĒ-thrăl	
ultrasonography (115)	ŭl-tră-sŏ-NŎG-ră-fē	
unilateral (115)	ū-nē-LĂT-ĕr-ăl	

REVIEW SHEET

Write the meanings of each word part in the space provided and test yourself. Check your answers with the information in the chapter or in the Glossary (Medical Word Parts—English) at the end of the book.

4

PREFIXES

Prefix	Meaning	Prefix	Meaning
a-, an-	_____	hypo-	_____
ab-	_____	in-	_____
ad-	_____	infra-	_____
ana-	_____	inter-	_____
ante-	_____	intra-	_____
anti-	_____	macro-	_____
auto-	_____	mal-	_____
bi-	_____	meta-	_____
brady-	_____	micro-	_____
cata-	_____	neo-	_____
con-	_____	pan-	_____
contra-	_____	para-	_____
de-	_____	per-	_____
dia-	_____	peri-	_____
dys-	_____	poly-	_____
ec-, ecto-	_____	post-	_____
en-, endo-	_____	supra-	_____
epi-	_____	syn-, sym-	_____
eu-	_____	tachy-	_____
ex-	_____	trans-	_____
hemi-	_____	ultra-	_____
hyper-	_____	uni-	_____

COMBINING FORMS

Combining Form	Meaning	Combining Form	Meaning
carp/o	_____	nect/o	_____
cib/o	_____	norm/o	_____
cost/o	_____	ophthalm/o	_____
cutane/o	_____	ox/o	_____
dactyl/o	_____	pub/o	_____
duct/o	_____	ren/o	_____
flex/o	_____	seps/o	_____
furc/o	_____	somn/o	_____
gloss/o	_____	son/o	_____
glyc/o	_____	the/o	_____
immun/o	_____	thyr/o	_____
later/o	_____	top/o	_____
morph/o	_____	tox/o	_____
mort/o	_____	trache/o	_____
nat/i	_____	urethr/o	_____
necr/o	_____	ven/o	_____

SUFFIXES

Combining Form	Meaning	Combining Form	Meaning
-blast	_____	-partum	_____
-crine	_____	-phoria	_____
-cyesis	_____	-physis	_____
-drome	_____	-plasia	_____
-fusion	_____	-plasm	_____
-gen	_____	-pnea	_____
-lapse	_____	-ptosis	_____
-lysis	_____	-rrhea	_____
-mission	_____	-stasis	_____
-or	_____	-trophy	_____
-meter	_____		

PREFIXES WITH SIMILAR MEANINGS

Prefix	Meaning	Prefix	Meaning
a- (an-), in-	_____	ec- (ecto-), ex-	_____
ante-, pre-, pro-	_____	en- (endo-), -in-, intra	_____
anti-, contra-	_____	epi-, hyper-, supra-	_____
con-, syn- (sym-)	_____	hypo-, infra-, sub-	_____
de-, cata-	_____	re-, retro-, post-	_____
dia-, per-, trans-	_____	ultra-, meta-	_____
dys-, mal-	_____		

 Please refer to the enclosed CD for additional exercises and images related to this chapter.

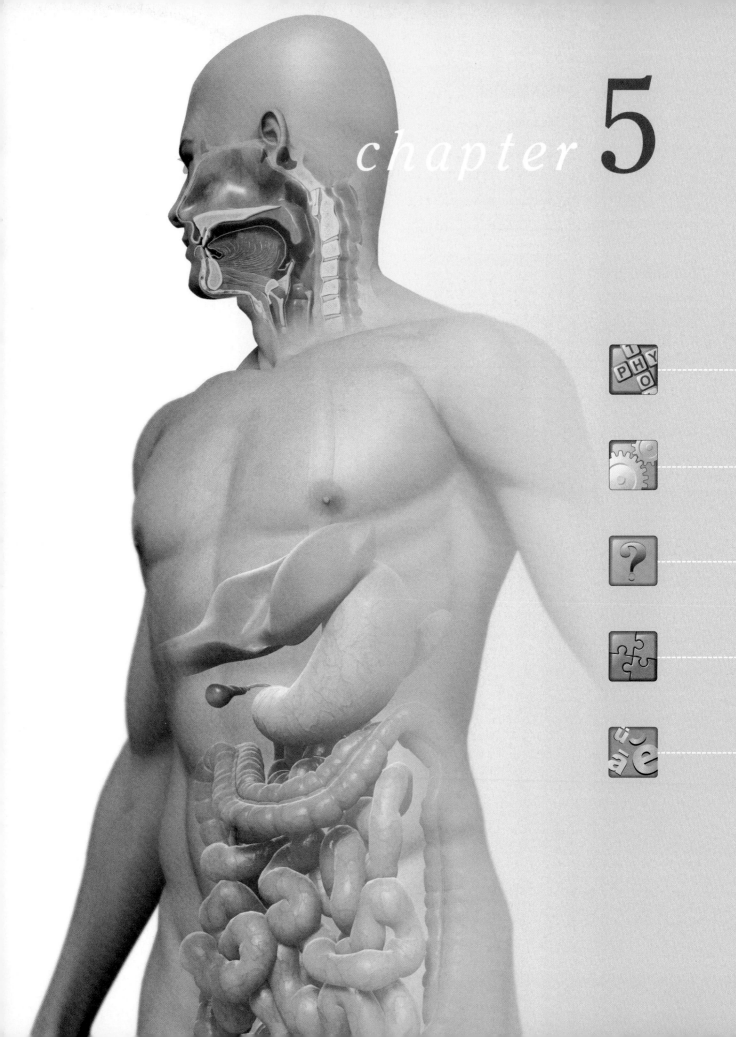

chapter 5

Digestive System

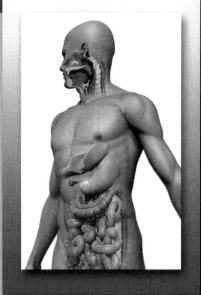

In this chapter you will

- Name the organs of the digestive system and describe their locations and functions.
- Describe disease processes and symptoms that affect these organs.
- Define combining forms for organs and the meaning of related terminology using these word parts.

Students and teachers ask why I begin study of body system terminology with the digestive system, rather than with the more traditional musculoskeletal system. After many years of teaching, both my students and I found it easier to start with the digestive system because it was more familiar. Also, the anatomy and physiology of the system was easier to explain and understand. The gastrointestinal tract resembles a long conveyor belt, with the mouth at the entrance and the anus at the exit.

Remember, however, that the text is organized so that you may begin study of the body systems with any chapter and create the order that best reflects your interests.

Image Description: The digestive tract within a male torso.

INTRODUCTION

The digestive or **gastrointestinal** tract begins with the mouth, where food enters, and ends with the anus, where solid waste material leaves the body. The three functions of the system are **digestion, absorption,** and **elimination.**

First, complex food material taken into the mouth is **digested,** or broken down, mechanically and chemically, as it travels through the gastrointestinal tract. Digestive **enzymes** speed up chemical reactions and aid the breakdown (digestion) of complex nutrients. Complex proteins are digested to simpler **amino acids**; complicated sugars are reduced to simple sugars, such as **glucose**; and large fat or lipid molecules **(triglycerides)** are broken down to **fatty acids** and glycerol.

Second, via **absorption** digested food passes into the bloodstream through the walls of the small intestine. Thus, valuable nutrients (sugar, fatty acids, and amino acids) travel to all cells of the body. Cells then catabolize (burn) nutrients in the presence of oxygen to release energy stored within the food. Cells also use amino acid nutrients to anabolize (build) large protein molecules needed for growth and development. Although the walls of the small intestine also absorb fatty acids and glycerol, these nutrients enter lymphatic vessels rather than blood vessels. Digested fats eventually enter the bloodstream as lymph vessels join with blood vessels in the upper chest region.

The third function of the digestive system is **elimination** of the solid waste materials that cannot be absorbed into the bloodstream. The large intestine concentrates these solid wastes, called **feces,** and the wastes finally pass out of the body through the anus.

ANATOMY AND PHYSIOLOGY

ORAL CAVITY

The gastrointestinal tract begins with the oral cavity. Oral means pertaining to the mouth (or/o). Label Figure 5–1 as you learn the major parts of the oral cavity.

The **cheeks** [1] form the walls of the oval-shaped oral cavity, and the **lips** [2] surround the opening to the cavity.

The **hard palate** [3] forms the anterior portion of the roof of the mouth, and the muscular **soft palate** [4] lies posterior to it. **Rugae** are irregular ridges in the mucous membrane covering the anterior portion of the hard palate. The **uvula** [5], a small soft tissue projection, hangs from the soft palate. It aids production of sounds and speech.

The **tongue** [6] extends across the floor of the oral cavity, and muscles attach it to the lower jaw bone. It moves food around during **mastication** (chewing) and **deglutition** (swallowing). **Papillae,** small raised areas on the tongue, contain taste buds that are sensitive to the chemical nature of foods and allow discrimination of different tastes as food moves across the tongue.

Absorption/Adsorption
Absorption means passing into tissues, while *adsorption* means adhering to the surface of tissues.

COMBINING FORMS
1. bucc/o
2. cheil/o, labi/o
3. palat/o
4. palat/o
5. uvul/o
6. gloss/o, lingu/o
7. tonsill/o
8. gingiv/o
9. dent/i, odont/o

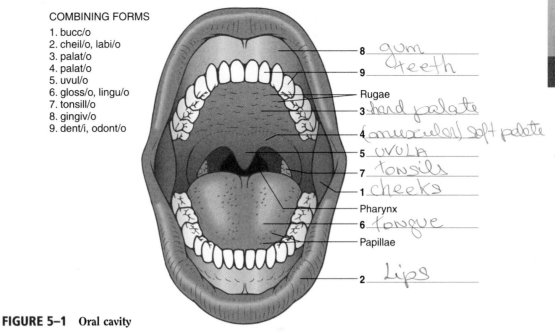

8 _gum_
9 _teeth_
— Rugae
3 _hard palate_
4 _(muscular) soft palate_
5 _UVULA_
7 _tonsils_
1 _cheeks_
— Pharynx
6 _tongue_
— Papillae
2 _Lips_

FIGURE 5–1 Oral cavity

The **tonsils** [7], masses of lymphatic tissue located in depressions of the mucous membranes, lie on both sides of the oropharynx (part of the throat near the mouth). They are filters to protect the body from the invasion of microorganisms and they produce lymphocytes, disease-fighting white blood cells.

The **gums** [8] are the fleshy tissue surrounding the sockets of the **teeth** [9]. Figure 5–2 shows a dental arch with 16 permanent teeth (there are 32 permanent teeth in the entire oral cavity). Label the figure with the following names of teeth:

Central **incisor** [1]   Second **premolar** [5]
Lateral **incisor** [2]   First **molar** [6]
Canine [3]   Second **molar** [7]
First **premolar** [4]   Third **molar** (wisdom tooth) [8]

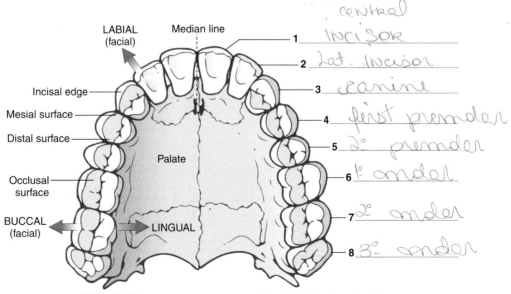

LABIAL (facial)   Median line

Incisal edge —
Mesial surface —
Distal surface —

Palate

Occlusal surface —

BUCCAL (facial)   LINGUAL

1 _central incisor_
2 _lat. incisor_
3 _canine_
4 _first premolar_
5 _2° premolar_
6 _1° molar_
7 _2° molar_
8 _3° molar_

FIGURE 5–2 Upper permanent teeth within the dental arch.

Dentists use special terms to describe the surfaces of teeth (see Fig. 5–2). The **labial** surface (labi/o means lip), for incisor and canine teeth, is nearest the lips. The **buccal** surface (bucc/o means cheek), for premolar and molar teeth, lies adjacent to the cheek, as illustrated in Figure 5–2. Dentists refer to both the labial and the buccal surfaces of a tooth as the **facial** surface (faci/o means face). On the side of the tooth directly opposite the facial surface is the **lingual** surface (lingu/o means tongue). The **mesial** surface of a tooth lies nearer to the median line, and the **distal** surface lies farther from the medial line. Premolars and molars have an additional **occlusal** surface (occlusion means to close) that comes in contact with a corresponding tooth in the opposing arch (i.e., "matching" top and bottom teeth). The incisors and canines have a sharp **incisal** edge.

Figure 5–3 shows the inner anatomy of a tooth. Label it as you read the following description:

A tooth consists of a **crown** [1], which shows above the gum line, and a **root** [2], which lies within the bony tooth socket. The outermost protective layer of the crown, the **enamel** [3], protects the tooth. Enamel is a dense, hard, white substance—the hardest substance in the body. **Dentin** [4], the main substance of the tooth, lies beneath the enamel and extends throughout the crown. Yellow in color, dentin is composed of bony tissue that is softer than enamel. The **cementum** covers, protects, and supports the dentin in the root. A **periodontal membrane** surrounds the cementum and holds the tooth in place in the tooth socket.

The **pulp** [5] lies underneath the dentin. This soft and delicate tissue fills the center of the tooth. Blood vessels, nerve endings, connective tissue, and lymphatic vessels are within the pulp canal (also called the **root canal**). Root canal therapy often is necessary when disease or abscess (pus collection) occurs in the pulp canal. A dentist opens the tooth from above and cleans the canal of infected tissue, nerves, and blood vessels. The canal is then disinfected and filled with material to prevent the entrance of microorganisms that could cause decay.

Three pairs of **salivary glands** (Fig. 5–4) surround the oral cavity. These exocrine glands produce **saliva,** which contains important digestive **enzymes** as well as healing

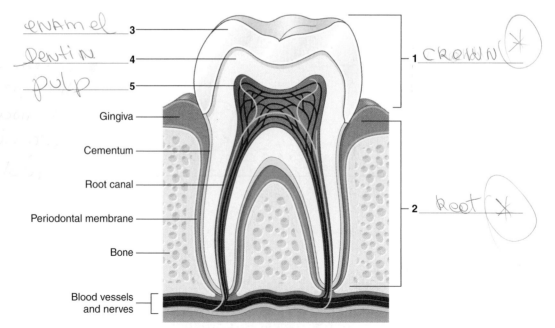

FIGURE 5–3 Anatomy of a tooth.

to know

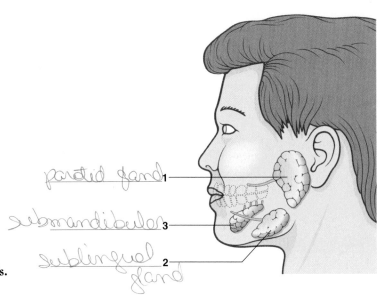

parotid gland 1

submandibular 3

sublingual 2
gland

FIGURE 5–4   Salivary glands.

growth factors such as cytokines and proteins. Saliva is released from the **parotid gland** [1], **submandibular gland** [2], and **sublingual gland** [3] on both sides of the mouth. Narrow ducts carry saliva into the oral cavity. The glands produce about 1.5 liters daily

PHARYNX

Refer to Figure 5–5. The **pharynx** or **throat** is a muscular tube, about 5 inches long, lined with a mucous membrane. It serves as a passageway both for air traveling from the nose (nasal cavity) to the windpipe (trachea) and for food traveling from the oral cavity to the **esophagus.** When swallowing **(deglutition)** occurs, a flap of tissue, the epiglottis, covers the trachea so that food cannot enter and become lodged there. See Figure 5–5, *A* and *B*.

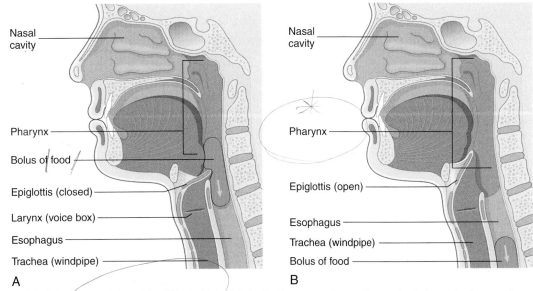

Nasal cavity

Pharynx

Bolus of food

Epiglottis (closed)

Larynx (voice box)

Esophagus

Trachea (windpipe)

A

Nasal cavity

Pharynx

Epiglottis (open)

Esophagus

Trachea (windpipe)

Bolus of food

B

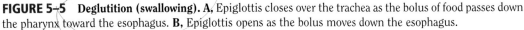

FIGURE 5–5   **Deglutition (swallowing). A,** Epiglottis closes over the trachea as the bolus of food passes down the pharynx toward the esophagus. **B,** Epiglottis opens as the bolus moves down the esophagus.

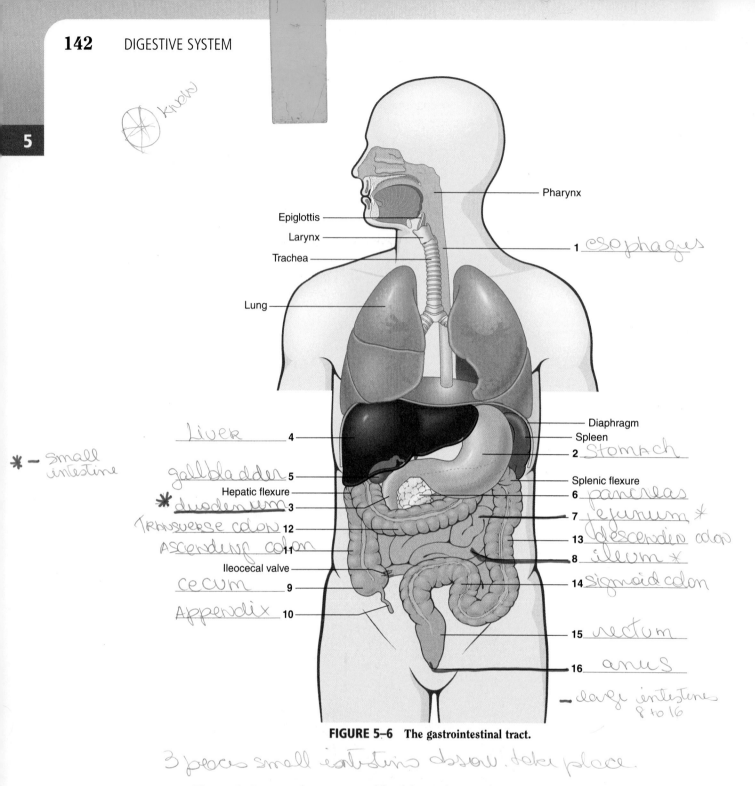

know

Pharynx

Epiglottis

Larynx

Trachea

Lung

Diaphragm
Spleen

Splenic flexure

Liver — 4
small intestine

gallbladder — 5
Hepatic flexure
* duodenum — 3
Transverse colon — 12
Ascending colon — 11
Ileocecal valve
cecum — 9
Appendix — 10

1 esophagus
2 Stomach
6 pancreas
7 jejunum *
13 descending colon
8 ileum *
14 sigmoid colon
15 rectum
16 anus
— large intestine 8 to 16

FIGURE 5–6 The gastrointestinal tract.

3 places small intestine absorb. take place.

Figure 5–6 traces the passage of food from the esophagus through the gastrointestinal tract. Label it as you read the following paragraphs.

ESOPHAGUS

The **esophagus** [1] is a 9- to 10-inch muscular tube extending from the pharynx to the stomach. **Peristalsis** is the involuntary, progressive, rhythmic contraction of muscles in the wall of the esophagus (and other gastrointestinal organs) propelling a **bolus** (mass of food) toward the stomach. The process is like squeezing a marble through a rubber tube.

STOMACH

Food passes from the esophagus into the **stomach** [2]. The stomach (Fig. 5–7) has three main parts: **fundus** (upper portion), **body** (middle section), and **antrum** (lower portion). Rings of muscle called **sphincters** control the openings into and leading out of the stomach. The **lower esophageal sphincter (cardiac sphincter)** relaxes and contracts to move food from the esophagus into the stomach; the **pyloric sphincter** allows food to leave the stomach when it is ready. Folds in the mucous membrane **(mucosa)** lining the stomach are called **rugae.** The rugae contain digestive glands that produce the enzyme **pepsin** (to begin digestion of proteins) and **hydrochloric acid.**

The stomach prepares food for the small intestine, where digestion and absorption into the bloodstream take place. The stomach controls passage of foods into the first part of the small intestine so that it proceeds only when it is chemically ready and in small amounts. Food leaves the stomach in 1 to 4 hours or longer, depending on the amount and type of food eaten.

SMALL INTESTINE (SMALL BOWEL)

(Continue labeling Fig. 5–6 on page 142.)

The **small intestine (small bowel)** extends for 20 feet from the pyloric sphincter to the first part of the large intestine. It has three parts. The first section, the **duodenum** [3], is only 1 foot long. It receives food from the stomach as well as **bile** from the **liver** [4] and **gallbladder** [5] and pancreatic juice from the **pancreas** [6]. Enzymes and bile help digest food before it passes into the second part of the small intestine, the **jejunum** [7], about 8 feet long. The jejunum connects with the third section, the **ileum** [8], about 11 feet long. The ileum attaches to the first part of the large intestine.

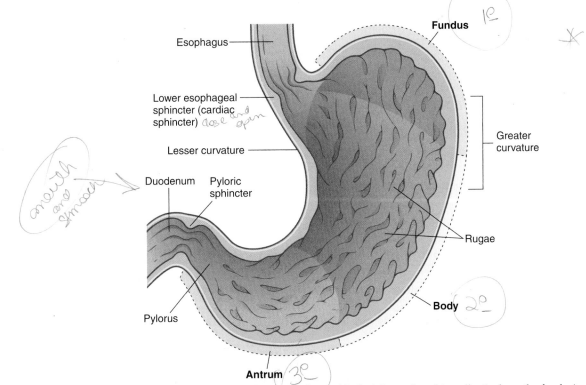

FIGURE 5–7 **Parts of the stomach.** The **fundus** and **body** (often referred to collectively as the fundus) are a reservoir for ingested food and an area for action by acid and pepsin (gastric enzyme). The **antrum** is a muscular grinding chamber that pulverizes food and feeds it gradually into the duodenum.

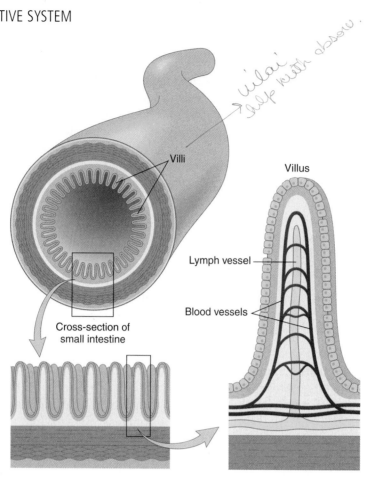

Villi

Villus

Lymph vessel

Blood vessels

Cross-section of
small intestine

FIGURE 5–8 Villi in the lining
of the small intestine.

Millions of tiny, microscopic projections called **villi** line the walls of the small intestine. The tiny capillaries (microscopic blood vessels) in the villi absorb the digested nutrients into the bloodstream and lymph vessels. Figure 5–8 shows several different views of villi in the lining of the small intestine.

LARGE INTESTINE (LARGE BOWEL)

(Continue labeling Fig. 5–6 on page 142.)

The **large intestine** extends from the end of the ileum to the anus. It has three main components: the cecum, the colon, and the rectum. The **cecum** [9] is a pouch on the right side that connects to the ileum at the ileocecal valve (sphincter). The **appendix** [10] hangs from the cecum. The appendix has no clear function and can become inflamed and infected when clogged or blocked. The **colon**, about 5 feet long, has four named segments: ascending, descending, transverse, and sigmoid. The **ascending colon** [11] extends from the cecum to the undersurface of the liver, where it turns to the left (hepatic flexure) to become the **transverse colon** [12]. The transverse colon passes horizontally to the left toward the spleen and then turns downward (splenic flexure) into the **descending colon** [13]. The **sigmoid colon** [14], shaped like an S (sigmoid means resembling the Greek letter sigma, which curves like the letter S), begins at the distal end of the descending colon and leads into the **rectum** [15]. The rectum terminates in the lower opening of the gastrointestinal tract, the **anus** [16].

The large intestine receives the fluid waste products of digestion (the material unable to pass into the bloodstream) and stores these wastes until they can be released from the body. Because the large intestine absorbs most of the water within the waste material, the body can expel solid **feces** (stools). **Defecation** is the expulsion or passage of feces from the body through the anus. Diarrhea, or passage of watery stools, results from reduced water absorption into the bloodstream through the walls of the large intestine.

LIVER, GALLBLADDER, AND PANCREAS

Three important additional organs of the digestive system—the liver, gallbladder, and pancreas—play crucial roles in the proper digestion and absorption of nutrients. Label Figure 5–9 as you study the following:

The **liver** [1], located in the right upper quadrant (RUQ) of the abdomen, manufactures a thick, orange-black, sometimes greenish, fluid called **bile.** Bile contains cholesterol (a fatty substance), bile acids, and several bile pigments. One of these pigments, **bilirubin,** is produced from the breakdown of hemoglobin during normal red blood cell destruction. Bilirubin travels via the bloodstream to the liver, where it is conjugated (combined) with another substance and added to bile. Thus, conjugated bilirubin enters the intestine with bile. Bacteria in the colon degrade bilirubin into a variety of pigments that give feces a brownish color. Bilirubin and bile leave the body in feces.

If bilirubin cannot leave the body, it remains in the bloodstream, causing **jaundice (hyperbilirubinemia)**—yellow discoloration of the skin, whites of the eyes, and mucous membranes. Figure 5–10 reviews the path of bilirubin from red blood cell destruction (hemolysis) to elimination with bile in the feces.

(Continue labeling Figure 5–9.)

The liver continuously releases bile, which then travels through the **hepatic duct** to the **cystic duct.** The cystic duct leads to the **gallbladder** [2], a pear-shaped sac under the liver, which stores and concentrates the bile for later use. After meals, in response to the presence of food in the stomach and duodenum, the gallbladder contracts, forcing the bile out the cystic duct into the **common bile duct** [3]. Meanwhile, the **pancreas** [4] secretes pancreatic juices (enzymes) that are released into the **pancreatic duct** [5], which joins with the common bile duct just as it enters the **duodenum** [6]. The duodenum thus receives a mixture of bile and pancreatic juices.

Bile has a detergent-like effect on fats in the duodenum. In the process of **emulsification,** bile breaks apart large fat globules, creating more surface area so that enzymes from the

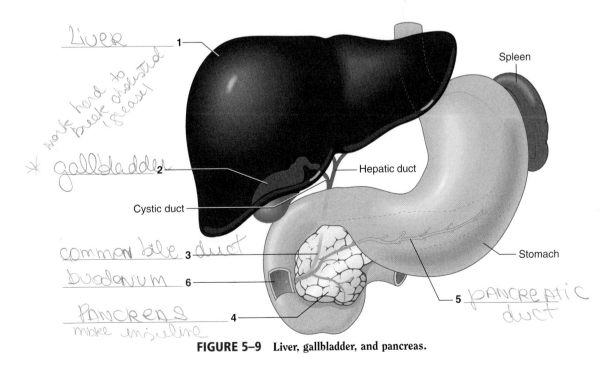

FIGURE 5–9 Liver, gallbladder, and pancreas.

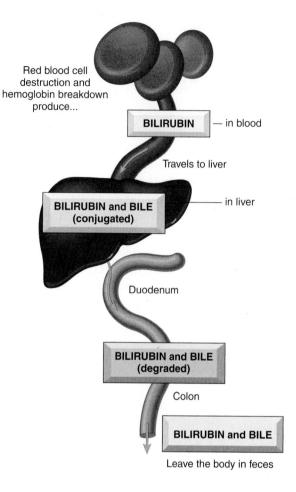

Red blood cell destruction and hemoglobin breakdown produce...

BILIRUBIN — in blood

Travels to liver

BILIRUBIN and BILE (conjugated) — in liver

Duodenum

BILIRUBIN and BILE (degraded)

Colon

BILIRUBIN and BILE

Leave the body in feces

FIGURE 5–10 Bilirubin pathway from bloodstream to elimination in feces.

pancreas can digest the fats. Without bile, most of the fat taken into the body remains undigested.

Besides producing bile, the liver has several other vital and important functions:

1. Maintaining normal blood **glucose** (sugar) levels. The liver removes excess glucose from the bloodstream and stores it as **glycogen** (starch) in liver cells. When the blood sugar level becomes dangerously low, the liver converts stored glycogen back into glucose via a process called **glycogenolysis.** In addition, the liver can also convert proteins and fats into glucose, when the body needs sugar, by a process called **gluconeogenesis.**
2. Manufacturing blood proteins, particularly those necessary for blood clotting
3. Releasing bilirubin, a pigment in bile
4. Removing poisons (toxins) from the blood

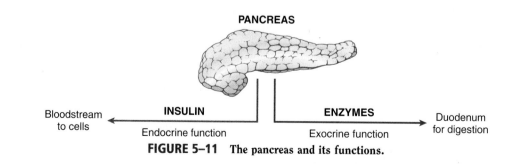

PANCREAS

Bloodstream to cells ← **INSULIN** | **ENZYMES** → Duodenum for digestion

Endocrine function | Exocrine function

FIGURE 5–11 The pancreas and its functions.

The **portal vein** brings blood to the liver from the intestines. Digested foods pass into the portal vein directly after being absorbed into the bloodstream from the small intestine, thus giving the liver the first chance to use the nutrients.

The **pancreas** (Fig. 5–11) is both an exocrine and an endocrine organ. As an exocrine gland, it produces enzymes to digest starch, such as **amylase** (amyl/o = starch, -ase = enzyme), to digest fat, such as **lipase** (lip/o = fat), and to digest proteins, such as **protease** (prote/o = protein). These pass into the duodenum through the pancreatic duct.

As an endocrine gland (secreting into the bloodstream), the pancreas secretes **insulin.** This hormone, needed to help release sugar from the blood, acts as a carrier to bring glucose into cells of the body to be used for energy.

Figure 5–12 is a flow chart that traces the pathway of food through the gastrointestinal tract.

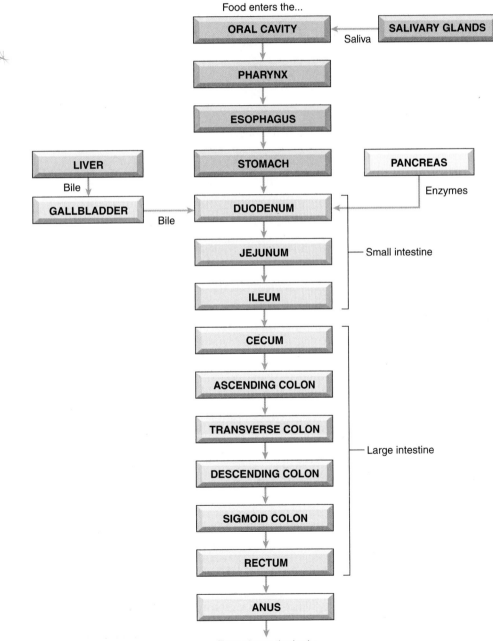

FIGURE 5–12   **Pathway of food through the gastrointestinal tract.**

VOCABULARY

The following list reviews many of the terms introduced in this chapter. Short definitions and additional information reinforce your understanding of the terms. All of the terms are included in the Pronunciation of Terms section later in the chapter.

absorption	Passage of materials through the walls of the small intestine into the bloodstream.
amino acids	Building blocks of proteins, produced when proteins are digested.
amylase	Enzyme secreted by the pancreas to digest starch.
anus	Opening of the digestive tract to the outside of the body.
appendix	Blind pouch hanging from the cecum (in the right lower quadrant [RLQ]). It literally means hanging (pend/o) on (ap-).
bile	Digestive juice made in the liver and stored in the gallbladder. It breaks up (emulsifies) large fat globules. Bile originally was called gall (Latin *bilis* meaning gall or anger), probably because it has a bitter taste. It is composed of bile pigments, cholesterol, and bile salts.
bilirubin	Pigment released by the liver in bile.
bowel	Intestine.
canine teeth	Pointed, "dog tooth"–like (canine) teeth, next to (distal to) the incisors. Also called cuspids or eyeteeth.
cecum	First part of the large intestine.
colon	Large intestine, consisting of the cecum; the ascending, transverse, and descending segments of the colon; and the rectum.
common bile duct	Carries bile from the liver and gallbladder to the duodenum. Also called the choledochus.
defecation	Elimination of feces from the digestive tract through the rectum.
deglutition	Swallowing.
dentin	Major tissue composing teeth, covered by the enamel in the crown and a protective layer of cementum in the root.
digestion	Breakdown of complex foods to simpler forms.
duodenum	First part of the small intestine. Duo = 2, den = 10; the duodenum measures 12 inches long.
elimination	Act of removal of materials from the body; in the digestive system, the removal of indigestible materials.
emulsification	Physical process of breaking up large fat globules into smaller globules, thereby increasing the surface area that enzymes can use to digest the fat.
enamel	Hard, outermost layer of a tooth.
enzyme	A chemical that speeds up a reaction between substances. Digestive enzymes break down complex foods to simpler substances. Enzymes are given names that end in -ase.
esophagus	Tube connecting the throat to the stomach. Eso- means inward; phag/o means swallowing.

fatty acids	Substances produced when fats are digested.
feces	Solid wastes; stools.
gallbladder	Small sac under the liver; stores bile. Remember: gallbladder is one word!
glucose	Simple sugar.
glycogen	Starch; glucose is stored in the form of glycogen in liver cells.
hydrochloric acid	Substance produced by the stomach; necessary for digestion of food.
ileum	Third part of the small intestine; from the Greek *eilos*, meaning twisted. When the abdomen was viewed at autopsy, the intestine appeared twisted, and the ileum often was an area of obstruction.
incisor	One of four front teeth in the dental arch.
insulin	Hormone produced by the endocrine cells of the pancreas. It transports sugar from the blood into cells and stimulates glycogen formation by the liver.
jejunum	Second part of the small intestine. The Latin *jejunus* means empty; this part of the intestine was always empty when a body was examined after death.
lipase	Pancreatic enzyme necessary to digest fats.
liver	A large organ located in the RUQ of the abdomen. The liver secretes bile; stores sugar, iron, and vitamins; produces blood proteins; and destroys worn-out red blood cells. The normal adult liver weighs about 2½ to 3 pounds.
lower esophageal sphincter (LES)	Ring of muscles between the esophagus and the stomach. Also called cardiac sphincter.
mastication	Chewing.
molar teeth	The sixth, seventh, and eighth teeth from the middle on either side of the dental arch. **Premolar teeth** are the fourth and fifth teeth, before the molars.
palate	Roof of the mouth. The hard palate lies anterior to the soft palate and is supported by the upper jaw bone (maxilla). The soft palate is the posterior fleshy part between the mouth and the throat.
pancreas	Organ under the stomach; produces insulin (for transport of sugar into cells) and enzymes (for digestion of foods).
papillae (*singular:* **papilla**)	Small elevations on the tongue. A papilla is a nipple-like elevation.
parotid gland	Salivary gland within the cheek, just anterior to the ear.
peristalsis	Rhythmic contractions of the tubes of the gastrointestinal (GI) tract and other tubular structures. Peristalsis moves the contents through the GI tract at different rates: stomach, 0.5 to 2 hours; small intestine, 2 to 6 hours; and colon, 6 to 72 hours. Peri- means surrounding; -stalsis is constriction.
pharynx	Throat, the common passageway for food from the mouth and for air from the nose.
portal vein	Large vein bringing blood to the liver from the intestines.
protease	Enzyme that digests protein.

5

pulp	Soft tissue within a tooth, containing nerves and blood vessels.
pyloric sphincter	Ring of muscle at the end of the stomach, near the duodenum. From the Greek *pyloros,* meaning gatekeeper. It is normally closed, but opens when a wave of peristalsis passes over it.
pylorus	Distal region of the stomach, opening to the duodenum.
rectum	Last section of the large intestine, connecting the end of the colon and the anus.
rugae	Ridges on the hard palate and the wall of the stomach.
saliva	Digestive juice produced by salivary glands.
salivary glands	Parotid, sublingual, and submandibular glands.
sigmoid colon	Fourth and last S-shaped segment of the colon, just before the rectum; empties into the rectum.
sphincter	Circular ring of muscle that constricts a passage or closes a natural opening.
stomach	Muscular organ that receives food from the esophagus. The stomach's parts are the fundus (proximal section), body (middle section), and antrum (distal section).
triglycerides	Large fat molecules composed of three parts fatty acid and one part glycerol.
uvula	Soft tissue hanging from the middle of the soft palate. The Latin *uva* means grape.
villi (*singular:* **villus**)	Microscopic projections in the wall of the small intestine that absorb nutrients into the bloodstream.

COMBINING FORMS, SUFFIXES, AND TERMINOLOGY

Write the meaning of the medical term in the space provided. Check the Pronunciation of Terms section later in the chapter for any unfamiliar words.

PARTS OF THE BODY

Combining Form	Meaning	Terminology	Meaning
an/o	anus	perianal _____	
append/o	appendix	appendectomy *Removal of the appendix*	
appendic/o	appendix	appendicitis *inflammation of the appendix* See Figure 5–13.	
bucc/o	cheek	buccal mucosa *pertaining to the cheek* *All types of mucosa are composed of epithelial cells.*	

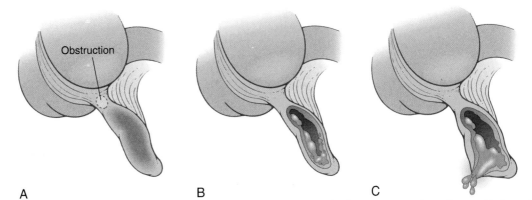

A B C

FIGURE 5–13 **Stages of appendicitis. A,** Obstruction and bacterial infection cause red, swollen, and inflamed appendix. **B,** Pus and bacteria invade the wall of the appendix. **C,** Pus perforates (ruptures through) the wall of the appendix into the abdomen, leading to peritonitis (inflammation of the peritoneum). (Modified from Damjanov I: Pathology for the Health-Related Professions, 3rd ed. Philadelphia, WB Saunders, 2006, p. 260.)

Combining Form	Meaning	Terminology	Meaning
cec/o	cecum	cecal _pertaining to the cecum_	
celi/o	belly, abdomen	celiac _pertaining to the abdomen_	
		Abdomin/o and lapar/o also mean abdomen. When more than one combining form have the same meaning, no rule exists for the proper usage of one or the other. You will learn to recognize each in its proper context.	
cheil/o	lip	cheilosis	
		Labi/o also means lip.	
cholecyst/o	gallbladder	cholecystectomy	
		Don't confuse cholecyst/o with cyst/o, which means urinary bladder!	
choledoch/o	common bile duct	choledochotomy	
col/o	colon, large intestine	colostomy	
		*The suffix -stomy, when used with a combining form for an organ, means an opening to the outside of the body. A **stoma** is an opening between an organ and the surface of the body (Fig. 5–14).*	
colon/o	colon	colonic	
		colonoscopy	
dent/i	tooth	dentibuccal _tooth. pertaining to the buccal._	
		Odont/o also means tooth.	
duoden/o	duodenum	duodenal	

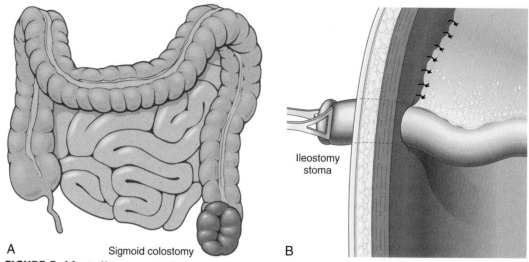

FIGURE 5–14 Different types of stomas. A, Sigmoid colostomy after resection of the rectum and part of the sigmoid colon. The stoma is at the end of the colon attached to the abdominal wall. **B,** Ileostomy after resection of the entire colon. The ileum is pulled out through the abdominal wall to form an ileostomy stoma.

Combining Form	Meaning	Terminology	Meaning
enter/o	intestines, usually small intestine	enterocolitis ___ *When two combining forms for gastrointestinal organs are in a term, the one for the organ closer to the mouth appears first.*	
		enterocolostomy ___ *-stomy, when used with two or more combining forms for organs, means the surgical creation of an opening between those organs inside the body. This is an **anastomosis,** which is any surgical connection between two parts, such as vessels, ducts, or bowel segments (ana = up, stom = opening, -sis = state of) (Fig. 5–15, A).*	
		mesentery ___ *Part of the double fold of peritoneum that stretches around the organs in the abdomen, the mesentery holds the organs in place. Literally, it lies in the middle (mes-) of the intestines, a membrane attaching the intestines to the muscle wall at the back of the abdomen (Fig. 5–15, B).*	
		parenteral ___ *Par (from para-) means apart from in this term. An intravenous line brings parenteral nutrition directly into the bloodstream, bypassing the intestinal tract (**enteral** nutrition). Parenteral injections may be subcutaneous or intramuscular as well.*	
esophag/o	esophagus	esophageal ___ Note: *Changing the suffix from -al to -eal softens the final g (ĕ-sŏf-a-JĒ-ăl).*	
faci/o	face	facial ___	

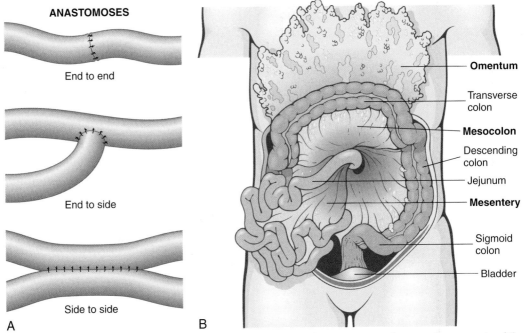

FIGURE 5–15   A, Three types of anastomoses. B, Mesentery. The **omentum** and **mesocolon** are parts of the mesentery. The omentum (raised in this figure) actually hangs down like an apron over the intestines.

Combining Form	Meaning	Terminology	Meaning
gastr/o	stomach	gastrostomy _____	
gingiv/o	gums	gingivitis _____	
gloss/o	tongue	hypoglossal _____ _Lingu/o also means tongue._	
hepat/o	liver	hepatoma _____ _Also called hepatocellular carcinoma._	
		hepatomegaly _____	
ile/o	ileum	ileocecal sphincter _____ _Also called the ileocecal valve._	
		ileitis _____	
		ileostomy _____ _See Figure 5–14, B._	
jejun/o	jejunum	choledochojejunostomy _____ _An anastomosis_	
		gastrojejunostomy _____ _This is part of a gastric bypass procedure._	

5

Combining Form	Meaning	Terminology	Meaning
labi/o	lip	labial _____	
lapar/o	abdomen	laparoscopy _____	
		A form of minimally invasive surgery (MIS). Examples are laparoscopic cholecystectomy and laparoscopic appendectomy.	
lingu/o	tongue	sublingual _____	
mandibul/o	lower jaw, mandible	submandibular _____	
odont/o	tooth	orthodontist _____	
		Orth/o means straight.	
		periodontist _____	
		endodontist _____	
		Performs root canal therapy.	
or/o	mouth	oral _____	
		Stomat/o also means mouth.	
palat/o	palate	palatoplasty _____	
		Procedure to repair cleft palate and cleft lip; repair of a cleft palate.	
pancreat/o	pancreas	pancreatitis _____	
peritone/o	peritoneum	peritonitis _____	
		The e of the root has been dropped in this term.	
pharyng/o	throat	pharyngeal _____	
		palatopharyngoplasty _____	
		Used to treat cases of snoring or sleep apnea caused by obstructions in the throat or nose.	
proct/o	anus and rectum	proctologist _____	
pylor/o	pyloric sphincter	pyloroplasty _____	
rect/o	rectum	rectocele _____	
sialaden/o	salivary gland	sialadenitis *enflam. of salivary gland.*	
sigmoid/o	sigmoid colon	sigmoidoscopy _____	
stomat/o	mouth	stomatitis _____	
uvul/o	uvula	uvulectomy _____	

SUBSTANCES

Combining Form	Meaning	Terminology	Meaning
amyl/o	starch	amylase _____ *The suffix -ase means enzyme.*	
bil/i	gall, bile	biliary _____ *The **biliary tract** includes the organs (liver and gallbladder) and ducts (hepatic, cystic, and common bile ducts) that secrete, store, and empty bile into the duodenum.*	
bilirubin/o	bilirubin (bile pigment)	hyperbilirubinemia _____	
chol/e	gall, bile	cholelithiasis _____ *Lith/o means stone or calculus; -iasis means abnormal condition.*	
chlorhydr/o	hydrochloric acid	achlorhydria _____ *Absence of gastric juice is associated with gastric carcinoma.*	
gluc/o	sugar	gluconeogenesis _____ *Liver cells make new sugar from fats and proteins.*	
glyc/o	sugar	hyperglycemia _____	
glycogen/o	glycogen, animal starch	glycogenolysis _____ *Liver cells change glycogen back to glucose when blood sugar levels drop*	
lip/o	fat, lipid	lipoma _____	
lith/o	stone	lithogenesis _____	
prote/o	protein	protease _____	
sial/o	saliva, salivary	sialolith _____	
steat/o	fat	steatorrhea _____ *Improperly digested (malabsorbed) fats will appear in the feces.*	

SUFFIXES

Suffix	Meaning	Terminology	Meaning
-ase	enzyme	lipase *Help digestion of fats* *Enzymes speed up chemical reactions. Lipase aids in the digestion of fats.*	
-chezia	defecation, elimination of wastes	hematochezia *defecation with stool* *(hē-mă-tō-KĒ-zē-ă). Bright red blood is found in the feces.*	
-iasis	abnormal condition	choledocholithiasis _____	
-prandial	meal	postprandial _____ ***Post cibum** (p.c.) also means after meals.*	

5

PATHOLOGY OF THE DIGESTIVE SYSTEM

This section presents medical terms that describe signs and symptoms (clinical indications of illness) and pathologic conditions of the gastrointestinal tract. Sentences following each definition describe the **etiology** (eti/o = cause) of the illness and treatment. When the etiology (cause) is not understood, the condition is said to be **idiopathic** (idi/o = unknown). You can find a list of drugs prescribed to treat gastrointestinal signs and symptoms and conditions on page 866 in Chapter 21, Pharmacology.

SYMPTOMS

anorexia

Lack of appetite (-orexia = appetite).

Anorexia often is a sign of malignancy or liver disease. Anorexia nervosa involves loss of appetite associated with emotional problems such as anger, anxiety, and irrational fear of weight gain. It is an eating disorder and is discussed, along with a similar disorder, bulimia nervosa, in Chapter 22.

ascites

Abnormal accumulation of fluid in the abdomen.

This condition occurs when fluid passes from the bloodstream and collects in the peritoneal cavity. It can be a symptom of neoplasm or inflammatory disorders in the abdomen, venous hypertension (high blood pressure) caused by liver disease (cirrhosis), and heart failure (Fig. 5–16). Treatment for ascites includes administration of diuretic drugs and paracentesis to remove abdominal fluid.

borborygmus
(pl. borborygmi)

Rumbling or gurgling noise produced by the movement of gas, fluid, or both in the gastrointestinal tract.

A sign of hyperactive intestinal peristalsis, borborygmi (bowel sounds) often are present in cases of gastroenteritis and diarrhea.

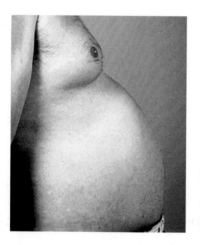

FIGURE 5–16 **Ascites in a male patient.** The photograph was taken after a paracentesis (puncture to remove fluid from the abdomen) was performed. Notice the gynecomastia (condition of female breasts) in this patient due to an excess of estrogen, which can accompany cirrhosis, especially in persons with alcoholism. (From Lewis SM, Heitkemper MM, Dirksen SR: Medical-Surgical Nursing, 6th ed. St. Louis, Mosby, 2004, p. 1119.)

Signs and Symptoms
A **sign** is an **objective** finding—such as a fever, rash, or a sound heard when listening to the chest—indicating the presence of a disease as perceived by an examiner. However, a **symptom** is a **subjective** sensation or change in health—such as itching, pain, fatigue, and nausea—as experienced by the patient. Clearly, the same feature may be noticed by both doctor and patient, which makes it at once both a sign and a symptom!

constipation	**Difficulty in passing stools (feces).** *rhythmic contractions of tubes (G. intestinal)* When peristalsis is slow, stools are dry and hard. A diet of fruit, vegetables, and water is helpful. **Laxatives** and **cathartics** are medications to promote movement of stools.
diarrhea	**Frequent passage of loose, watery stools.** Abrupt onset of diarrhea immediately after eating suggests acute infection or toxin in the gastrointestinal tract. Untreated, severe diarrhea may lead to dehydration. Antidiarrheal drugs are helpful.
dysphagia	**Difficulty in swallowing.** This sensation feels like a lump in the throat when a swallowed bolus fails to progress, either because of a physical obstruction (obstructive dysphagia) or because of a motor disorder in which esophageal peristalsis is not coordinated (motor dysphagia). **Odynophagia** is when swallowing causes pain (odyn/o).
eructation	**Gas expelled from the stomach through the mouth.** Eructation produces a characteristic sound and also is called **belching.**
flatus	**Gas expelled through the anus.** **Flatulence** is the presence of excessive gas in both the stomach and the intestines.
hematochezia	**Passage of fresh, bright red blood from the rectum.** The cause of hematochezia usually is bleeding due to colitis or from ulcers or polyps in the colon or rectum.
jaundice (icterus)	**Yellow-orange coloration of the skin and whites of the eyes caused by high levels of bilirubin in the blood (hyperbilirubinemia).** Jaundice can occur when (1) excessive destruction of erythrocytes, as in **hemolysis,** causes excess bilirubin in the blood; (2) malfunction of liver cells (hepatocytes) due to **liver disease** prevents the liver from excreting bilirubin with bile; or (3) **obstruction of bile flow,** such as from choledocholithiasis or tumor, prevents bilirubin in bile from being excreted into the duodenum.
melena	**Black, tarry stools; feces containing digested blood.** This symptom usually reflects a condition in which blood has had time to be digested (acted on by intestinal juices) and results from bleeding in the upper gastrointestinal tract (duodenal ulcer). A positive stool guaiac test (see page 189) indicates blood in the stool.
nausea	**Unpleasant sensation in the stomach associated with a tendency to vomit.** Common causes are sea and motion sickness and early pregnancy. Nausea and vomiting may be symptomatic of a perforation (hole in the wall) of an abdominal organ; obstruction of a bile duct, stomach, or intestine; or exposure to toxins (poisons).
steatorrhea	**Fat in the feces; frothy, foul-smelling fecal matter.** Improper digestion or absorption of fat can cause fat to remain in the intestine. This may occur with disease of the pancreas (pancreatitis) when pancreatic enzymes are not excreted. It also is a sign of intestinal disease that involves malabsorption of fat.

5

PATHOLOGIC CONDITIONS
Oral Cavity and Teeth

aphthous stomatitis

Inflammation of the mouth with small, painful ulcers.

Commonly called **canker** (KĂNK-ĕr) **sores;** its cause is unknown.

dental caries

Tooth decay (caries means decay).

Dental plaque results from the accumulation of foods, proteins from saliva, and necrotic debris on the tooth enamel. Bacteria grow in the plaque and cause production of acid that dissolves the tooth enamel, resulting in a cavity (area of decay). If the bacterial infection reaches the pulp of the tooth (causing pulpitis), root canal therapy may be necessary.

herpetic stomatitis

Inflammation of the mouth (gingiva, lips, palate, and tongue) **by infection with the herpesvirus.**

This condition is marked by painful fluid-filled blisters on skin and mucous membranes, commonly called **fever blisters** or **cold sores.** It is caused by herpes simplex virus type 1 (HSV1). Treatment is medication to relieve symptoms. Herpes genitalis (due to HSV2) occurs on the reproductive organs. Both conditions are highly contagious.

oral leukoplakia

White plaques or patches (-plakia means plaque) **on the mucosa of the mouth.**

This precancerous lesion can result from chronic tobacco use (pipe smoking or chewing tobacco). Malignant potential is assessed by microscopic study of biopsied tissue.

periodontal disease

Inflammation and degeneration of gums, teeth, and surrounding bone.

Chronic inflammation of gums (gingivitis) occurs as a result of accumulation of **dental plaque** (noncalcified collection of oral microorganisms and their products) and **dental calculus** or **tartar** (a white, brown, or yellow-brown calcified deposit at or below the gingival margin of teeth). In gingivectomy, after a periodontist uses a metal instrument to scrape away plaque and tartar from teeth, pockets of pus are removed to allow new tissue to form. Localized infections are treated with systemic antibiotics.

Upper Gastrointestinal Tract

achalasia

Failure of the lower esophagus sphincter (LES) muscle to relax.

Achalasia (-chalasia means relaxation) results from the loss of peristalsis so that food cannot pass easily through the esophagus. Both failure of the LES to relax and the loss of peristalsis cause dilatation (widening) of the esophagus above the constriction (Fig. 5–17, A). Physicians recommend a bland diet low in bulk and dilation of the LES to relieve symptoms (Fig. 5–17, B).

esophageal varices

Swollen, varicose veins at the lower end of the esophagus.

Liver disease (such as cirrhosis and chronic hepatitis) causes increased pressure in veins near and around the liver **(portal hypertension).** This leads to enlarged, tortuous esophageal veins with danger of hemorrhage (bleeding). Treatment includes drug therapy to lower portal hypertension and banding or tying off the swollen esophageal veins (Fig. 5–18, A).

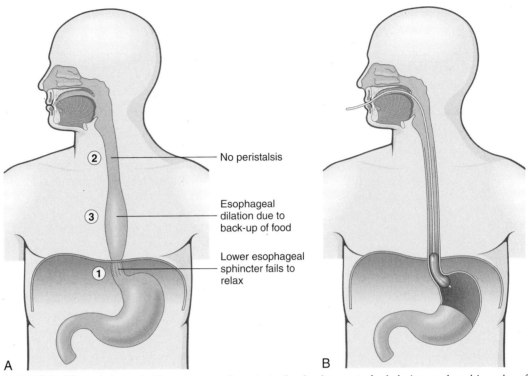

No peristalsis

Esophageal
dilation due to
back-up of food

Lower esophageal
sphincter fails to
relax

A   B

FIGURE 5–17   Achalasia. A, The sequence of events in the development of achalasia, numbered in order of
occurrence. **B, Balloon dilation (dilatation)** of the lower esophageal sphincter (LES) is a treatment for achalasia.

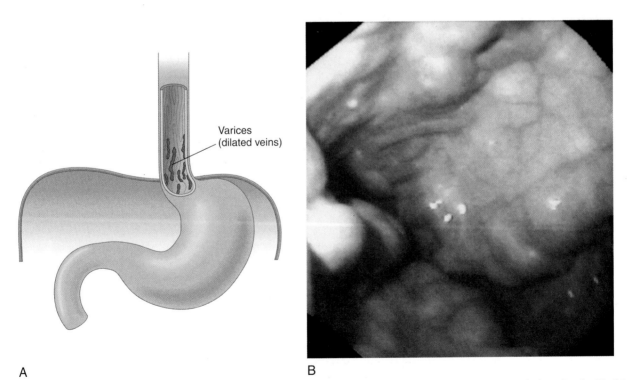

Varices
(dilated veins)

A   B

FIGURE 5–18   A, Esophageal varices. B, Endoscopic view of esophageal varices. (**A** from Damjanov I: Pathology for the Health-
Related Professions, 3rd ed. Philadelphia, WB Saunders, 2006, p. 246. **B** from Gould BE: Pathophysiology for Health Professions, 3rd
ed. Philadelphia, WB Saunders, 2006, p. 466.)

5

gastric carcinoma	**Malignant tumor of the stomach.**

Chronic gastritis associated with *Helicobacter pylori* (bacterial) infection is a major risk factor for gastric carcinoma. Gastric endoscopy and biopsy diagnose the condition. Cure depends on early detection and surgical removal of the cancerous tissue.

gastroesophageal reflux disease (GERD)	**Solids and fluids return to the mouth from the stomach.**

Heartburn is the burning sensation caused by regurgitation of hydrochloric acid from the stomach to the esophagus. Chronic exposure of esophageal mucosa to gastric acid and pepsin (an enzyme that digests protein) leads to **reflux esophagitis**. Drug treatment for GERD includes antacid (acid-suppressive) agents and medication to increase the tone of the LES.

hernia	**Protrusion of an organ or part through the muscle normally containing it.**

A **hiatal hernia** occurs when the upper part of the stomach protrudes upward through the diaphragm (Fig. 5–19, *A*). This condition can lead to GERD. An **inguinal hernia** occurs when a small loop of bowel protrudes through a weak lower abdominal muscle (Fig. 5–19, *B*). Surgical repair of inguinal hernias is known as herniorrhaphy (-rrhaphy means suture).

peptic ulcer	**Open sore or lesion of the mucous membrane of the stomach or duodenum.**

A bacterium, *H. pylori*, is responsible for peptic ulcer disease. The combination of bacteria, hyperacidity, and gastric juice damages epithelial linings. Drug treatment includes antibiotics, antacids, and agents to protect the lining of the stomach and intestine.

Lower Gastrointestinal Tract (Small and Large Intestine)

anal fistula	**Abnormal tube-like passageway near the anus.**

The fistula often results from a break or **fissure** in the wall of the anus or rectum, or from an abscess (infected area) there (Fig. 5–20, *A*).

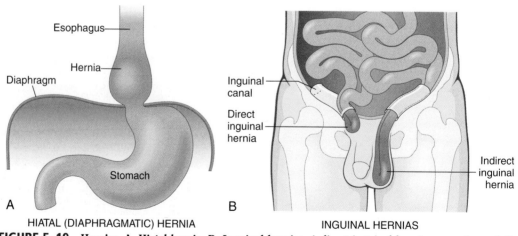

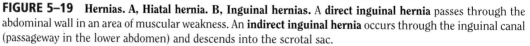

FIGURE 5–19 Hernias. A, Hiatal hernia. B, Inguinal hernias. A direct inguinal hernia passes through the abdominal wall in an area of muscular weakness. An **indirect inguinal hernia** occurs through the inguinal canal (passageway in the lower abdomen) and descends into the scrotal sac.

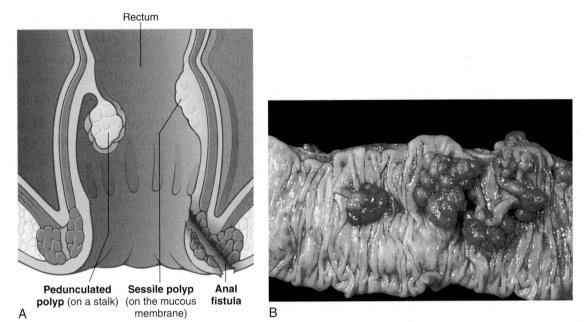

Rectum

Pedunculated **Sessile polyp** **Anal**
polyp (on a stalk) (on the mucous **fistula**
                        membrane)
A   B

FIGURE 5–20 **Anal fistula and intestinal polyps. A,** Anal fistula and two types of polyps. **B,** Multiple polyps of the colon. (**B** from Damjanov I: Pathology for the Health-Related Professions, 3rd ed. Philadelphia, WB Saunders, 2006, p. 266.)

colonic polyposis

Polyps (benign growths) protrude from the mucous membrane of the colon.

Figure 5–20, *A,* illustrates two types of polyps: **pedunculated** (attached to the membrane by a stalk) and **sessile** (sitting directly on the mucous membrane). Figure 5–20, *B,* shows multiple polyps of the colon. Polyps often are removed (polypectomy) for biopsy and to prevent growth leading to malignancy

colorectal cancer

Adenocarcinoma of the colon or rectum, or both.

Colorectal cancer (Fig. 5–21) can arise from polyps in the colon or rectal region. Diagnosis is determined by detecting melena (blood in stool) and by colonoscopy. Prognosis depends on the stage (extent of spread) of the tumor, including size, depth of invasion, and involvement of lymph nodes. Surgical treatment may require wide resection with colostomy. Chemotherapy and radiotherapy are administered as needed.

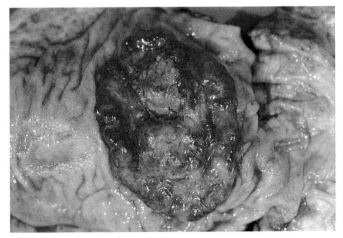

FIGURE 5–21 **Adenocarcinoma of the colon.** This tumor has heaped-up edges and an ulcerated central portion. (From Damjanov I: Pathology for the Health-Related Professions, 3rd ed. Philadelphia, WB Saunders, 2006, p. 268.)

5

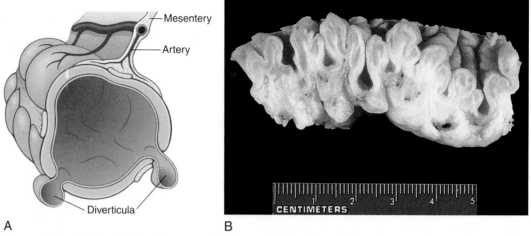

A   B

FIGURE 5–22 **Diverticula and diverticulosis. A, A diverticulum is** formed when the mucous membrane lining of the colon bulges through the muscular wall. **B, Diverticulosis** can result when fecal material lodges in diverticula. Avoidance of foods with seeds and nuts decreases the risk of this condition. (**B** from Kumar V, Cotran RS, Robbins SL: Basic Pathology, 7th ed. Philadelphia, WB Saunders, 2003, p. 577.)

Crohn disease (Crohn's)	**Chronic inflammation of the intestinal tract (terminal ileum and colon).**
	Signs and symptoms include diarrhea, severe abdominal pain, fever, anorexia, weakness, and weight loss. Both Crohn disease (Crohn's) and ulcerative colitis are forms of **inflammatory bowel disease (IBD).** Treatment is with drugs to control symptoms or by surgical removal of diseased portions of the intestine, with anastomosis of remaining parts.
diverticulosis	**Abnormal side pockets (outpouchings) in the intestinal wall.**
	Diverticula (Fig. 5–22, *A*) are pouch-like herniations through the muscular wall of the colon. When fecal matter becomes trapped in diverticula, **diverticulitis** can occur. Pain and rectal bleeding are symptoms. Figure 5–22, *B,* shows diverticulosis in a section through the sigmoid colon.
dysentery	**Painful, inflamed intestines.**
	Commonly occurring in the colon, dysentery usually results from the ingestion of food or water containing bacteria (salmonellae or shigellae), amebae (one-celled organisms), or viruses. Symptoms are bloody stools and abdominal pain.
hemorrhoids	**Swollen, twisted, varicose veins in the rectal region.**
	Varicose veins can be internal (within the rectum) or external (outside the anal sphincter). Pregnancy and chronic constipation, which put pressure on anal veins, often cause hemorrhoids.
ileus	**Failure of peristalsis with resulting obstruction of the intestines.**
	Mechanical obstruction of the bowel (by adhesions, tumor, or stones) is a cause. Surgery, trauma, or bacterial injury to the peritoneum can lead to a **paralytic ileus** (acute, transient loss of peristalsis).

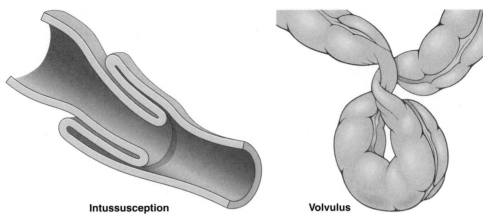

Intussusception   Volvulus

FIGURE 5–23 Intussusception and volvulus. (From Damjanov I: Pathology for the Health-Related Profession, 3rd ed. Philadelphia, WB Saunders, 2006, p. 261.)

intussusception	**Telescoping of the intestines.**
	In this condition, one segment of the bowel collapses into the opening of another segment (Fig. 5–23). It often occurs in children and at the ileocecal region. Intestinal obstruction with pain and vomiting can occur. Surgical removal of the affected segment of bowel with anastomosis frequently is necessary to correct the obstruction.
irritable bowel syndrome (IBS)	**Group of gastrointestinal symptoms associated with stress and tension.**
	Gastrointestinal symptoms are diarrhea, constipation, bloating, and lower abdominal pain. On extensive examination, the intestines appear normal, yet symptoms persist. Treatment is symptomatic, with a diet high in bran and fiber to soften stools and establish regular bowel habits.
ulcerative colitis	**Chronic inflammation of the colon with presence of ulcers.**
	This idiopathic, chronic, recurrent diarrheal disease (an **inflammatory bowel disease**) presents with rectal bleeding and pain. Often beginning in the colon, the inflammation spreads proximally, involving the entire colon. Drug treatment and careful attention to diet are recommended. Resection of diseased bowel with ileostomy may be necessary. Patients with ulcerative colitis have a higher risk of colon cancer.
volvulus	**Twisting of the intestine on itself.**
	Volvulus causes intestinal obstruction. Severe pain, nausea and vomiting, and absence of bowel sounds are symptoms. Surgical correction is necessary to prevent necrosis of the affected segment of the bowel (see Fig. 5–23).

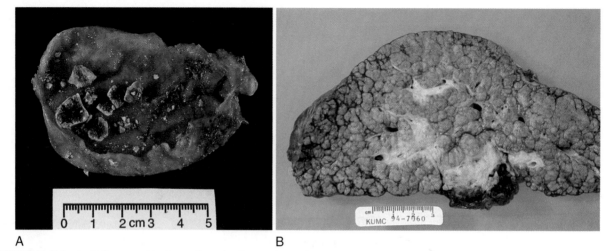

A   B

FIGURE 5–24 A, Gallstones. Mechanical manipulation during laparoscopic cholecystectomy has caused fragmentation of several cholesterol gallstones, revealing interiors that are pigmented because of entrapped bile pigments. The gallbladder mucosa is reddened and irregular as result of coexistent acute and chronic cholecystitis. **B, Liver with alcoholic cirrhosis.** The normal liver cells (hepatocytes) have been replaced by nodules that are yellow because of their high fat content. (**A** from Kumar V, Cotran RS, Robbins S: Basic Pathology, 7th ed. Philadelphia, WB Saunders, 2003, p. 629. **B** from Damjanov I: Pathology for the Health-Related Professions, 3rd ed. Philadelphia, WB Saunders, 2006, p. 286.)

Liver, Gallbladder, and Pancreas

cholelithiasis

Gallstones in the gallbladder (Fig. 5–24, A).

Calculi (stones) prevent bile from leaving the gallbladder and bile ducts (Fig. 5–25). Many patients remain asymptomatic and do not require treatment; however, if a patient experiences episodes of **biliary colic** (pain from blocked cystic or common bile duct), treatment may be required. Currently, laparoscopic or

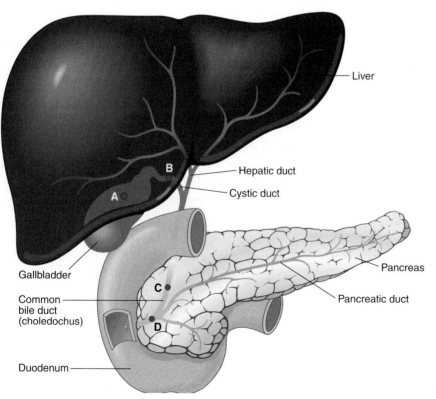

FIGURE 5–25 Gallstone positions. A, Stone in the gallbladder, causing mild or no symptoms. **B,** Stone obstructing the cystic duct, causing pain. **C,** Stone obstructing the common bile duct, causing pain and jaundice. **D,** Stone at the lower end of the common bile duct and pancreatic duct, causing pain, jaundice, and pancreatitis.

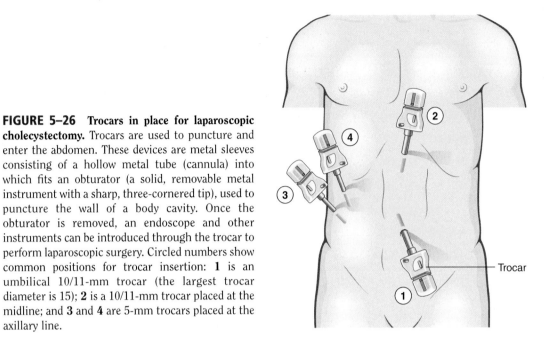

FIGURE 5–26 **Trocars in place for laparoscopic cholecystectomy.** Trocars are used to puncture and enter the abdomen. These devices are metal sleeves consisting of a hollow metal tube (cannula) into which fits an obturator (a solid, removable metal instrument with a sharp, three-cornered tip), used to puncture the wall of a body cavity. Once the obturator is removed, an endoscope and other instruments can be introduced through the trocar to perform laparoscopic surgery. Circled numbers show common positions for trocar insertion: **1** is an umbilical 10/11-mm trocar (the largest trocar diameter is 15); **2** is a 10/11-mm trocar placed at the midline; and **3** and **4** are 5-mm trocars placed at the axillary line.

minimally invasive surgery **(laparoscopic cholecystectomy)** is performed to remove the gallbladder and stones (Fig. 5–26).

cirrhosis	**Chronic degenerative disease of the liver.**

Cirrhosis is commonly the result of chronic alcoholism and often malnutrition, hepatitis, or other causes. Lobes of the liver become covered with fibrous tissue, hepatic cells degenerate, and the liver is infiltrated with fat. Cirrh/o means yellow-orange, which describes the liver's color caused by fat accumulation (see Fig. 5–24, *B*). Treatment is dependent on the cause.

pancreatitis	**Inflammation of the pancreas.**

Digestive enzymes attack pancreatic tissue and damage the gland. Other etiologic factors include chronic alcoholism, drug toxicity, gallstone obstruction of the common bile duct, and viral infections. Treatment includes medications to relieve epigastric pain, intravenous fluids, and subtotal pancreatectomy if necessary.

viral hepatitis	**Inflammation of the liver caused by a virus.**

Hepatitis A is viral hepatitis caused by the hepatitis A virus (HAV). It is a benign disorder spread by contaminated food or water and characterized by slow onset of symptoms. Complete recovery is expected. **Hepatitis B** is caused by the hepatitis B virus (HBV) and is transmitted by blood transfusion, sexual contact, or the use of contaminated needles or instruments. Severe infection can cause destruction of liver cells, cirrhosis, or death. A vaccine that provides immunity is available and recommended for persons at risk for exposure. **Hepatitis C** is caused by the hepatitis C virus (HCV) and is transmitted by blood transfusions or needle inoculation (such as among intravenous drug users sharing needles). The acute illness may progress to chronic hepatitis.

In all types, liver enzyme levels may be elevated, indicating damage to liver cells. Signs and symptoms include malaise, anorexia, hepatomegaly, jaundice, and abdominal pain.

? EXERCISES

Remember to check your answers carefully with those given in the Answers to Exercises, page 174.

A. Match the following digestive system structures with their meanings below.

anus	esophagus	liver
cecum	gallbladder	pancreas
colon	ileum	pharynx
duodenum	jejunum	sigmoid colon

1. large intestine ___*colon*___

2. small sac under the liver; stores bile ___*gallbladder*___

✗ 3. first part of the large intestine ___*cecum*___

4. opening of the digestive tract to the outside of the body ___*anus*___

✗ 5. second part of the small intestine ___*jejunum*___

6. tube connecting the throat to the stomach ___*esophagus*___

7. third part of the small intestine ___*ileum*___

8. large organ located in the RUQ; secretes bile, stores sugar, produces blood proteins ___*liver*___

9. throat ___*pharynx*___

10. lower part of the colon ___*sigmoid colon*___

11. first part of the small intestine ___*duodenum*___

12. organ under the stomach; produces insulin and digestive enzymes ___*pancreas*___

B. Circle the term that fits the given definition. You should be able to define the other terms as well!

1. **microscopic projections in the walls of the small intestine:**
   papillae (villi) rugae *stomach*
   tongue

2. **salivary gland near the ear:**
   submandibular sublingual (parotid)

3. **ring of muscle at the end of the stomach:**
   pyloric sphincter uvula lower esophageal sphincter
   bace *esophego and stomach*

4. **soft, inner section of a tooth:**
   dentin enamel (pulp)

5. **chemical that speeds up reactions and helps digest foods:**
   triglyceride amino acid (enzyme)

6. **pigment released with bile:**
   glycogen (bilirubin) melena

7. **hormone produced by endocrine cells of the pancreas:**

insulin   amylase   lipase

8. **rhythm-like movement of the muscles in the walls of the gastrointestinal tract:**

deglutition   mastication   peristalsis

9. **breakdown of large fat globules:**

absorption   emulsification   anabolism

10. **pointed, dog-like tooth medial to premolars:**

incisor   canine   molar

C. Complete the following.

1. Labi/o and cheil/o both mean _lip_.

2. Gloss/o and lingu/o both mean _tongue_.

3. Or/o and stomat/o both mean _mouth_.

4. Dent/i and odont/o both mean _tooth_.

5. Lapar/o and celi/o both mean _abdomen_.

6. Gluc/o and glyc/o both mean _sugar_.

7. Lip/o, steat/o, and adip/o all mean _fat_.

8. The suffixes -iasis and -osis both mean _abnormal condition_.

9. Chol/e and bil/i both mean _gall, bile_.

10. Resection and -ectomy both mean _removal, excision_.

D. Build medical terms based on the given definitions.

1. removal of a salivary gland _sialadenectomy_

2. pertaining to the throat _pharyngeal_

3. hernia of the rectum _rectocele_

4. enlargement of the liver _hepatomegaly_

5. surgical repair of the roof of the mouth _palatoplasty_

6. after meals _____

7. visual examination of the anal and rectal region _proctoscopy_

8. study of the cause (of disease) _____

9. incision of the common bile duct _____

10. pertaining to tooth and cheek (the surface of a tooth against the cheek) _____

11. disease condition of the small intestine _____

12. new opening between the common bile duct and the jejunum _____

13. pertaining to surrounding the anus _____

14. new opening from the colon to the outside of the body _____

15. pertaining to under the lower jaw _____

16. pertaining to the face _____

E. Match the following doctors or dentists with their specialties.

colorectal surgeon   nephrologist   periodontist
endodontist   oral surgeon   proctologist
gastroenterologist   orthodontist   urologist

1. diagnoses and treats disorders of the anus and rectum _proctologist_

2. operates on the organs of the urinary tract _urologist_

3. straightens teeth _orthdontist_

4. performs root canal therapy _endodontist_

5. operates on the mouth and teeth _oral surgeon_

6. diagnoses and uses drugs to treat kidney disorders _nephrologist_

7. diagnoses and treats gastrointestinal tract disorders _gastroenterologist_

8. treats gum disease _periodontist_

9. operates on the intestinal tract _colorectal surgeon_

F. Build medical terms to describe the following inflammations.

1. inflammation of the appendix _appendicitis_

2. inflammation of the large intestine _colitis_

3. inflammation of the tube from the throat to the stomach _esophagitis_

4. inflammation of the membrane surrounding the abdomen _peritonitis_

5. inflammation of the gallbladder _cholecystitis_

6. inflammation of the third part of the small intestine _____

7. inflammation of the pancreas _____

8. inflammation of the gums _____

9. inflammation of the liver _____

10. inflammation of the mouth _____

11. inflammation of the salivary gland _____

12. inflammation of the small and large intestines _____

G. Match the following terms with their meanings below.

anastomosis	gluconeogenesis	mesentery
biliary	glycogenolysis	mucosa
defecation	hyperbilirubinemia	parenteral
cheilitis	hyperglycemia	portal vein

1. high level of blood sugar *hyperglycemia*

2. inflammation of the lip _____

3. pertaining to administration other than through the intestinal tract _____

4. a mucous membrane _____

5. expulsion of feces from the body through the anus _____

6. breakdown (conversion) of animal starch to sugar _____

7. membrane that connects the small intestine to the abdominal wall _____

8. large vessel that takes blood to the liver from the intestines _____

9. new surgical connection between two previously unconnected structures or organs

_____

10. pertaining to bile ducts and organs _____

11. process of forming new sugar from proteins and fats _____

12. high levels of a bile pigment in the bloodstream _____

H. Give the names of the following gastrointestinal symptoms based on their descriptions.

1. passage of bright red blood from the rectum _____

2. lack of appetite _____

3. fat in the feces _____

4. black, tarry stools; feces containing digested blood _____

5. abnormal accumulation of fluid in the abdomen _____

6. rumbling noise produced by gas in the GI tract _____

7. gas expelled through the anus _____

8. an unpleasant sensation in the stomach and a tendency to vomit _____

9. loose, watery stools _____

10. difficulty in passing stools (feces) _____

11. difficulty in swallowing _____

12. painful swallowing _____

5

I. Write short answers for the following questions.

1. What is jaundice? _____

2. List three ways in which a patient can become jaundiced:

   a._____

   b._____

   c._____

3. What does it mean when a disease is described as *idiopathic?*_____

   _____

J. Select from the list of pathologic conditions to make a diagnosis.

achalasia	colorectal cancer	herpetic stomatitis
anal fistula	Crohn's disease	oral leukoplakia
aphthous stomatitis	dental caries	periodontal disease
colonic polyposis		

1. Ms. Jones complained of pain during swallowing. Her physician explained that the pain was caused by a failure of muscles in her lower esophagus to relax during swallowing. Diagnosis: _____.

2. An abnormal tube-like passageway near his anus caused Mr. Rosen's proctalgia. His doctor performed surgery to close off the abnormality. Diagnosis: _____.

3. Bebe's dentist informed her that the enamel of three teeth was damaged by bacteria-producing acid. Diagnosis: _____.

4. Paola's symptoms of chronic diarrhea, abdominal cramps, and fever led her doctor to suspect that she suffered from an inflammatory bowel disease affecting the distal portion of her ileum. The doctor prescribed steroid drugs to heal her condition. Diagnosis: _____.

5. Mr. Hart learned that his colonoscopy showed the presence of small benign growths protruding from the mucous membrane of his large intestine. Diagnosis: _____.

6. During a routine dental checkup, Dr. Friedman discovered white plaques on Mr. Longo's buccal mucosa. He advised Mr. Longo, who was a chronic smoker and heavy drinker, to have these precancerous lesions removed. Diagnosis: _____.

7. Every time Carl had a stressful time at work, he developed a fever blister (cold sore) on his lip, resulting from reactivation of a previous viral infection. His doctor told him that there was no treatment 100% effective in preventing the reappearance of these lesions. Diagnosis: _____.

8. Mr. Green had a biopsy of a neoplastic lesion in his ascending colon. The pathology report indicated a malignancy. Radical (complete) colectomy followed by ileostomy was necessary. Diagnosis: _____.

9. After irritating her mouth with vigorous tooth brushing, small ulcers (canker sores) appeared on Diane's gums. They were painful and annoying. Diagnosis: _____.

10. Sharon's failure to floss her teeth and remove dental plaque regularly led to development of gingivitis. Her dentist advised consulting a specialist, who could treat her condition. Diagnosis: _____.

K. Match the following pathologic diagnoses with their definitions.

cholecystolithiasis   hemorrhoids   pancreatitis
cirrhosis   hiatal hernia   peptic ulcer
diverticulosis   ileus   ulcerative colitis
dysentery   intussusception   viral hepatitis
esophageal varices   irritable bowel syndrome volvulus

1. protrusion of the upper part of the stomach through the diaphragm _____

2. painful, inflamed intestines caused by bacterial infection _____

3. swollen, twisted veins in the rectal region_____

4. open sore or lesion of the mucous membrane of the stomach or duodenum_____

5. failure of peristalsis with obstruction of intestines _____

6. twisting of the intestine on itself _____

7. swollen, varicose veins in the distal portion of the esophagus _____

8. abnormal side pockets (outpouchings) in the intestinal wall_____

9. chronic inflammation of the colon with ulcers_____

10. telescoping of the intestines _____

11. inflammation of the liver caused by type A, type B, or type C virus_____

12. inflammation of the pancreas_____

13. calculi in the sac that stores bile _____

14. chronic degenerative liver disease resulting from alcoholism and malnutrition _____

15. a group of symptoms (diarrhea and constipation, abdominal pain, bloating) associated with

    stress and tension, but without inflammation of the intestine _____

L. Complete the following terms from their meanings given below.

1. membrane (peritoneal fold) that holds the intestines together: mes_____

2. removal of the gallbladder: _____ectomy

3. black or dark brown, tarry stools containing blood: mel_____

4. high levels of pigment in the blood (jaundice): hyper_____

5. pertaining to under the tongue: sub_____

6. twisting of the intestine on itself: vol_____

7. organ under the stomach that produces insulin and digestive enzymes: pan_____

8. lack of appetite: an_____

9. swollen, twisted veins in the rectal region: _____oids

10. new connection between two previously unconnected tubes: ana_____

11. absence of acid in the stomach: a_____

12. return of solids and fluids to the mouth from the stomach: gastro_____

    re_____ disease

13. removal of soft tissue hanging from the roof of the mouth _____ectomy

14. formation of stones _____genesis.

MEDICAL SCRAMBLE

Unscramble the letters to form suffixes from the clues. Use the letters in squares to complete the bonus term.

1. *Clue:* Yellow discoloration of skin

___ ___ ___ [ ] ___ ___ ___ ___   ICNAJUED

2. *Clue:* Discharge of watery waste from colon

___ [ ] ___ ___ ___ ___ ___ [ ]   AERDHRAI

3. *Clue:* Fluid-filled enlargement of the abdomen

[ ] [ ] ___ ___ [ ] ___ [ ]   TASSEIC

4. *Clue:* Rumbling, gurgling sounds from the GI tract

___ [ ] ___ [ ] ___ ___ [ ] ___ [ ]   YROMOSGBRUB

BONUS TERM: *Clue:* Surgical reconnection of gastrointestinal organs.

[ ] [ ] [ ] [ ] [ ] [ ] [ ] [ ] [ ] [ ]

ANSWERS TO EXERCISES

A

1. colon
2. gallbladder
3. cecum
4. anus
5. jejunum
6. esophagus
7. ileum
8. liver
9. pharynx
10. sigmoid colon
11. duodenum
12. pancreas

B

1. Villi. Papillae are nipple-like projections in the tongue where taste buds are located, and rugae are folds in the mucous membrane of the stomach and hard palate.
2. Parotid. The submandibular gland is under the lower jaw, and the sublingual gland is under the tongue.
3. Pyloric sphincter. The uvula is soft tissue hanging from the soft palate, and the lower esophageal sphincter is a ring of muscle between the esophagus and stomach.
4. Pulp. Dentin is the hard part of the tooth directly under the enamel and in the root, and enamel is the hard, outermost part of the tooth composing the crown.
5. Enzyme. A triglyceride is a large fat molecule, and an amino acid is a substance produced when proteins are digested.
6. Bilirubin. Glycogen is animal starch that is produced in liver cells from sugar, and melena is dark, tarry stools.
7. Insulin. Amylase and lipase are digestive enzymes produced by the exocrine cells of the pancreas.
8. Peristalsis. Deglutition is swallowing, and mastication is chewing.
9. Emulsification. Absorption is the passage of materials through the walls of the small intestine into the bloodstream, and anabolism is the process of building up proteins in a cell (protein synthesis).
10. Canine. An incisor is one of the four front teeth in the dental arch (not pointed or like a dog's tooth), and a molar is one of three large teeth just behind (distal to) the two premolar teeth.

C

1. lip
2. tongue
3. mouth
4. tooth
5. abdomen
6. sugar
7. fat
8. abnormal condition
9. gall, bile
10. removal, excision

D

1. sialadenectomy
2. pharyngeal
3. rectocele
4. hepatomegaly
5. palatoplasty
6. postprandial (post cibum—cib/o refers to meals or feeding)
7. proctoscopy
8. etiology
9. choledochotomy
10. dentibuccal
11. enteropathy
12. choledochojejunostomy
13. perianal
14. colostomy
15. submandibular
16. facial

E

1. proctologist
2. urologist
3. orthodontist
4. endodontist
5. oral surgeon
6. nephrologist
7. gastroenterologist
8. periodontist
9. colorectal surgeon

F

1. appendicitis
2. colitis
3. esophagitis
4. peritonitis (note that the e is dropped)
5. cholecystitis
6. ileitis
7. pancreatitis
8. gingivitis
9. hepatitis
10. stomatitis
11. sialadenitis
12. enterocolitis (when two combining forms for gastrointestinal organs are in a term, use the one that is closest to the mouth first)

G

1. hyperglycemia
2. cheilitis
3. parenteral
4. mucosa
5. defecation
6. glycogenolysis
7. mesentery
8. portal vein
9. anastomosis
10. biliary
11. gluconeogenesis
12. hyperbilirubinemia

H

1. hematochezia
2. anorexia
3. steatorrhea
4. melena
5. ascites
6. borborygmus
7. flatus
8. nausea
9. diarrhea
10. constipation
11. dysphagia
12. odynophagia

I

1. yellow-orange coloration of the skin and other tissues (hyperbilirubinemia)
2. **a.** any liver disease (hepatopathy—such as cirrhosis, hepatoma, or hepatitis), so that bilirubin is not processed into bile and cannot be excreted in feces
   b. obstruction of bile flow, so that bile and bilirubin are not excreted and accumulate in the bloodstream
   c. excessive hemolysis leading to overproduction of bilirubin and high levels in the bloodstream
3. cause is not known.

J

1. achalasia
2. anal fistula
3. dental caries
4. Crohn disease (Crohn's)
5. colonic polyposis
6. oral leukoplakia
7. herpetic stomatitis
8. colorectal cancer
9. aphthous stomatitis
10. periodontal disease

K

1. hiatal hernia
2. dysentery
3. hemorrhoids
4. peptic ulcer
5. ileus
6. volvulus
7. esophageal varices
8. diverticulosis
9. ulcerative colitis
10. intussusception
11. viral hepatitis
12. pancreatitis
13. cholecystolithiasis (gallstones)
14. cirrhosis
15. irritable bowel syndrome

L

1. mesentery
2. cholecystectomy
3. melena
4. hyperbilirubinemia
5. sublingual
6. volvulus
7. pancreas
8. anorexia
9. hemorrhoids
10. anastomosis
11. achlorhydria
12. gastroesophageal reflux disease
13. uvulectomy
14. lithogenesis

ANSWERS TO MEDICAL SCRAMBLE

1. JAUNDICE   2. DIARRHEA   3. ASCITES   4. BORBORYGMUS

BONUS TERM: ANASTOMOSIS

PRONUNCIATION OF TERMS

PRONUNCIATION GUIDE

ā as in āpe   ă as in ăpple
ē as in ēven   ĕ as in ĕvery
ī as in īce   ĭ as in ĭnterest
ō as in ōpen   ŏ as in pŏt
ū as in ūnit   ŭ as in ŭnder

To test your understanding of the terminology in this chapter, write the meaning of each term in the space provided. In addition, you may wish to cover the terms and write them by looking at your definitions. Make sure your spelling is correct. The page number after each term indicates where it is defined or used in the book, so you can easily check your responses. You will find complete definitions for all of these terms and their audio pronunciations on the CD.

VOCABULARY AND TERMINOLOGY

Term	Pronunciation	Meaning
absorption (148)	ăb-SŎRP-shŭn	_____
achlorhydria (155)	ā-chlōr-HĬD-rē-ă	_____
amino acids (148)	ă-MĒ-nō ĂS-ĭdz	_____
amylase (148)	ĂM-ĭ-lās	_____
anastomosis (152)	ă-năs-tō-MŌ-sĭs	_____
anus (148)	Ā-nŭs	_____
appendectomy (150)	ăp-ĕn-DĔK-tō-mē	_____
appendicitis (150)	ă-pĕn-dĭ-SĪ-tĭs	_____
appendix (148)	ă-PĔN-dĭks	_____
bile (148)	bīl	_____
biliary (155)	BĬL-ē-ăr-ē	_____
bilirubin (148)	bĭl-ĭ-ROO-bĭn	_____
bowel (148)	BŎW-ĕl	_____
buccal mucosa (150)	BŬK-ăl mū-KŌ-să	_____
canine teeth (148)	KĀ-nīn tēth	_____
cecal (151)	SĒ-kăl	_____
cecum (148)	SĒ-kŭm	_____
celiac (151)	SĒ-lē-ăk	_____
cheilitis (151)	kī-LĪ-tĭs	_____
cholecystectomy (151)	kō-lĕ-sĭs-TĔK-tō-mē	_____
choledocholithiasis (155)	kō-lĕ-dō-kō-lĭ-THĪ-ă-sĭs	_____
choledochojejunostomy (153)	kō-lĕ-dō-kō-jĭ-jū-NŎS-tō-mē	_____
choledochotomy (151)	kō-lĕ-dō-KŎT-ō-mē	_____
cholelithiasis (155)	kō-lē-lĭ-THĪ-ă-sĭs	_____

Term	Pronunciation	Meaning
colon (148)	KŌ-lŏn	_____
colonic (151)	kō-LŎN-ĭk	_____
colonoscopy (151)	kō-lŏn-ŎS-kō-pē	_____
colostomy (151)	kŏ-LŎS-tō-mē	_____
common bile duct (148)	KŎM-ŏn bīl dŭkt	_____
defecation (148)	dĕf-ĕ-KĀ-shŭn	_____
deglutition (148)	dē-gloo-TĬSH-ŭn	_____
dentibuccal (151)	dĕn-tĭ-BŬK-ăl	_____
dentin (148)	DĔN-tĭn	_____
digestion (148)	dī-JĔST-yŭn	_____
duodenal (151)	dū-ō-DĒ-năl *or* dū-ŎD-ĕ-năl	_____
duodenum (148)	dū-ō-DĒ-nŭm *or* dū-ŎD-ĕ-nŭm	_____
elimination (148)	ē-lĭm-ĭ-NĀ-shŭn	_____
emulsification (148)	ē-mŭl-sĭ-fĭ-KĀ-shŭn	_____
enamel (148)	ē-NĂM-ĕl	_____
endodontist (154)	ĕn-dō-DŎN-tĭst	_____
enterocolitis (152)	ĕn-tĕr-ō-kō-LĪ-tĭs	_____
enterocolostomy (152)	ĕn-tĕr-ō-kō-LŎS-tō-mē	_____
enzyme (148)	ĔN-zīm	_____
esophageal (152)	ĕ-sŏf-ă-JĒ-ăl	_____
esophagus (148)	ĕ-SŎF-ă-gŭs	_____
fatty acid (149)	FĂT-tē Ă-sĭd	_____
facial (152)	FĀ-shŭl	_____
feces (149)	FĒ-sēz	_____
gallbladder (149)	găwl-BLĂ-dĕr	_____
gastrointestinal tract (138)	găs-trō-ĭn-TĔS-tĭn-ăl trăct	_____
gastrojejunostomy (153)	găs-trō-jĕ-jū-NŎS-tō-mē	_____
gastrostomy (153)	găs-TRŎS-tō-mē	_____
gingivitis (153)	jĭn-jĭ-VĪ-tĭs	_____
gluconeogenesis (155)	gloo-kō-nē-ō-JĔN-ĕ-sĭs	_____
glucose (149)	GLOO-kōs	_____
glycogen (149)	GLĪ-kō-jĕn	_____
glycogenolysis (155)	glī-kō-jĕ-NŎL-ĭ-sĭs	_____

5

Term	Pronunciation	Meaning
hepatoma (153)	hĕ-pă-TŌ-mă	
hepatomegaly (153)	hĕ-pă-tō-MĔG-ă-lē	
hydrochloric acid (149)	hī-drō-KLŌR-ĭk Ă-sĭd	
hyperbilirubinemia (155)	hī-pĕr-bĭl-ĭ-roo-bĭ-NĒ-mē-ă	
hyperglycemia (155)	hī-pĕr-glī-SĒ-mē-ă	
hypoglossal (153)	hī-pō-GLŎ-săl	
ileitis (153)	ĭl-ē-Ī-tĭs	
ileocecal sphincter (153)	ĭl-ē-ō-SĒ-kăl SFĬNK-tĕr	
ileostomy (153)	ĭl-ē-ŎS-tō-mē	
ileum (149)	ĬL-ē-ŭm	
incisor (149)	ĭn-SĪ-zŏr	
insulin (149)	ĬN-sŭ-lĭn	
jejunum (149)	jĕ-JOO-nŭm	
labial (154)	LĀ-bē-ăl	
laparoscopy (154)	lă-pă-RŎS-kō-pē	
lipase (149)	LĪ-pās	
lithogenesis (155)	lĭth-ō-JĔN-ĕ-sĭs	
liver (149)	LĬ-vĕr	
lower esophageal sphincter (149)	LŌW-ĕr ĕ-sŏf-ă-JĒ-ăl SFĬNGK-tĕr	
mastication (149)	măs-tĭ-KĀ-shŭn	
mesentery (152)	MĔS-ĕn-tĕr-ē	
molar teeth (149)	MŌ-lăr tēth	
oral (154)	ŎR-ăl	
orthodontist (154)	ŏr-thō-DŎN-tĭst	
palate (149)	PĂL-ăt	
palatopharyngoplasty (154)	păl-ă-tō-fă-RĬNG-gō-plăs-tē	
palatoplasty (154)	PĂL-ă-tō-plăs-tē	
pancreas (149)	PĂN-krē-ăs	
pancreatitis (154)	păn-krē-ă-TĪ-tĭs	
papillae (149)	pă-PĬL-ē	
parenteral (152)	pă-RĔN-tĕr-ăl	
parotid gland (149)	pă-RŎT-ĭd glănd	

Term	Pronunciation	Meaning
perianal (150)	pĕ-rē-Ā-năl	_____
periodontist (154)	pĕr-ē-ō-DŎN-tĭst	_____
peritonitis (154)	pĕr-ĭ-tō-NĪ-tĭs	_____
peristalsis (149)	pĕr-ĭ-STĂL-sĭs	_____
pharyngeal (154)	făr-ăn-JĒ-ăl _or_ fă-RĬN-jē-ăl	_____
pharynx (149)	FĂR-ĭnks	_____
portal vein (149)	PŎR-tăl vān	_____
postprandial (155)	pōst-PRĂN-dē-ăl	_____
premolar teeth (149)	prē-MŌ-lăr tēth	_____
proctologist (154)	prŏk-TŎL-ō-jĭst	_____
protease (149)	PRŌ-tē-āse	_____
pulp (150)	pŭlp	_____
pyloric sphincter (150)	pī-LŎR-ĭk SFĬNK-tĕr	_____
pyloroplasty (154)	pī-LŎR-ō-plăs-tē	_____
pylorus (150)	pī-LŎR-ŭs	_____
rectocele (154)	RĔK-tō-sēl	_____
rectum (150)	RĔK-tŭm	_____
rugae (150)	ROO-gē	_____
saliva (150)	să-LĪ-vă	_____
salivary glands (150)	SĂL-ĭ-vār-ē glăndz	_____
sialadenitis (154)	sī-ăl-ă-dĕ-NĪ-tĭs	_____
sialolith (155)	sī-ĂL-ō-lĭth	_____
sigmoid colon (150)	SĬG-moyd KŌ-lŏn	_____
sigmoidoscopy (154)	sĭg-moyd-ŎS-kō-pē	_____
sphincter (150)	SFĬNGK-tĕr	_____
steatorrhea (157)	stē-ă-tō-RĒ-ă	_____
stomatitis (154)	stō-mă-TĬ-tĭs	_____
sublingual (154)	sŭb-LĬNG-wăl	_____
submandibular (154)	sŭb-măn-DĬB-ū-lăr	_____
triglycerides (150)	trī-GLĬ-sĕ-rīdz	_____
uvula (150)	Ū-vū-lă	_____
uvulectomy (154)	ū-vū-LĔK-tō-mē	_____
villi (150)	VĬL-ī	_____

5

PATHOLOGIC TERMINOLOGY

Term	Pronunciation	Meaning
achalasia (158)	ăk-ăh-LĀ-zē-ă	_____
anal fistula (160)	Ā-năl FĬS-tū-lă	_____
anorexia (156)	ăn-ō-RĔK-sē-ă	_____
aphthous stomatitis (158)	ĂF-thŭs stō-mă-TĪ-tĭs	_____
ascites (156)	ă-SĪ-tēz	_____
borborygmus (156)	bŏr-bō-RĬG-mŭs	_____
cholelithiasis (164)	kō-lĕ-lĭ-THĪ-ă-sĭs	_____
cirrhosis (165)	sĭr-RŌ-sĭs	_____
colonic polyposis (161)	kō-LŎN-ĭk pŏl-ĭ-PŌ-sĭs	_____
colorectal cancer (161)	kō-lō-RĔK-tăl KĂN-sĕr	_____
constipation (157)	cŏn-stĭ-PĀ-shŭn	_____
Crohn's disease (162)	krōnz dĭ-ZĒZ	_____
dental caries (158)	DĔN-tăl KĂR-ēz	_____
diarrhea (157)	dī-ăh-RĒ-ă	_____
diverticula (162)	dī-vĕr-TĬK-ū-lă	_____
diverticulitis (162)	dī-vĕr-tĭk-ū-LĪ-tĭs	_____
diverticulosis (162)	dī-vĕr-tĭk-ū-LŌ-sĭs	_____
dysentery (162)	DĬS-ĕn-tĕr-ē	_____
dysphagia (157)	dĭs-PHĀ-jē-ă	_____
eructation (157)	ē-rŭk-TĀ-shŭn	_____
esophageal varices (158)	ĕ-sŏf-ă-JĒ-ăl VĂR-ĭ-sēz	_____
etiology (156)	ē-tē-ŎL-ō-jē	_____
flatus (157)	FLĀ-tŭs	_____
gastric carcinoma (160)	GĂS-trĭk kăr-sĭ-NŌ-mă	_____
gastroesophageal reflux disease (160)	găs-trō-ĕ-sŏf-ă-JĒ-ăl RĒ-flŭx dĭ-ZĒZ	_____
hematochezia (157)	hē-mă-tō-KĒ-zē-ă	_____
hemorrhoids (162)	HĔM-ō-roydz	_____
herpetic stomatitis (158)	hĕr-PĔT-ĭk stō-mă-TĪ-tĭs	_____
hiatal hernia (160)	hī-Ā-tăl HĔR-nē-ă	_____
icterus (157)	ĬK-tĕr-ŭs	_____
idiopathic (156)	ĭd-ē-ō-PĂTH-ĭk	_____

5

Term	Pronunciation	Meaning
ileus (162)	ĬL-ē-ŭs	_____
inflammatory bowel disease (162)	ĭn-FLĂ-mă-tō-rē BŎW-ĕl dĭ-ZĒZ	_____
inguinal hernia (160)	ĬNG-wĭ-năl HĔR-nē-ă	_____
intussusception (163)	ĭn-tŭs-sŭs-SĔP-shŭn	_____
irritable bowel syndrome (163)	ĬR-ĭ-tă-b'l BŎW-ĕl SĬN-drōm	_____
jaundice (157)	JĂWN-dĭs	_____
melena (157)	MĔL-ĕ-nă *or* mĕ-LĒ-nă	_____
nausea (157)	NĂW-zē-ă	_____
odynophagia (157)	ō-dĭn-ō-FĀ-jă	_____
oral leukoplakia (158)	ŎR-ăl lū-kō-PLĀ-kē-ă	_____
pancreatitis (165)	păn-krē-ă-TĪ-tĭs	_____
peptic ulcer (160)	PĔP-tĭc ŬL-sĕr	_____
periodontal disease (158)	pĕr-ē-ō-DŎN-tăl dĭ-ZĒZ	_____
ulcerative colitis (163)	ŬL-sĕr-ă-tĭv kō-LĪ-tĭs	_____
viral hepatitis (165)	VĪ-răl hĕp-ă-TĪ-tĭs	_____
volvulus (163)	VŎL-vū-lŭs	_____

Note: The review sheet for this chapter is combined with the review sheet for Chapter 6 on page 208.

 Please refer to the enclosed CD for additional exercises and images related to this chapter.

chapter 6

Additional Suffixes and Digestive System Terminology

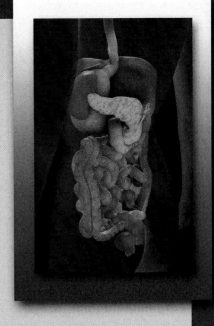

THIS CHAPTER IS DIVIDED INTO THE FOLLOWING SECTIONS

In this chapter you will

- Define new suffixes and use them with digestive system combining forms.
- List and explain laboratory tests, clinical procedures, and abbreviations relevant to the digestive system.
- Apply your new knowledge to understanding medical terms in their proper context, such as in medical reports and records.

Image Description: Posterior view, angled to the left side, of a female torso containing the digestive system.

INTRODUCTION

This chapter gives you practice in word building, while not introducing a large number of new terms. It uses many familiar terms from Chapter 5, which should give you a breather after your hard work.

Study the new suffixes first and complete the meanings of the terms. Checking the meanings of the terms with a dictionary may prove helpful and add another dimension to your understanding.

The information included under Laboratory Tests and Clinical Procedures and in the Abbreviations section relates to the gastrointestinal system and will be useful for work in clinical or laboratory medical settings.

The Practical Applications section gives you examples of medical language in context. Congratulate yourself as you decipher medical sentences, operative reports, case studies, and other material.

SUFFIXES

Write the meaning of the medical term in the space provided.

Suffix	Meaning	Terminology	Meaning
-ectasis, -ectasia	stretching, dilation, dilatation; widening	bronchiectasis _____ *Bronchi/o means bronchial tubes. Often the result of chronic infection or obstruction of bronchial tubes.* lymphangiectasia _____ *Dilation of smaller lymphatic vessels usually results from obstruction in larger vessels.*	
-emesis	vomiting	hematemesis _____ *Bright red blood is vomited, often associated with esophageal varices or peptic ulcer.*	
-lysis	destruction, breakdown, separation	hemolysis _____ *Red blood cells are destroyed.*	
-pepsia	digestion	dyspepsia _____	
-phagia	eating, swallowing	polyphagia *deficult to swallowing* _____ *Excessive appetite and uncontrolled eating.* dysphagia _____ *Difficulty in swallowing. Often associated with obstruction or motor (movement) disorder of the esophagus.* odynophagia _____ *Pain (odyn/o) caused by swallowing.*	

Dysphagia/Dysphasia/Dysplasia
Don't confuse *dysphagia* with *dysplasia,* which is abnormal formation (plas/o = formation).

Suffix	Meaning	Terminology	Meaning
-plasty	surgical repair	rhinoplasty _____	
		The structure of the nose is changed.	
		enteroplasty _____	
		A STEP (serial transverse enteroplasty) procedure lengthens a short bowel so that enteral feeding is possible.	
		blepharoplasty _____	
-ptosis	droop; sag; protrude	proptosis _____	
		Pro- means before, forward. This term refers to the forward protrusion of the eye (exophthalmos).	
-ptysis	spitting	hemoptysis _____	
		From the respiratory tract and lungs.	
-rrhage, -rrhagia	bursting forth (of blood)	hemorrhage _feist_ _____	
		Loss of a large amount of blood in a short period.	
		menorrhagia _____	
		Excessive bleeding at the time of menstruation. Men/o means menstrual flow or menstruation.	
-rrhaphy	suture	herniorrhaphy _____	
		Repair (as in stitching or suturing) of a hernia. Herni/o means hernia.	
-rrhea	flow, discharge	dysmenorrhea _____	
		Pain associated with menstruation.	
-spasm	sudden, involuntary contraction of muscles	pylorospasm _____	
		bronchospasm _____	
		A chief characteristic of bronchitis and asthma.	
-stasis	to stop; control	cholestasis _____	
		Flow of bile from the liver to the duodenum is interrupted.	
		hemostasis _____	
		Bleeding is stopped by mechanical or chemical means, or by the coagulation process of the body.	
-stenosis	tightening, stricture, narrowing	pyloric stenosis _____	
		This is a congenital defect in newborns blocking the flow of food into the small intestine. Pyloromyotomy can correct the condition.	
-tresia	opening	atresia _____	
		Absence of a normal opening.	
		esophageal atresia _____	
		A congenital anomaly in which the esophagus does not connect with the stomach. A tracheoesophageal fistula often accompanies this abnormality (Fig. 6–1).	
		biliary atresia _____	
		Congenital hypoplasia or nonformation of bile ducts causes neonatal cholestasis and jaundice.	

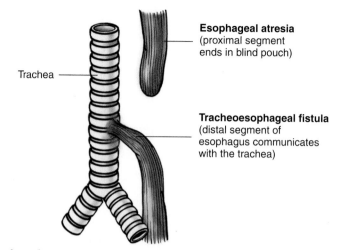

FIGURE 6–1   **Esophageal atresia with tracheoesophageal fistula.** (From Cotran RS, Kumar V, Collins T [eds]: Robbins Pathologic Basis of Disease, 6th ed. Philadelphia, WB Saunders, 1999, p. 777.)

Suffixes listed on pages 184 and 185 also are used alone as separate terms. Here are examples of such terms as used in a sentence.

emesis (emetic)	If a child swallows poison, physicians prescribe a drug to induce **emesis.** An example of an emetic is a strong solution of salt or ipecac syrup.
lysis	The disease caused **lysis** of liver cells.
ptosis	Mr. Smith's weakened eyelid muscles caused **ptosis** of his lids.
spasm	Eating spicy foods can lead to **spasm** of gastric sphincters.
stasis	Overgrowth of bacteria within the small intestine causes **stasis** of the intestinal contents.
stenosis	Projectile vomiting in an infant during feeding is a symptom of pyloric **stenosis.**

COMBINING FORMS AND TERMINOLOGY

Write the meaning of the combining form and then the meaning of the term that includes that combining form in the spaces provided.

Combining Form	Meaning	Terminology	Meaning
bucc/o	_____	buccal	_pertaining to the cheek_
cec/o	_____	cecal volvulus	_____
celi/o	_____	celiac disease	_____
		*This is an inherited autoimmune disease. Villi in the small intestine are damaged from eating gluten found in barley and rye. Malabsorption and malnutrition occur. Treatment consists of a lifelong gluten-free diet. Also called **celiac sprue.***	

Combining Form	Meaning	Terminology	Meaning
cheil/o	_____	cheilosis _____ _Characterized by scales and fissures on the lips and resulting from a deficiency of vitamin B_2 in the diet._	
chol/e	_____	cholelithiasis _____	
cholangi/o	_____	cholangiectasis _____ _Bile vessels are bile ducts._	
cholecyst/o	_____	cholecystectomy _____	
choledoch/o	_____	choledochal _____	
col/o	_____	colectomy _____ _Surgeons perform laparoscopic assisted colectomy (LAC) as an alternative to open colectomy to remove nonmetastatic colorectal carcinomas._	
colon/o	_____	colonoscopy _____	
dent/i	_____	dentalgia _____	
duoden/o	_____	gastroduodenal anastomosis _____	
enter/o	_____	gastroenteritis _____	
esophag/o	_____	esophageal atresia _____ _This congenital anomaly must be corrected surgically._	
gastr/o	_____	gastrojejunostomy _stomach_ _____	
		gastrostomy _____ _A PEG (percutaneous endoscopic gastrostomy) tube is inserted (laparoscopically) through the abdomen into the stomach to deliver food and liquids when swallowing is impossible. Also called a G tube._	
gingiv/o	_____	gingivectomy _____	
gloss/o	_____	glossopharyngeal _____	
glyc/o	_____	glycolysis _____	
hepat/o	_____	hepatomegaly _____	
herni/o	_____	herniorrhaphy _____	
ile/o	_____	ileostomy _____	
jejun/o	_____	cholecystojejunostomy _____	
labi/o	_____	labioglossopharyngeal _____	
lingu/o	_____	sublingual _____	

colncysts

6

Combining Form	Meaning	Terminology	Meaning
lip/o		lipase	
lith/o	stone	cholecystolithiasis	
odont/o		periodontal membrane	
or/o	oral	oropharynx	
		The tonsils are located in the oropharynx.	
palat/o		palatoplasty	
		Also called palatorrhaphy, this procedure corrects cleft (split) palate, a congenital anomaly.	
pancreat/o		pancreatic	
proct/o		proctosigmoidoscopy	
pylor/o		pyloric stenosis	
rect/o	rectum	rectocele	
sialaden/o		sialadenectomy	
splen/o		splenic flexure	
		The downward bend in the transverse colon near the spleen.	
steat/o		steatorrhea	
stomat/o	mouth	aphthous stomatitis	

LABORATORY TESTS AND CLINICAL PROCEDURES

LABORATORY TESTS

liver function tests (LFTs)   **Tests for the presence of enzymes and bilirubin in serum** (clear fluid that remains after blood has clotted).

Examples are the aminotransferase enzymes **ALT** (*al*anine *t*ransaminase) and **AST** (*a*spartate *t*ransaminase). ALT was formerly called SGPT (*s*erum *g*lutamic-*p*yruvic *t*ransaminase), and AST was called SGOT (*s*erum *g*lutamic-*o*xaloacetic *t*ransaminase). ALT and AST are present in many tissues, and levels are elevated in the serum of patients with liver disease. High ALT and AST levels indicate damage to liver cells (as in hepatitis).

Alkaline phosphatase (alk phos) is another enzyme that may be elevated in patients with liver, bone, and other diseases.

Serum bilirubin levels are elevated in patients with liver disease and jaundice. A **direct bilirubin test** measures conjugated bilirubin (combined with a substance in the liver). High levels indicate liver disease or biliary obstruction. An **indirect bilirubin test** measures unconjugated bilirubin. Increased levels mean excessive hemolysis, as may occur in a newborn.

stool culture	**Test for microorganisms present in feces.** Feces are placed in a growth medium and examined microscopically.
stool guaiac or Hemoccult test	**Detection of occult (hidden) blood in feces.** This is an important screening test for colon cancer. **Guaiac** (GWĪ-ăk) is a chemical from the wood of trees. When added to a stool sample, it reacts with any blood present in the feces.

CLINICAL PROCEDURES

X-Ray Tests

lower gastrointestinal series (barium enema)	**X-ray images of the colon and rectum obtained after injection of barium into the rectum.** Radiologists inject barium, a contrast medium (substance that x-rays cannot penetrate), by enema into the rectum. Figure 6–2A shows a barium enema study of a colon with diverticulosis.
upper gastrointestinal series	**X-ray images of the esophagus, stomach, and small intestine obtained after administering barium by mouth.** Often performed immediately after an upper gastrointestinal series, a **small bowel follow-through** shows sequential x-ray pictures of the small intestine as barium passes through (Fig. 6–2B). A **barium swallow** is a study of the esophagus.

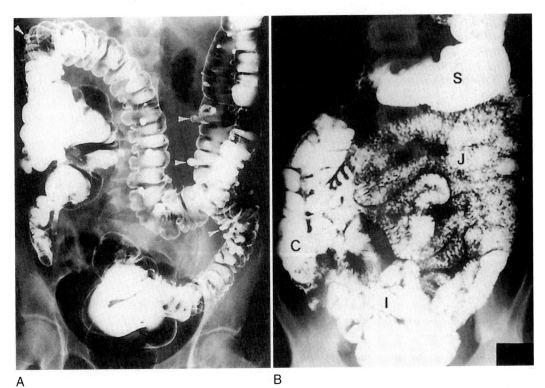

A   B

FIGURE 6–2 A, Barium enema. This x-ray record of a barium enema with air contrast demonstrates diverticulosis. The *arrowheads* point to the diverticula throughout the colon. A majority of patients with diverticula are asymptomatic, but complications (diverticulitis, perforated diverticulum, obstruction, or hemorrhage) may occur. **B,** An x-ray record of a **small bowel follow-through** study demonstrating the normal appearance of the jejunum (J) in the upper left abdomen and of the ileum (I) in the right lower abdomen. Notice the contrast material within the stomach (S) and cecum (C). (From Heuman DM, Mills AS, McGuire HH: Gastroenterology. Philadelphia, WB Saunders, 1997, pp. 120 and 110.)

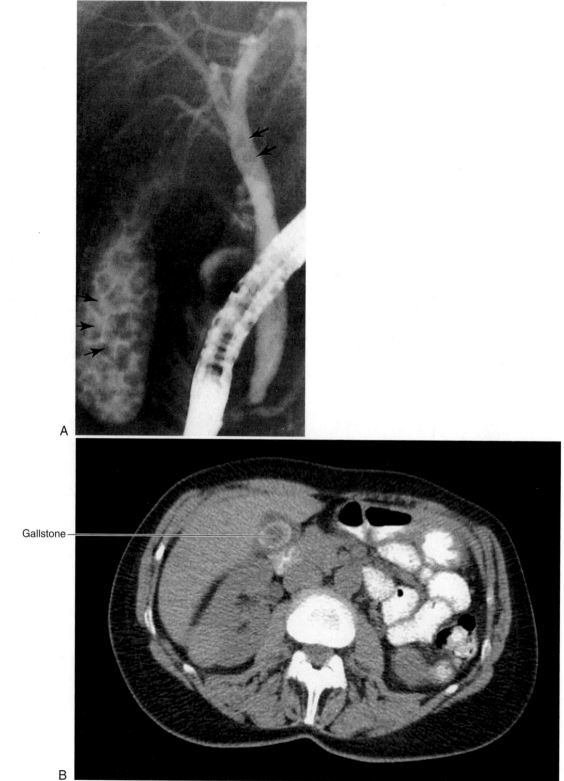

A

Gallstone

B

FIGURE 6–3 **A, Endoscopic retrograde cholangiopancreatography (ERCP) showing choledocholithiasis** in a patient with biliary colic (pain). Multiple stones are visible in the gallbladder and common bile duct. The stones (*arrows*) are seen as filling defects in the contrast-opacified gallbladder and duct. This patient was treated with open (via laparotomy) cholecystectomy and choledocholithotomy. **B, Computed tomography scan** with contrast showing large "porcelain stone" in the gallbladder. The patient was asymptomatic, but a therapeutic option with this type of stone is removal of her gallbladder (using laparoscopy) to prevent any future problems (cholecystitis or gallbladder carcinoma). (**A** from Heuman DM, Mills AS, McGuire HH: Gastroenterology. Philadelphia, WB Saunders, 1997, p. 87; **B** courtesy Radiology Department, Massachusetts General Hospital, Boston.)

cholangiography	**X-ray examination of the biliary system performed after injection of contrast into the bile ducts.**

In **percutaneous transhepatic cholangiography,** the contrast medium enters via a needle through the abdominal wall into the liver. In **endoscopic retrograde cholangiopancreatography (ERCP)** (Figure 6–3, *A*), contrast medium is injected via catheter (tube) through the mouth, esophagus, stomach, and duodenum and then into bile ducts.

computed tomography (CT)	**Imaging technique in which a series of x-ray films are obtained to visualize internal organs in multiple views including in cross section.**

A CT scan is performed using a circular array of x-ray beams to produce the cross-sectional image based on differences in tissue densities. Use of contrast material allows visualization of the GI tract, blood vessels, and organs (Figs. 6–3, *B*, and 6–4, *A, B,* and *C*). **Tomography** (tom/o means to cut) produces a *series* of x-ray

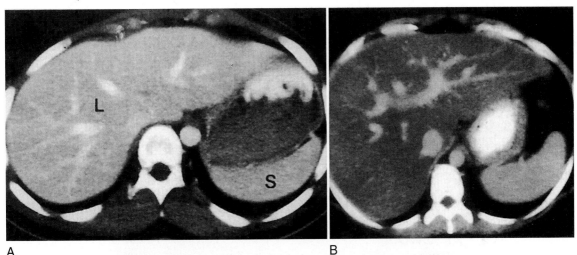

A   B

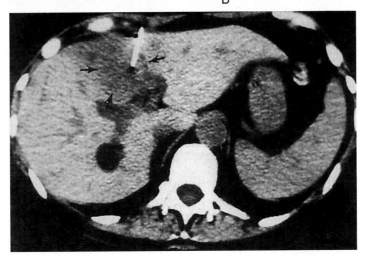

C

FIGURE 6–4   Computed tomography (CT) images of normal and diseased liver. **A, Normal liver.** Contrast material has been injected intravenously, making blood vessels appear bright. The liver (L) and spleen (S) have the same density on this CT image. **B, Fatty liver.** The radiodensity of the liver tissue is reduced because of the large volume of fat contained in the tissue, making it appear darker than normal. Compare the appearance of the spleen. **C, CT-guided needle aspiration biopsy of a liver lesion.** The lesion (*arrows*) has a lower density than that of the surrounding liver. A needle has been placed into the liver tissue, and its tip can be seen in the center of the lesion. Microscopic examination of material aspirated from the lesion revealed it to be a hepatocellular carcinoma. CT-guided needle placement also can be used to insert a catheter for drainage of a liver abscess (a collection of infection and pus). (From Heuman DM, Mills AS, McGuire HH: Gastroenterology. Philadelphia, WB Saunders, 1997, p. 166.)

pictures showing multiple views of an organ. (An earlier name for a CT scan is "CAT scan" [computerized axial tomography scan].)

Ultrasound Examination

abdominal ultrasonography (ultrasound examination or sonography)

Sound waves beamed into the abdomen produce an image of abdominal viscera.

Ultrasonography is especially useful for examination of fluid-filled structures such as the gallbladder.

Magnetic Resonance Techniques

magnetic resonance imaging (MRI)

Magnetic and radio waves produce images of organs and tissues in all three planes of the body.

This technique does not use x-rays and shows subtle differences in tissue composition.

Radionuclide Studies

liver scan

Image of the liver after injecting radioactive material into the blood stream.

Radioactive material (a pharmaceutical radionuclide) is injected intravenously and taken up by the liver cells. An image of the liver (scintiscan) is made using a special scanner (gamma camera) that records radioisotope uptake by the liver cells.

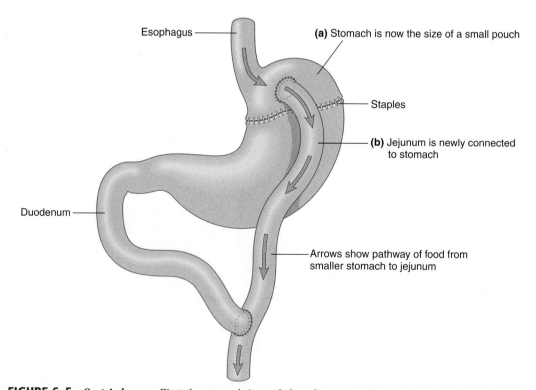

FIGURE 6–5 **Gastric bypass.** First the stomach is stapled so that it is reduced to the size of a small pouch **(a)**. Next, a shortened jejunum is brought up to connect with the smaller stomach **(b)**. This diverts food so that it has a shorter travel time through the intestine and less food is absorbed into the bloodstream.

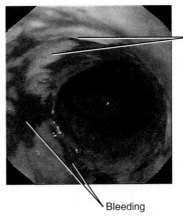

Erosion/inflammation of esophageal mucosa

Bleeding

FIGURE 6–6 Esophagogastroduodenoscopy. This endoscopic view shows severe esophagitis in a patient who had gastroesophageal reflux disease (GERD). (From Black JM, Hawks JH: Medical-Surgical Nursing: Clinical Management for Positive Outcomes, 7th ed. Philadelphia, WB Saunders, 2005.)

Other Procedures

gastric bypass

Reducing the size of the stomach and diverting food to the jejunum (gastrojejunostomy).

This is bariatric (bar/o = weight) surgery for severe obesity. The Roux-en-Y gastric bypass procedure reduces the size of the stomach to a volume of 2 tablespoons and bypasses a large section of the small intestine. See Figure 6–5.

gastrointestinal endoscopy

Visual examination of the gastrointestinal tract using an endoscope.

A physician places a flexible fiberoptic tube through the mouth or the anus to view parts of the gastrointestinal tract. Examples are **esophagogastroduodenoscopy** (Fig. 6–6), **colonoscopy** (Figs. 6–7 and 6–8), **sigmoidoscopy, proctoscopy,** and **anoscopy.**

Virtual colonoscopy (CT colonography) combines CT scanning and computer technology to enable physicians to examine the entire length of the colon noninvasively in just minutes. Because this is only a screening procedure, patients with positive findings require conventional colonoscopy afterward.

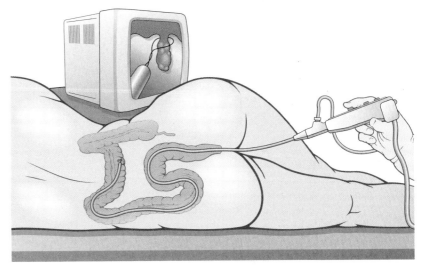

FIGURE 6–7 Colonoscopy with polypectomy. Before the procedure, the patient ingests agents to clean the bowel of feces. The patient is sedated and the gastroenterologist advances the instrument in retrograde fashion, guided by images from a video camera on the tip of the colonoscope. When a polyp is located, a wire snare is passed through the endoscope and looped around the stalk. After the loop is gently tightened, an electric current is applied to cut through the stalk. The polyp is removed for microscopic tissue examination (biopsy).

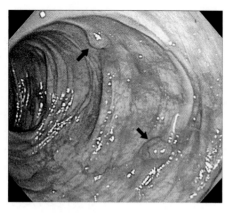

FIGURE 6–8 Colonoscopy case report. A 60-year-old man with a history of multiple and prominent colon adenomas (some high-grade dysplasia) underwent colonoscopy. The endoscope was passed through the anus and advanced to the cecum. Two pedunculated polyps were found at the hepatic flexure. Polypectomy was performed with a hot snare. Resection and retrieval were complete. (From Weinstein WM, Hawkey CJ, Bosch J: Clinical Gastroenterology and Hepatology, St. Louis, Mosby, 2005.)

laparoscopy

Visual (endoscopic) examination of the abdomen with a laparoscope inserted through small incisions in the abdomen.

Laparoscopic cholecystectomy (see Fig. 5–26, page 165) and laparoscopic appendectomy are performed by gastrointestinal and general surgeons.

liver biopsy

Removal of liver tissue followed by microscopic visualization.

A physician inserts a needle through the skin to remove a small piece of tissue for microscopic examination. The average sample is less than 1 inch long. The procedure helps doctors diagnose cirrhosis, chronic hepatitis, and tumors of the liver.

nasogastric intubation

Insertion of a tube through the nose into the stomach.

Physicians use a nasogastric (NG) tube to remove fluid postoperatively and to obtain gastric or intestinal contents for analysis. See Figure 6-9.

paracentesis (abdominocentesis)

Surgical puncture to remove fluid from the abdomen.

This procedure is necessary to drain fluid (accumulated in ascites) from the peritoneal (abdominal) cavity.

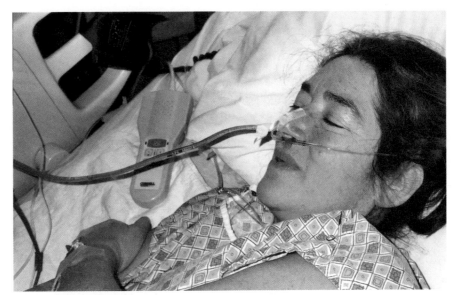

FIGURE 6–9 **Nasogastric intubation.** This patient is recovering from surgery, and the nasogastric tube is suctioning secretions from the stomach postoperatively.

ABBREVIATIONS

alk phos	alkaline phosphatase
ALT, AST	alanine transaminase, aspartate transaminase—enzymes measured to evaluate liver function
BE	barium enema
BM	bowel movement
BRBPR	bright red blood per rectum—hematochezia (Latin *per* means through)
CT	computed tomography
EGD	esophagogastroduodenoscopy
ERCP	endoscopic retrograde cholangiopancreatography
FOBT	fecal occult blood test
G tube	gastrostomy tube; also called stomach tube and PEG tube—used to introduce nutrients into the stomach after insertion through the abdominal wall with laparoscopic instruments
GB	gallbladder
GERD	gastroesophageal reflux disease
GI	gastrointestinal
HBV	hepatitis B virus
IBD	inflammatory bowel disease
LAC	laparoscopic assisted colectomy
LFTs	liver function tests—alk phos, bilirubin, AST (SGOT), ALT (SGPT)
MRI	magnetic resonance imaging
NG tube	nasogastric tube
NPO	nothing by mouth (Latin *nil per os*)
PEG tube	percutaneous endoscopic gastrostomy tube—feeding tube
PEJ tube	percutaneous endoscopic jejunostomy tube—feeding tube
PTHC	percutaneous transhepatic cholangiography
PUD	peptic ulcer disease
STEP	serial transverse enteroplasty
TPN	total parenteral nutrition
	Intravenous TPN solutions typically contain sugar (dextrose), proteins (amino acids), electrolytes (sodium, potassium, chloride), and vitamins.
T tube	tube placed in the biliary tract for drainage

PRACTICAL APPLICATIONS

Reproduced here is an actual medical report using terms that you have studied in this and previous chapters. Explanations of more difficult terms are added in brackets. Questions based on your reading of the report follow. Check your answers on page 205 in the Answers to Exercises section.

COLONOSCOPY REPORT

The patient is a 73-year-old female who underwent colonoscopy and polypectomy on June 10, 1997. Biopsy revealed an invasive carcinoma, and on June 12, 1997, she underwent a low anterior resection and coloproctostomy. Sixteen months later, on August 2, 1998, she was seen in the office for flexible sigmoidoscopy, and a polyp was detected. Colonoscopy was scheduled.

Description of Procedure. The fiberoptic colonoscope was introduced, and I could pass it to about 15 cm, at which point there appeared to be an anastomosis. The colonoscope passed easily through a wide-open anastomosis to 30 cm, at which point a very friable [easily crumbled] polyp, irregular, on a short little stalk, was encountered. This was snared, the coagulating [blood-clotting] current was applied, and the pedicle [stalk of the polyp] was severed and recovered and sent to pathology for histological identification. The colonoscope was then reintroduced and passed through the rectum to the sigmoid colon. Again the anastomosis was seen, and proximal to this, the fulgurated [destroyed by high-frequency electric current] base of the removed polyp could be seen. No bleeding was encountered, and I continued to advance the colonoscope through the descending colon. I proceeded to advance the colonoscope through the splenic flexure in the transverse colon. Despite vigorous mechanical bowel preparation and the shortened colon from the previous resection, she had a considerable amount of stool, and it became progressively more difficult to visualize as I approached the hepatic flexure. Finally, at the hepatic flexure, I abandoned further evaluation and began to withdraw the colonoscope. The colonoscope passed through the transverse colon, splenic flexure, descending colon, sigmoid colon, rectum, and anus and was withdrawn. She tolerated the procedure well, but had some nausea. I will await the results of pathology, and in the event that it is not an invasive carcinoma, I would recommend a repeat colonoscopy in 6 months, at which time we will use a 48-hour, more vigorous mechanical bowel preparation.

Questions about the Colonoscopy Report

1. On June 10, the initial procedure that the patient underwent was
   a. Anastomosis of two parts of the colon
   b. Visual examination of the rectum and anus
   c. Visual examination of the large bowel and removal of a growth
   d. Resection of a portion of the colon

2. On June 12 the patient had additional surgery to
   a. Remove a portion of the colon and reattach the cut end to the rectum.
   b. Join two parts of the small intestine.
   c. Reconnect the colon to the small intestine.
   d. Remove a portion of the distal end of the small intestine.

3. Which term in the report refers to an anastomosis?
   a. Sigmoidoscopy
   b. Colonoscopy
   c. Low anterior resection
   d. Coloproctostomy

4. Why was it impossible to visualize the entire colon?
   a. The patient experienced nausea.
   b. Feces were blocking the colon.
   c. Tumor was blocking the colon.
   d. The hepatic flexure was twisted.

? EXERCISES

6

Remember to check your answers carefully with those given in the Answers to Exercises, page 204.

A. Give the meanings of the following suffixes.

1. -pepsia ___digestion___

2. -ptysis ___breakdown / separation___

3. -emesis ___vomiting___

4. -phagia ___eating / swallowing___

5. -ptosis ___prolapse___

6. -rrhea ___discharge___

7. -rrhagia ___bursting forth___

8. -rrhaphy ___suture___

9. -plasty ___surgical___

10. -lysis ___breakdown___

11. -ectasis ___dilatation___

12. -stenosis ___thightening___

13. -stasis ___contraction___

14. -spasm ___sudden contraction of muscle___

15. -ectasia ___dilatation___

B. Using the suffixes from exercise A and the combining forms below, build medical terms.

blephar/o   hemat/o   men/o
bronch/o   herni/o   pylor/o
chol/e   lymphangi/o   rhin/o
hem/o

1. painful menstrual flow _____

2. stoppage of bile (flow) _____

3. suture of a hernia _____

4. dilation of lymph vessels _____

5. spitting up blood (from the respiratory tract) _____

6. vomiting blood (from the digestive tract) _____

7. dilation of tubes leading from the windpipe into the lungs _____

8. surgical repair of eyelids _____

9. stopping blood flow _____

10. surgical repair of the nose _____

11. destruction of blood (red blood cells) _____

12. sudden, involuntary contraction of muscles at the distal region of the stomach _____

13. excessive bleeding (bursting forth of blood) during menstruation _____

14. sudden, involuntary contraction of muscles within the bronchial tubes _____

C. Give the meanings of the following terms.

1. dysphagia _____

2. polyphagia _____

3. dyspepsia _____

4. biliary atresia _____

5. proptosis _____

6. cholestasis _____

7. esophageal atresia _____

8. odynophagia _____

9. splenorrhagia _____

10. proctosigmoidoscopy _____

D. Match the following surgical procedures with their meanings below.

blepharoplasty	colectomy	ileostomy
cecostomy	gastroduodenal anastomosis	paracentesis
cholecystectomy	gingivectomy	rectocele
cholecystojejunostomy	herniorrhaphy	sphincterotomy

1. removal of the gallbladder _____

2. large bowel resection ____*colectomy*_____

3. suture of a weakened muscular wall (hernia) _____

4. new opening of the first part of the colon to the outside of the body ___*cecostomy*___

5. surgical repair of the eyelid _____

6. incision of a ring of muscles _____

7. new surgical connection between the stomach and the first part of the small intestine

   _____*gastroduodenal anastomosis*_____

8. opening of the third part of the small intestine to the outside of the body _____

9. removal of gum tissue _____

10. new surgical connection between the gallbladder and the second part of the small intestine

   _____

11. surgical puncture of the abdomen for withdrawal of fluid _____

12. hernia of the rectum _____

6

E. Use the given meanings to complete the following terms.

1. discharge of fat: steat_____

2. difficulty in swallowing: dys_____

3. abnormal condition of gallstones: chole_____

4. pertaining to the cheek: _____al

5. pain in a tooth: dent_____

6. prolapse of an eyelid: blepharo_____

7. enlargement of the liver: hepato_____

8. pertaining to under the tongue: sub_____

9. removal of the gallbladder: _____ectomy

10. pertaining to the common bile duct: chole_____

F. Give the meanings of the following terms.

1. cecal volvulus_____

2. aphthous stomatitis_____

3. celiac disease _____

4. lipase _____

5. cheilosis _____

6. oropharynx _____

7. glycolysis _____

8. glossopharyngeal _____

9. sialadenectomy _____

10. periodontal membrane _____

G. Match the name of the laboratory test or clinical procedure with its description.

- abdominal ultrasonography
- barium enema
- CT of the abdomen
- endoscopic retrograde cholangiopancreatography
- gastric bypass
- gastrostomy
- laparoscopy
- liver biopsy
- liver scan
- nasogastric intubation
- percutaneous transhepatic cholangiography
- serum bilirubin
- small bowel follow-through
- stool culture
- stool guaiac (Hemoccult)

1. measurement of bile pigment in the blood _____Serum bilirubin_____

2. placement of feces in a growth medium for bacterial analysis _____Stool culture_____

3. x-ray examination of the lower gastrointestinal tract _____barium enema_____

4. imaging of abdominal viscera via sound waves _abdominal ultresonography_

5. test to reveal hidden blood in feces _stool guaiac_

6. sequential x-ray images of the small intestine _small bowel follow-through_

7. injection of contrast material through the skin into the liver, to obtain x-ray images of bile vessels
percutaneous transhepatic cholangiography

8. insertion of a tube through the nose into the stomach _nasogastric intubation_

9. transverse x-ray pictures of the abdominal organs _CT scan of the abdomen_

10. injection of contrast material via endoscope to obtain x-ray images of the pancreas and bile ducts
endoscopy retrograde

11. reduction of stomach size and gastrojejunostomy _gastric bypass_

12. injection of radioactive material intravenously, and production of an image of liver cells as they
take up the radioactivity _Liver scan_

13. percutaneous removal of liver tissue followed by microscopic examination _Liver biopsy_

14. visual examination (endoscopic) of abdominal viscera through small abdominal incisions
laparoscopy

15. new opening of the stomach to the outside of the body for feeding _gastrostomy_

H. Give the meanings of the abbreviations in Column I. Then select the letter of the correct description from Column II.

Column I

1. TPN _____ ____

2. PUD _____ ____

3. EGD _____ ____

4. IBD _____ ____

5. BE _____ ____

6. BRBPR _____ ____

7. LFTs _____ ____

8. GERD _____ ____

9. HBV _____ ____

10. CT _____ ____

Column II

A. Tests such as measurement of ALT, AST, alk phos, and serum bilirubin.
B. Heartburn is a symptom of this condition.
C. This general condition includes Crohn disease and ulcerative colitis.
D. *H. pylori* causes this condition.
E. Intravenous injection of nutrition.
F. This is a lower gastrointestinal series.
G. X-ray procedure that produces a series of cross-sectional images.
H. This infectious agent causes chronic inflammation of the liver.
I. Hematochezia describes this gastrointestinal symptom.
J. Endoscopic visualization of the upper gastrointestinal tract.

6

I. Give the suffixes for the following terms.

1. bursting forth _____
2. flow, discharge _____
3. suture _____
4. dilation _____
5. narrowing, stricture _____
6. vomiting _____
7. spitting _____
8. prolapse _____
9. excision _____
10. digestion _____

11. eating, swallowing _____
12. hardening _____
13. to stop; control _____
14. surgical repair _____
15. opening _____
16. surgical puncture _____
17. involuntary contraction _____
18. new opening _____
19. incision _____
20. destruction, breakdown _____

J. Circle the correct term in parentheses to complete each sentence.

1. When Mrs. Smith began to have diarrhea and crampy abdominal pain, she consulted a **(urologist, nephrologist, gastroenterologist)** and worried that the cause of her symptoms might be **(inflammatory bowel disease, esophageal varices, achalasia)**.

2. After taking a careful history and performing a thorough physical examination, Dr. Blakemore diagnosed Mr. Bean, a long-time drinker, with **(hemorrhoids, pancreatitis, appendicitis)**. Mr. Bean had complained of sharp midepigastric pain and a change in bowel habits.

3. Many pregnant women cannot lie flat after eating because of a burning sensation in their chest and throat. Doctors call this condition **(volvulus, dysentery, gastroesophageal reflux)**.

4. Pediatric surgeons must be wary of **(inguinal hernia, pyloric stenosis, oral leukoplakia)** in young infants who display projectile vomiting.

5. Boris had terrible problems with his teeth. He needed not only a periodontist for his **(anorexia, ascites, gingivitis)** but also an **(endodontist, oral surgeon, orthodontist)** to straighten his teeth.

6. After 6 weeks of radiation therapy to her throat, Betty experienced severe esophageal irritation and inflammation. She complained to her doctor about her **(dyspepsia, odynophagia, hematemesis)**.

7. Barbara had cramping and bloating before otherwise normal menstrual periods. Her physician prescribed pain medication to alleviate her **(dyspepsia, dysmenorrhea, menorrhagia)**.

8. Chris had been a heavy alcohol drinker all of his adult life. His wife noticed worsening yellow discoloration of the whites of his eyes and skin. After a physical examination and blood tests, his family physician told him his **(colon, skin, liver)** was diseased. The yellow discoloration was **(jaundice, exophthalmos, proptosis)**, and his condition was **(cheilosis, cirrhosis, hemostasis)**.

9. When Carol was working as a phlebotomist, she accidentally cut her finger while drawing a patient's blood. Unfortunately, the patient had (**pancreatitis, hemoptysis, hepatitis**), and HBV was transmitted to Carol. Blood tests and (**liver biopsy, gastrointestinal endoscopy, stool culture**) confirmed Carol's unfortunate diagnosis. Her doctor told her that her condition was chronic and that she might be a candidate for a (**bone marrow, liver, kidney**) transplant in the future.

10. Operation Smile is a rescue project that performs (**herniorrhaphy, oral leukopenia, palatoplasty**) on children with a congenital cleft in the roof of the mouth.

MEDICAL SCRAMBLE

Unscramble the letters to form suffixes from the clues. Use the letters in squares to complete the bonus term. Answers are found on page 205.

1. *Clue*: Narrowing

  – ___ ___ ___ ☐ ☐ ___ ___ ___   OTSESSNI

2. *Clue*: Bursting forth of blood

  – ☐ ___ ☐ ___ ___ ___ ___   GRAIRAH

3. *Clue*: Spitting

  – ☐ ___ ☐ ___ ___ ___   SPSTIY

4. *Clue*: Vomiting

  – ☐ ___ ___ ___ ☐ ___   SMIESE

5. *Clue*: Flow, discharge

  – ☐ ☐ ☐ ___ ___   HARER

6. *Clue*: Eating or swallowing

  – ___ ☐ ☐ ___ ___ ___   AGPAHI

BONUS TERM: *Clue*: This common surgical procedure fixes a bulge or protrusion.

☐ ☐ ☐ ☐ ☐ ☐ ☐ ☐ ☐ ☐ ☐ ☐ ☐

6

ANSWERS TO EXERCISES

A

1. digestion
2. spitting (from the respiratory tract)
3. vomiting
4. eating, swallowing
5. prolapse, falling, sagging
6. flow, discharge
7. bursting forth of blood
8. suture
9. surgical repair
10. destruction, breakdown, separation
11. stretching, dilation, dilatation
12. tightening, narrowed lumen, stricture
13. to stop; control
14. sudden, involuntary contraction of muscles
15. dilation, stretching, dilatation; widening

B

1. dysmenorrhea
2. cholestasis
3. herniorrhaphy
4. lymphangiectasis
5. hemoptysis
6. hematemesis
7. bronchiectasis
8. blepharoplasty
9. hemostasis
10. rhinoplasty
11. hemolysis
12. pylorospasm
13. menorrhagia
14. bronchospasm

C

1. difficulty in swallowing
2. excessive (much) eating
3. difficult digestion
4. biliary ducts are not open (congenital anomaly)
5. forward prolapse (bulging) of the eyes (exophthalmos)
6. stoppage of flow of bile
7. esophagus is not open (closed off) at birth (congenital anomaly)
8. pain caused by swallowing
9. bursting forth of blood (hemorrhage) from the spleen
10. visual (endoscopic) examination of the rectum and sigmoid colon

D

1. cholecystectomy
2. colectomy
3. herniorrhaphy
4. cecostomy
5. blepharoplasty
6. sphincterotomy
7. gastroduodenal anastomosis (gastroduodenostomy)—both are acceptable
8. ileostomy
9. gingivectomy
10. cholecystojejunostomy (cholecystojejunal anastomosis)
11. paracentesis (abdominocentesis)
12. rectocele

E

1. steatorrhea
2. dysphagia
3. cholelithiasis
4. buccal
5. dentalgia
6. blepharoptosis
7. hepatomegaly
8. sublingual
9. cholecystectomy
10. choledochal

F

1. twisted intestine in the area of the cecum
2. inflammation of the mouth with small ulcers
3. inherited autoimmune disorder in which the lining of the small
intestine (villi) is damaged from eating gluten found in wheat, barley, and rye.
4. enzyme to digest fat
5. abnormal condition of lips
6. the part of the throat near the mouth
7. breakdown of sugar
8. pertaining to the tongue and the throat
9. removal of a salivary gland
10. membrane surrounding a tooth

G

1. serum bilirubin
2. stool culture
3. barium enema cholangiography
4. abdominal ultrasonography
5. stool guaiac (Hemoccult)
6. small bowel follow-through
7. percutaneous transhepatic cholangiopancreatography (ERCP)
8. nasogastric intubation
9. CT scan of the abdomen
10. endoscopic retrograde
11. gastric bypass
12. liver scan
13. liver biopsy
14. laparoscopy (form of minimally invasive surgery)
15. gastrostomy (G tube)

H

1. total parenteral nutrition: E
2. peptic ulcer disease: D
3. esophagoduodenoscopy: J
4. inflammatory bowel disease: C
5. barium enema: F
6. bright red blood per rectum: I
7. liver function tests: A
8. gastroesophageal reflux disease: B
9. hepatitis B virus: H
10. computed tomography: G

I

1. -rrhagia, -rrhage	8. -ptosis	15. -tresia
2. -rrhea	9. -ectomy	16. -centesis
3. -rrhaphy	10. -pepsia	17. -spasm
4. -ectasis, -ectasia	11. -phagia	18. -stomy
5. -stenosis	12. -sclerosis	19. -tomy
6. -emesis	13. -stasis	20. -lysis
7. -ptysis	14. -plasty	

J

1. gastroenterologist; inflammatory	5. gingivitis; orthodontist	8. liver; jaundice; cirrhosis
2. pancreatitis	6. odynophagia	9. hepatitis; liver biopsy; liver
3. gastroesophageal reflux	7. dysmenorrhea	10. palatoplasty
4. pyloric stenosis		

ANSWERS TO PRACTICAL APPLICATIONS

1. c
2. a
3. d
4. b

ANSWERS TO MEDICAL SCRAMBLE

1. -STENOSIS   2. -RRHAGIA   3. -PTYSIS   4. -EMESIS   5. -RRHEA   6. -PHAGIA

BONUS TERM: HERNIORRHAPHY

PRONUNCIATION OF TERMS

PRONUNCIATION GUIDE

ā as in āpe   ă as in ăpple
ē as in ēven   ě as in ěvery
ī as in īce   ĭ as in ĭnterest
ō as in ōpen   ŏ as in pŏt
ū as in ūnit   ŭ as in ŭnder

To test your understanding of the terminology in this chapter, write the meaning of each term in the space provided. In addition, you may wish to cover the terms and write them by looking at your definitions. Make sure your spelling is correct. The page number after each term indicates where it is defined in the text, so you can easily check your responses. You will find complete definitions for all of these terms and their audio pronunciations on the CD.

Term	Pronunciation	Meaning
abdominal ultrasonography (192)	ăb-DŎM-ĭn-ăl ŭl-tră-sō-NŎG-ră-fē	_____
aphthous stomatitis (188)	ĂF-thŭs stō-mă-TĪ-tĭs	_____
atresia (185)	ā-TRĒ-zē-ă	_____
biliary atresia (185)	BĬL-ē-ĕr-ē ā-TRĒ-zē-ă	_____
bronchiectasis (184)	brŏng-kē-ĔK-tă-sĭs	_____
bronchospasm (185)	BRŎNG-kō-spăsm	_____
buccal (186)	BŬK-ăl	_____
cecal volvulus (186)	SĒ-kăl VŎL-vū-lŭs	_____
celiac disease (186)	SĒ-lē-ăk dĭ-ZĒZ	_____
cheilosis (187)	kī-LŌ-sĭs	_____
cholangiectasis (187)	kōl-ăn-jē-ĔK-tă-sĭs	_____

6

Term	Pronunciation	Meaning
cholangiography (191)	kōl-ăn-jē-ŎG-ră-fē	
cholangiopancreatography (191)	kōl-ăn-jē-ō-păn-krē-ă-TŎG-ră-fē	
cholecystectomy (187)	kō-lē-sĭs-TĔK-tō-mē	
cholecystojejunostomy (187)	kō-lē-sĭs-tō-jĕ-jŭ-NŎS-tō-mē	
cholecystolithiasis (188)	kō-lē-sĭs-tō-lĭ-THĪ-ă-sĭs	
choledochal (187)	kō-lē-DŌK-ăl	
cholelithiasis (187)	kō-lē-lĭ-THĪ-ă-sĭs	
cholestasis (185)	kō-lē-STĀ-sĭs	
colectomy (187)	kō-LĔK-tō-mē	
colonoscopy (187)	kō-lŏn-ŎS-kō-pē	
computed tomography (191)	kŏm-PŪ-tĕd tō-MŎG-ră-FĒ	
dentalgia (187)	dĕn-TĂL-jă	
dysmenorrhea (185)	dĭs-mĕn-ŏr-RĒ-ă	
dyspepsia (184)	dĭs-PĔP-sē-ă	
dysphagia (184)	dĭs-FĀ-jē-ă	
enteroplasty (185)	ĕn-tĕr-ō-PLĂS-tē	
esophageal atresia (185)	ĕ-sŏf-ă-JĒ-ăl ā-TRĒ-zē-ă	
gastric bypass (193)	GĂS-trĭk BĪ-păs	
gastroduodenal anastomosis (187)	găs-trō-dū-ō-DĒ-năl ă-nă-stō-MŌ-sĭs	
gastroenteritis (187)	găs-trō-ĕn-tĕ-RĪ-tĭs	
gastrointestinal endoscopy (193)	găs-trō-ĭn-TĔS-tĭn-ăl ĕn-DŎS-kō-pē	
gastrojejunostomy (187)	găs-trō-jĕ-jū-NŎS-tō-mē	
gastrostomy (187)	găs-TRŎS-tō-mē	
gingivectomy (187)	gĭn-gĭ-VĔK-tō-mē	
glossopharyngeal (187)	glŏs-ō-fă-rĭn-GĒ-ăl	
glycolysis (187)	glī-KŎL-ĭ-sĭs	
hematemesis (184)	hē-mă-TĔM-ĕ-sĭs	
hemolysis (184)	hē-MŎL-ĭ-sĭs	
hemoptysis (185)	hē-MŎP-tĭ-sĭs	
hemorrhage (185)	HĔM-ŏr-ĭj	
hemostasis (185)	hē-mō-STĀ-sĭs	
hepatomegaly (187)	hĕp-ă-tō-MĔG-ă-lē	

Term	Pronunciation	Meaning
herniorrhaphy (187)	hĕr-nē-ŎR-ă-fē	
ileostomy (187)	ĭl-ē-ŎS-tō-mē	
labioglossopharyngeal (187)	lā-bē-ō-glŏs-ō-fă-RĬN-jē-ăl	
laparoscopy (194)	lă-păr-ŎS-kō-pē	
lipase (188)	LĪ-pās	
liver biopsy (194)	LĬ-vĕr BĪ-ŏp-sē	
liver function tests (188)	LĬ-vĕr FUNG-shŭn tests	
liver scan (192)	LĬ-vĕr scăn	
lower gastrointestinal series (189)	LŎW-ĕr găs-trō-ĭn-TĔS-tĭ-năl SĔR-ēz	
lymphangiectasia (184)	lĭm-făn-jē-ĕk-TĀ-zē-ă	
magnetic resonance imaging (192)	măg-NĔT-ĭk rĕ-zō-NĂNS ĬM-ă-gĭng	
menorrhagia (185)	mĕn-ŏr-RĀ-jă	
nasogastric intubation (194)	nā-zō-GĂS-trĭk ĭn-tū-BĀ-shŭn	
odynophagia (184)	ō-dĭn-ō-FĀ-jē-ă	
oropharynx (188)	ŏr-ō-FĂR-ĭnks	
palatoplasty (188)	PĂL-ă-tō-plăs-tē	
pancreatic (188)	păn-krē-ĂH-tĭk	
paracentesis (194)	păr-ă-sĕn-TĒ-sĭs	
periodontal membrane (188)	pĕr-ē-ō-DŎN-tăl MĔM-brān	
polyphagia (184)	pŏl-ē-FĀ-jē-ă	
proctosigmoidoscopy (188)	prŏk-tō-sĭg-mŏyd-ŎS-kō-pē	
proptosis (185)	prŏp-TŌ-sĭs	
pyloric stenosis (185)	pī-LŎR-ĭk stĕ-NŌ-sĭs	
pylorospasm (185)	pī-LŎR-ō-spăsm	
rectocele (188)	RĔK-tō-sēl	
rhinoplasty (185)	rī-nō-PLĂS-tē	
sialadenectomy (188)	sī-ăl-ă-dĕ-NĔK-tō-mē	
splenic flexure (188)	SPLĔ-nĭk FLĔK-shŭr	
steatorrhea (188)	stē-ă-tō-RĒ-ă	
stool culture (189)	stool KŬL-chŭr	
stool guaiac (189)	stool GWĪ-ăk	
sublingual (187)	sŭb-LĬNG-wăl	

REVIEW SHEET

Write meanings for combining forms and suffixes in the spaces provided. Check your answers with information in Chapter 5 and this chapter or in the Glossary (Medical Word Parts–English) at the end of the book.

COMBINING FORMS

Combining Form	Meaning	Combining Form	Meaning
amyl/o		gastr/o	
an/o		gingiv/o	
append/o		gloss/o	
appendic/o		gluc/o	
bil/i		glyc/o	
bilirubin/o		glycogen/o	
bronch/o		hem/o	
bucc/o		hemat/o	
cec/o		hepat/o	
celi/o		herni/o	
cervic/o		idi/o	
cheil/o		ile/o	
chlorhydr/o		pancreat/o	
chol/e		peritone/o	
cholangi/o		pharyng/o	
cholecyst/o		proct/o	
choledoch/o		prote/o	
cib/o		pylor/o	
cirrh/o		rect/o	
col/o		sialaden/o	
colon/o		sigmoid/o	
dent/i		splen/o	
duoden/o		steat/o	
enter/o		stomat/o	
esophag/o		tonsill/o	
eti/o			

SUFFIXES

Suffix	Meaning	Suffix	Meaning
-ase		-orexia	
-centesis		-rrhage	
-chezia		-rrhagia	
-ectasia		-rrhaphy	
-ectasis		-rrhea	
-ectomy		-scopy	
-emesis		-spasm	
-emia		-stasis	
-genesis		-stenosis	
-graphy		-stomy	
-iasis		-tomy	
-lysis		-tresia	
-megaly			

 Please refer to the enclosed CD for additional exercises and images related to this chapter.

chapter 7

Urinary System

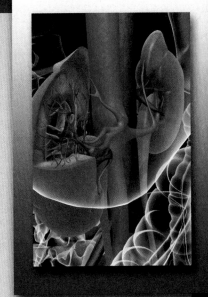

THIS CHAPTER IS DIVIDED INTO THE FOLLOWING SECTIONS

In this chapter you will

- Name the organs of the urinary system and describe their locations and functions.
- Give the meaning of various pathologic conditions affecting the urinary system.
- Recognize the uses and interpretation of urinalysis as a diagnostic test.
- Define combining forms, prefixes, and suffixes of urinary system terminology.
- List and explain some clinical procedures, laboratory tests, and abbreviations that pertain to the urinary system.
- Apply your new knowledge to understanding medical terms in their proper contexts, such as medical reports and records.

Image Description: Anterior view of the kidneys showing a partially sectioned right kidney.

211

INTRODUCTION

When foods containing proteins are used by cells in the body, waste products containing **nitrogen** are released into the bloodstream. These **nitrogenous wastes** are urea, creatinine, and uric acid, which the urinary system removes from the blood so that they do not accumulate and become harmful. As blood passes through the kidneys, the kidneys filter nitrogenous wastes to form **urine** (composed also of water, salts, and acids), which leaves the body through the ureters, urinary bladder, and urethra.

Besides removing urea and other nitrogenous wastes from the blood, the kidneys maintain the proper balance of water, electrolytes, and acids in body fluids. **Electrolytes** are small molecules that conduct an electrical charge. Examples are **sodium** (Na^+) and **potassium** (K^+). Electrolytes are necessary for proper functioning of muscle and nerve cells. The kidney adjusts the amounts of water and electrolytes by secreting some substances into the urine and holding back others in the bloodstream for use in the body.

In addition to forming and excreting (eliminating) urine from the body, the kidneys secrete substances such as renin (RĒ-nĭn) and erythropoietin (ĕ-rĭth-rō-PŌ-ĕ-tĭn). **Renin** is an enzymatic hormone important in adjusting blood pressure (raising pressure to keep blood moving through the kidney). **Erythropoietin** (-poietin means substance that forms) is a hormone that stimulates red blood cell production in bone marrow. The kidneys also secrete an active form of vitamin D, necessary for the absorption of calcium from the intestine. In addition, hormones such as insulin and parathyroid hormone are degraded and extracted from the bloodstream by the kidney.

ANATOMY OF THE MAJOR ORGANS

The following paragraphs describe the organs of the urinary system. Label Figure 7–1 as you identify each organ.

The **kidney** [1] is one of two bean-shaped organs behind the abdominal cavity (retroperitoneal) on either side of the spine in the lumbar region. The kidneys are embedded in a cushion of adipose tissue and surrounded by fibrous connective tissue for protection. These fist-sized organs weigh about 4 to 6 ounces each.

The kidneys consist of an outer **cortex** region (cortex means bark, as the bark of a tree) and an inner **medulla** region (medulla means marrow). The **hilum** is a depression on the medial border of the kidney. Blood vessels and nerves pass through the hilum.

The **ureter** [2] is one of two muscular tubes (16 to 18 inches long) lined with mucous membrane. The ureters carry urine in peristaltic waves from the kidneys to the urinary bladder.

The **urinary bladder** [3] is a hollow, muscular sac in the pelvic cavity. It is a temporary reservoir for urine. The **trigone** is a triangular region at the base of the bladder where the ureters enter and the urethra exits.

The **urethra** [4] is a membranous tube that carries urine from the urinary bladder to the outside of the body. The process of expelling **(voiding)** urine through the urethra is **urination** or **micturition.** The external opening of the urethra is the urinary **meatus.** The female urethra, about 1½ inches long, lies anterior to the vagina and vaginal meatus. The male urethra, about 8 inches long, extends downward through the prostate gland to the meatus at the tip of the penis. Figure 7–2 illustrates the female urinary system. Compare it with Figure 7–1, which shows the male urinary system.

FIGURE 7–1 Organs of the urinary system in a male.

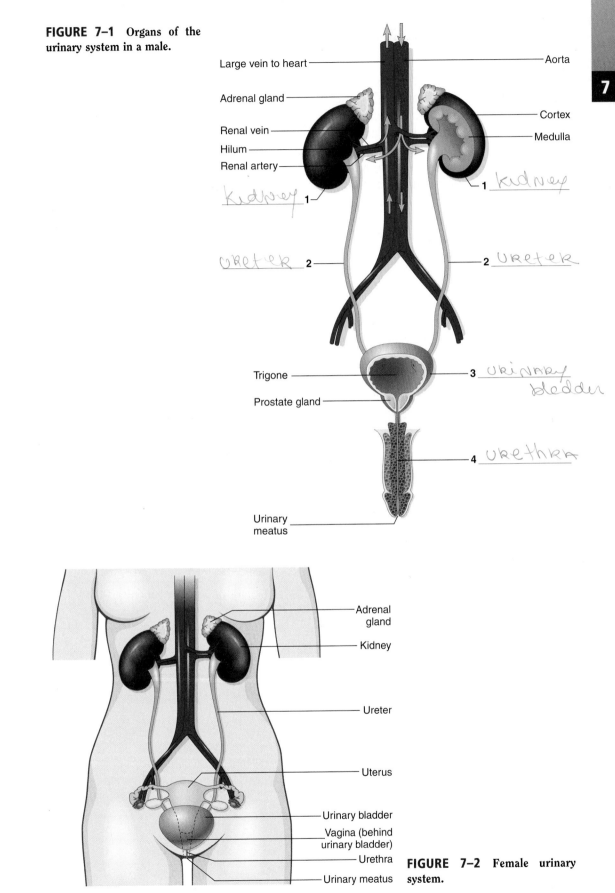

Large vein to heart

Adrenal gland

Renal vein

Hilum

Renal artery

Kidney 1

ureter 2

Aorta

Cortex

Medulla

1 *kidney*

2 *Ureter*

Trigone

Prostate gland

3 *urinary bladder*

4 *urethra*

Urinary meatus

Adrenal gland

Kidney

Ureter

Uterus

Urinary bladder

Vagina (behind urinary bladder)

Urethra

Urinary meatus

FIGURE 7–2 Female urinary system.

7

PHYSIOLOGY: HOW THE KIDNEYS PRODUCE URINE

Blood enters each kidney from the aorta by way of the right and left **renal arteries.** After the renal artery enters the kidney (at the hilum), the artery branches into smaller and smaller arteries. The smallest arteries, called **arterioles,** are located throughout the cortex of the kidney (Fig. 7–3, *A*).

Because the arterioles are small, blood passes through them slowly but constantly. Blood flow through the kidney is so essential that the kidneys have their own special device for maintaining blood flow. If blood pressure falls in the vessels of the kidney, so that blood flow diminishes, the kidney produces **renin** and discharges it into the blood. Renin promotes the formation of a substance that stimulates the contraction of arterioles. This increases blood pressure and restores blood flow in the kidneys to normal.

Each arteriole in the cortex of the kidney leads into a mass of very tiny, coiled, and intertwined smaller blood vessels called **capillaries.** The collection of capillaries, shaped in the form of a tiny ball, is a **glomerulus.** There are about 1 million glomeruli in the cortex region of each kidney.

The kidneys produce urine by **filtration.** As blood passes through the many glomeruli, the thin walls of each glomerulus (the filter) permit water, salts, sugar, and **urea** (with other nitrogenous wastes such as **creatinine** and **uric acid**) to leave the bloodstream. These materials collect in a tiny, cup-like structure, a **Bowman capsule,** which surrounds each glomerulus (Fig. 7–3, *B*). The walls of the glomeruli prevent large substances, such as proteins and blood cells, from filtering into the Bowman capsule. These substances remain in the blood and normally do not appear in urine.

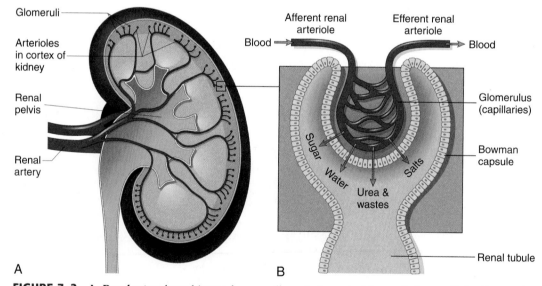

FIGURE 7–3 A, Renal artery branching to form smaller arteries, arterioles, and glomeruli. **B, Glomerulus** and **Bowman capsule.** Afferent arteriole carries blood toward (in this term, af- is a form of ad-) the glomerulus. Efferent arteriole carries blood away (ef- is a form of ex-) from the glomerulus.

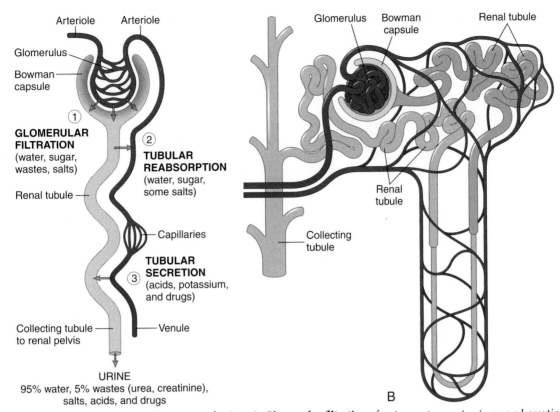

FIGURE 7–4   **A, Three steps in the formation of urine. 1, Glomerular filtration** of water, sugar, wastes (urea and creatinine), and salts. **2, Tubular reabsorption** of water, sugar, and some salts. **3, Tubular secretion** of acids, potassium, and drugs. **B,** Nephron.

Attached to each Bowman capsule is a long, twisted tube called a **renal tubule** (Figs. 7–3, *B,* and 7–4). As water, sugar, salts, urea, and other wastes pass through the renal tubule, most of the water, all of the sugar, and some salts (such as sodium) return to the bloodstream through tiny capillaries surrounding each tubule. This active process of **reabsorption** ensures that the body retains essential substances such as sugar (glucose), water, and salts. The final process in the formation of urine is **secretion** of some substances from the bloodstream into the renal tubule. These waste products of metabolism become toxic if allowed to accumulate in the body. Thus, acids, drugs (such as penicillin), and potassium (as a salt) leave the body in urine.

Only wastes, water, salts, acids, and some drugs (often as metabolites—partially broken down forms of the original drug) remain in the renal tubule. Each renal tubule, now containing urine (95 percent water and 5 percent urea, creatinine, salts, acids, and drugs), ends in a larger collecting tubule. See Figure 7–4, *A,* which reviews the steps involved in urine formation. The combination of a glomerulus and a renal tubule is a unit called a **nephron** (Fig. 7–4, *B*). There are more than 1 million nephrons in a kidney.

All collecting tubules lead to the **renal pelvis,** a basin-like area in the central part of the kidney. Small, cup-like regions of the renal pelvis are called **calyces** or **calices** (singular: **calyx** or **calix**). Figure 7–5 illustrates a section of the kidney and shows the renal pelvis and calyces.

7

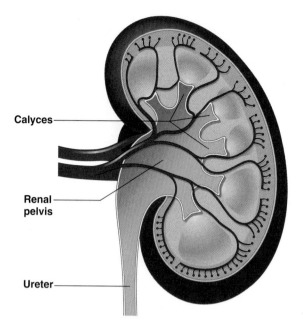

Calyces

Renal pelvis

Ureter

FIGURE 7–5 Section of the kidney showing renal pelvis, calyces, and ureter.

The renal pelvis narrows into the **ureter,** which carries the urine to the **urinary bladder** where the urine is temporarily stored. Sphincters control the exit area of the bladder to the **urethra.** These muscular rings do not permit urine to leave the bladder. As the bladder fills up and pressure increases at the base of the bladder, the person notices a need to urinate and voluntarily relaxes the sphincter muscles.

Study the flow diagram in Figure 7–6 to trace the process of forming urine and expelling it from the body.

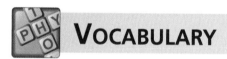 # VOCABULARY

arteriole	Small artery.
Bowman capsule	Enclosing structure surrounding each glomerulus.
calyx *or* **calix** (*plural:* **calyces** or **calices**)	Cup-like collecting region of the renal pelvis.
catheter	Tube for injecting or removing fluids.
cortex	Outer region; the renal cortex is the outer region of the kidney (**cortical** means pertaining to the cortex).
creatinine	Waste product of muscle metabolism; nitrogenous waste excreted in urine. **Creatinine clearance** is a measure of the efficiency of the kidneys in removing creatinine from the blood.
electrolyte	A chemical element that carries an electrical charge when dissolved in water. Examples are potassium (K^+) and sodium (Na^+), each carrying a positive charge. The most important negatively charged electrolytes are bicarbonate (HCO_3^-) and chloride (Cl^-). Electrolytes are essential to cellular function and transmission of impulses in nerve and muscle fibers.

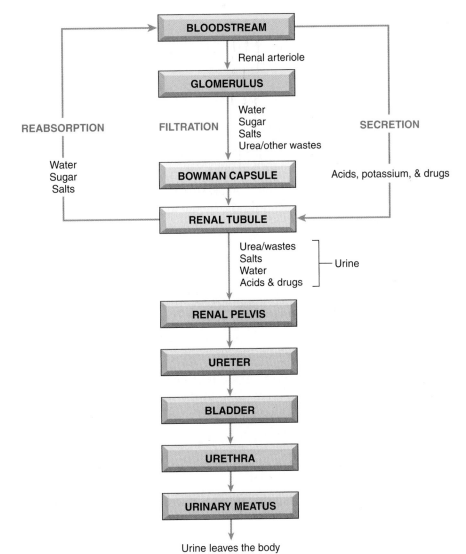

FIGURE 7–6   Flow diagram illustrating the process of forming and expelling urine.

erythropoietin (EPO)	A hormone secreted by the kidney to stimulate the production of red blood cells by bone marrow.
filtration	Passive process whereby some substances, but not all, pass through a filter or other material. In the kidney, blood pressure forces materials through the filter (glomerulus). About 180 quarts of fluid are filtered from the blood daily, but the kidney returns 98 to 99 percent of the water and salts. Only about 1½ quarts (1500 mL) of urine are excreted daily.
glomerulus (*plural:* **glomeruli**)	Tiny ball of capillaries (microscopic blood vessels) in cortex of kidney.
hilum	Depression or hollow in that part of an organ where blood vessels and nerves enter and leave.
kidney	One of two bean-shaped organs behind the abdominal cavity on either side of the backbone in the lumbar region.
meatus	Opening or canal.
medulla	Inner region; the renal medulla is the inner region of the kidney (**medullary** means pertaining to the medulla).

7

micturition	Urination; the act of voiding.
nephron	Combination of glomerulus and renal tubule where filtration, reabsorption, and secretion take place in the kidney. It is the functional unit of the kidney, each capable of forming urine by itself. There are about 1 million nephrons in a kidney
nitrogenous waste	Substance containing nitrogen and excreted in urine.
potassium (K⁺)	An electrolyte important to body processes. The kidney regulates the balance of potassium concentration within the blood.
reabsorption	In this process, the renal tubules return materials necessary to the body back into the bloodstream.
renal artery	Blood vessel that carries blood to the kidney.
renal pelvis	Central collecting region in the kidney.
renal tubule	Microscopic tube in the kidney in which urine is formed after filtration. In the renal tubule, the composition of urine is altered by the processes of reabsorption and secretion.
renal vein	Blood vessel that carries blood away from the kidney and toward the heart.
renin	An enzymatic hormone synthesized, stored, and secreted by the kidney; it raises blood pressure by influencing vasoconstriction (narrowing of blood vessels).
sodium (Na⁺)	An electrolyte regulated in the blood and urine by the kidneys.
trigone	Triangular area in the urinary bladder in which the ureters enter and the urethra exits.
urea	Major nitrogenous waste product excreted in urine.
ureter	Tube leading from each kidney to the urinary bladder.
urethra	Tube leading from the urinary bladder to the outside of the body.
uric acid	A nitrogenous waste excreted in the urine.
urinary bladder	Hollow muscular sac that holds and stores urine.
urination	Process of expelling urine; also called micturition.
voiding	Emptying of urine from the urinary bladder; urination or micturition.

TERMINOLOGY: STRUCTURES, SUBSTANCES, AND URINARY SYMPTOMS

7

Write the meanings of the medical terms in the spaces provided.

STRUCTURES

Combining Form	Meaning	Terminology	Meaning
cali/o, calic/o	calyx (calix)	caliectasis _____	
		caliceal _____	
cyst/o	urinary bladder	cystitis _____	
		Bacterial infections often cause acute or chronic cystitis. In acute cystitis, the bladder contains blood as a result of mucosal hemorrhage (Fig. 7–7).	
		cystectomy _____	
		cystostomy _____	
		An opening is made into the urinary bladder from the outside of the body. A catheter is placed into the bladder for drainage.	
glomerul/o	glomerulus	glomerular _____	
meat/o	meatus	meatal stenosis _____	
		meatotomy _____	

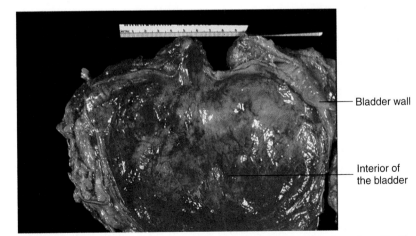

FIGURE 7–7   Acute cystitis. Notice that the mucosa of the bladder is red and swollen. Bladder and urinary tract infections are more common in women because of the shorter urethra, which allows easier bacterial colonization of the urinary bladder. They usually occur without a known cause but may be acquired during sexual intercourse ("honeymoon cystitis") or after surgical procedures and urinary catheterization. (From Damjanov I: Pathology for the Health-Related Professions, 3rd ed. Philadelphia, WB Saunders, 2006, p. 329.)

7

Combining Form	Meaning	Terminology	Meaning
nephr/o	kidney	para<u>nephr</u>ic _____	
		<u>nephr</u>opathy _____ (ně-FRŎ-pă-thē)	
		<u>nephr</u>optosis _____ *Downward displacement or dropping of a kidney when its anatomic supports are weakened.*	
		<u>nephr</u>olithotomy _____ *Incision (percutaneous) into the kidney to remove a stone.*	
		<u>nephr</u>osclerosis _____ *Arterioles in the kidney are affected.*	
		hydro<u>nephr</u>osis _____ *Obstruction of urine flow may be caused by renal calculi (Fig. 7–8), compression of the ureter by tumor, or hyperplasia of the prostate gland at the base of the bladder in males.*	
		<u>nephr</u>ostomy _____ *Surgical opening to the outside of the body (from the renal pelvis). This is necessary when a ureter becomes obstructed and the obstruction cannot be removed easily. The renal pelvis becomes distended with urine (hydronephrosis), making nephrostomy necessary.*	

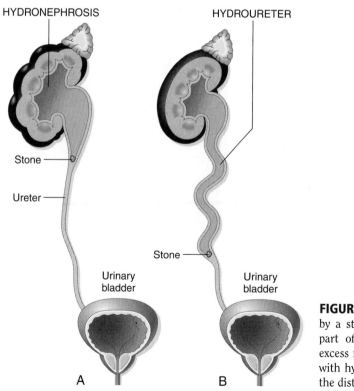

FIGURE 7–8 A, Hydronephrosis caused by a stone (obstruction) in the proximal part of a ureter. Notice the buildup of excess fluid in the kidney. **B, Hydroureter** with hydronephrosis caused by a stone in the distal part of the ureter.

Combining Form	Meaning	Terminology	Meaning
pyel/o	renal pelvis	pyelolithotomy _____	
		Removal of a large calculus (stone) contributing to blockage of urine flow and development of infection. The renal pelvis is surgically opened.	
		pyelogram _____	
ren/o	kidney	renal ischemia _____	
		renal colic _____	
		Colic is intermittent spasms of pain caused by inflammation and distention of a hollow organ. In renal colic, pain results from calculi in the kidney or ureter.	
trigon/o	trigone (region of the bladder)	trigonitis _____	
ureter/o	ureter	ureteroplasty _____	
		ureterolithotomy _____	
		ureteroileostomy _____	
		After cystectomy, the urologic surgeon forms a pouch from a segment of the ileum, used in place of the bladder to carry urine from the ureters out of the body. It is an **ileal conduit**.	
urethr/o	urethra	urethritis _____	
		urethroplasty _____	
		urethral stricture _____	
		A **stricture** is an abnormal narrowing of an opening or passageway.	
vesic/o	urinary bladder	perivesical _____	
		Do not confuse the term **vesical** with the term **vesicle**, which is a small blister on the skin.	
		vesicoureteral reflux _____	

SUBSTANCES AND SYMPTOMS

Combining Form or Suffix	Meaning	Terminology	Meaning
albumin/o	albumin (a protein in the blood)	albuminuria _____	
		The suffix -uria means urine condition. This finding can indicate malfunction of the kidney as protein leaks out of damaged glomeruli.	
azot/o	nitrogen	azotemia _____	
		This toxic condition is characteristic of uremia. It is indicated by an elevated BUN (blood urea nitrogen) test.	

7

Combining Form or Suffix	Meaning	Terminology	Meaning
bacteri/o	bacteria	bacteriuria _____ *Usually a sign of **urinary tract infection (UTI)**. The bacteria in the urine are cultured (grown in a special nutrient environment), and then tested with antibiotics to determine which antibiotic will inhibit growth. This is known as **culture and sensitivity testing (C&S)**.*	
dips/o	thirst	polydipsia _____ *A sign of diabetes insipidus or diabetes mellitus.*	
ket/o, keton/o	ketone bodies (ketoacids and **acetone**)	ketosis _____ *Often called **ketoacidosis** because acids accumulate in the blood and tissues. The breath of a patient with ketosis has a sweet or "fruity" odor. This is produced by acetone (a ketone body) released from the blood in the lungs and exhaled through the mouth.*	
		ketonuria _____	
lith/o	stone	nephrolithiasis _____	
noct/o	night	nocturia _____ *Frequent, excessive urination at night.*	
olig/o	scanty	oliguria _____	
-poietin	substance that forms	erythropoietin _____	
py/o	pus	pyuria _____	
-tripsy	to crush	lithotripsy _____	
ur/o	urine (urea)	uremia _____ *This toxic state results when nitrogenous waste products accumulate greatly in the blood.*	
		enuresis _____ *Literally, a condition of being "in urine"; bed-wetting.*	
		diuresis _____ *Di- (from dia-) means complete. Caffeine and alcohol are well-known **diuretics**—they induce increased formation and secretion of urine (diuresis).*	
		antidiuretic hormone _____ *This substance (a hormone from the pituitary gland, and literally meaning against diuresis) normally acts on the renal tubules to cause water to be reabsorbed into the bloodstream. Abbreviated **ADH**.*	

Enuresis/Nocturia

Enuresis is the involuntary discharge of urine or bed-wetting, while *nocturia* is voluntary, frequent urination at night.

Combining Form or Suffix	Meaning	Terminology	Meaning
urin/o	urine	urinary incontinence _____	
		Incontinence literally means not (in-) able to hold (tin) together (con-). This is loss of control of the passage of urine from the bladder. **Stress incontinence** *occurs with strain on the bladder opening during coughing or sneezing.* **Urgency incontinence** *occurs with inability to hold back urination when feeling the urge to void.*	
		urinary retention _____	
		This symptom results with blockage to the outflow of urine from the bladder.	
-uria	urination; urine condition	dysuria _____	
		anuria _____	
		Commonly caused by renal dysfunction or failure or urinary tract obstruction.	
		hematuria _____	
		glycosuria _____	
		A symptom of diabetes mellitus.	
		polyuria _____	
		A symptom of both diabetes insipidus and diabetes mellitus.	

URINALYSIS

Urinalysis is an examination of urine to determine the presence of abnormal elements that may indicate various pathologic conditions.

The following are some of the tests included in a urinalysis:

1. **Color**—Normal urine color is yellow (amber) or straw-colored. A colorless, pale urine indicates a large amount of water in the urine, whereas a smoky-red or brown color of urine indicates the presence of large amounts of blood. Foods such as beets and certain drugs also can produce a red coloration of urine.

2. **Appearance**—Normally, urine should be clear. If it is cloudy **(turbid),** this often indicates a urinary tract infection with **pus (pyuria)** and bacteria (bacteriuria) in urine.

3. **pH**—Determination of pH reveals the chemical nature of urine. It indicates to what degree a solution (such as urine or blood) is **acidic** or **alkaline (basic).** The pH range is between 0 (very acid) and 14 (very alkaline). Normal urine is slightly acidic (6.5). However, in infections of the bladder, the urine pH may be alkaline, owing to the actions of bacteria in the urine that break down the urea and release an alkaline substance called ammonia.

4. **Protein**—Small amounts of protein are normally found in the urine but not in sufficient quantity to produce a positive result by ordinary methods of testing. When urinary tests for protein become positive, **albumin** is usually responsible. Albumin is the major protein in blood plasma. If it is detected in urine

7

(albuminuria), it may indicate a leak in the glomerular membrane, which allows albumin to enter the renal tubule and pass into the urine.

Through more sensitive testing, abnormal amounts of albumin may be detected (microalbuminuria) when ordinary tests are negative. Microalbuminuria is recognized as the earliest sign of renal involvement in diabetes mellitus (see page 227) and essential hypertension (see pages 226–227).

5. **Glucose**—Sugar is not normally found in the urine. In most cases, when it does appear **(glycosuria),** it indicates **diabetes mellitus.** In diabetes mellitus, there is excess sugar in the bloodstream (hyperglycemia), which leads to the "spilling over" of sugar into the urine. The renal tubules cannot reabsorb all the sugar that filters out through the glomerular membrane.

6. **Specific gravity**—The specific gravity of urine reflects the amounts of wastes, minerals, and solids in the urine. It is a comparison of the density of urine with that of water. The urine of patients with diabetes mellitus has a higher-than-normal specific gravity because of the presence of sugar.

7. **Ketone bodies**—Ketones (or **acetones,** which are a type of ketone body) are breakdown products resulting from increased delivery of free fatty acids to the liver, and from catabolism of the fatty acids. Ketones accumulate in large quantities in blood and urine when the body breaks down fat, instead of sugar, for fuel. Ketonuria occurs in diabetes mellitus when cells deprived of sugar must use up their available fat for energy. In starvation, when sugar is not available, ketonuria and ketosis (ketones in the blood) occur as fat is catabolized abnormally.

The presence of ketones in the blood is quite dangerous because ketones increase the acidity of the blood **(acidosis).** This can lead to coma (unconsciousness) and death.

8. **Sediment** and **casts**—The presence of abnormal particles in the urine is a sign of a pathologic condition. Such particles, which may settle to the bottom of a urine sample as sediment, may include cells (epithelial cells, white blood cells, or red blood cells), bacteria, crystals, and casts (cylindrical structures of protein often containing cellular elements).

9. **Phenylketonuria (PKU)**—Phenylketones are substances that accumulate in the urine of infants born lacking the important enzyme phenylalanine hydroxylase. Normally, this enzyme changes the amino acid phenylalanine to another amino acid, tyrosine. Lack of the enzyme causes phenylalanine to reach high levels in the infant's bloodstream, which will eventually lead to mental retardation. The PKU test, done just after birth, detects the phenylketonuria or phenylalanine in the blood. If it is detected, the infant is fed a low-protein diet that excludes phenylalanine to prevent mental retardation. The child remains on this diet until adulthood.

10. **Bilirubin**—This pigment substance, which results from hemoglobin breakdown, may be present in the urine, producing a darker appearance, as an indication of liver or gallbladder disease or excessive hemolysis (breakdown of hemoglobin is too rapid for the liver to clear). When the liver has difficulty removing bilirubin from blood, **hyperbilirubinemia** occurs and **bilirubinuria** follows.

Pathologic Terminology: Kidney, Bladder, and Associated Conditions

KIDNEY

glomerulonephritis

Inflammation of the kidney glomerulus.

Acute glomerulonephritis may develop as part of a systemic disorder (a condition that affects many organs in the body) or may be idiopathic. It can also occur after an acute infection, as in poststreptococcal glomerulonephritis. In this condition, which appears 10 to 14 days after a streptococcal infection, no bacteria are actually found in the kidney, but inflammation results from an immune (antigen and antibody) reaction in the glomerulus. Most patients recover spontaneously, but in some cases the disease becomes chronic. Chronic glomerulonephritis can result in hypertension (high blood pressure), albuminuria (due to seepage of protein through damaged glomerular walls), renal failure, and uremia. Drugs may be useful to control inflammation, and dialysis or renal transplantation may be necessary if uremia occurs.

interstitial nephritis

Inflammation of the renal interstitium (connective tissue that lies between the renal tubules).

Acute interstitial nephritis, an increasingly common disorder, may develop after the administration of drugs. This condition is characterized by fever, skin rash, eosinophils in the blood and urine, and poor renal function; recovery may occur when the patient discontinues using the offending agent. Recovery is helped with corticosteroids (anti-inflammatory agents).

nephrolithiasis

Kidney stones (renal calculi).

Kidney stones usually are composed of uric acid or calcium salts. Although the etiology often remains unclear, conditions associated with an increase in the concentration of calcium (parathyroid gland tumors) or high levels of uric acid in the blood (**hyperuricemia**—associated with gouty arthritis) may contribute to the formation of calculi. Stones often lodge in the ureter or bladder, as well as in the renal pelvis, and may require removal by **lithotripsy** or surgery.

nephrotic syndrome (nephrosis)

A group of clinical signs and symptoms caused by excessive protein loss in the urine.

In addition to marked proteinuria, clinical manifestations include **edema** (swelling caused by fluid in tissue spaces), **hypoalbuminemia,** hypercholesterolemia, hypercoagulability (tendency of the blood to clot more than normal), and susceptibility to infections. Nephrotic syndrome may follow glomerulonephritis, exposure to toxins or certain drugs, and other pathologic conditions, such as diabetes mellitus and malignant disease. Particular drugs may be useful to heal the leaky glomerulus.

polycystic kidney disease (PKD)

Multiple fluid-filled sacs (cysts) within and on the kidney.

This hereditary condition usually remains **asymptomatic** (without symptoms) until adult life. Cysts progressively develop in both kidneys, leading to nephromegaly, hematuria, urinary tract infection, hypertension, and uremia. Figure 7–9, *A,* shows polycystic kidney disease.

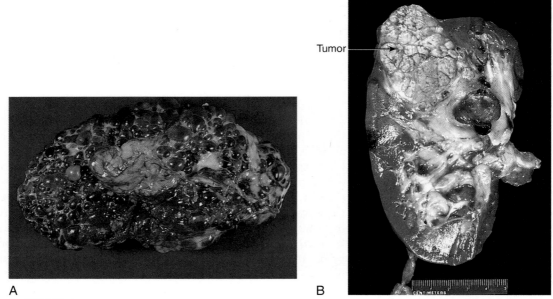

Tumor

FIGURE 7–9 **A, Polycystic kidney disease.** The kidneys contain masses of cysts. Typically, polycystic kidneys weigh 20 times more than their usual weight (150 to 200 grams). **B, Renal cell carcinoma.** (**A** from Damjanov I: Pathology for Health-Related Professions, 3rd ed. Philadelphia, WB Saunders, 2006, p. 321. **B** from Kumar V, Abbas AK, Fausto N: Robbins and Cotran Pathologic Basis of Disease, 7th ed. Philadelphia, WB Saunders, 2005, p. 1017.)

pyelonephritis	**Inflammation of the renal pelvis and renal medulla.**
	Bacterial infection causes this urinary tract infection. In acute pyelonephritis, many small **abscesses** (collections of pus) form in the renal pelvis and adjacent medulla. Urinalysis reveals pyuria. Treatment consists of antibiotics and surgical correction of any obstruction to urine flow.
renal cell carcinoma (hypernephroma)	**Cancerous tumor of the kidney in adulthood.**
	This tumor (see Fig. 7–9, *B*) accounts for 2 percent of all cancers in adults. Hematuria is the primary abnormal finding, and the tumor often metastasizes to bones and lungs. Likelihood of survival depends on the extent of spread of the tumor. Nephrectomy is the treatment of choice. There are now effective treatments using anti-angiogenic drugs that block the growth of new blood vessels.
renal failure	**Failure of the kidney to excrete wastes and maintain its filtration function.**
	The kidney stops excreting nitrogenous waste products and acids derived from diet and body metabolism. Renal failure may be acute or chronic, reversible or progressive, mild or severe. A new classification of **chronic kidney disease (CKD)** stages patients according to the level of creatinine clearance, ranging from normal (stage 1) to end-stage renal failure (stage 5). Erythropoietin is used to treat patients with CKD (stages 3 to 5). This substance increases red blood cells, resulting in marked improvement in energy levels. Hemodialysis, peritoneal dialysis, and renal transplantation are advised when medical measures have been exhausted.
renal hypertension	**High blood pressure resulting from kidney disease.**
	Renal hypertension is the most common type of **secondary hypertension** (high blood pressure caused by an abnormal condition, such as glomerulonephritis or renal artery stenosis). If the cause of high blood pressure is not known, it is called

essential hypertension. Chronic essential hypertension causes arterial and arteriolar damage, potentially resulting in stroke, myocardial infarction (heart attack), heart failure, and renal failure.

Wilms tumor	**Malignant tumor of the kidney occurring in childhood.**
	This tumor may be treated with surgery, radiation therapy, and chemotherapy.

URINARY BLADDER

bladder cancer	**Malignant tumor of the urinary bladder.**
	The bladder is the most common site of malignancy of the urinary system. It occurs more frequently in men (often smokers) and in persons older than 50 years of age, especially industrial workers exposed to dyes and leather tanning agents. Signs and symptoms include gross (visible to the naked eye) or microscopic hematuria and dysuria and increased urinary frequency. Cystoscopy with biopsy is the most common diagnostic procedure. Staging of the tumor is based on the depth to which the bladder wall (urothelium) has been penetrated and the extent of metastasis. Superficial tumors are removed by electrocauterization (burning). Cystectomy, chemotherapy, and radiation therapy are helpful for more invasive disease.

ASSOCIATED CONDITIONS

diabetes insipidus	**Inadequate secretion or resistance of the kidney to the action of antidiuretic hormone (ADH).**
	Two major symptoms of this condition are polydipsia and polyuria. Lack of ADH prevents water from being reabsorbed into the blood through the renal tubules. Insipidus means tasteless, reflecting very dilute and watery urine, not sweet as in diabetes mellitus. The term **diabetes** comes from the Greek *diabainein*, meaning to pass through. Both types of diabetes (insipidus and mellitus) are marked by polyuria (excessive excretion of urine).
diabetes mellitus	**Inadequate secretion or improper utilization of insulin.**
	The major signs and symptoms of diabetes mellitus are glycosuria, hyperglycemia, polyuria, and polydipsia. Without insulin, sugar cannot leave the bloodstream and be available to body cells for energy. Sugar remains in the blood (hyperglycemia) and spills over into the urine (glycosuria) when the kidney cannot reabsorb it through the renal tubules. Mellitus means sweet, reflecting the content of the urine. The term diabetes, when used alone, refers to the more common condition diabetes mellitus, rather than diabetes insipidus. See Chapter 18 for more information about diabetes mellitus.

LABORATORY TESTS AND CLINICAL PROCEDURES

LABORATORY TESTS

blood urea nitrogen (BUN)	**Measurement of urea levels in blood.**
	Normally, the blood urea level is low because urea is excreted in the urine continuously. However, when the kidney is diseased or fails, urea accumulates in the blood (uremia), leading to unconsciousness and death.

creatinine clearance	**Measures the rate at which creatinine is cleared from the blood by the kidney.**
	A blood sample is drawn and the creatinine concentration is compared with the amount of creatinine excreted in the urine during a fixed time period. If the kidney is not functioning well in its job of clearing creatinine from the blood, the amount of creatinine in the blood will be high relative to the amount in urine. This is the most widely used test to assess excretory function of the kidneys.

CLINICAL PROCEDURES
X-Ray Studies

CT scan	**X-ray image showing a detailed cross-sectional view of organs and tissues.**
	Transverse x-ray views of the kidney, taken with or without contrast material, are useful in the diagnosis of tumors, cysts, abscesses, and hydronephrosis. See Figure 7–10, A.
kidneys, ureters, and bladder (KUB)	**X-ray examination (without contrast) of the kidneys, ureters, and bladder.**
	A KUB study demonstrates the size and location of the kidneys in relation to other organs in the abdominopelvic region.
renal angiography	**X-ray examination (with contrast) of the vascular system (blood vessels) of the kidney.**
	This procedure helps diagnose kidney tumors and outline renal vessels in hypertensive patients.
retrograde pyelogram (RP)	**X-ray imaging of the kidneys, ureters, and bladder after injection of contrast through a urinary catheter into the ureters.**
	This technique is useful in locating urinary stones and obstructions.

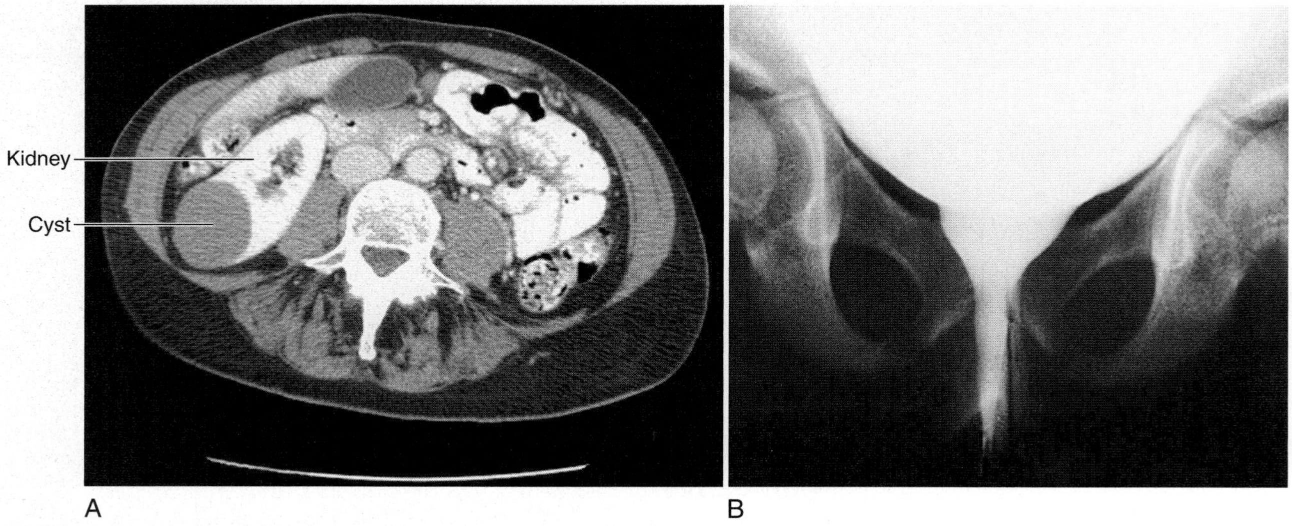

Kidney

Cyst

A   B

FIGURE 7–10 A, Computed tomography (CT) scan with contrast shows a benign cyst on the kidney. It does not take up the contrast and is smooth and round. **B, Voiding cystourethrogram** showing a normal female urethra. (Courtesy of William H. Bush, Jr., MD, University of Washington, Seattle.)

| voiding cystourethrogram (VCUG) | **X-ray record (with contrast) of the urinary bladder and urethra obtained while the patient is voiding urine.** |
| | The bladder is filled with contrast material, followed by x-ray imaging. See Figure 7–10, *B*. The ureters may be seen when there is reflux of urine into the lower end of the ureters. |

Ultrasound Examination

| ultrasonography | **Process of imaging urinary tract structures using high-frequency sound waves.** |
| | Kidney size, tumors, hydronephrosis, polycystic kidney disease, and ureteral and bladder obstruction can be diagnosed using ultrasound techniques. |

Radioactive Studies

| radioisotope scan | **Image of the kidney after injecting into the bloodstream a radioactive substance (radioisotope) that concentrates in the kidney.** |
| | Pictures show the size and shape of the kidney (**renal scan**) and its functioning (**renogram**). These studies can indicate size of blood vessels, diagnose obstruction, and determine the individual functioning of each kidney. |

Magnetic Imaging

| magnetic resonance (MR) | **A magnetic field and radio waves produce images of the kidney and surrounding structures in all three planes of the body.** |
| | The patient lies within a cylindrical magnetic resonance machine, and images are made of the pelvic and retroperitoneal regions using magnetic and radio waves. |

Other Procedures

| cystoscopy | **Direct visual examination of urinary bladder with an endoscope (cystoscope).** |
| | A urologist introduces a hollow metal tube into the urinary meatus and passes it through the urethra into the bladder. Using a light source, special lenses, and mirrors, the bladder mucosa is examined for tumors, calculi, or inflammation. When a catheter is placed through the cystoscope, urine samples are withdrawn and contrast material is injected into the bladder. See Figure 7–11. A **panendoscope** is a cystoscope that gives a wide-angle view of the bladder. |

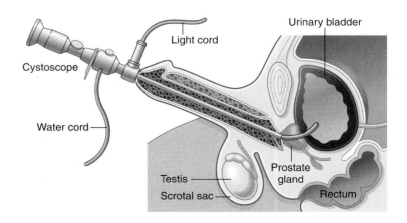

FIGURE 7–11   Cystoscopy.

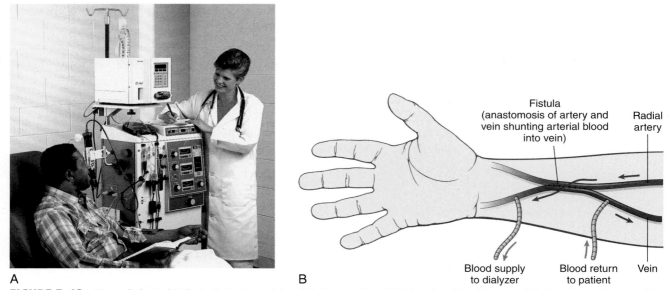

A   B

Fistula
(anastomosis of artery and
vein shunting arterial blood
into vein)

Radial
artery

Blood supply
to dialyzer

Blood return
to patient

Vein

FIGURE 7–12 **Hemodialysis (HD). A,** Patient receiving HD. Conventional HD involves 3 to 4 hours of dialysis three times weekly. Newer alternative modalities include slower and longer dialysis, nocturnal HD, and daily short HD. **B,** Arteriovenous fistula for HD. (**A** from Lewis SM, Heitkemper MM, Dirksen SR: Medical-Surgical Nursing: Assessment and Management of Clinical Problems, 5th ed. St. Louis, Mosby, 2000, p. 1328.)

dialysis

Process of separating nitrogenous waste materials from the bloodstream when the kidneys no longer function.

There are two methods:

1. **Hemodialysis** (HD) uses an artificial kidney machine that receives waste-filled blood from the patient's bloodstream, filters it, and returns the dialyzed blood to the patient's body. See Figure 7–12, *A*. An **arteriovenous fistula** (communication between an artery and vein) is created surgically to provide access for hemodialysis. See Figure 7–12, *B*.

2. **Peritoneal dialysis** (PD) uses a peritoneal **catheter** (tube) to introduce fluid into the peritoneal (abdominal) cavity. Chemical properties of the fluid cause wastes in the capillaries of the peritoneum to pass out of the bloodstream and into the fluid. The fluid (with wastes) is then removed by catheter. When used to treat patients with chronic kidney disease, PD may be performed continuously by the patient without mechanical support (CAPD—continuous ambulatory PD; see Figure 7–13) or with the aid of a mechanical apparatus at night during sleep (CCPD—continuous cycling PD).

lithotripsy

Urinary tract stones are crushed and either removed or pass from the body in urine.

The **extracorporeal** method uses shock waves directed toward the stone from the outside of the body. The patient receives light sedation or an analgesic (pain medication). The **endoscopic** method uses an endoscope in the ureter and a laser to crush the stone under direct vision. A basket is used to retrieve larger pieces of stone.

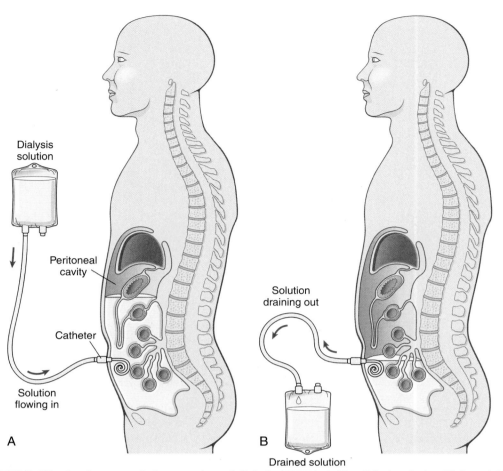

FIGURE 7–13 **Continuous ambulatory peritoneal dialysis (CAPD). A,** The dialysis solution (dialysate) flows from a collapsible plastic bag through a catheter (a Tenckhoff peritoneal catheter) into the patient's peritoneal cavity. The empty bag is then folded and inserted into undergarments. **B,** After 4 to 8 hours, the bag is unfolded, and the fluid is allowed to drain into it by gravity. The full bag is discarded, and a new bag of fresh dialysate is attached.

renal angioplasty	**Dilation of narrowed areas in renal arteries.**
	A balloon attached to a catheter is inserted into the artery and then inflated to enlarge the vessel diameter. Afterward, stents (metal meshed tubes) may be inserted to keep the vessel open.
renal biopsy	**Removal of kidney tissue for microscopic examination by a pathologist.**
	Biopsy may be performed at the time of surgery (open) or through the skin (percutaneous, or closed). When the latter technique is used, the patient lies in the prone position and, after administration of local anesthesia to the overlying skin and muscles of the back, the physician inserts a biopsy needle downward into the kidney.

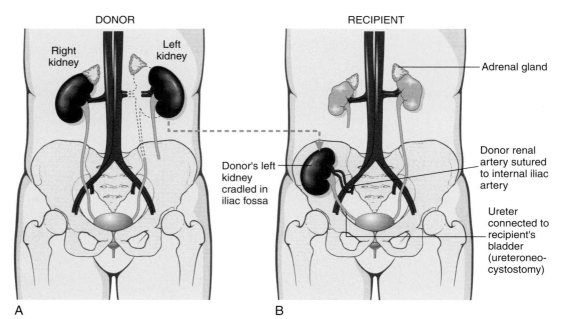

FIGURE 7–14 **Renal (kidney) transplantation. A,** Left kidney of donor is removed for transplantation. **B,** Kidney is transplanted to right pelvis of the recipient. The renal artery and vein of the donor kidney are joined to the recipient kidney's artery and vein, and the lower end of the donor ureter is connected to the recipient's bladder (ureteroneocystostomy). The health of the donor is not affected by losing one kidney. In fact, the remaining kidney enlarges (hypertrophies) to take over almost full function.

renal transplantation

Surgical transfer of a complete kidney from a donor to a recipient.

Patients with renal failure may receive a kidney from a living donor, such as an identical twin (isograft) or other person (allograft), or from a cadaver (dead body). Best results occur when the donor is closely related to the recipient—better than 90 percent of the kidneys survive for 1 year or longer (Fig. 7–14).

urinary catheterization

Passage of a flexible, tubular instrument through the urethra into the urinary bladder.

Catheters are used primarily for short- or long-term drainage of urine. A **Foley catheter** is an indwelling (left in the bladder) catheter held in place by a balloon inflated with air or liquid (Fig. 7–15).

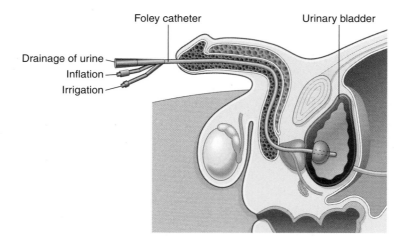

FIGURE 7–15 A **Foley catheter** in place in the urinary bladder. The three-way catheter has three separate lumens: for drainage of urine, for inflation of balloons in the bladder, and for introduction of irrigating solutions into the bladder.

ABBREVIATIONS

ADH	antidiuretic hormone—vasopressin
ARF	acute renal failure
BILI	bilirubin
BUN	blood urea nitrogen
CAPD	continuous ambulatory peritoneal dialysis
Cath	catheter, catheterization
CCPD	continuous cycling peritoneal dialysis
CKD	chronic kidney disease—a condition during which serum creatinine and BUN levels rise, which may result in impairment of all body systems
Cl⁻	chloride—an electrolyte excreted by the kidney
CRF	chronic renal failure—progressive loss of kidney function
C&S	culture and sensitivity testing—to determine antibiotic effectiveness against bacteria grown from a patient's specimen
cysto	cystoscopic examination
ESRD	end-stage renal disease—see CKD

HCO₃⁻	bicarbonate—an electrolyte conserved by the kidney
HD	hemodialysis
IC	interstitial cystitis—chronic inflammation of the bladder wall; not caused by bacterial infection and not responsive to conventional antibiotic therapy.
K⁺	potassium—an electrolyte
KUB	kidney, ureter, and bladder
Na⁺	sodium—an electrolyte
PD	peritoneal dialysis
pH	symbol for degree of acidity or alkalinity
PKD	polycystic kidney disease
PKU	phenylketonuria
PUL	percutaneous ultrasonic lithotripsy
RP	retrograde pyelogram
sp gr	specific gravity
UA	urinalysis
UTI	urinary tract infection
VCUG	voiding cystourethrogram

PRACTICAL APPLICATIONS

Answers to the questions about the case report and the urinalysis findings are on page 243.

UROLOGIC CASE REPORT

The patient, a 50-year-old woman, presented herself at the clinic complaining of dysuria. This symptom was followed by sudden onset of hematuria and clots. There had been no history of urolithiasis, pyuria, or previous hematuria. Nocturia had been present about 5 years earlier. Panendoscopy revealed a carcinoma located about 2 cm from the left ureteral orifice. A partial cystectomy was carried out and the lesion cleared. No ileal conduit was necessary. A metastatic workup was negative. Bilateral pelvic lymphadenectomy revealed no positive nodes.

Questions about the Case Report

1. Urologic refers to which system of the body?
   a. Digestive
   b. Reproductive
   c. Excretory

2. What was the patient's reason for appearing at the clinic?
   a. Scanty urination
   b. Inability to urinate
   c. Painful urination

3. What acute symptom followed?
   a. Blood in the feces
   b. Blood in the urine
   c. Excessive urea in the blood

4. Which of the following was a previous symptom?
   a. Pus in the urine
   b. Blood in the urine
   c. Excessive urination at night

5. What diagnostic procedure was carried out?
   a. Lithotripsy
   b. Cystoscopy using a wide-angle view of the bladder
   c. Urinalysis

6. The patient's diagnosis was
   a. Malignant tumor of the bladder
   b. Tumor in the proximal ureter
   c. Lymph nodes affected by tumor

7. Treatment was
   a. Ureteroileostomy
   b. Removal of tumor and subtotal removal of the bladder
   c. Not necessary because of negative lymph nodes

URINALYSIS FINDINGS

Test	Normal	Abnormal
Color	Amber-yellow	Smoky-red (blood in urine): renal calculi; tumor; kidney disease; cystitis; urinary obstruction
Appearance	Clear	Cloudy (pyuria): urinary tract infection (UTI)
pH	4.6–8.0	Alkaline: UTI
Protein	None or small amt	Proteinuria: nephritis; renal failure
Glucose	None	Glycosuria: diabetes mellitus
Ketones	None	Ketonuria: diabetes mellitus
Bilirubin	None	Bilirubinuria: hepatitis or gallbladder disease
Specific gravity	1.003–1.030	*High:* renal calculi; diabetes mellitus *Low:* diabetes insipidus
Sediment	None	Casts: nephritis; renal disease

Name the appropriate test for detecting or evaluating each of the following:

1. Sugar in urine _____

2. Level of bile pigment in urine _____

3. Hematuria _____

4. Albumin in urine _____

5. Structures in the shape of renal tubules in urine _____

6. Chemical reaction of urine _____

7. Dilution or concentration of urine _____

8. Acetones in urine _____

9. Pus in urine _____

EXERCISES

Remember to check your answers carefully with those given in the Answers to Exercises, page 242.

A. Using the following terms, trace the path of urine from the renal arterioles (bloodstream) to the point at which urine leaves the body. The first answer is provided.

Bowman capsule	renal pelvis	ureter	urinary bladder
glomerulus	renal tubule	urethra	urinary meatus

1. _glomerulus_ _____

2. _____

3. _____

4. _____

5. _____

6. _____

7. _____

8. _____

B. Match the term in Column I with its definition or a term of similar meaning in Column II. Write the correct letter in the spaces provided.

Column I

1. voiding _____

2. trigone _____

3. renal cortex _____

4. renal medulla _____

5. urea _____

6. erythropoietin _____

7. renin _____

8. electrolyte _____

9. hilum _____

10. calyx (calix) _____

Column II

A. A hormone secreted by the kidney that stimulates formation of red blood cells.
B. Notch on the surface of the kidney where blood vessels and nerves enter.
C. Micturition; urination.
D. Nitrogenous waste.
E. Cup-like collecting region of the renal pelvis.
F. A small molecule that carries an electric charge in solution.
G. Inner region of the kidney.
H. Enzymatic hormone made by the kidney; increases blood pressure.
I. Triangular area in the bladder.
J. Outer section of the kidney.

C. Give the meanings of the following medical terms.

1. caliceal _____

2. uric acid _____

3. urinary meatal stenosis _____

4. cystocele _____

5. pyelolithotomy _____

6. trigonitis _____

7. ureteroileostomy _____

8. urethrostenosis _____

9. vesicoureteral reflux _____

10. creatinine _____

11. medullary _____

12. cortical _____

D. The following terms all contain the suffix *-uria*, meaning urination. Write their meanings in the spaces provided.

1. nocturia _____

2. dysuria _____

3. oliguria _____

4. polyuria _____

5. anuria _____

E. In the following terms, *-uria* means urine condition (substance in the urine). What's in the urine?

1. pyuria _____   4. glycosuria _____

2. albuminuria _____   5. ketonuria _____

3. hematuria _____   6. bacteriuria _____

F. Give the meanings of the following terms that relate to urinary symptoms.

1. azotemia _____

2. polydipsia _____

3. urinary incontinence _____

4. enuresis _____

5. urinary retention _____

6. ketosis _____

G. Give short answers for the following.

1. What is the difference between hematuria and uremia? _____

2. What is diuresis? _____

3. What is a diuretic? _____

4. What is antidiuretic hormone? _____

H. Match the following terms that pertain to urinalysis with their meanings below.

albuminuria	hematuria	phenylketonuria	sediment
bilirubinuria	ketonuria	pyuria	specific gravity
glycosuria	pH		

1. Abnormal particles present in the urine—cells, bacteria, casts, and crystals.

   _____

2. High levels of a substance appear in urine when a baby is born with a deficiency of an enzyme. The infant can become mentally retarded if not immediately put on a strict diet that prevents the substance from accumulating in the blood and urine. _____

3. Smoky-red color of urine caused by the presence of blood. _____

4. Turbid (cloudy) urine caused by the presence of polymorphonuclear leukocytes and pus.

   _____

5. Sugar in the urine; a symptom of diabetes mellitus and a result of hyperglycemia.

   _____

6. This urine test reflects the acidity or alkalinity of the urine. _____

7. High levels of acids and acetones accumulate in the urine as a result of abnormal fat catabolism.

   _____

8. Dark pigment accumulates in urine as a result of liver or gallbladder disease.

   _____

9. This urine test reflects the concentration of the urine. _____

10. Leaky glomeruli can produce accumulation of protein in the urine. _____

I. Describe the following abnormal conditions that affect the kidney.

1. renal failure _____

2. polycystic kidney _____

3. interstitial nephritis _____

4. glomerulonephritis _____

5. nephrolithiasis _____

6. renal cell carcinoma _____

7. pyelonephritis _____

8. Wilms tumor _____

9. nephrotic syndrome _____

10. renal hypertension _____

J. Match the following terms with their meanings below.

abscess   edema   renal colic
catheter   essential hypertension   secondary hypertension
diabetes insipidus   nephroptosis   stricture
diabetes mellitus

1. idiopathic high blood pressure _____

2. swelling, fluid in tissues _____

3. narrowed area in a tube _____

4. collection of pus _____

5. inadequate secretion of insulin or improper utilization of insulin leads to this condition

   _____

6. high blood pressure caused by kidney disease or another disease _____

7. tube for withdrawing or giving fluid _____

8. inadequate secretion or resistance of the kidney to the action of antidiuretic hormone

   _____

9. prolapse of a kidney _____

10. severe pain resulting from a stone that is blocking a ureter or a kidney

   _____

K. Give the meanings of the following abbreviations. Then select the letter of the sentence that is the best association for each.

Column I

1. CAPD _____ ____

2. BUN _____ ____

3. RP _____ ____

4. cysto _____ ____

5. UA _____ ____

6. UTI _____ ____

7. CKD _____ ____

8. K+ _____ ____

9. VCUG _____ ____

10. HD _____ ____

Column II

A. Bacterial invasion leads to this condition; acute cystitis is an example.

B. This electrolyte is secreted by renal tubules into the urine.

C. A machine removes nitrogenous wastes from the patient's blood.

D. High levels measured on this test lead to the suspicion of renal disease.

E. This endoscopic procedure is used to examine the interior of the urinary bladder.

F. Dialysate (fluid) is injected into the peritoneal cavity and then drained out.

G. Contrast is injected into the urinary bladder and ureters and x-ray pictures of the urinary tract are taken.

H. X-ray pictures of the urinary bladder and urethra are taken while the patient urinates.

I. The parts of this test include specific gravity, color, protein, glucose, and pH.

J. This condition includes mild to severe kidney failure.

L. Match the following procedures with their meanings below.

cystectomy   nephrectomy   ureterolithotomy
cystostomy   nephrolithotomy   urethroplasty
lithotripsy   nephrostomy
meatotomy   ureteroileostomy (ileal conduit)

1. Excision of a kidney_____

2. Surgical incision into the kidney to remove a stone_____

3. Incision of the urinary meatus for enlargement _____

4. Crushing of stones_____

5. New opening of the ureters to a segment of ileum (in place of the bladder)

_____

6. Surgical repair of the urethra_____

7. Creation of an artificial opening into the kidney (via catheter) from the outside of the body

_____

8. Surgical formation of an opening from the bladder to the outside of the body

_____

9. Removal of the urinary bladder _____

10. Incision of a ureter to remove a stone _____

M. Circle the correct term to complete the following sentences.

1. After diagnosis of renal cell carcinoma (made by renal biopsy), Dr. Davis advised Donna that **(nephrostomy, meatotomy, nephrectomy)** would be necessary.

2. Ever since Bill's condition of gout was diagnosed, he has been warned that uric acid crystals could accumulate in his blood and tissues, leading to **(pyuria, renal calculi, cystocele)**.

3. The voiding cystourethrogram demonstrated blockage of urine flow from Jim's bladder and **(hydronephrosis, renal ischemia, azotemia)**.

4. Narrowed arterioles in the kidney increase blood pressure, so **(urinary incontinence, urinary retention, nephrosclerosis)** is often associated with hypertension.

5. Eight-year-old Willy continually wet his bed at night while sleeping. His pediatrician instructed his mother to limit Willy's intake of fluids in the evening to discourage his **(nocturia, oliguria, enuresis)**.

6. David's chronic type 1 diabetes eventually resulted in **(nephropathy, meatal stenosis, urolithiasis)**, which led to renal failure.

7. After Sue's bilateral renal failure, her doctor advised dialysis and possible **(cystostomy, nephrolithotomy, renal transplantation)**.

7

8. When Maria's left kidney stopped functioning, her contralateral kidney overdeveloped or **(metastasized, atrophied, hypertrophied)** to meet the increased workload.

9. A popular diet program recommends eating foods high in fats and protein. People on this diet check their urine for the presence of **(ketones, glucose, amino acids)**.

10. Andrea's urinalysis revealed proteinuria, and her ankles began to swell, demonstrating pitting, a condition known as **(ascites, edema, stricture)**. Her **(gastroenterologist, urologist, nephrologist)** diagnosed Andrea's condition as **(polycystic kidneys, nephrotic syndrome, bladder carcinoma)** and recommended drugs to heal leaky glomeruli and diuretics to reduce swelling.

MEDICAL SCRAMBLE

Unscramble the letters to form urinary system terms from the clues. Use the letters in squares to complete the bonus term. Answers are found on page 243.

1. *Clue:* Pus in the urine

___ ☐ ___ ☐ ___ ☐   RAPIYU

2. *Clue:* Blood in the urine

___ ___ ___ ___ ___ ___ ☐ ___   TAMIHUERA

3. *Clue:* Sugar in the urine

___ ☐ ___ ___ ___ ☐ ☐ ___ ___ ___   CILASGUYRO

4. *Clue:* Protein in the urine

___ ___ ___ ___ ___ ___ ☐ ___ ___ ☐ ___   NLIBAIMURAU

5. *Clue:* An electrolyte

☐ ___ ___ ___ ___ ___   MIDOSU

BONUS TERM: *Clue:* Examination of urine to determine its contents.

☐ ☐ ☐ ☐ ☐ ☐ ☐ ☐ ☐ ☐

7

ANSWERS TO EXERCISES

A

1. glomerulus
2. Bowman capsule
3. renal tubule
4. renal pelvis
5. ureter
6. urinary bladder
7. urethra
8. urinary meatus

B

1. C
2. I
3. J
4. G
5. D
6. A
7. H
8. F
9. B
10. E

C

1. pertaining to a calix (collecting cup of renal pelvis)
2. nitrogenous waste excreted in urine; high levels of uric acid in the blood are associated with gouty arthritis
3. narrowing of the urinary meatus
4. hernia of the urinary bladder
5. incision to remove a stone from the renal pelvis
6. inflammation of the trigone (triangular area in the bladder in which the ureters enter and urethra exits)
7. new opening between the ureter and the ileum (an anastomosis); urine then leaves the body through an ileostomy; this surgery is performed when the bladder has been resected
8. narrowing (narrowed portion) of the urethra
9. backflow of urine from the bladder into the ureter
10. nitrogenous waste produced as a result of muscle metabolism and excreted in the urine
11. pertaining to the inner, middle section (of the kidney)
12. pertaining to the outer section (of the kidney)

D

1. frequent urination at night
2. painful urination
3. scanty urination
4. excessive urination
5. no urination

E

1. pus
2. protein
3. blood
4. sugar
5. ketones or acetones
6. bacteria

F

1. excess nitrogenous waste in the bloodstream
2. condition of much thirst
3. inability to hold urine in the bladder
4. bedwetting
5. inability to release urine from the bladder
6. abnormal condition of ketone bodies (acids and acetones) in the blood and body tissues

G

1. Hematuria is the presence of blood in the urine, and uremia is a toxic condition of excess urea (nitrogenous waste) in the bloodstream. Hematuria is a symptomatic condition of the urine (-uria), and uremia is an abnormal condition of the blood (-emia).
2. Diuresis is the excessive production of urine (polyuria).
3. A diuretic is a drug or chemical (caffeine or alcohol) that causes diuresis to occur.
4. Antidiuretic hormone is a hormone produced by the pituitary gland that normally helps the renal tubules to reabsorb water back into the bloodstream. It works against diuresis to help retain water in the blood.

H

1. sediment
2. phenylketonuria (phenylketones in the urine)
3. hematuria (blood in the urine)
4. pyuria (pus in the urine)
5. glycosuria (sugar in the urine)
6. pH
7. ketonuria (ketone bodies in the urine)
8. bilirubinuria (high levels of bilirubin in the urine)
9. specific gravity
10. albuminuria

I

1. kidney does not excrete wastes
2. multiple fluid-filled sacs form in and on the kidney
3. inflammation of the connective tissue (interstitium) lying between the renal tubules
4. inflammation of the glomerulus of the kidney (may be a complication following a streptococcal infection)
5. condition of kidney stones (renal calculi)
6. malignant tumor of the kidney in adults
7. inflammation of the kidney and renal pelvis (caused by a bacterial infection, such as with *Escherichia coli,* that spreads to the urinary tract from the gastrointestinal tract)
8. malignant tumor of the kidney in children
9. group of symptoms (proteinuria, edema, hypoalbuminemia) that appears when the kidney is damaged by disease; also called nephrosis
10. high blood pressure caused by kidney disease

J

1. essential hypertension
2. edema
3. stricture
4. abscess
5. diabetes mellitus
6. secondary hypertension
7. catheter
8. diabetes insipidus
9. nephroptosis
10. renal colic

K

1. continuous ambulatory peritoneal dialysis: F
2. blood, urea, nitrogen: D
3. retrograde pyelogram: G
4. cystoscopy: E
5. urinalysis: I
6. urinary tract infection: A
7. chronic kidney disease: J
8. potassium: B
9. voiding cystourethrogram: H
10. hemodialysis: C

L

1. nephrectomy
2. nephrolithotomy
3. meatotomy
4. lithotripsy
5. ureteroileostomy
6. urethroplasty
7. nephrostomy
8. cystostomy
9. cystectomy
10. ureterolithotomy

M

1. nephrectomy
2. renal calculi—don't confuse a calculus (stone) with dental calculus, which is an accumulation of dental plaque that has hardened
3. hydronephrosis
4. nephrosclerosis
5. enuresis
6. nephropathy
7. renal transplantation
8. hypertrophied
9. ketones
10. edema, nephrologist, nephrotic syndrome

ANSWERS TO PRACTICAL APPLICATIONS

Case Report
1. c
2. c
3. b
4. c
5. b
6. a
7. b

Urinalysis Findings
1. glucose
2. bilirubin
3. color
4. protein
5. sediment
6. pH
7. specific gravity
8. ketones
9. appearance

ANSWERS TO MEDICAL SCRAMBLE

1. PYURIA　　2. HEMATURIA　　3. GLYCOSURIA　　4. ALBUMINURIA　　5. SODIUM
BONUS TERM: URINALYSIS

PRONUNCIATION OF TERMS

To test your understanding of the terminology in this chapter, write the meaning of each term in the space provided. In addition, you may wish to cover the terms and write them by looking at your definitions. Make sure your spelling is correct. The page number after each term indicates where it is defined or used in the book, so you can easily check your responses. You will find complete definitions for all of these terms and audio pronunciations on the CD.

Term	Pronunciation	Meaning
abscess (226)	ĂB-sĕs	_____
acetone (222)	ĂS-ĕ-tōn	_____
albuminuria (221)	ăl-bū-mĭn-Ū-rē-ă	_____
antidiuretic hormone (222)	ăn-tĭ-dī-ū-RĔ-tĭk HŎR-mōn	_____
anuria (223)	ăn-Ū-rē-ă	_____
arteriole (216)	ăr-TĔR-ē-ōl	_____
azotemia (221)	ă-zō-TĒ-mē-ă	_____
bacteriuria (222)	băk-tē-rē-Ū-rē-ă	_____
Bowman capsule (216)	BŌ-măn KĂP-sŭl	_____
caliceal (219)	kā-lĭ-SĒ-ăl	_____
caliectasis (219)	kā-lē-ĔK-tă-sĭs	_____
calyx (calix); *plural:* calyces (calices) (216)	KĀ-lĭks; KĀ-lĭ-sēz	_____
catheter (216)	KĂ-thĕ-tĕr	_____
cortex (216)	KŎR-tĕks	_____
cortical (216)	KŎR-tĭ-kăl	_____
creatinine (216)	krē-ĂT-ĭ-nēn	_____
creatinine clearance test (216)	krē-ĂT-ĭ-nēn KLĔR-ăns tĕst	_____
cystectomy (219)	sĭs-TĔK-tō-mē	_____
cystitis (219)	sĭs-TĪ-tĭs	_____
cystoscopy (229)	sĭs-TŎS-kō-pē	_____
cystostomy (219)	sĭs-TŎS-tō-mē	_____
diabetes insipidus (227)	dī-ă-BĒ-tēz ĭn-SĬP-ĭ-dŭs	_____
diabetes mellitus (227)	dī-ă-BĒ-tēz MĔL-ĭ-tŭs	_____
diuresis (222)	dī-ūr-RĒ-sĭs	_____
dysuria (223)	dĭs-Ū-rē-ă	_____

Term	Pronunciation	Meaning
edema (225)	ĕ-DĒ-mă	_____
electrolyte (216)	ē-LĔK-trō-līt	_____
enuresis (222)	ĕn-ū-RĒ-sĭs	_____
erythropoietin (222)	ĕ-rĭth-rō-PŌ-ĕ-tĭn	_____
essential hypertension (227)	ē-SĔN-shŭl hī-pĕr-TĔN-shŭn	_____
filtration (217)	fĭl-TRĀ-shŭn	_____
glomerular (219)	glō-MĔR-ū-lăr	_____
glomerulonephritis (225)	glō-mĕr-ū-lō-nĕ-FRĪ-tĭs	_____
glomerulus; glomeruli (217)	glō-MĔR-ū-lŭs; glō-MĔR-ū-lī	_____
glycosuria (223)	glī-kōs-Ū-rē-ă	_____
hematuria (223)	hēm-ă-TŪ-rē-ă	_____
hemodialysis (230)	hē-mō-dī-ĂL-ĭ-sĭs	_____
hilum (217)	HĪ-lŭm	_____
hydronephrosis (220)	hī-drō-nĕ-FRŌ-sĭs	_____
interstitial nephritis (225)	ĭn-tĕr-STĬ-shŭl nĕ-FRĪ-tĭs	_____
ketonuria (222)	kē-tōn-Ū-rē-ă	_____
ketosis (222)	kē-TŌ-sĭs	_____
kidney (217)	KĬD-nē	_____
lithotripsy (222)	LĬTH-ō-trĭp-sē	_____
meatal stenosis (219)	mē-Ā-tăl stĕ-NŌ-sĭs	_____
meatotomy (219)	mē-ā-TŎT-ō-mē	_____
meatus (217)	mē-Ā-tŭs	_____
medulla (217)	mĕ-DŪL-ă or mĕ-DŬL-ă	_____
medullary (217)	MĔD-ū-lăr-ē	_____
micturition (218)	mĭk-tū-RĬSH-ŭn	_____
nephrolithiasis (225)	nĕf-rō-lĭ-THĪ-ă-sĭs	_____
nephrolithotomy (220)	nĕf-rō-lĭ-THŎT-ō-mē	_____
nephron (218)	NĔF-rŏn	_____
nephropathy (220)	nĕ-FRŎ-pă-thē	_____
nephroptosis (220)	nĕf-rŏp-TŌ-sĭs	_____
nephrosclerosis (220)	nĕf-rō-sklĕ-RŌ-sĭs	_____
nephrostomy (220)	nĕ-FRŎS-tō-mē	_____
nephrotic syndrome (225)	nĕ-FRŎT-ĭk SĬN-drōm	_____

7

Term	Pronunciation	Meaning
nitrogenous waste (218)	nĭ-TRŎJ-ĕ-nŭs wāst	
nocturia (222)	nŏk-TŪ-rē-ă	
oliguria (222)	ŏl-ĭ-GŪ-rē-ă	
paranephric (220)	pă-ră-NĔF-rĭk	
peritoneal dialysis (230)	pĕr-ĭ-tō-NĒ-ăl dī-ĂL-ĭ-sĭs	
perivesical (221)	pĕ-rē-VĔS-ĭ-kăl	
phenylketonuria (224)	fē-nĭl-kē-tōn-ŪR-ē-ă	
polycystic kidney disease (225)	pŏl-ē-SĬS-tĭk KĬD-nē dĭ-ZĒZ	
polydipsia (222)	pŏl-ē-DĬP-sē-ă	
polyuria (223)	pŏl-ē-Ū-rē-ă	
potassium (218)	pō-TĂ-sē-ŭm	
pyelogram (221)	PĪ-ĕ-lo-grăm	
pyelolithotomy (221)	pī-ĕ-lō-lĭ-THŎT-ō-mē	
pyelonephritis (226)	pī-ĕ-lō-nĕf-RĪ-tĭs	
pyuria (222)	pī-Ū-rē-ă	
reabsorption (218)	rē-ăb-SŎRP-shŭn	
renal angiography (228)	RĒ-năl ăn-jē-ŎG-ră-fē	
renal angioplasty (231)	RĒ-năl ĂN-jē-ō-plăs-tē	
renal artery (218)	RĒ-năl ĂR-tĕ-rē	
renal calculi (225)	RĒ-năl KĂL-kū-lī	
renal cell carcinoma (226)	RĒ-năl sĕl kăr-sĭ-NŌ-mă	
renal colic (221)	RĒ-năl KŎL-ĭk	
renal failure (226)	RĒ-năl FĀL-ūr	
renal hypertension (226)	RĒ-năl hī-pĕr-TĔN-shŭn	
renal ischemia (221)	RĒ-năl ĭs-KĒ-mē-ă	
renal pelvis (218)	RĒ-năl PĔL-vĭs	
renal transplantation (232)	RĒ-năl trăns-plăn-TĀ-shŭn	
renal tubule (218)	RĒ-năl TŪ-būl	
renal vein (218)	RĒ-năl vān	
renin (218)	RĒ-nĭn	
retrograde pyelogram (228)	RĔ-trō-grād PĪ-ĕ-lō-grăm	
secondary hypertension (226)	SĔ-kŏn-dă-rē hī-pĕr-TĔN-shŭn	
sodium (218)	SŌ-dē-ŭm	

Term	Pronunciation	Meaning
stricture (221)	STRĬK-shŭr	_____
trigone (218)	TRĪ-gōn	_____
trigonitis (221)	trī-gō-NĪ-tĭs	_____
urea (218)	ū-RĒ-ă	_____
uremia (222)	ū-RĒ-mē-ă	_____
ureter (218)	ū-RĒ-tĕr _or_ ŪR-ĕ-tĕr	_____
ureteroileostomy (221)	ū-rē-tĕr-ō-ĭl-ē-ŎS-tō-mē	_____
ureterolithotomy (221)	ū-rē-tĕr-ō-lĭ-THŎT-ō-mē	_____
ureteroneocystostomy (232)	ū-rē-tĕr-ō-nē-ō-sĭs-TŎS-tō-mē	_____
ureteroplasty (221)	ū-rē-tĕr-ō-PLĂS-tē	_____
urethra (218)	ū-RĒ-thră	_____
urethral stricture (221)	ū-RĒ-thrăl STRĬK-shŭr	_____
urethritis (221)	ū-rē-THRĪ-tĭs	_____
urethroplasty (221)	ū-rē-thrō-PLĂS-tē	_____
uric acid (218)	Ū-rĭk ĂS-ĭd	_____
urinalysis (223)	ū-rĭn-ĂL-ĭ-sĭs	_____
urinary bladder (218)	ŪR-ĭ-năr-ē BLĂ-dĕr	_____
urinary catheterization (232)	ŪR-ĭ-năr-ē kă-thĕ-tĕr-ĭ-ZĀ-shŭn	_____
urinary incontinence (223)	ŪR-ĭ-năr-ē ĭn-KŎN-tĭ-nĕns	_____
urinary retention (223)	ŪR-ĭ-năr-ē rē-TĔN-shŭn	_____
urination (218)	ūr-ĭ-NĀ-shŭn	_____
vesicoureteral reflux (221)	vĕs-ĭ-kō-ū-RĒ-tĕr-ăl RĒ-flŭks	_____
voiding (218)	VOY-dĭng	_____
voiding cystourethrogram (229)	VOY-dĭng sĭs-tō-ū-RĒ-thrō-grăm	_____
Wilms tumor (227)	wĭlmz TŪ-mŭr	_____

REVIEW SHEET

Write the meanings of the combining forms, suffixes, and prefixes in the spaces provided. Check your answers with the information in the chapter or in the glossary (Medical Word Parts—English) at the end of the book.

COMBINING FORMS

Combining Form	Meaning	Combining Form	Meaning
albumin/o		meat/o	
angi/o		necr/o	
azot/o		nephr/o	
bacteri/o		noct/o	
cali/o		olig/o	
calic/o		py/o	
cyst/o		pyel/o	
dips/o		ren/o	
glomerul/o		trigon/o	
glycos/o		ur/o	
hydr/o		ureter/o	
isch/o		urethr/o	
ket/o		urin/o	
keton/o		vesic/o	
lith/o			

SUFFIXES

Suffix	Meaning	Suffix	Meaning
-ectasis		-pathy	
-ectomy		-plasty	
-emia		-poietin	
-esis		-ptosis	
-gram		-rrhea	
-lithiasis		-sclerosis	
-lithotomy		-stenosis	
-lysis		-stomy	
-megaly		-tomy	
-ole		-tripsy	
-osis		-uria	

PREFIXES

Prefix	Meaning	Prefix	Meaning
a-, an-	_____	en-	_____
anti-	_____	peri-	_____
dia-	_____	poly-	_____
dys-	_____	retro-	_____

ANATOMIC TERMS

Match the locations/functions in Column I with the urinary system structures in Column II. Write the number of the correct structure in the blanks provided.

Column I

Tiny structure surrounding each glomerulus; receives filtered materials from blood.

Tubes carrying urine from kidney to urinary bladder.

Tubules leading from the Bowman capsule. Urine is formed there as water, sugar, and salts are reabsorbed into the bloodstream.

Inner (middle) region of the kidney.

Muscular sac that serves as a reservoir for urine.

Cup-like divisions of the renal pelvis that receive urine from the renal tubules.

Tube carrying urine from the bladder to the outside of the body.

Central urine-collecting basin in the kidney that narrows into the ureter.

Collection of capillaries through which materials from the blood are filtered into the Bowman capsule.

Outer region of the kidney.

Column II

1. urethra
2. cortex
3. Bowman capsule
4. calices
5. renal pelvis
6. glomerulus
7. medulla
8. renal tubules
9. urinary bladder
10. ureters

Please refer to the enclosed CD for additional exercises and images related to this chapter.

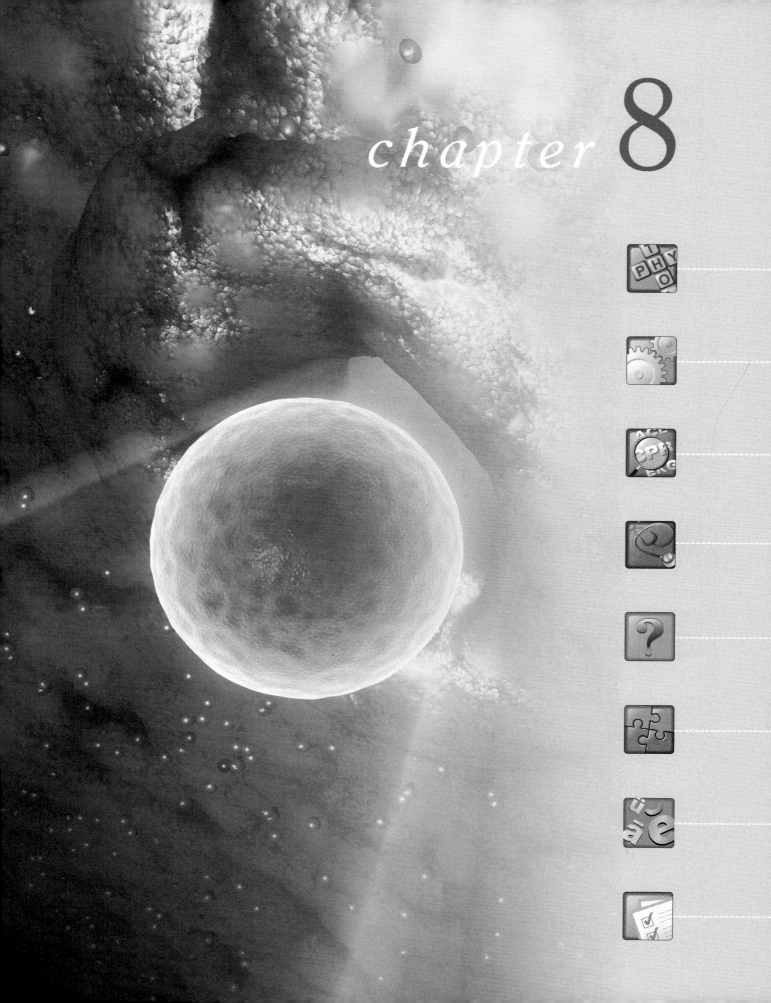

chapter 8

Female Reproductive System

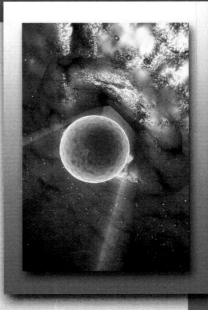

THIS CHAPTER IS DIVIDED INTO THE FOLLOWING SECTIONS

In this chapter you will

- Name the organs of the female reproductive system, their locations, and combining forms.
- Explain how these organs and their hormones function in the normal processes of ovulation, menstruation, and pregnancy.
- Identify abnormal conditions of the female reproductive system and of the newborn child.
- Describe important laboratory tests and clinical procedures used in gynecology and obstetrics, and recognize related abbreviations.
- Apply your new knowledge to understanding medical terms in their proper contexts, such as medical reports and records.

Image Description: Cellular conceptual visualization of the moment when an ovum is released into the fallopian tube.

8

INTRODUCTION

Sexual reproduction is the union of the nuclei of the female sex cell **(ovum)** and the male sex cell **(sperm cell)** that results in the creation of an embryo, the forerunner of a new individual. The ovum and the sperm cell are specialized cells differing primarily from normal body cells in one important way: Each sex cell **(gamete)** contains exactly half the number of chromosomes of a normal body cell. When the nuclei of ovum and sperm cell unite, the cell produced receives half of its genetic material from its female parent and half from its male parent; thus, it contains a full, normal complement of hereditary material.

Gametes are produced in special organs called **gonads** in both males and females. The female gonads are the **ovaries,** and the male gonads are the **testes.** After an ovum leaves the ovary, it travels down a duct **(fallopian tube)** leading to the **uterus** (womb). If **coitus** (copulation, sexual intercourse) has occurred and sperm cells are present in the fallopian tube, union of the ovum and sperm may take place. This union is **fertilization.** The fertilized egg divides to form a ball of cells, called a **zygote** and then an **embryo** (2 to 6 weeks) and **fetus** (6 to 38 weeks). The period of development within the uterus is **gestation** or **pregnancy.**

The female reproductive system consists of organs that produce **ova** and provide a place for the growth of the embryo. In addition, the female reproductive organs supply important hormones that contribute to the development of female secondary sex characteristics (body hair, breast development, structural changes in bones and fat).

The eggs, or ova, are present from birth in the female ovary but begin to mature and are released from the ovary in a 21- to 28-day cycle when secondary sex characteristics develop. This cycle continues until **menopause** (cessation of fertility and diminishing of hormone production). If fertilization occurs at any time during the years between puberty and menopause, the fertilized egg may grow and develop within the uterus. A new, blood vessel–rich lining called a **placenta** develops to nourish the embryo, which implants in the uterine lining. Various hormones are secreted from the ovary and from the placenta to stimulate the expansion of the placenta. If fertilization does not occur, hormone changes result in shedding of the uterine lining, and bleeding, or **menstruation,** occurs.

The hormones of the ovaries, **estrogen** and **progesterone,** play important roles in the processes of menstruation and pregnancy, and in the development of secondary sex characteristics. The **pituitary gland,** located at the base of the brain, secretes other hormones that govern the reproductive functions of the ovaries, breasts, and uterus.

Gynecology is the study of the female reproductive system (organs, hormones, and diseases); **obstetrics** (Latin *obstetrix* means midwife) is a specialty concerned with pregnancy and the delivery of the fetus; and **neonatology** is the study of the care and treatment of the newborn child.

ORGANS OF THE FEMALE REPRODUCTIVE SYSTEM

UTERUS, OVARIES, AND ASSOCIATED ORGANS

Label Figures 8–1 and 8–3 as you read the following description of the female reproductive system.

Figure 8–1 is a side view of the female reproductive organs and shows their relationship to the other organs in the pelvic cavity. The **ovaries** [1] (only one ovary is shown in this lateral view) are a pair of small, almond-shaped organs located in the pelvis. The **fallopian tubes** [2] (only one is shown in this view) lead from each ovary to the **uterus** [3], which is a hollow muscular organ situated between the urinary bladder and the rectum. The uterus (womb) normally is the size and shape of a pear and about

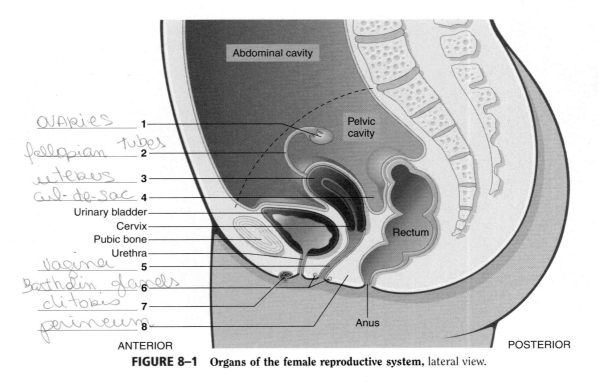

ovaries — 1
fallopian tubes — 2
uterus — 3
cul-de-sac — 4
Urinary bladder —
Cervix —
Pubic bone —
Urethra —
vagina — 5
Bartholin glands — 6
clitoris — 7
perineum — 8

Abdominal cavity

Pelvic cavity

Rectum

Anus

ANTERIOR   POSTERIOR

FIGURE 8–1 Organs of the female reproductive system, lateral view.

3 inches long in a nonpregnant woman. Midway between the uterus and the rectum is a region in the abdominal cavity known as the **cul-de-sac** [4].

The **vagina** [5] is a tubular structure extending from the uterus to the exterior of the body. **Bartholin glands** [6] are two small, rounded glands on either side of the vaginal orifice. These glands produce a mucous secretion that lubricates the vagina. The **clitoris** [7] is an organ of sensitive, erectile tissue located anterior to the vaginal orifice and in front of the urethral meatus. The region between the vaginal orifice and the anus is the **perineum** [8].

The external genitalia (the structures associated with sexual activity) of the female are collectively called the **vulva.** Figure 8–2 shows the various structures that are part of the vulva. The **labia majora,** the outer lips of the vagina, surround the smaller, inner lips, which are the **labia minora.** The **hymen,** a thin membrane partially covering the entrance to the vagina, is broken apart during the first episode of intercourse. The clitoris and Bartholin glands also are parts of the vulva.

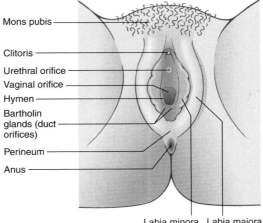

Mons pubis
Clitoris
Urethral orifice
Vaginal orifice
Hymen
Bartholin glands (duct orifices)
Perineum
Anus

Labia minora   Labia majora

FIGURE 8–2 **Female external genitalia (vulva).** The mons pubis (Latin *mons*, mountain) is a pad of tissue overlying the pubic symphysis. After puberty it is covered with pubic hair.

8

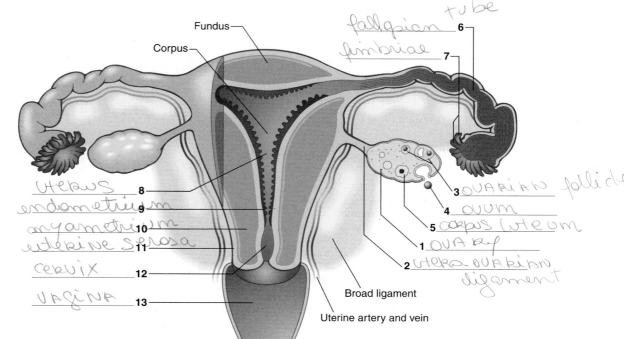

Handwritten annotations on the figure:

Fundus

Corpus

6 — fallopian tube

7 — fimbriae

3 — OVARIAN follicle

4 — OVUM

5 — corpus luteum

1 — OVARy

2 — utero-ovARIAN ligament

8 — uterus

9 — endometrium

10 — myometrium

11 — uterine serosa

12 — cervix

13 — vagina

Broad ligament

Uterine artery and vein

FIGURE 8–3 **Organs of the female reproductive system,** anterior view.

Figure 8–3 is an anterior view of the female reproductive system. Each **ovary** [1] is held in place on either side of the uterus by a **utero-ovarian ligament** [2].

Within each ovary are thousands of small sacs—the **ovarian follicles** [3]. Each follicle contains an **ovum** [4]. When an ovum matures, its follicle ruptures through the surface and releases the ovum from the ovary. This is **ovulation.** A ruptured follicle fills first with blood and then with a yellow, fat-like material. It is then the **corpus luteum** [5], meaning yellow body. The corpus luteum secretes a hormone to maintain the very first stages of pregnancy.

A fallopian tube [6] is about 5½ inches long and lies near each ovary. Collectively, the fallopian tubes, ovaries, and supporting ligaments are the **adnexa** (accessory structures) of the uterus. The egg, after its release from the ovary, is caught up by the finger-like ends of the fallopian tube. These ends are the **fimbriae** [7]. The tube itself is lined with cilia (small hairs) that, through their motion, sweep the ovum along. It usually takes the ovum about 2 to 3 days to pass through the fallopian tube.

If sperm cells are present in the fallopian tube, fertilization may occur. If sperm cells are not present, the ovum remains unfertilized and eventually disintegrates.

The fallopian tubes, one on either side, lead into the **uterus** [8], a pear-shaped organ with muscular walls and a mucous membrane lining filled with a rich supply of blood vessels. The rounded upper portion of the uterus is the **fundus,** and the larger, central section is the **corpus** (body of the organ). The specialized epithelial mucosa of the uterus (its inner layer) is the **endometrium** [9]; the middle, muscular layer of the uterine wall is the **myometrium** [10]; and the outer, membranous tissue layer is the **uterine serosa** [11]. The outermost layer of an organ in the abdomen or thorax is known as a serosa.

The narrow, lowermost portion of the uterus is the **cervix** [12] (Latin *cervix* means neck). The cervical opening leads into a 3-inch-long muscular, mucosa-lined canal called the **vagina** [13], which opens to the outside of the body.

THE BREAST (ACCESSORY ORGAN OF REPRODUCTION)

Label Figure 8–4 as you read the following description of breast structures.

The breasts are two **mammary glands** located in the upper anterior region of the chest. The **glandular tissue** [1] contains milk glands or lobules that develop in response to hormones from the ovaries during puberty. The breasts also contain **fibrous** and **fatty tissue** [2], special **lactiferous** (milk-carrying) **ducts** [3], and **sinuses** (cavities) [4] that carry milk to the nipple, which has small openings for the ducts to release their milk. The breast nipple is the **mammary papilla** [5], and the dark pigmented area around the mammary papilla is the **areola** [6].

During pregnancy, the hormones from the ovaries and the placenta stimulate glandular tissues in the breasts to their full development. After **parturition** (giving birth), hormones from the pituitary gland stimulate the normal secretion of milk **(lactation)**.

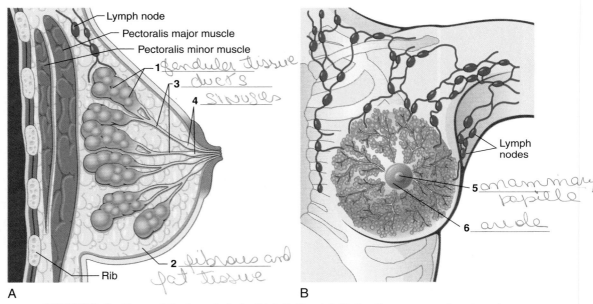

FIGURE 8–4   **Views of the breast. A,** Sagittal. **B,** Frontal. Notice the numerous lymph nodes.

8

MENSTRUATION AND PREGNANCY

MENSTRUAL CYCLE (Fig. 8–5)

Menarche, or the first menstrual cycle, occurs at the onset of puberty. An average menstrual cycle lasts for 28 days but may be shorter or longer, and cycles may be irregular in length. These days can be divided into four time periods, useful in describing the events of the cycle. The approximate time periods are as follows:

Days 1 to 5 (menstrual period)	Discharge of bloody fluid containing disintegrated endometrial cells, glandular secretions, and blood cells.
Days 6 to 12	After bleeding ceases, the endometrium begins to repair itself. The maturing follicle in the ovary releases **estrogen,** which aids in the repair. The ovum grows in the follicle during this period.
Days 13 and 14 (ovulatory period)	On about the 14th day of the cycle, the follicle ruptures **(ovulation)** and the egg leaves the ovary, passing through the fallopian tube.
Days 15 to 28	The empty follicle fills with a yellow material and is now the **corpus luteum.** The corpus luteum functions as an endocrine organ and secretes the hormone **progesterone** into the bloodstream. This hormone stimulates the building up of the lining of the uterus in anticipation of fertilization of the egg and pregnancy.
	If fertilization does *not* occur, the corpus luteum in the ovary stops producing progesterone and regresses. At this time, lowered levels of progesterone and estrogen probably are responsible for some women's symptoms of depression, breast

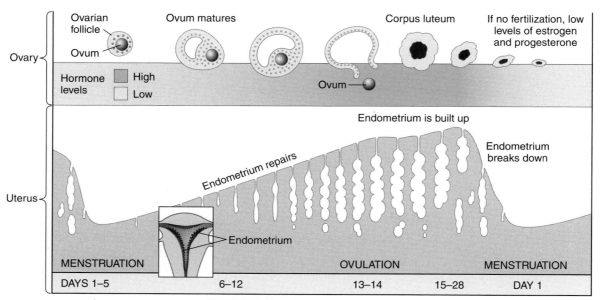

FIGURE 8–5 The menstrual cycle.

tenderness, and irritability before menstruation. These symptoms are known as **premenstrual syndrome (PMS).** After 2 days of decrease in hormones, the uterine endometrium breaks down and the menstrual period begins (days 1 to 5).

Note: Cycles vary in length, ranging from 21 to 42 days or longer. Ovulation typically occurs 14 days before the end of the cycle. A woman with a 42-day cycle ovulates on day 28, whereas a woman with a 21-day cycle ovulates on day 7.

PREGNANCY

If fertilization does occur in the fallopian tube, the fertilized egg travels to the uterus and implants in the uterine endometrium. The corpus luteum in the ovary continues to produce progesterone and estrogen. This supports the vascular and glandular development of the uterine lining.

The **placenta,** a vascular organ, now forms within the uterine wall. The placenta is derived from maternal endometrium and from the **chorion,** the outermost membrane that surrounds the developing embryo. The **amnion,** the innermost of the embryonic membranes, holds the fetus suspended in an amniotic cavity surrounded by a fluid called the **amniotic fluid.** The amnion with its fluid also is known as the "bag of waters" or amniotic sac, which ruptures (breaks) during labor.

The maternal blood and the fetal blood never mix during pregnancy, but important nutrients, oxygen, and wastes are exchanged as the blood vessels of the fetus (coming from the umbilical cord) lie side by side with the mother's blood vessels in the placenta. Figure 8–6, *A* and *B,* shows implantation in the uterus and the embryo's relationship to the placenta and enveloping membranes (chorion and amnion).

As the placenta develops in the uterus, it produces its own hormone, **human chorionic gonadotropin (hCG).** When women test their urine with a pregnancy test kit, hCG confirms or denies that they are pregnant. hCG stimulates the corpus luteum to continue producing hormones until about the third month of pregnancy, when the placenta takes over the endocrine function and releases estrogen and progesterone. Progesterone maintains the development of the placenta. Low levels of progesterone can lead to spontaneous abortion in pregnant women and menstrual irregularities in nonpregnant women.

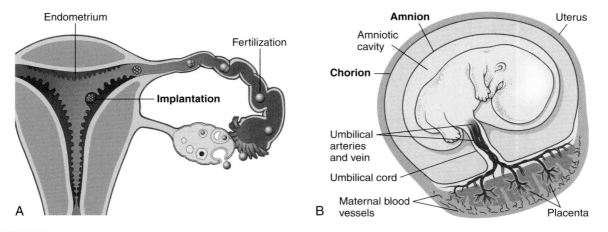

FIGURE 8–6   **A,** Implantation of the embryo in the endometrium. **B,** The placenta and membranes (chorion and amnion).

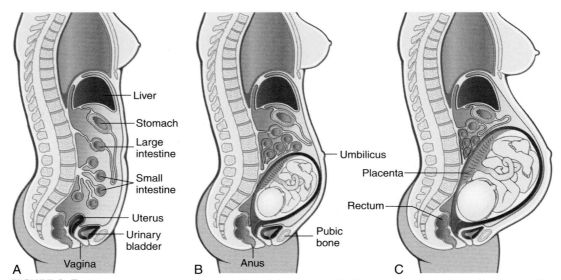

FIGURE 8–7   The growing uterus changes the pelvic anatomy during pregnancy, as shown here in sagittal section. **A,** In a nonpregnant woman. **B,** In a woman 20 weeks pregnant. **C,** In a woman 30 weeks pregnant.

The uterus normally lies within the pelvis. During pregnancy, the uterus expands as the fetus grows, and the superior part rises out of the pelvic cavity. By about 28 to 30 weeks, it occupies a large part of the abdominopelvic cavity and reaches the epigastric region (Fig. 8–7).

The onset of true labor is marked by rhythmic contractions, dilation of the cervix, and a discharge of bloody mucus from the cervix and vagina (the "show"). In a normal delivery position, the baby's head appears first (cephalic presentation) and helps to dilate the cervix. After vaginal delivery of the baby, the placenta follows, and the physician (or family member) cuts the umbilical cord (Fig. 8–8). Figure 8–9, *A* and *B,* are photographs of a newborn and the placenta with attached cord, minutes after birth. The expelled placenta is the **afterbirth.**

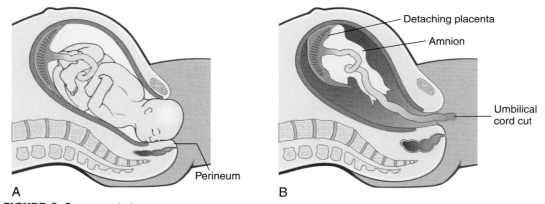

FIGURE 8–8   A, Cephalic presentation ("crowning") of the fetus during delivery from the vaginal (birth) canal. **B,** Between 10 and 15 minutes after parturition (birth), the placenta separates from the uterine wall. Forceful contractions expel the placenta and attached membranes, also called the afterbirth. The three phases of labor are (I) dilation of the cervix, (II) expulsion or birth of the infant, and (III) delivery of the placenta.

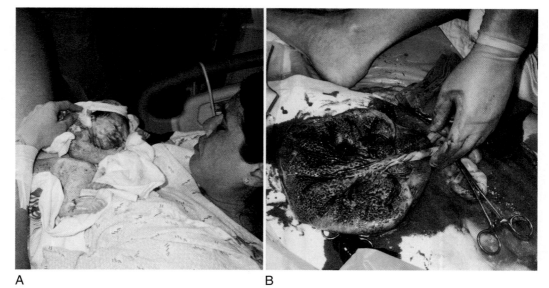

A   B

FIGURE 8–9   A, My newborn granddaughter, Beatrix Bess (Bebe) Thompson, and her mother, Dr. Elizabeth Chabner Thompson, minutes after Bebe's birth. Notice that Bebe's skin is covered with vernix caseosa, a mixture of a fatty secretion from fetal sebaceous (oil) glands and dead skin. The vernix protects the fetus's delicate skin from abrasions, chapping, and hardening as a result of being bathed in amniotic fluid. **B,** The placenta and umbilical cord just after expulsion from the uterus.

HORMONAL INTERACTIONS

The events of menstruation and pregnancy depend not only on hormones from the ovaries (estrogen and progesterone) but also on hormones from the **pituitary gland.** The pituitary gland secretes **follicle-stimulating hormone (FSH)** and **luteinizing hormone (LH)** after the onset of menstruation. In the hypothalamus (a region of the brain), "pulses" of a hormone called gonadotropin-releasing hormone (GnRH) lead to an upsurge of FSH and LH. As their levels rise in the bloodstream, FSH and LH stimulate maturation of the ovum and ovulation. After ovulation, LH in particular influences the maintenance of the corpus luteum and its production of estrogen and progesterone.

During pregnancy, the high levels of estrogen and progesterone coming from the ovary and placenta cause the pituitary gland to stop producing FSH and LH. Therefore, while a woman is pregnant, additional eggs do not mature and ovulation cannot occur. This hormonal interaction wherein a high level of hormones (estrogen and progesterone) shuts off production of another set of hormones (FSH and LH) is **negative feedback.** Oral contraceptives (birth control pills) work by negative feedback. The pills contain variable amounts of estrogen and progesterone, which causes blood levels of these hormones to rise. Negative feedback occurs, and the pituitary does not release FSH or LH. Low blood concentration of FSH means that ovarian follicles do not mature and ovulation does not occur. Subdermal birth control implants containing progesterone-like drugs (progestins) are effective for up to 5 years.

Another female reversible birth control measure is use of an **IUD (intrauterine device).** A physician inserts the IUD, a small device designed to remain inside the uterus. Some IUDs release progestins, which prevent implantation and also decrease heavy menstrual periods. A series of patches called Ortho Evra and a NuvaRing (vaginal ring) are other contraceptive devices containing hormones that work like birth control pills.

When all of the ova are used up and secretion of estrogen from the ovaries lessens, **menopause** begins. Menopause signals the gradual ending of the menstrual cycle. Premature menopause occurs before age 45, whereas delayed menopause occurs after age 55. Artificial menopause occurs if the ovaries are removed by surgery or made nonfunctional as a result of radiation therapy or some forms of chemotherapy.

During menopause, when estrogen levels fall, the most common signs and symptoms are hot flashes (temperature regulation in the brain is disturbed), insomnia, and vaginal atrophy (lining of the vagina dries and thins, predisposing it to irritation and discomfort during sexual intercourse). **Estrogen replacement therapy (ERT),** given orally or as a transdermal patch or vaginal ring, relieves the symptoms of menopause and delays the development of weak bones (osteoporosis). ERT use may be associated with an increased risk of breast cancer, stroke, or heart attack. This therapy should be used only after careful consideration of potential risks and benefits.

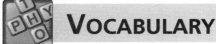 # VOCABULARY

The following list reviews many of the new terms introduced in the text. Short definitions reinforce your understanding of the terms.

adnexa uteri	Fallopian tubes, ovaries, and supporting ligaments.
amnion	Innermost membranous sac surrounding the developing fetus.
areola	Dark-pigmented area surrounding the breast nipple.
Bartholin glands	Small mucus-secreting exocrine glands at the vaginal orifice (opening to outside of the body).
cervix	Lower, neck-like portion of the uterus.
chorion	Outermost layer of the two membranes surrounding the embryo; it forms the fetal part of the placenta.
clitoris	Organ of sensitive erectile tissue anterior to the opening of the female urethra.
coitus	Sexual intercourse; copulation. Pronunciation is KŌ-ĭ-tus.
corpus luteum	Empty ovarian follicle that secretes progesterone after release of the egg cell; literally means yellow (luteum) body (corpus).
cul-de-sac	Region in the lower abdomen, midway between the rectum and the uterus.
embryo	Stage in prenatal development from 2 to 6 weeks.
endometrium	Inner, mucous membrane lining of the uterus.
estrogen	Hormone produced by the ovaries; promotes female secondary sex characteristics.
fallopian tube	One of a pair of ducts through which the ovum travels to the uterus.
fertilization	Union of the sperm cell and ovum from which the embryo develops.
fetus	Stage in prenatal development from 6 to 39 or 40 weeks.
fimbriae *(plural)*	Finger- or fringe-like projections at the end of the fallopian tubes.
follicle-stimulating hormone (FSH)	Secreted by the pituitary gland to stimulate maturation of the egg cell (ovum).

8

gamete	Male or female sexual reproductive cell; sperm cell or ovum.
genitalia	Reproductive organs; also called genitals.
gestation	Period from fertilization of the ovum to birth.
gonad	Female or male reproductive organ that produces sex cells and hormones; ovary or testis.
gynecology	Study of the female reproductive organs including the breasts.
human chorionic gonadotropin (hCG)	Hormone produced by the placenta to sustain pregnancy by stimulating (-tropin) the mother's ovaries to produce estrogen and progesterone.
hymen	Mucous membrane partially or completely covering the opening to the vagina.
labia	Lips of the vagina; labia majora are the larger, outermost lips, and labia minora are the smaller, innermost lips.
lactiferous ducts	Tubes that carry milk within the breast.
luteinizing hormone (LH)	Hormone produced by the pituitary gland; promotes ovulation.
mammary papilla	Nipple of the breast. A papilla is any small nipple-shaped projection.
menarche	Beginning of the first menstrual period during puberty.
menopause	Gradual ending of menstruation.
menstruation	Monthly shedding of the uterine lining. The flow of blood and tissue normally discharged during menstruation is called the **menses** (Latin *mensis* means month).
myometrium	Muscle layer of the uterus.
neonatology	Branch of medicine that studies the disorders and care of the newborn (neonate).
obstetrics	Branch of medicine concerned with pregnancy and childbirth.
orifice	An opening.
ovarian follicle	Developing sac enclosing each ovum within the ovary. Only about 400 of these sacs mature in a woman's lifetime.
ovary	One of a pair of female organs (gonads) on each side of the pelvis. Ovaries are almond-shaped, about the size of large walnuts, and produce egg cells (ova) and hormones.
ovulation	Release of the ovum from the ovary.
ovum (*plural:* **ova**)	Egg cell; female gamete.
parturition	Act of giving birth.
perineum	In females, the area between the anus and the vagina.
pituitary gland	Endocrine gland at the base of the brain. It produces hormones to stimulate the ovaries.
placenta	Vascular organ that develops in the uterine wall during pregnancy. It serves as a communication between maternal and fetal bloodstreams.
pregnancy	Condition in a female of having a developing embryo and fetus in her uterus for about 40 weeks.

progesterone	Hormone produced by the corpus luteum in the ovary and the placenta of pregnant women.
puberty	Point in the life cycle at which the ability to reproduce begins; secondary sex characteristics appear and gametes are produced.
uterine serosa	Outermost layer surrounding the uterus.
uterus	Hollow, pear-shaped muscular female organ in which the embryo and fetus develop, and from which menstruation occurs. The upper portion is the fundus; the middle portion is the corpus; and the lowermost, neck-like portion is the cervix (see Fig. 8–3).
vagina	Muscular, mucosa-lined canal extending from the uterus to the exterior of the body.
vulva	External female genitalia; includes the labia, hymen, clitoris, and vaginal orifice.
zygote	Stage in prenatal development from fertilization and implantation to 2 weeks.

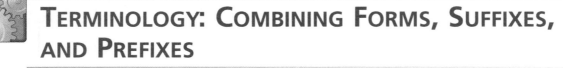

TERMINOLOGY: COMBINING FORMS, SUFFIXES, AND PREFIXES

Write the meanings of the medical terms in the spaces provided.

COMBINING FORMS

Combining Form	Meaning	Terminology	Meaning
amni/o	amnion	amniocentesis _____	
		amniotic fluid _____ *Produced by fetal membranes and the fetus.*	
cervic/o	cervix, neck	endocervicitis _____	
chori/o, chorion/o	chorion	choriogenesis _____	
		chorionic _____	
colp/o	vagina	colposcopy _____	
culd/o	cul-de-sac	culdocentesis _____ *A needle is placed through the posterior wall of the vagina and fluid is withdrawn for diagnostic purposes.*	
episi/o	vulva	episiotomy _____ *An incision through the skin of the perineum enlarges the vaginal orifice for delivery. The incision is repaired by perineorrhaphy.*	

Combining Form	Meaning	Terminology	Meaning
galact/o	milk	galactorrhea _____ *Abnormal, persistent discharge of milk, commonly seen with pituitary gland tumors.*	
gynec/o	woman, female	gynecomastia _____ *Enlargement of one or both breasts in a male. It often occurs with puberty or aging, or the condition can be drug related.*	
hyster/o	uterus, womb	hysterectomy _____ *A **total abdominal hysterectomy (TAH)** is removal of the entire uterus (including the cervix) through an abdominal incision (Fig. 8–10). A **total vaginal hysterectomy (TVH)** is removal through the vagina.*	
		hysteroscopy _____ *A gynecologist uses an endoscope (passed through the vagina) to view the uterine cavity.*	
lact/o	milk	lactogenesis _____	
		lactation _____ *The normal secretion of milk.*	
mamm/o	breast	mammary _____	
		mammoplasty _____ *Includes reduction and augmentation (enlargement) operations.*	
mast/o	breast	mastitis _____ *Usually caused by streptococcal or staphylococcal infection.*	
		mastectomy _____ *Mastectomy procedures are discussed under carcinoma of the breast (see page 270).*	

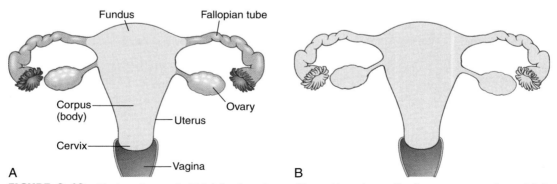

FIGURE 8–10   Hysterectomy. A, Total hysterectomy. The entire uterus (fundus, corpus, and cervix) is removed *(gray area),* but the ovaries and fallopian tubes remain. **B, Total hysterectomy with bilateral salpingo-oophorectomy** (fallopian tubes and ovaries are removed with uterus). In a radical hysterectomy, the entire uterus, ovaries, fallopian tubes, lymph nodes, and the top half of the vagina are removed (mostly performed for cervical cancer).

8

Combining Form	Meaning	Terminology	Meaning
men/o	menses, menstruation	amenorrhea _____ *Absence of menses for 6 months or for longer than 3 of the patient's normal menstrual cycles.*	
		dysmenorrhea _____	
		oligomenorrhea _____ *Infrequent or scanty menstrual periods.*	
		menorrhagia _____ *Abnormally heavy or long menstrual periods. Fibroids (see page 268) are a leading cause of menorrhagia.*	
metr/o, metri/o	uterus	metrorrhagia _____ *Bleeding between menses. Possible causes of metrorrhagia include ectopic pregnancy, cervical polyps, and ovarian and uterine tumors.*	
		menometrorrhagia _____ *Excessive uterine bleeding during and between menstrual periods.*	
		endometriosis _____ *See page 268.*	
my/o, myom/o	muscle, muscle tumor	myometrium _____	
		myomectomy _____ *Removal of fibroids from the uterus.*	
nat/i	birth	new neonatal _____	
obstetr/o	pregnancy and childbirth	obstetrics _____ *From the Latin* obstetrix, *midwife.*	
o/o	egg	oogenesis _____	
oophor/o	ovary	bilateral oophorectomy _____ *Oophor/o means to bear (phor/o) eggs (o/o). Bilateral is both sides (both ovaries are removed).*	
ov/o	egg	ovum _____	
ovari/o	ovary	ovarian _____	
ovul/o	egg	anovulatory _____	
perine/o	perineum	perineorrhaphy _____	
phor/o	to bear	oophoritis _____	
salping/o	fallopian tubes	salpingectomy _____ *Figure 8–10, B, shows a total hysterectomy with bilateral salpingo-oophorectomy (BSO). TAH-BSO and TVH-BSO are surgical options.*	

8

Combining Form	Meaning	Terminology	Meaning
uter/o	uterus	uterine prolapse _____	
vagin/o	vagina	vaginal orifice _____	
		An orifice is an opening.	
		vaginitis _____	
		Bacteria and yeast (Candida) commonly cause this infection. Use of antibiotics can change the internal environment (pH) of the vagina and destroy normally occurring bacteria, allowing yeast to grow.	
vulv/o	vulva	vulvovaginitis _____	

SUFFIXES

Suffix	Meaning	Terminology	Meaning
-arche	beginning	menarche _____	
-cyesis	pregnancy	pseudocyesis _____	
		Pseudo- means false. No pregnancy exists, but physical changes such as weight gain and amenorrhea occur.	
-gravida	pregnant	primigravida _____	
		A woman during her first pregnancy (primi- means first). Gravida also is used to designate a pregnant woman often followed by a number to indicate the number of pregnancies (gravida 1, 2, 3).	
-parous	bearing, bringing forth	primiparous _____	
		An adjective describing a woman who has given birth to at least one child. Para also is used as a noun, often followed by a number to indicate the number of deliveries after the 20th week of gestation (para 1, 2, 3). When a woman arrives in the birthing facility, her gravidity and parity are important facts to include in the medical and surgical history. For example, a G2 P2 is a woman who has had 2 pregnancies and 2 deliveries.	
-rrhea	discharge	leukorrhea _____	
		This nonbloody vaginal discharge may be mucoid or purulent (containing pus) and a sign of infection or cervicitis.	
		menorrhea _____	
-salpinx	uterine tube	pyosalpinx _____	
-tocia	labor, birth	dystocia _____	
		oxytocia _____	
		*Oxy- means rapid. The pituitary gland releases **oxytocin,** which stimulates the pregnant uterus to contract (labor begins). It also stimulates milk secretion from mammary glands.*	

8

Suffix	Meaning	Terminology	Meaning
-version	act of turning	cephalic version _____	
		The fetus turns so that the head is the body part closest to the cervix (version can occur spontaneously or can be performed by the obstetrician). **Fetal presentation** *is the manner in which the fetus appears to the examiner during delivery. A breech presentation is buttocks first, or feet first in a footling breech; a cephalic presentation is head first.*	

PREFIXES

Prefix	Meaning	Terminology	Meaning
dys-	painful	dyspareunia _____	
		(dĭs-pă-ROO-nē-ă.) Pareunia means sexual intercourse.	
endo-	within	endometritis _____	
		Usually caused by a bacterial infection.	
in-	in	involution of the uterus _____	
		Vol- means to roll. The uterus returns to its normal nonpregnant size.	
intra-	within	intrauterine device _____	
		Figure 8–11, A, shows an IUD.	
multi-	many	multipara _____	
		multigravida _____	
		A woman who has been pregnant more than once.	
nulli-	no, not, none	nulligravida _____	
		nullipara _____	
		Para 0. Figure 8–11, B, shows the cervix of a nulliparous woman and the cervix of a parous woman (who has had a vaginal delivery).	

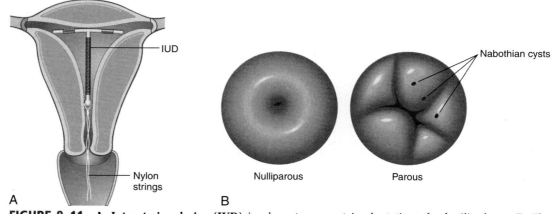

A   B

FIGURE 8–11   A, Intrauterine device (IUD) in place, to prevent implantation of a fertilized egg. **B,** The cervix of a **nulliparous** woman (the os, or opening, is small and perfectly round) and the cervix of a **parous** woman (the os is wide and irregular). Nabothian cysts are normal plugged glands of the cervix, common in women who have borne children. These views would be visible under colposcopic examination.

Prefix	Meaning	Terminology	Meaning
pre-	before	prenatal _____	
primi-	first	primipara _____	
retro-	backward	retroversion _____ *The uterus is abnormally tilted backward. This occurs in 30% of women.*	

PATHOLOGY: GYNECOLOGIC/BREAST, PREGNANCY, AND NEONATAL

GYNECOLOGIC/BREAST

Uterus

carcinoma of the cervix

Malignant cells within the cervix (cervical cancer).

Cervical carcinoma occurs more commonly in women who have sexual intercourse at an early age, multiple sexual partners, a history of sexually transmitted diseases (STDs), and evidence of **human papillomavirus (HPV)** infection. HPV is one of the most common causes of sexually transmitted infection in the world. Some types of HPV cause genital warts—benign growths on the vulva, cervix, vagina, or anus. Although most HPV infections do not progress to cervical cancer, early neoplastic changes in the cervix can range from **dysplasia** (abnormal cell growth) to **carcinoma in situ (CIS)** (localized cancer growth). See Figure 8-12. Biopsy and resection **(conization)** may be necessary to diagnose and treat CIS. Surgery (hysterectomy) and radiation therapy combined with chemotherapy are used to treat more extensive and metastatic disease.

cervicitis

Inflammation of the cervix.

This condition can become chronic because the lining of the cervix is not renewed each month as is the uterine lining during menstruation.

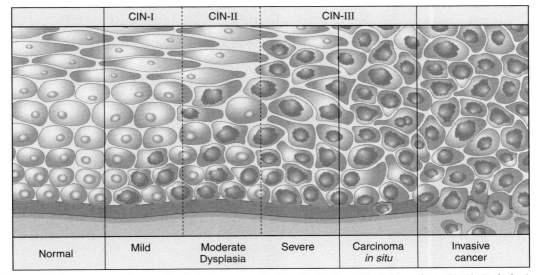

FIGURE 8–12 Preinvasive neoplastic lesions are called **cervical intraepithelial neoplasia (CIN).** Pathologists diagnose such lesions from a Pap smear (microscopic examination of cells scraped from cervical epithelium) and grade them as CIN I to CIN III.

Bacteria such as *Chlamydia trachomatis* and *Neisseria gonorrhoeae* commonly cause cervicitis. Acute cervicitis, marked by **cervical erosions,** or ulcers, appears as raw, red patches on the cervical mucosa. **Leukorrhea** (clear, white, or yellow pus-filled vaginal discharge) also is a symptom of cervical erosion.

After the presence of malignancy has been excluded (by Pap smear or biopsy), **cryocauterization** (destroying tissue by freezing) of the eroded area and treatment with antibiotics may be indicated.

carcinoma of the endometrium (endometrial cancer)

Malignant tumor of the uterus (adenocarcinoma).

The major sign of endometrial cancer is postmenopausal bleeding. This malignancy occurs more often in women exposed to high levels of estrogen, either from either exogenous estrogen (pills) or estrogen-producing tumors or with obesity (estrogen is produced by fat tissue) and in nulliparous women. Physicians perform endometrial biopsy, hysteroscopy, and **dilation** (opening the cervical canal) and **curettage** (scraping the inner lining of the uterus) for diagnosis. When the cancer is confined to the uterus, surgery (hysterectomy) is curative. Radiation oncologists administer radiation therapy for patients with more advanced disease. Progesterone treatment often causes regression of endometrial cancer.

endometriosis

Endometrial tissue located outside the uterus.

Endometrial tissue found in ovaries, fallopian tubes, supporting ligaments or small intestine causes inflammation and scar tissue, with dysmenorrhea, pelvic pain, infertility (inability to become pregnant), and dyspareunia (painful intercourse). Most cases develop as a result of bits of menstrual endometrium that pass backward through the **lumen** (opening) of the fallopian tube and into the peritoneal cavity. Often, when disease affects the ovaries, large blood-filled cysts (endometriomas, or "chocolate cysts") develop. Treatment ranges from symptomatic relief of pain and hormonal drugs that suppress the menstrual cycle to surgical removal of ectopic endometrial tissue and hysterectomy.

fibroids

Benign tumors in the uterus.

Fibroids, also called **leiomyomata** or **leiomyomas** (lei/o = smooth, my/o = muscle, and -oma = tumor), are composed of fibrous tissue and muscle. If fibroids grow too large and cause symptoms such as metrorrhagia, pelvic pain, or menorrhagia, hysterectomy or myomectomy is indicated. Fibroid removal without surgery includes uterine artery embolization (UAE), in which tiny pellets are injected into

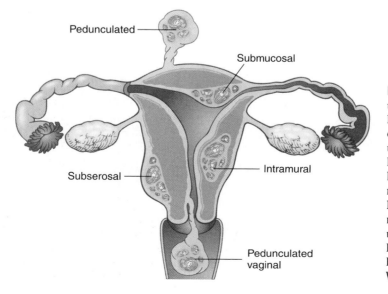

FIGURE 8–13 Location of uterine fibroids (leiomyomas). Pedunculated growths protrude on stalks. A **subserosal** mass lies under the serosal (outermost) layer of the uterus. A **submucosal** leiomyoma grows under the mucosal (innermost) layer. **Intramural** (mural means wall) masses arise within the muscular uterine wall. (From Damjanov I: Pathology for the Health-Related Professions, 3rd ed. Philadelphia, WB Saunders, 2006, p. 369.)

a uterine artery supplying blood to fibroids. Blood flow is blocked by the pellets (emboli), causing fibroids to shrink in size. Figure 8–13 shows the location of uterine fibroids.

Ovaries

ovarian carcinoma

Malignant tumor of the ovary (adenocarcinoma).

Carcinomas of the ovary account for more deaths than those of cancers of the cervix and of the uterus together. The tumor, which may be cystic or solid in consistency, usually is discovered in an advanced stage as an abdominal mass and may produce few symptoms in its early stages. In most patients, the disease metastasizes beyond the ovary before diagnosis and often causes abdominal ascites (accumulation of fluid in the abdominal cavity). Surgery (oophorectomy and salpingectomy) and chemotherapy are used as therapeutic measures. A protein marker produced by tumor cells, CA 125, can be measured in the bloodstream to assess effectiveness of treatment.

ovarian cysts

Collections of fluid within a sac (cyst) in the ovary.

Some cysts are lined by cells that are typical, normal lining cells of the ovary. These cysts originate in unruptured ovarian follicles (follicular cysts) or in follicles that have ruptured and have immediately been sealed (luteal cysts). Other cysts are lined with tumor cells (**cystadenomas** and **cystadenocarcinomas**). Physicians decide to remove these cysts to distinguish between benign and malignant tumors.

   Dermoid cysts are lined with a variety of cell types, including skin, hair, teeth, and cartilage, and arise from immature egg cells in the ovary. Because of the strange assortment of tissue types in the tumor (Fig. 8–14), this tumor often is called benign cystic **teratoma** (terat/o = monster) or a **mature teratoma**. Surgical removal of the cyst is curative.

Fallopian Tubes

pelvic inflammatory disease (PID)

Inflammation and infection of organs in the pelvic region; salpingitis, oophoritis, endometritis, endocervicitis.

The leading causes of PID are bacterial infections such as gonorrhea and chlamydial infection (common STDs). Repetitive episodes of these infections lead to formation of adhesions and scarring within the fallopian tubes. After PID, women have an increased risk of ectopic pregnancy and infertility. Signs and symptoms include fever, foul-smelling vaginal discharge, abdominal pain in the left and right lower quadrants (LLQ and RLQ), and tenderness to **palpation** (examining by touch) of the cervix. Antibiotics are used as treatment. More information on STDs in women and men can be found in Chapter 9 (page 312).

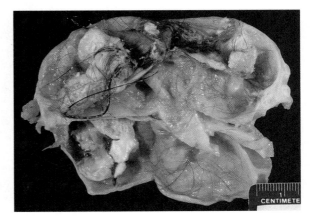

FIGURE 8–14   Dermoid cyst of the ovary with hair, skin, and teeth. (Courtesy of Dr. Elizabeth Chabner Thompson.)

8

Breast

carcinoma of the breast

Malignant tumor of the breast (arising from milk glands and ducts).

The most common type of breast cancer is **invasive ductal carcinoma.** Figure 8–15, *A*, shows the tumor on a mammogram. Figure 8–15, *B*, shows a cut section of an invasive ductal carcinoma. Other histopathologic (histo- means tissue) types are medullary carcinoma and lobular carcinoma.

Breast cancer spreads first to lymph nodes in the axilla (armpit) adjacent to the affected breast and then to the skin and chest wall. From the lymph nodes it also may metastasize to other body organs, including bone, liver, lung, or brain. The diagnosis is first established by biopsy, either needle core or needle aspiration biopsy, or surgical removal of a specimen.

For small primary tumors, the lump with immediately surrounding tissue is removed **(lumpectomy).** To determine whether the tumor has spread to lymph nodes, a **sentinel node biopsy (SNB)** is performed. For this procedure, a blue dye or a radioisotope is injected into the tumor site and tracks to the axillary (underarm) lymph nodes. By visualizing the path of the dye or radioactivity, it is possible to identify the lymph nodes most likely to contain tumor. These lymph nodes, the sentinel nodes, are removed first, and if tissue studies give negative results, the procedure can be stopped at this point. Radiation therapy to the breast and to any involved lymph nodes then follows, to kill remaining tumor cells.

An alternative surgical procedure is **mastectomy** (Fig. 8–16), which is removal of the breast. After either lumpectomy or mastectomy if lymph nodes are involved with cancer, adjuvant (aiding) chemotherapy is given to prevent recurrence of the tumor.

After surgery, further treatment (adjuvant therapy) may be indicated to prevent recurrence. To determine what kind of treatment to use, it is important to

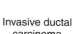

Invasive ductal carcinoma

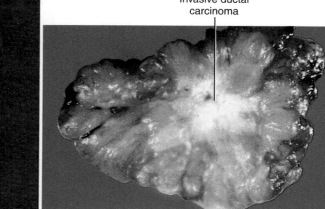

A   B

FIGURE 8–15   **A,** *Arrows* in mammogram point to invasive carcinoma of the breast. A dense white fragment of calcium is seen at 2 o'clock in the mass; calcifications like this frequently are a sign of cancer. **B,** Cut section of invasive ductal carcinoma of the breast. (From Kumar V, Abbas AK, Fausto N: Robbins and Cotran Pathologic Basis of Disease, 7th ed. Philadelphia, WB Saunders, 2005, p. 1143.)

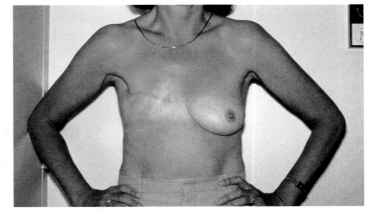

FIGURE 8–16 Surgical scar, mastectomy, right breast. A modified radical mastectomy removes the breast and axillary lymph nodes (usually 20 to 30 nodes). (Courtesy of Dr. Elizabeth Chabner Thompson.)

test the breast cancer tumor for the presence of **estrogen receptors (ERs).** These receptor proteins indicate that the tumor will respond to hormonal therapy. If metastases should subsequently develop, this information will be valuable in selecting further treatment. There are two types of drugs that block the effects of estrogen and thereby kill ER-positive breast cancer cells. Drugs of the first type directly block the ER reception. An example is **tamoxifen.** Drugs of the second type block the production of estrogen by inhibiting the enzyme aromatase. These **aromatase inhibitors (AIs)** are particularly useful in treating post-menopausal women. Examples of AIs are anastrozole (Arimidex) and letrozole (Femara).

A second receptor protein, her-2/neu, is found in some breast cancers and signals a high risk of tumor recurrence. **Herceptin,** an antibody that binds to and blocks her-2/neu, is effective in stopping growth when used with chemotherapy.

fibrocystic disease	**Numerous small sacs of fibrous connective tissue and fluid in the breast.**

Women with this common benign condition notice a nodular (lumpy) consistency of the breast, often associated with premenstrual tenderness and fullness. Mammography and surgical biopsy are indicated to differentiate fibrocystic changes from carcinoma of the breast.

PREGNANCY

abruptio placentae

Premature separation of the implanted placenta.

Abruptio placentae (Latin *ab*, away from; *rumpere*, to rupture) occurs because of trauma, such as a fall, or secondary to vascular insufficiency resulting from hypertension or preeclampsia (see page 272). Signs and symptoms include a sudden searing (burning) abdominal pain and bleeding. It is an obstetric emergency.

choriocarcinoma

Malignant tumor of the placenta.

The tumor may appear with signs of enlarged ovaries, bleeding and a positive pregnancy test. It may spread to lungs and other organs. Treatment is with dilation and curettage (D&C) and chemotherapy.

ectopic pregnancy

Implantation of the fertilized egg in any site other than the normal uterine location.

The condition occurs in 15 percent of pregnancies, and 90 percent of these occur in the fallopian tubes **(tubal pregnancy).** Rupture of the ectopic implant within the fallopian tube can lead to massive abdominal bleeding and death. Surgeons can remove the implant, or treatment with medication (methotrexate) can destroy it, thereby preserving the fallopian tube before rupture occurs. Other sites of

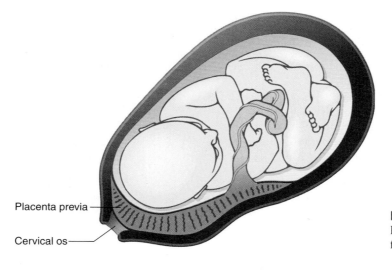

Placenta previa

Cervical os

FIGURE 8–17 Placenta previa. Previa means before or in the front of.

ectopic pregnancy include the ovaries and abdominal cavity; wherever the location, ectopic pregnancy always constitutes a surgical emergency.

placenta previa

Placental implantation over the cervical os (opening) or in the lower region of the uterine wall (Fig. 8–17).

This condition can result in less oxygen supply to the fetus and increased risk of hemorrhage and infection for the mother. Maternal signs and symptoms include painless bleeding, hemorrhage, and premature labor. Cesarean delivery usually is recommended.

preeclampsia

Abnormal condition associated with pregnancy, marked by high blood pressure, proteinuria (loss of protein in urine), and edema.

Mild preeclampsia can be managed by bed rest and close monitoring of blood pressure. Women with severe preeclampsia need treatment with medications such as magnesium sulfate to prevent seizures, and the baby is delivered as quickly as possible. The Greek word *eklampein* means to shine forth, referring to the convulsions and hypertension—typically with visual symptoms of flashing lights—that accompany the condition.

NEONATAL

The following terms describe conditions or symptoms that can affect the newborn. The **Apgar score** is a system of scoring an infant's physical condition 1 and 5 minutes after birth. **Heart rate, respiration, color, muscle tone,** and **response to stimuli** each are rated 0, 1, or 2. The maximum total score is 10. Infants with low Apgar scores require prompt medical attention (Fig. 8–18).

Down syndrome

Chromosomal abnormality (trisomy 21) results in mental retardation, retarded growth, a flat face with a short nose, low-set ears, and slanted eyes.

erythroblastosis fetalis

Hemolytic disease in the newborn caused by a blood group (Rh factor) incompatibility between the mother and the fetus. See page 116.

APGAR SCORING CHART

SIGN	0	1	2
Heart rate	Absent	Below 100	Over 100
Respiratory effort	Absent	Slow, irregular	Good, crying
Muscle tone	Limp	Some flexion of extremities	Active motion
Response to catheter in nostril (tested after oropharynx is clear)	No response	Grimace	Cough or sneeze
Color	Blue, pale	Body pink, extremities blue	Completely pink

FIGURE 8–18 **Apgar scoring chart.** This test is named for anesthesiologist Virginia Apgar (1909–1974), who devised it in 1953. Dr. Joseph Butterfield, in 1963, introduced an acronym (APGAR) as a mnemonic (memory device): **A**ppearance (color), **P**ulse (heart rate), **G**rimace (response to catheter in nostril), **A**ctivity (muscle tone), **R**espiration (respiratory effort) (Modified from O'Toole M [ed]: Miller-Keane Encyclopedia and Dictionary of Medicine, Nursing & Allied Health, 7th ed. Philadelphia, WB Saunders, 2003, p. 136.)

hyaline membrane disease	**Acute lung disease commonly seen in the premature newborn.**
	This condition, also called **respiratory distress syndrome of the newborn,** is caused by deficiency of **surfactant,** a protein necessary for proper lung function. Surfactant can be administered to the newborn to cure the condition. Hyaline refers to the shiny (hyaline means glassy) membrane that forms in the lung sacs.
hydrocephalus	**Accumulation of fluid in the spaces of the brain.**
	In an infant, the entire head can enlarge because the bones of the skull do not completely fuse together at birth. The soft spot, normally present between the cranial bones of the fetus, is called a **fontanelle.** Hydrocephalus occurs because of a problem in the circulation of fluid within the brain and spinal cord.
meconium aspiration syndrome	**Abnormal inhalation of meconium (first stools) produced by a fetus or newborn.**
	Meconium is a thick, sticky, greenish to black substance that forms the first stools of the fetus and newborn. Meconium can block air passages and cause respiratory distress as the lungs fail to expand. **Meconium ileus** is obstruction of the small intestine in the newborn caused by impaction of thick, dry meconium near the ileocecal valve.
pyloric stenosis	**Narrowing of the opening of the stomach to the duodenum.**
	Present at birth; surgical repair of the pyloric opening may be necessary.

CLINICAL TESTS AND PROCEDURES

CLINICAL TESTS

Pap smear (test)	**Microscopic examination of stained cells removed from the vagina and cervix.**

After inserting a vaginal **speculum** (instrument to hold apart the vaginal walls), the physician uses a small spatula to remove exfoliated (peeling and sloughing off) cells from the cervix and vagina (Fig. 8–19). Microscopic analysis of the cell smear (spread on a glass slide) detects cervical or vaginal cellular abnormalities.

pregnancy test	**Blood or urine test to detect the presence of hCG.**

PROCEDURES

X-Ray Studies

hysterosalpingography	**X-ray imaging of the uterus and fallopian tubes after injection of contrast material.**

This radiologic procedure is used to evaluate tubal patency (adequate opening) and uterine cavity abnormalities.

mammography	**X-ray imaging of the breast.**

Women are advised to have a baseline mammogram at 50 years of age for later comparison if needed. A mammogram every 1 to 2 years is recommended for women older than 50, to screen for breast cancer. Figure 8–20 illustrates mammography. Full-field digital mammography is faster than traditional mammography and displays images on a computer screen.

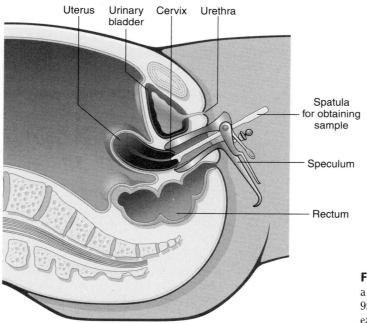

FIGURE 8–19 Method of obtaining a sample for a **Pap smear.** The test is 95 percent accurate in diagnosing early carcinoma of the cervix.

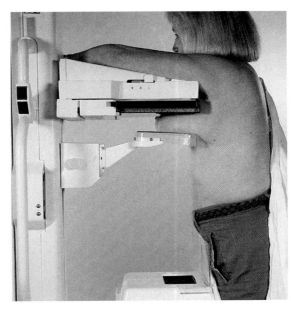

FIGURE 8–20 Mammography. The machine compresses the breast, and x-ray pictures (top to bottom and lateral) are taken. (From Ballinger PW, Frank ED: Merrill's Atlas of Radiographic Positions and Radiologic Procedures, 10th ed. St. Louis, Mosby, 2003, vol. 2, p. 510.)

Ultrasound Examination and MRI

breast ultrasound imaging and breast MRI

Technologies using sound waves and magnetic waves to create images of breast tissue.

These imaging techniques confirm the presence of a mass and can distinguish a benign cyst from a malignancy. MRI is very useful in detecting masses in young women with dense breasts. Breast ultrasound is useful to evaluate a specific area of cancer on a mammogram.

pelvic ultrasonography

Recording images of sound waves as they bounce off organs in the pelvic region.

This technique can evaluate fetal size, maturity, and organ development, as well as fetal and placental position. Uterine tumors and other pelvic masses, including abscesses, also are diagnosed by ultrasonography. **Transvaginal ultrasound** allows the radiologist a closer, sharper look at organs within the pelvis. The sound probe is placed in the vagina, instead of across the pelvis or abdomen; this method is best used to evaluate fluid-filled cysts.

Gynecologic Procedures

aspiration

Withdrawal of fluid from a cavity or sac with an instrument using suction.

Aspiration needle biopsy is a valuable evaluation technique for patients with breast disease.

cauterization

Destruction of tissue by burning.

Destruction of abnormal tissue with chemicals (silver nitrate), dry ice, or an electrically heated instrument. Cauterization is used to treat cervical dysplasia or cervical erosion. The loop electrocautery excision procedure (**LEEP**) is used to biopsy abnormal cervical tissue.

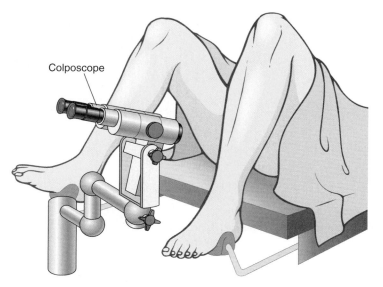

Colposcope

FIGURE 8–21 **Colposcopy** is used to evaluate a patient with an abnormal Pap smear. For this examination, the woman lies in the dorsal lithotomy position. This is the same position used to remove a urinary tract stone (lithotomy means incision to remove a stone).

colposcopy

Visual examination of the vagina and cervix using a colposcope.

A colposcope is a lighted magnifying instrument resembling a small, mounted pair of binoculars. Gynecologists prefer colposcopy for pelvic examination when cervical dysplasia is present because it identifies the specific areas of abnormal cells. A biopsy specimen can then be taken for more accurate diagnosis (Fig. 8–21).

conization

Removal of a cone-shaped section (cone biopsy) of the cervix.

The physician resects the tissue with a **LEEP (loop electrocautery excision procedure),** or carbon dioxide laser, or surgical knife (scalpel). Figure 8–22, *A,* shows conization with LEEP, and Figure 8–22, *B,* shows the cone biopsy specimen removed.

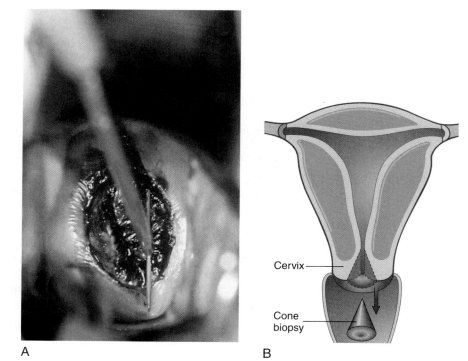

Cervix

Cone biopsy

A   B

FIGURE 8–22 **A,** Cervical loop electrocautery excision procedure (LEEP) for cone biopsy. **B,** Removal of conical biopsy specimen. (**A** courtesy Dr. A.K. Goodman, Massachusetts General Hospital, Boston, Massachusetts.)

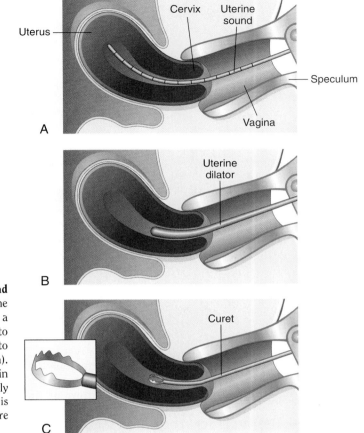

FIGURE 8–23 Dilation and curettage (D&C) of the uterus. A, The uterine cavity is explored with a **uterine sound** (a slender instrument to measure the depth of the uterus to prevent perforation during dilation). **B, Uterine dilators** (Hanks or Hagar) in graduated sizes are used to gradually dilate the cervix. **C,** The uterus is gently curetted and specimens are collected.

cryosurgery

Use of cold temperatures to destroy tissue.

A liquid nitrogen probe produces the freezing (cry/o means cold) temperature. Also called **cryocauterization.**

culdocentesis

Needle aspiration of fluid from the cul-de-sac.

The physician inserts a needle through the vagina into the cul-de-sac. The presence of blood may indicate a ruptured ectopic pregnancy.

dilation (dilatation) and curettage (D&C)

Widening of the cervix and scraping the endometrium of the uterus.

Dilation is accomplished by inserting a series of probes of increasing size. A **curet** (metal loop at the end of a long, thin handle) is then used to sample the uterine lining. This procedure helps diagnose uterine disease and can temporarily halt prolonged or heavy uterine bleeding. When necessary, a D&C is used to remove the tissue during a spontaneous or therapeutic abortion (Fig. 8–23).

exenteration

Removal of internal organs.

Pelvic exenteration is removal of the organs and adjacent structures of the pelvis.

laparoscopy

Visual examination of the abdominal cavity using an endoscope (laparoscope).

In this procedure, a form of **minimally invasive surgery (MIS)**, small incisions (5 to 10 mm) are made near a woman's navel for introduction of the laparoscope and other instruments. Uses of laparoscopy include inspection and removal of

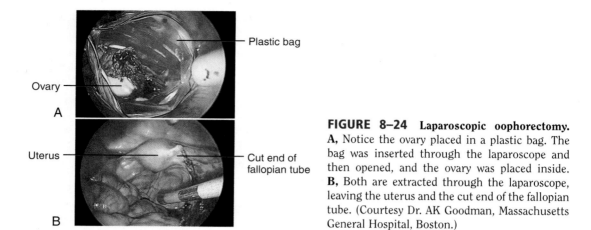

FIGURE 8–24 **Laparoscopic oophorectomy. A,** Notice the ovary placed in a plastic bag. The bag was inserted through the laparoscope and then opened, and the ovary was placed inside. **B,** Both are extracted through the laparoscope, leaving the uterus and the cut end of the fallopian tube. (Courtesy Dr. AK Goodman, Massachusetts General Hospital, Boston.)

ovaries and fallopian tubes, diagnosis and treatment of endometriosis, and removal of fibroids. Laparoscopy also is used to perform subtotal (cervix is left in place) and total hysterectomies. See Figure 8–24.

tubal ligation	**Blocking the fallopian tubes to prevent fertilization from occurring.**

This **sterilization** procedure (making an individual incapable of reproduction) is performed using laparoscopy or through a hysteroscope inserted into an incision in the cervix. Ligation means to tie and doesn't pertain solely to tying off the fallopian tubes—which may be "tied" using clips or bands, or by surgically cutting or burning through the tissue.

Procedures Related to Pregnancy

abortion	**Spontaneous or induced termination of pregnancy before the embryo or fetus can exist on its own.**

Major methods for abortion include vaginal evacuation by D&C or vacuum aspiration (suction) and stimulation of uterine contractions by injection of saline (salt solution) into the amniotic cavity (in second-trimester pregnancies).

amniocentesis	**Needle puncture of the amniotic sac to withdraw amniotic fluid for analysis** (Fig. 8–25).

The cells of the fetus, found in the fluid, are cultured (grown), and cytologic and biochemical studies are performed to check fetal chromosomes, concentrations of proteins and bilirubin, and fetal maturation.

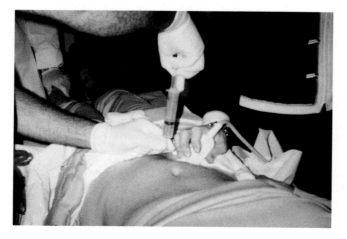

FIGURE 8–25 **Amniocentesis.** The obstetrician places a long needle through the pregnant woman's abdominal wall into the amniotic cavity. Needle placement (avoiding the fetus and the placenta) is guided by concurrent ultrasound images produced by the transducer in the hand of the radiologist. The yellow amniotic fluid is aspirated into the syringe attached to the needle. This procedure took place in the 16th week of pregnancy. The indication for the amniocentesis was a low AFP (alpha-fetoprotein) level. This suggested a higher risk that the baby had Down syndrome. Karyotype analysis (received 10 days later) showed normal chromosome configuration.

cesarean section	**Surgical incision of the abdominal wall and uterus to deliver a fetus.**
	Indications for cesarean section include cephalopelvic disproportion (the baby's head is too big for the mother's birth canal), abruptio placentae or placenta previa, fetal distress (fetal hypoxia), and breech or shoulder presentation. The name comes from a law during the time of Julius Caesar requiring removal of a fetus before a deceased pregnant woman could be buried.
chorionic villus sampling (CVS)	**Sampling of placental tissues (chorionic villi) for prenatal diagnosis.**
	The sample of tissue is removed with a catheter inserted into the uterus. The procedure can be performed earlier than amniocentesis, at about 9 to 12 weeks of gestation.
fetal monitoring	**Continuous recording of the fetal heart rate and maternal uterine contractions to reduce fetal distress during labor.**
in vitro fertilization (IVF)	**Egg and sperm cells are combined outside the body in a laboratory dish (in vitro) to facilitate fertilization.**
	After an incubation period of 48 to 72 hours, the fertilized ova are injected into the uterus through the cervix. (Latin *in vitro* means in glass, as used for laboratory containers.)
pelvimetry	**Measurement of the dimensions of the maternal pelvis.**
	Pelvimetry helps determine if the mother's pelvis will allow passage of the fetus through the birth canal. This examination is important during protracted labor or with breech presentation.

ABBREVIATIONS

AB	abortion			indicates a higher risk for invasive ductal breast cancer
AFP	alpha-fetoprotein—high levels in amniotic fluid of fetus or maternal serum indicate increased risk of neurologic birth defects in the infant.		**DES**	diethylstilbestrol—an estrogen compound used in the treatment of menopausal problems involving estrogen deficiency; if administered during pregnancy, it has been found to be related to subsequent tumors in the daughters (rarely in sons) of mothers so treated.
ASCUS	atypical squamous cells of unknown significance—abnormal Pap smear but does not meet the criteria for a lesion			
BSE	breast self-examination		**DUB**	dysfunctional uterine bleeding
CA 125	protein marker elevated in ovarian cancer (normal range of values is 0–35)		**ECC**	endocervical curettage
			EDC	estimated date of confinement
			EMB	endometrial biopsy
C-section	cesarean section		**FHR**	fetal heart rate
CIN	cervical intraepithelial neoplasia		**FSH**	follicle-stimulating hormone
CIS	carcinoma in situ		**G**	gravida (pregnant)
CS	cesarean section		**GnRH**	gonadotropin-releasing hormone—secreted by the hypothalamus to stimulate release of FSH and LH from the pituitary gland
CVS	chorionic villus sampling			
Cx	cervix			
D&C	dilation (dilatation) and curettage		**GYN**	gynecology
DCIS	ductal carcinoma in situ; a precancerous breast lesion that		**hCG** *or* **HCG**	human chorionic gonadotropin

HDN	hemolytic disease of the newborn	**Pap smear**	Papanicolaou smear—test for cervical or vaginal cancer
HPV	human papillomavirus	**Path**	pathology
HRT	hormone replacement therapy	**PID**	pelvic inflammatory disease
HSG	hysterosalpingography	**PMS**	premenstrual syndrome
IUD	intrauterine device; contraceptive	**primip**	primipara; primiparous
IVF	in vitro fertilization	**RDS**	respiratory distress syndrome of the newborn
LAVH	laparoscopically assisted vaginal hysterectomy	**SLN biopsy or SNB**	sentinel lymph node biopsy—blue dye or radioisotopes (or both) identifies the first lymph node draining the breast lymphatics
LEEP	loop electrocautery excision procedure		
LH	luteinizing hormone	**TAH-BSO**	total abdominal hysterectomy with bilateral salpingo-oophorectomy
LMP	last menstrual period		
multip	multipara; multiparous	**TRAM flap**	trans–rectus abdominis musculocutaneous flap—for breast reconstruction
OB	obstetrics		
OCPs	oral contraceptive pills		
para 2-0-1-2	woman's reproductive history: 2 full-term infants, 0 preterm, 1 abortion, and 2 living children	**TVH**	total vaginal hysterectomy
		UAE	uterine artery embolization

PRACTICAL APPLICATIONS

This section contains an actual operative report and brief excerpts from other medical records using words that you have studied in this and previous chapters. Explanations of more difficult terms are added in brackets. Answers for the matching exercise are on page 292.

OPERATIVE REPORT

Preoperative diagnosis: Menorrhagia, leiomyomata
   Anesthetic: General
   Material forwarded to laboratory for examination:
      A. Endocervical curettings
      B. Endometrial curettings
   Operation performed: Dilation and curettage of the uterus
   With the patient in the dorsal lithotomy position [legs are flexed on the thighs, thighs flexed on the abdomen and abducted] and sterilely prepped and draped, manual examination of the uterus revealed it to be 6- to 8-week size, retroflexed; no adnexal masses noted. The anterior lip of the cervix was then grasped with a tenaculum [a hook-like surgical instrument for grasping and holding parts]. The cervix was dilated up to a #20 Hank's dilator. The uterus was sounded [depth measured] up to 4 inches. A sharp curettage of the endocervix showed only a scant amount of tissue. With a sharp curet, the uterus was curetted in a clockwise fashion with an irregularity noted in the posterior floor. A large amount of endometrial tissue was removed. The patient tolerated the procedure well.

Operative diagnosis: Leiomyomata uteri

Recommendation: Hysterectomy for myomectomy

SENTENCES USING MEDICAL TERMINOLOGY

1. Mammogram report: The breast parenchyma [essential tissue] is symmetrical bilaterally. There are no abnormal masses or calcifications in either breast. The axillae are normal.

2. This is a 43-year-old gravida 3 para 2 with premature ovarian failure and now on HRT. She has history of endocervical atypia [cells are not normal or typical] secondary to chlamydial infection, which is now being treated.

3. The patient is a 40-year-old gravida 3, para 2, white female admitted for exploratory laparotomy to remove and evaluate 10-cm left adnexal mass. Discharge diagnosis: (1) endometriosis, left ovary; (2) benign cystic teratoma [dermoid cyst], left ovary.

4. History: 51-year-old G3 P3; LMP early 40's; on HRT until age 49 when diagnosed with carcinoma of breast; treated with mastectomy and tamoxifen. Followed by ultrasounds showing slightly thickened 9-10 mm endometrium seen. No bleeding.

   Operative findings: office endometrial biopsy, scant tissue

   Clinical diagnosis: rule out hyperplasia

OPERATING ROOM SCHEDULE

The operating room schedule for one day in a large general hospital listed six different gynecologic procedures. Match the surgical procedures in Column I with the indications for surgery in Column II. Write the letter of the indication in the blanks provided.

Column I		*Column II*
1. Conization of the cervix	_____	A. LLQ pain; ovarian mass on pelvic ultrasound
2. Vaginal hysterectomy with colporrhaphy	_____	B. Fibroids
3. TAH-BSO, pelvic and periaortic lymphadenectomy	_____	C. Endometrial carcinoma
4. Exploratory laparotomy for uterine myomectomy	_____	D. Small invasive ductal carcinoma of the breast
5. Left oophorectomy	_____	E. Suspected cervical cancer
6. Lumpectomy with SLN biopsy	_____	F. Uterine prolapse

8

? EXERCISES

Remember to check your answers carefully with those given in the Answers to Exercises, page 290.

A. Match the following terms for structures or tissues with their meanings below.

amnion   clitoris   labia   placenta
areola   endometrium   mammary papilla   uterine serosa
cervix   fallopian tubes   ovaries   vagina
chorion   fimbriae   perineum   vulva

1. inner lining of the uterus _____

2. area between the anus and the vagina in females _____

3. dark-pigmented area around the breast nipple _____

4. finger-like ends of the fallopian tube _____

5. ducts through which the egg travels into the uterus from the ovary _____

6. organ of sensitive erectile tissue in females; anterior to urethral orifice _____

7. nipple of the breast _____

8. blood vessel–filled organ that develops during pregnancy in the uterine wall and serves as a

   communication between maternal and fetal bloodstreams _____

9. lower, neck-like portion of the uterus _____

10. innermost membrane around the developing embryo _____

11. outermost layer of the membranes around the developing embryo and forming part of the placenta

    _____

12. membrane surrounding the uterus _____

13. lips of the vulva _____

14. female gonads; producing ova and hormones _____

15. includes the perineum, labia, clitoris, and hymen; external genitalia _____

16. mucosal tube extending from the uterus to the exterior of the body _____

B. Identify the following terms.

1. fetus _____

2. lactiferous ducts _____

3. gametes _____

4. gonads _____

8

5. adnexa uteri _____

6. cul-de-sac _____

7. genitalia _____

8. Bartholin glands _____

9. ovarian follicle _____

10. corpus luteum _____

C. Match the terms below with their descriptions.

coitus	human chorionic	myometrium
estrogen	gonadotropin	prenatal
fertilization	luteinizing hormone	progesterone
follicle-stimulating hormone	menarche	

1. a hormone produced by the ovaries; responsible for femaleness and buildup of the uterine lining during the menstrual cycle_____

2. a hormone produced by the pituitary gland to stimulate the maturation of the ovarian follicle and ovum in the ovary _____

3. sexual intercourse _____

4. before birth _____

5. beginning of the first menstrual period during puberty_____

6. hormone produced by the placenta to sustain pregnancy by stimulating the ovaries to produce estrogen and progesterone _____

7. muscle layer of the uterus _____

8. hormone produced by the corpus luteum in the ovary and also by the placenta of a pregnant woman _____

9. hormone produced by the pituitary gland to promote ovulation_____

10. fusion of the nuclei of the sperm and ovum _____

D. Supply definitions to complete the following sentences.

1. galact/o and lact/o both mean _____.

2. colp/o and vagin/o both mean _____.

3. mamm/o and mast/o both mean _____.

4. metr/o, uter/o, and hyster/o all mean _____.

5. oophor/o and ovari/o both mean _____.

6. o/o, ov/o, and ovul/o all mean _____.

7. in- and endo- both mean _____.

8. -cyesis and -gravida both mean _____.

9. salping/o and -salpinx both mean _____.

10. episi/o and vulv/o both mean _____.

E. Match the following terms with their meanings below.

bilateral salpingo-oophorectomy   lactogenesis   oxytocin
cervicitis   neonatology   total hysterectomy
culdocentesis   obstetrics   vulvovaginitis
chorion

1. study of the newborn _____

2. hormone that stimulates the pregnant uterus to contract _____

3. production of milk _____

4. removal of the entire uterus _____

5. inflammation of the neck of the uterus _____

6. branch of medicine concerned with pregnancy and childbirth _____

7. outermost membrane surrounding the fetus _____

8. removal of both fallopian tubes and both ovaries _____

9. inflammation of the external female genitalia and vagina _____

10. needle puncture to remove fluid from the cul-de-sac _____

F. Give the meanings of the following symptoms.

1. amenorrhea _____

2. dysmenorrhea _____

3. leukorrhea _____

4. metrorrhagia _____

5. galactorrhea _____

6. menorrhagia _____

7. pyosalpinx _____

8. dyspareunia _____

9. menometrorrhagia _____

10. oligomenorrhea _____

G. State whether the following sentences are true or false, and explain your answers.

1. After a total (complete) hysterectomy, a woman still has regular menstrual periods.

   _____

2. After a total hysterectomy, a woman may still produce estrogen and progesterone.

   _____

3. Birth control pills prevent pregnancy by keeping levels of estrogen and progesterone high.

   _____

4. After a total hysterectomy with bilateral salpingo-oophorectomy, a doctor may advise hormone

   replacement therapy._____

5. Human papillomavirus can cause genital warts and ovarian cancer.

   _____

6. A Pap smear can detect CIN._____

7. Human chorionic gonadotropin is produced by the ovaries during pregnancy.

   _____

8. Gynecomastia is a common condition in pregnant women.

   _____

9. Treatment for endometriosis is uterine myomectomy.

   _____

10. A gravida 3, para 2 is a woman who has given birth 3 times.

    _____

11. A nulligravida is a woman who has had several pregnancies.

    _____

12. Pseudocyesis is the same condition as a tubal pregnancy.

    _____

13. Fibrocystic changes in the breast are a malignant condition.

    _____

14. Cystadenomas occur in the ovaries.

    _____

15. FSH and LH are ovarian hormones.

    _____

8

H. Give the meanings of the following terms.

1. parturition _____

2. menopause _____

3. menarche _____

4. ovulation _____

5. gestation _____

6. anovulatory _____

7. dilatation _____

8. lactation _____

9. nulliparous _____

10. oophoritis _____

I. Match the following terms with their meanings as given below.

abruptio placentae   choriocarcinoma   leiomyoma
carcinoma in situ   cystadenocarcinoma   placenta previa
cervical carcinoma   endometrial carcinoma   preeclampsia
cervicitis   endometriosis

1. malignant tumor of the ovary _____

2. chlamydial infection causing inflammation in the lower, neck-like portion of the uterus

   _____

3. condition during pregnancy or shortly thereafter, marked by hypertension, proteinuria, and edema

   _____

4. uterine tissue located outside the uterus; for example, in the ovaries, cul-de-sac, fallopian tubes,

   or peritoneum _____

5. premature separation of a normally implanted placenta _____

6. placenta implantation over the cervical opening _____

7. malignant tumor of the placenta _____

8. malignant condition that can be diagnosed by a Pap smear, revealing dysplastic changes in cells

   _____

9. malignant condition of the inner lining of the uterus _____

10. benign muscle tumor in the uterus _____

J. Name the appropriate test or procedure for each of the following descriptions.

1. burning of abnormal tissue with chemicals or an electrically heated instrument

   _____

2. contrast material is injected into the uterus and fallopian tubes, and x-ray images are obtained

   _____

3. cold temperature is used to destroy tissue_____

4. visual examination of the vagina and cervix _____

5. widening the cervical opening and scraping the lining of the uterus _____

6. withdrawal of fluid by suction with a needle _____

7. process of recording x-ray images of the breast _____

8. removal of a cone-shaped section of the cervix for diagnosis or treatment of cervical dysplasia

   _____

9. surgical puncture to remove fluid from the cul-de-sac_____

10. echoes from sound waves create an image of structures in the pelvic region

    _____

11. blocking the fallopian tubes to prevent fertilization from occurring

    _____

12. visual examination of the abdominal cavity with an endoscope

    _____

13. hCG is measured in the urine or blood _____

14. cells are scraped from the cervix or vagina for microscopic analysis_____

15. removal of internal gynecologic organs and adjacent structures in the pelvis

    _____

K. Match the obstetrical and neonatal terms with the descriptions given below.

abortion
Apgar score
cephalic version
cesarean section
erythroblastosis fetalis

fetal monitoring
fetal presentation
fontanelle
hydrocephalus
in vitro fertilization

meconium aspiration syndrome
pelvimetry
pyloric stenosis
respiratory distress syndrome of
  the newborn

1. Turning the fetus so that the head presents during birth_____

2. Measurement of the dimensions of the maternal pelvic bone _____

3. The soft spot between the newborn's cranial bones _____

4. The evaluation of the newborn's physical condition _____

5. Premature termination of pregnancy is known as _____

6. Removal of the fetus by abdominal incision of the uterus _____

7. Acute lung disease in the premature newborn: surfactant deficiency _____

8. Use of a machine to electronically record fetal heart rate during labor_____

9. Narrowing of the opening of the stomach to the small intestine in the infant

_____

10. Hemolytic disease of the newborn _____

11. Accumulation of fluid in the spaces of a neonate's brain _____

12. Manner in which the fetus appears to the examiner during delivery_____

13. Condition resulting from inhalation of a thick, sticky black substance by the newborn

_____

14. Union of the egg and sperm cell in a laboratory dish _____

L. Give medical terms for the following definitions. Pay careful attention to spelling.

1. benign muscle tumors in the uterus _____

2. no menses _____

3. removal of an ovary_____

4. condition of female breasts (in a male) _____

5. ovarian hormone that sustains pregnancy_____

6. nipple-shaped elevation on the breast _____

M. Give the meanings of the abbreviations in Column I. Then select the letter of the correct description from Column II.

Column I

1. CIN_____ _____

2. FSH _____ _____

3. D&C_____ _____

4. multip _____ _____

5. C-section _____ _____

6. AFP_____ _____

7. DCIS_____ _____

8. TAH-BSO _____ _____

9. primip _____ _____

10. OB _____ _____

Column II

A. This woman has given birth to more than one infant.

B. Elevated levels of the protein may be a sign of fetal spinal cord abnormalities.

C. This woman has given birth for the first time.

D. Secretion from the pituitary gland stimulates the ovaries.

E. This procedure may be used to diagnose uterine disease.

F. Preinvasive changes in the cervix.

G. Surgical procedure to remove the uterus, fallopian tubes, and ovaries.

H. Surgical delivery of an infant through an abdominal incision.

I. Branch of medicine dealing with pregnancy and delivery of infants.

J. Precancerous breast lesion

N. Circle the term in parentheses that best completes the meaning of each sentence.

1. Dr. Hanson felt that it was important to do a **(culdocentesis, Pap smear, amniocentesis)** once yearly on each of her GYN patients to screen for abnormal cells.

2. When Doris missed her period, her doctor checked for the presence of **(LH, IUD, hCG)** in Doris' urine to see if she was pregnant.

3. Ellen was 34 weeks' pregnant and experiencing bad headaches and blurry vision, with a 10-pound weight gain in 2 days. Dr. Murphy told her to go to the obstetric emergency room because she suspected **(preeclampsia, pelvic inflammatory disease, fibroids)**.

4. Dr. Harris felt a breast mass when examining Mrs. Clark. She immediately ordered a **(dilation and curettage, hysterosalpingogram, mammogram)** for her 42-year-old patient.

5. Clara knew that she should not ignore her fevers and yellow vaginal discharge and the pain in her side. She had previous episodes of **(PMS, PID, DES)** treated with IV antibiotics. She worried that she might have a recurrence.

6. After years of trying to become pregnant, Jill decided to speak to her **(hematologist, gynecologist, urologist)** about in vitro **(gestation, parturition, fertilization)**.

7. To harvest her ova, Jill's physician prescribed hormones to stimulate egg maturation and **(coitus, lactation, ovulation)**. Ova were surgically removed and fertilized with sperm cells in a petri dish.

8. Next, multiple embryos were implanted into Jill's **(fallopian tube, vagina, uterus)**, and she received hormones to ensure the survival of at least one embryo.

9. The IVF was successful and after **(abdominal CT, ultrasound examination, pelvimetry)**, Jill was told that she would have twins in 8½ months.

10. At 37 weeks, Jill went into labor. Under continuous **(chorionic villus sampling, culdocentesis, fetal monitoring)**, two healthy infants were delivered vaginally.

MEDICAL SCRAMBLE

Unscramble the letters to form medical terms from the clues. Use the letters in squares to complete the bonus term. Answers are found on page 292.

1. *Clue:* Neck-like region of the womb ___ ___ ☐ ___ ☐ ___ RIVXEC

2. *Clue:* Lips of the vagina ___ ☐ ___ ___ ___ BALIA

3. *Clue:* Produces eggs and hormones ☐ ___ ___ ☐ ___ RAOYV

4. *Clue:* Womb ☐ ☐ ___ ___ ___ ___ TUSREU

5. *Clue:* Region between the anus and the vagina

☐ ___ ___ ☐ ☐ ___ ___ ___ ENMPREIU

6. *Clue:* Sperm cell or ovum ___ ___ ___ ☐ ___ TMAGEE

BONUS TERM: *Clue:* The act of giving birth.

☐ ☐ ☐ ☐ ☐ ☐ ☐ ☐ ☐ ☐

ANSWERS TO EXERCISES

A

1. endometrium
2. perineum
3. areola
4. fimbriae
5. fallopian tubes
6. clitoris
7. mammary papilla
8. placenta
9. cervix
10. amnion
11. chorion
12. uterine serosa
13. labia
14. ovaries
15. vulva
16. vagina

B

1. embryo from the third month (after 8 weeks) to birth
2. tubes that carry milk within the breast
3. sex cells; the egg and sperm cells
4. organs (ovaries and testes) in the female and male that produce gametes
5. ovaries, fallopian tubes, and supporting ligaments (accessory parts of the uterus)
6. region of the abdomen between the rectum and the uterus
7. reproductive organs (genitals)
8. small exocrine glands at the vaginal orifice that secrete a lubricating fluid
9. developing sac in the ovary that encloses the ovum
10. empty follicle that secretes progesterone after ovulation

C

1. estrogen
2. follicle-stimulating hormone
3. coitus
4. prenatal
5. menarche
6. human chorionic gonadotropin
7. myometrium
8. progesterone
9. luteinizing hormone
10. fertilization

D

1. milk
2. vagina
3. breast
4. uterus
5. ovary
6. egg
7. in, within
8. pregnancy
9. fallopian tube
10. vulva (external female genitalia)

E

1. neonatology
2. oxytocin
3. lactogenesis
4. total hysterectomy
5. cervicitis
6. obstetrics
7. chorion
8. bilateral salpingo-oophorectomy
9. vulvovaginitis
10. culdocentesis

F

1. no menstrual flow
2. painful menstrual flow
3. white discharge (from the vagina and associated with cervicitis)
4. bleeding from the uterus at irregular intervals
5. abnormal discharge of milk from the breasts
6. profuse or prolonged menstrual bleeding occurring at regular intervals
7. pus in the fallopian (uterine) tubes
8. painful sexual intercourse
9. heavy bleeding at and between menstrual periods
10. scanty menstrual flow

G

1. False. Total hysterectomy means removal of the entire uterus so that menstruation does not occur.
2. True. Total hysterectomy does not mean that the ovaries have been removed.
3. True. Birth control pills contain estrogen and progesterone; high levels prevent ovulation and pregnancy.
4. True. This may be necessary to treat symptoms of estrogen loss (vaginal atrophy, hot flashes) and to prevent bone deterioration (osteoporosis).
5. False. HPV does produce genital warts but not ovarian cancer. In some cases, HPV infection may lead to cervical cancer.
6. True. A Pap smear can detect abnormal changes in the cervix from cervical dysplasia to cervical intraepithelial neoplasia (CIN) and CIS (carcinoma in situ).
7. False. HCG is produced by the *placenta* during pregnancy.
8. False. Gynecomastia is a condition of increased breast development in *males*.
9. False. Myomectomy means removal of muscle tumors (fibroids). Endometriosis is abnormal location of uterine tissue outside the uterine lining.
10. False. A gravida 3, para 2 is a woman who has had two children but is pregnant with her third.
11. False. A nulligravida has had no pregnancies. A multigravida has had many pregnancies.
12. False. A pseudocyesis is a false pregnancy (no pregnancy occurs), and a tubal pregnancy is an example of ectopic pregnancy (pregnancy occurs in the fallopian tube, not in the uterus).
13. False. Fibrocystic changes in the breast are a benign condition.
14. True. Cystadenomas are glandular sacs lined with tumor cells; they occur in the ovaries.
15. False. FSH and LH are pituitary gland hormones. Estrogen and progesterone are secreted by the ovaries.

H

1. act of giving birth
2. gradual ending of menstrual function
3. beginning of the first menstrual period at puberty
4. release of the ovum from the ovary
5. pregnancy
6. pertaining to no ovulation (egg is not released from the ovary)
7. widening
8. natural secretion of milk
9. a woman who has never given birth
10. inflammation of the ovaries

I

1. cystadenocarcinoma
2. cervicitis
3. preeclampsia
4. endometriosis
5. abruptio placentae
6. placenta previa
7. choriocarcinoma
8. cervical carcinoma
9. endometrial carcinoma
10. leiomyoma

J

1. cauterization
2. hysterosalpingography
3. cryosurgery or cryocauterization
4. colposcopy
5. dilation (dilatation) and curettage
6. aspiration
7. mammography
8. conization
9. culdocentesis
10. pelvic ultrasonography
11. tubal ligation
12. laparoscopy
13. pregnancy test
14. Pap smear
15. pelvic exenteration

K

1. cephalic version
2. pelvimetry
3. fontanelle
4. Apgar score
5. abortion
6. cesarean section
7. respiratory distress syndrome
8. fetal monitoring
9. pyloric stenosis
10. erythroblastosis fetalis
11. hydrocephalus
12. fetal presentation
13. meconium aspiration syndrome
14. in vitro fertilization

L

1. fibroids or leiomyomata
2. amenorrhea
3. oophorectomy
4. gynecomastia
5. progesterone
6. mammary papilla

M

1. cervical intraepithelial neoplasia: F
2. follicle-stimulating hormone: D
3. dilation (dilatation) and curettage: E
4. multipara: A
5. cesarean section: H
6. alpha-fetoprotein: B
7. ductal carcinoma in situ: J
8. total abdominal hysterectomy with bilateral salpingo-oophorectomy: G
9. primipara: C
10. obstetrics: I

N

1. Pap smear
2. hCG
3. preeclampsia
4. mammogram
5. PID
6. gynecologist; fertilization
7. ovulation
8. uterus
9. ultrasound examination
10. fetal monitoring

ANSWERS TO PRACTICAL APPLICATIONS

1. E
2. F
3. C
4. B
5. A
6. D

ANSWERS TO MEDICAL SCRAMBLE

1. CERVIX   2. LABIA   3. OVARY   4. UTERUS   5. PERINEUM   6. GAMETE
BONUS TERM: PARTURITION

PRONUNCIATION OF TERMS

PRONUNCIATION GUIDE

ā as in āpe   ă as in ăpple
ē as in ēven   ĕ as in ĕvery
ī as in īce   ĭ as in ĭnterest
ō as in ōpen   ŏ as in pŏt
ū as in ūnit   ŭ as in ŭnder

To test your understanding of the terminology in this chapter, write the meaning of each term in the space provided. In addition, you may wish to cover the terms and write them by looking at your definitions. Make sure your spelling is correct. The page number after each term indicates where it is defined or used in the book, so you can easily check your responses. You will find complete definitions for all of these terms and audio pronunciations on the CD.

VOCABULARY AND TERMINOLOGY

Term	Pronunciation	Meaning
adnexa uteri (260)	ăd-NĔK-să Ū-tĕ-rī	_____
amenorrhea (264)	āmĕn-ō-RĒ-ă	_____
amniocentesis (262)	ăm-nē-ō-sĕn-TĒ-sĭs	_____
amnion (260)	ĂM-nē-ŏn	_____
amniotic fluid (262)	ăm-nē-ŎT-ĭk FLOO-ĭd	_____

Term	Pronunciation	Meaning
anovulatory (264)	ăn-ŎV-ū-lă-tōr-ē	
areola (260)	ă-RĒ-ō-lă	
Bartholin glands (260)	BĂR-thō-lĭn glăndz	
bilateral oophorectomy (264)	bī-LĂ-tĕr-ăl ō-ŏf-ō-RĔK-tō-mē *or* oo-fō-RĔK-tō-mē	
cephalic version (266)	sē-FĂL-lĭk VĔR-shŭn	
cervix (260)	SĔR-vĭkz	
choriogenesis (262)	kŏr-ē-ō-JĔN-ĕ-sĭs	
chorion (260)	KŎ-rē-ŏn	
chorionic (262)	kŏ-rē-ŎN-ĭk	
clitoris (260)	KLĬ-tō-rĭs	
coitus (260)	KŌ-ĭ-tŭs	
colposcopy (262)	kŏl-PŎS-kō-pē	
corpus luteum (260)	KŎR-pŭs LOO-tē-ŭm	
cul-de-sac (260)	KŬL-dē-săk	
culdocentesis (262)	kŭl-dō-sĕn-TĒ-sĭs	
dysmenorrhea (264)	dĭs-mĕn-ō-RĒ-ă	
dyspareunia (266)	dĭs-pă-ROO-nē-ă	
dystocia (265)	dĭs-TŌ-sē-ă	
embryo (260)	ĔM-brē-ō	
endocervicitis (262)	ĕn-dō-sĕr-vĭs-SĪ-tĭs	
endometritis (266)	ĕn-dō-mĕ-TRĪ-tis	
endometrium (260)	ĕn-dō-MĒ-trē-ŭm	
episiotomy (262)	ĕ-pĭs-ē-ŎT-ō-mē	
estrogen (260)	ĔS-trō-jĕn	
fallopian tube (260)	fă-LŌ-pē-ăn tūb	
fertilization (260)	fĕr-tĭl-ĭ-ZĀ-shŭn	
fetal presentation (266)	FĒ-tăl prĕ-sĕn-TĀ-shŭn	
fetus (260)	FĒ-tŭs	
fimbriae (260)	FĬM-brē-ē	
follicle-stimulating hormone (260)	FŎL-lĭ-k'l STĬM-ū-lā-tĭng HŌR-mōn	
galactorrhea (263)	gă-lăk-tō-RĒ-ă	
gamete (261)	GĂM-ēt	

8

Term	Pronunciation	Meaning
genitalia (261)	jĕn-ĭ-TĀ-lē-ă	
gestation (261)	jĕs-TĀ-shŭn	
gonad (261)	GŌ-năd	
gynecology (261)	gī-nĕ-KŎL-ō-jē	
gynecomastia (263)	gī-nĕ-kō-MĂS-tē-ă	
human chorionic gonadotropin (261)	HŪ-măn kō-rē-ŎN-ĭk gō-nă-dō-TRŌ-pĭn	
hymen (261)	HĪ-mĕn	
hysterectomy (263)	hĭs-tĕr-ĔK-tō-mē	
hysteroscopy (263)	hĭs-tĕr-ŎS-kō-pē	
intrauterine device (266)	ĭn-tră-Ū-tĕ-rĭn dĕ-VĪS	
involution (266)	ĭn-vō-LOO-shŭn	
labia (261)	LĀ-bē-ă	
lactation (263)	lăk-TĀ-shŭn	
lactiferous ducts (261)	lăk-TĬ-fĕ-rŭs dŭkts	
lactogenesis (263)	lăk-tō-JĔN-ĕ-sĭs	
leukorrhea (265)	loo-kō-RĒ-ă	
luteinizing hormone (261)	LOO-tē-nī-zĭng HŎR-mōn	
mammary (263)	MĂM-ăr-ē	
mammary papilla (261)	MĂM-ăr-ē pă-PĬL-ă	
mammoplasty (263)	MĂM-ō-plăs-tē	
mastectomy (263)	măs-TĔK-tō-mē	
mastitis (263)	măs-TĪ-tĭs	
menarche (261)	mĕ-NĂR-kē	
menometrorrhagia (264)	mĕn-ō-mĕt-rō-RĀ-jă	
menopause (261)	MĔN-ō-păwz	
menorrhea (265)	mĕn-ō-RĒ-ă	
menorrhagia (264)	mĕn-ō-RĀ-jă	
menstruation (261)	mĕn-strū-Ā-shŭn	
metrorrhagia (264)	mĕ-trō-RĀ-jă	
multigravida (266)	mŭl-tĭ-GRĂV-ĭ-dă	
multipara (266)	mŭl-TĬP-ă-ră	
myomectomy (264)	mī-ō-MĔK-tō-mē	

Term	Pronunciation	Meaning
myometrium (261)	mī-ō-MĒ-trē-ŭm	
neonatal (264)	nē-ō-NĀ-tăl	
neonatology (261)	nē-ō-nā-TŎL-ō-jē	
nullipara (266)	nŭl-LĬP-ă-ră	
obstetrics (261)	ŏb-STĔT-rĭks	
oligomenorrhea (264)	ŏl-ĭ-gō-mĕn-ō-RĒ-ă	
oogenesis (264)	ō-ō-JĔN-ĕ-sĭs	
oophoritis (264)	ō-ŏf-ōr-Ī-tĭs	
orifice (261)	ŎR-ĭ-fĭs	
ovarian (264)	ō-VĂ-rē-an	
ovarian follicle (261)	ō-VĂ-rē-an FŎL-lĭ-k'l	
ovary (261)	Ō-vă-rē	
ovulation (261)	ŏv-ū-LĀ-shŭn	
ovum; ova (261)	Ō-vŭm; Ō-vă	
oxytocia (265)	ŏks-ē-TŌ-sē-ă	
oxytocin (265)	ŏks-ē-TŌ-sĭn	
parturition (261)	păr-tū-RĬSH-ŭn	
perineorrhaphy (264)	pĕ-rĭ-nē-ŎR-ră-fē	
perineum (261)	pĕ-rĭ-NĒ-ŭm	
pituitary gland (261)	pĭ-TOO-ĭ-tăr-ē glănd	
placenta (261)	plă-SĔN-tă	
pregnancy (261)	PRĔG-năn-sē	
prenatal (267)	prē-NĀ-tăl	
primigravida (265)	prī-mĭ-GRĂV-ĭ-dă	
primipara (267)	prī-MĬP-ă-ră	
primiparous (265)	prī-MĬP-ă-rŭs	
progesterone (262)	prō-JĔS-tĕ-rōn	
pseudocyesis (265)	sū-dō-sī-Ē-sĭs	
puberty (262)	PŪ-bĕr-tē	
pyosalpinx (265)	pī-ō-SĂL-pĭnks	
retroversion (267)	rĕ-trō-VĔR-zhŭn	
salpingectomy (264)	săl-pĭn-JĔK-tō-mē	
salpingitis (269)	săl-pĭn-JĪ-tĭs	

8

Term	Pronunciation	Meaning
uterine serosa (262)	Ū-tĕr-ĭn sē-RŌ-să	_____
uterus (262)	Ū-tĕr-ŭs	_____
vagina (262)	vă-JĪ-nă	_____
vaginal orifice (265)	VĂ-jĭ-năl ŎR-ĭ-fĭs	_____
vaginitis (265)	vă-jĭ-NĪ-tĭs	_____
vulva (262)	VŬL-vă	_____
vulvovaginitis (265)	vŭl-vō-vă-jĭ-NĪ-tĭs	_____
zygote (262)	ZĪ-gōt	_____

PATHOLOGIC CONDITIONS, CLINICAL TESTS, AND PROCEDURES

Term	Pronunciation	Meaning
abortion (278)	ă-BŎR-shŭn	_____
abruptio placentae (271)	ă-BRŬP-shē-ō plă-SĔN-tă	_____
Apgar score (272)	ĂP-găr skōr	_____
aspiration (275)	ăs-pĭ-RĀ-shŭn	_____
carcinoma in situ (267)	kăr-sĭ-NŌ-mă ĭn SĪ-tū	_____
carcinoma of the breast (270)	kăr-sĭ-NŌ-mă of the brĕst	_____
carcinoma of the cervix (267)	kăr-sĭ-NŌ-mă of the SĔR-vĭks	_____
carcinoma of the endometrium (268)	kăr-sĭ-NŌ-mă of the ĕn-dō-MĒ-trē-ŭm	_____
cauterization (275)	kăw-tĕr-ĭ-ZĀ-shŭn	_____
cervical dysplasia (267)	SĔR-vĭ-kăl dĭs-PLĀ-zē-ă	_____
cervicitis (267)	sĕr-vĭ-SĪ-tĭs	_____
cesarean section (279)	sē-ZĀ-rē-ăn SĔK-shŭn	_____
Chlamydia (268)	klă-MĬD-ē-ă	_____
choriocarcinoma (271)	kō-rē-ō-kăr-sĭ-NŌ-mă	_____
chorionic villus sampling (279)	kō-rē-ŎN-ik VĬL-us SĂMP-lĭng	_____
colposcopy (276)	kōl-PŎS-kō-pē	_____
conization (276)	kō-nĭ-ZĀ-shŭn	_____
cryocauterization (277)	krī-ō-kăw-tĕr-ĭ-ZĀ-shŭn	_____
culdocentesis (277)	kŭl-dō-sĕn-TĒ-sĭs	_____
cystadenocarcinoma (269)	sĭs-tăd-ĕ-nō-kăr-sĭ-NŌ-mă	_____
cystadenoma (269)	sĭs-tăd-ĕ-NŌ-mă	_____
dermoid cyst (269)	DĔR-moyd sĭst	_____

Term	Pronunciation	Meaning
dilatation (277)	dĭ-lă-TĀ-shŭn	
dilation and curettage (277)	dī-LĀ-shŭn and kŭr-ĕ-TĂZH	
ectopic pregnancy (271)	ĕk-TŎP-ĭk PRĔG-năn-sē	
endometriosis (268)	ĕn-dō-mē-trē-Ō-sĭs	
erythroblastosis fetalis (272)	ĕ-rĭth-rō-blăs-TŌ-sĭs fē-TĂ-lĭs	
exenteration (277)	ĕks-ĕn-tĕ-RĀ-shŭn	
fetal monitoring (279)	FĒ-tăl MŎN-ĭ-tŏ-rĭng	
fibrocystic disease (271)	fī-brō-SĬS-tĭk dĭ-ZĒZ	
fibroids (268)	FĬ-broydz	
hyaline membrane disease (273)	HĬ-ă-lĭn MĔM-brān dĭ-ZĒZ	
hydrocephalus (273)	hī-drō-SĔF-ă-lŭs	
hysterosalpingography (274)	hĭs-tĕr-ō-săl-pĭng-ŎG-ră-fē	
in vitro fertilization (279)	ĭn-VĒ-trō fĕr-tĭl-ĭ-ZĀ-shŭn	
laparoscopy (277)	lă-pă-RŎS-kō-pē	
leiomyomas (268)	lī-ō-mī-Ō-măz	
lumen (268)	LOO-mĕn	
mammography (274)	măm-MŎG-ră-fē	
meconium aspiration syndrome (273)	mĕ-KŌ-nē-um ăs-pĭ-RĀ-shŭn SĬN-drōm	
ovarian carcinoma (269)	ō-VĂR-ē-an kăr-sĭ-NŌ-mă	
ovarian cyst (269)	ō-VĂR-ē-an sĭst	
palpation (269)	păl-PĀ-shŭn	
Pap smear (274)	păp smēr	
pelvic inflammatory disease (269)	PĔL-vĭk ĭn-FLĂM-mă-tō-rē dĭ-ZĒZ	
pelvic ultrasonography (275)	PĔL-vĭk ŭl-tră-sŏn-ŎG-ră-fē	
pelvimetry (279)	pĕl-VĬM-ĭ-trē	
placenta previa (272)	plă-SĔN-tă PRĒ-vē-ă	
preeclampsia (272)	prē-ē-KLĂMP-sē-ă	
pyloric stenosis (273)	pī-LŎR-ĭk stĕ-NŌ-sĭs	
respiratory distress syndrome (273)	RĔS-pĭr-ă-tō-rē dĭs-STRĔS SĬN-drōm	
tubal ligation (278)	TOO-băl lī-GĀ-shŭn	

8

REVIEW SHEET

Write the meanings of the word parts in the spaces provided and test yourself. Check your answers with the information in the chapter or in the glossary (Medical Word Parts—English) at the end of the book.

COMBINING FORMS

Combining Form	Meaning	Combining Form	Meaning
amni/o	_____	my/o	_____
cephal/o	_____	myom/o	_____
cervic/o	_____	nat/i	_____
chori/o	_____	obstetr/o	_____
chorion/o	_____	olig/o	_____
colp/o	_____	o/o	_____
culd/o	_____	oophor/o	_____
episi/o	_____	ov/o	_____
galact/o	_____	ovari/o	_____
gynec/o	_____	ovul/o	_____
hyster/o	_____	perine/o	_____
lact/o	_____	phor/o	_____
mamm/o	_____	py/o	_____
mast/o	_____	salping/o	_____
men/o	_____	uter/o	_____
metr/o	_____	vagin/o	_____
metri/o	_____	vulv/o	_____

SUFFIXES

Suffix	Meaning	Suffix	Meaning
-arche	_____	-pareunia	_____
-cele	_____	-parous	_____
-cyesis	_____	-plasia	_____
-ectasis	_____	-plasty	_____
-ectomy	_____	-ptosis	_____
-flexion	_____	-rrhagia	_____
-genesis	_____	-rrhaphy	_____
-gravida	_____	-rrhea	_____
-itis	_____	-salpinx	_____

8

-scopy	_____	-tomy	_____
-stenosis	_____	-tresia	_____
-stomy	_____	-version	_____
-tocia	_____		

PREFIXES

Prefix	Meaning	Prefix	Meaning
bi-	_____	oxy-	_____
dys-	_____	peri-	_____
endo-	_____	pre-	_____
in-	_____	primi-	_____
intra-	_____	pseudo-	_____
multi-	_____	retro-	_____
nulli-	_____	uni-	_____

 Please refer to the enclosed CD for additional exercises and images related to this chapter.

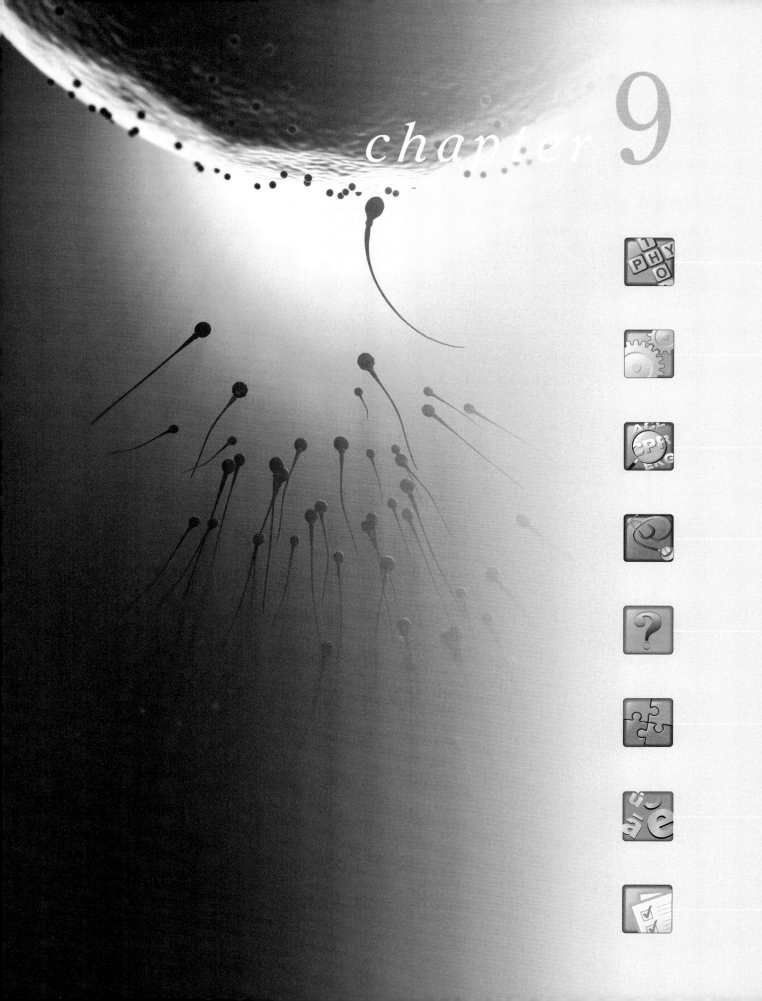

chapter 9

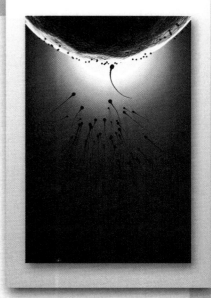

Male Reproductive System

THIS CHAPTER IS DIVIDED INTO THE FOLLOWING SECTIONS

In this chapter you will

- Name, locate, and describe the functions of the organs of the male reproductive system.
- Define some abnormal conditions and infectious diseases that affect the male reproductive system.
- Differentiate among several types of sexually transmitted diseases.
- Define many combining forms used to describe the structures of this system.
- Describe various laboratory tests and clinical procedures pertinent to disorders of the male reproductive system, and recognize related abbreviations.
- Apply your new knowledge to understanding medical terms in their proper contexts, such as medical reports and records.

Image Description: *Microscopic stylized view of sperm surrounding an ovum before fertilization.*

INTRODUCTION

The male sex cell, the **spermatozoon** (sperm cell), is microscopic—in volume, only one-third the size of a red blood cell and less than 1/100,000th the size of the female ovum. A relatively uncomplicated cell, the sperm is composed of a head region, containing nuclear hereditary material (chromosomes), and a tail region, consisting of a **flagellum** (hair-like process). The flagellum makes the sperm motile and makes it look somewhat like a tadpole. The spermatozoon cell contains relatively little food and cytoplasm, as it lives only long enough to travel from its point of release from the male to where the egg cell lies within the female reproductive tract (fallopian tube). Only one spermatozoon out of approximately 300 million sperm cells released during a single **ejaculation** (ejection of sperm and fluid from the male urethra) can penetrate a single ovum and result in fertilization of the ovum.

If more than one egg is passing down the fallopian tube when sperm are present, multiple fertilizations are possible, and twins, triplets, quadruplets, and so on may occur. Twins resulting from the fertilization of separate ova by separate sperm cells are called **fraternal twins.** Fraternal twins, developing with separate placentas, can be of the same sex or different sexes and resemble each other no more than ordinary brothers and sisters. Fraternal twinning is hereditary; the daughters of mothers of twins can carry the gene.

Identical twins result from fertilization of a single egg cell by a single sperm. As the fertilized egg cell divides and forms many cells, it somehow splits, and each part continues separately to undergo further division, each producing an embryo. Depending on when the embryo splits (day 1, 2, or 3), the fetuses will share the same gestational sac and/or placenta. Identical twins are always of the same sex and are very similar in form and feature.

The organs of the male reproductive system are designed to produce and release billions of spermatozoa throughout the lifetime of a male from puberty onward. In addition, the male reproductive system secretes a hormone called **testosterone.** Testosterone is responsible for the production of the bodily characteristics of the male (such as beard, pubic hair, and deeper voice) and for the proper development of male gonads **(testes)** and accessory organs **(prostate gland** and **seminal vesicles)** that secrete fluids to ensure the lubrication and viability of sperm.

ANATOMY

Label Figure 9–1 as you study the following description of the anatomy of the male reproductive system.

Each male gonad is a **testis** [1]. There are two **testes** (plural) or **testicles** that develop in the abdomen at about the level of the kidneys before descending during embryonic development into the **scrotum** [2], a sac enclosing the testes on the outside of the body.

The scrotum, lying between the thighs, exposes the testes to a lower temperature than that of the rest of the body. This lower temperature is necessary for the adequate maturation and development of sperm **(spermatogenesis).** Lying between the anus and the scrotum, at the floor of the pelvic cavity in the male, the **perineum** [3] is analogous to the perineal region in the female.

The interior of a testis is composed of a large mass of narrow, coiled tubules called the **seminiferous tubules** [4]. These tubules contain cells that manufacture spermatozoa. The seminiferous tubules are the **parenchymal tissue** of the testis, which means that they perform the essential work of the organ (formation of sperm). Other cells in the testis, called **interstitial cells,** manufacture an important male hormone, **testosterone.**

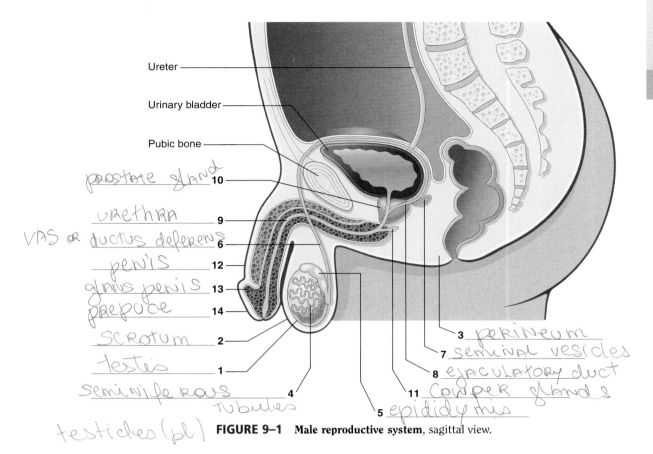

Ureter

Urinary bladder

Pubic bone

prostate gland 10

urethra 9

VAS or ductus deferens 6

penis 12

glans penis 13

prepuce 14

scrotum 2

testis 1

seminiferous tubules 4

testicles (pl.)

3 *perineum*
7 *seminal vesicles*
8 *ejaculatory duct*
11 *Cowper glands*
5 *epididymis*

FIGURE 9–1 **Male reproductive system**, sagittal view.

All body organs contain **parenchyma** (parenchymal cells or tissue), which perform the essential functions of the organ. Organs also contain supportive, connective, and framework tissue, such as blood vessels, connective tissues, and sometimes muscle as well. This supportive tissue is called **stroma (stromal tissue).**

After formation, sperm cells move through the seminiferous tubules and collect in ducts that lead to a large tube, the **epididymis** [5], at the upper part of each testis. The spermatozoa mature, become motile in the epididymis, and are temporarily stored there. An epididymis runs down the length of each testicle (the coiled tube is about 16 feet long) and then turns upward again and becomes a narrow, straight tube called the **vas deferens** [6] or **ductus deferens.** Figure 9–2 shows the internal structure of a testis and the epididymis. The vas deferens is about 2 feet long and carries the sperm up into the pelvic region, at the level of the urinary bladder, merging with ducts from the **seminal vesicles** [7] to form the **ejaculatory duct** [8] leading toward the urethra. During a **vasectomy** or **sterilization** procedure, the urologist cuts and ties off each vas deferens.

The seminal vesicles, two glands (only one is shown in Fig. 9–1) located at the base of the bladder, open into the ejaculatory duct as it joins the **urethra** [9]. They secrete a thick, sugary, yellowish substance that nourishes the sperm cells and forms much of the volume of ejaculated semen. **Semen** is a combination of fluid (seminal fluid) and spermatozoa (sperm cells account for less than 1 percent of the semen volume) that is ejected from the body through the urethra. In the male, as opposed to that in the female, the genital orifice combines with the urinary (urethral) opening.

The **prostate gland** [10] lies at the region where the vas deferens enters the urethra, almost encircling the upper end of the urethra. It secretes a thick fluid that, as part of semen, aids the motility of the sperm. The muscular tissue of the prostate aids in the expulsion of sperm during ejaculation. **Cowper (bulbourethral) glands** [11], lying below the prostate gland, also secrete fluid into the urethra.

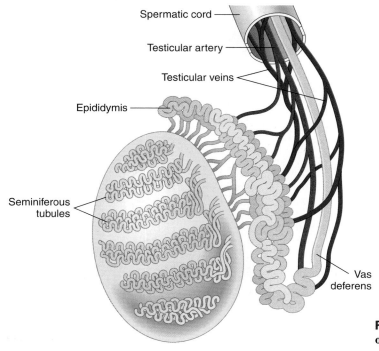

Spermatic cord

Testicular artery

Testicular veins

Epididymis

Seminiferous
tubules

Vas
deferens

FIGURE 9–2 Internal structure
of a testis and the epididymis.

The urethra passes through the **penis** [12] to the outside of the body. The penis is composed of erectile tissue and at its tip expands to form a soft, sensitive region called the **glans penis** [13]. Ordinarily, a fold of skin called the **prepuce,** or **foreskin** [14], covers the glans penis. During a circumcision the foreskin is removed, leaving the glans penis visible at all times.

Erectile dysfunction (impotence) is the inability of the adult male to achieve an erection. Viagra (sildenafil citrate) is a drug that increases blood flow to the penis, enhancing ability to have an erection.

The flow diagram in Figure 9–3 traces the path of spermatozoa from their formation in the seminiferous tubules of the testes to the outside of the body.

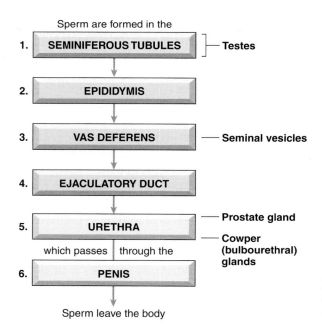

Sperm are formed in the

1. **SEMINIFEROUS TUBULES** — **Testes**

2. **EPIDIDYMIS**

3. **VAS DEFERENS** — **Seminal vesicles**

4. **EJACULATORY DUCT**

5. **URETHRA** — **Prostate gland**
— **Cowper (bulbourethral) glands**

which passes | through the

6. **PENIS**

Sperm leave the body

FIGURE 9–3 The **passage of sperm** from the seminiferous tubules in the testes to the outside of the body.

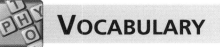

VOCABULARY

This list reviews new terms introduced in the text. Short definitions reinforce your understanding.

bulbourethral gland	One of a pair of exocrine glands near the male urethra.
Cowper gland	Bulbourethral gland.
ejaculation	Ejection of sperm and fluid from the male urethra.
ejaculatory duct	Tube through which semen enters the male urethra.
epididymis (*plural:* **epididymides**)	One of a pair of long, tightly coiled tubes lying on top of each testis. It carries sperm from the seminiferous tubules to the vas deferens.
erectile dysfunction	Inability of an adult male to achieve an erection; impotence.
flagellum	Hair-like projection on a sperm cell that makes it motile (able to move).
fraternal twins	Two infants born of the same pregnancy from two separate ova fertilized by two different sperm. See Figure 9–4.
glans penis	Sensitive tip of the penis.
identical twins	Two infants resulting from division of one fertilized egg into two distinct embryos. Conjoined ("Siamese") twins are incompletely separated identical twins.
impotence	Inability of an adult male to achieve an erection. From Latin *in/im*, not, and *potentia*, power.

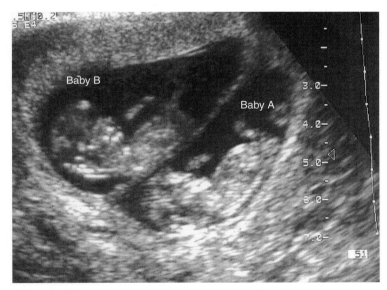

FIGURE 9–4   **Fraternal twins** (Marcos and Matheus Do Carmo). Notice the 6-week-old embryos in two separate amniotic sacs. (Courtesy Julianna Do Carmo.)

9

interstitial cells	In the testes, these cells lie between the seminiferous tubules and produce the hormone testosterone. A pituitary gland hormone (luteinizing hormone [LH]) stimulates interstitial cells to produce testosterone.
parenchyma	Tissue composed of essential and functional cells of organ. In the testis, the parenchymal tissue includes seminiferous tubules that produce sperm.
perineum	External region between the anus and scrotum in the male.
prepuce	Fold of skin covering the tip of the penis. Also called foreskin.
prostate gland	Exocrine gland, in men, at the base of the urinary bladder. The prostate gland secretes the fluid part of semen into the urethra during ejaculation.
scrotum	External sac that contains the testes.
semen	Spermatozoa (sperm cells) and seminal fluid (prostatic and other glandular secretions).
seminal vesicle	Either of paired sac-like male exocrine glands that secrete a fluid into the vas deferens. The seminal fluid is the major component of semen.
seminiferous tubules	Narrow, coiled tubules that produce sperm in the testes.
spermatozoon (*plural:* **spermatozoa**)	Sperm cell.
sterilization	Any procedure that removes an individual's ability to produce or release reproductive cells.
stroma	Supportive, connective tissue of an organ, as distinguished from its parenchyma.
testis (*plural:* **testes**)	Male gonad (testicle) that produces spermatozoa and the hormone testosterone. *Remember:* testis means one testicle, and testes are two testicles.
testosterone	Hormone secreted by the interstitial tissue of the testes; responsible for male sex characteristics.
vas deferens	Narrow tube (one on each side) that carries sperm from the epididymis into the body and toward the urethra. Also called ductus deferens.

Prostate/Prostrate
Don't confuse *prostate* with *prostrate*, which means lying down.

Semen/Sperm
Don't confuse *semen* with *sperm*. *Semen* is the thick, whitish secretion discharged from the urethra during ejaculation. It contains *sperm*, cells that develop in the testes.

COMBINING FORMS AND TERMINOLOGY

Write the meanings of the medical terms in the spaces provided.

Combining Form	Meaning	Terminology	Meaning
andr/o	male	androgen	
		Testosterone is an androgen. The testes in males and the adrenal glands in both men and women produce androgens.	
balan/o	glans penis (Greek *balanos*, acorn)	balanitis	
		Caused by overgrowth of organisms (bacteria and yeast). See Figure 9–5, A.	
cry/o	cold	cryogenic surgery	
		New techniques for prostate cancer treatment use cryosurgery to freeze and kill cells that radical prostatectomy cannot reach.	
crypt/o	hidden	cryptorchism	
		In this congenital condition, one or both testicles do not descend, by the time of birth, into the scrotal sac from the abdominal cavity. See Figure 9–5, B.	
epididym/o	epididymis	epididymitis	
		Symptoms are fever, chills, pain in the groin, tender, swollen epididymis.	
gon/o	seed (Greek *gone*, seed)	gonorrhea	
		See page 313.	
hydr/o	water, fluid	hydrocele	
		See page 310.	

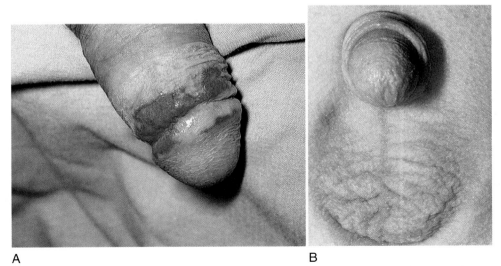

A   B

FIGURE 9–5   A, Balanitis. B, Cryptorchism. (A from Callen JP, et al: Color Atlas of Dermatology, 2nd ed. Philadelphia, WB Saunders, 2000. **B** from Zitelli BJ, Davis HW: Atlas of Pediatric Physical Diagnosis, 2nd ed. St. Louis, Mosby, 1992.)

Combining Form	Meaning	Terminology	Meaning
orch/o, orchi/o, orchid/o	testis, testicle (the botanical name for orchid, the flower, is derived from the Greek word *orchis*, testicle, describing the fleshy tubers on the rootstocks of the plant)	orchiectomy _____ *Castration in males. (Also called orchidectomy.)* anorchism _____ orchitis _____ *Caused by injury or by the mumps virus, which also infects the salivary glands.*	
prostat/o	prostate gland	prostatitis _____ *Bacterial (E. coli) prostatitis often is associated with urethritis and infection of the lower urinary tract.* prostatectomy _____	
semin/i	semen, seed	seminiferous tubules _____ *The suffix -ferous means pertaining to bearing, or bearing or carrying.* seminal vesicles _____	
sperm/o, spermat/o	spermatozoa, semen	spermolytic _____ *Noun suffixes ending in -sis, like -lysis, form adjectives by dropping the -sis and adding -tic.* oligospermia _____ aspermia _____ *Lack of formation or ejaculation of semen (sperm and fluid).*	
terat/o	monster (Greek *teras*, monster)	teratoma _____ *A benign tumor occurring in the testes composed of different types of tissue, such as bone, hair, cartilage, and skin cells.*	
test/o	testis, testicle	testicular _____ *The term testis originates from a Latin term meaning witness. In ancient times men would take an oath with one hand on their testes, swearing by their manhood to tell the truth.*	
varic/o	varicose veins	varicocele _____ *A collection of varicose (swollen, twisted) veins above the testis. See page 310.*	
vas/o	vessel, duct; vas deferens	vasectomy _____ *See page 360. Remember: in this term, vas/o refers to the vas deferens, and not to any other vessel or duct.*	
zo/o	animal life	azoospermia _____ *Lack of spermatozoa in the semen. Causes include testicular dysfunction, chemotherapy, blockage of the epididymis, and vasectomy.*	

SUFFIXES

Suffix	Meaning	Terminology	Meaning
-genesis	formation	spermatogenesis _____	
-one	hormone	testosterone _____	
		Ster/o indicates that this is a type of steroid compound.	
-pexy	fixation, put in place	orchiopexy _____	
		A surgical procedure to correct cryptorchism.	
-stomy	new opening	vasovasostomy _____	
		Reversal of vasectomy; a urologist rejoins the cut ends of the vas deferens.	

PATHOLOGIC CONDITIONS; SEXUALLY TRANSMITTED DISEASES

TUMORS AND ANATOMIC/STRUCTURAL DISORDERS

Testes

carcinoma of the testes (testicular cancer)

Malignant tumor of the testicles.

Testicular tumors are rare except in the 15- to 35-year-old age group. The most common tumor, a **seminoma,** arises from embryonic cells in the testes (see Fig. 9–6, *A*). Nonseminomatous tumors are **embryonal carcinoma** (see Fig. 9–6, *B*), **teratocarcinoma,** and **choriocarcinoma,** or combinations of the three. Teratomas (benign tumors) are composed of tissue such as bone, hair, cartilage, and skin cells (terat/o means monster).

Testicular cancers can be treated and cured with surgery (orchiectomy), radiotherapy, and chemotherapy. Tumors produce the proteins hCG and alpha-fetoprotein. Serum levels of these proteins are used as **tumor markers** to determine success of treatment.

cryptorchism; cryptorchidism

Undescended testicles.

Orchiopexy is performed to bring the testes into the scrotum, if they do not descend on their own by the age of 1 or 2 years. Undescended testicles are associated with a high risk for sterility and testicular cancer.

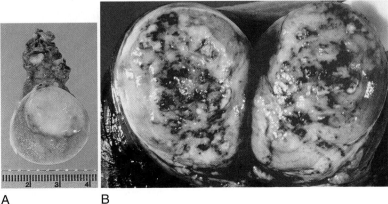

A   B

FIGURE 9–6   **A, Seminoma of a testis. B, Embryonal carcinoma** of a testis. (From Kumar V, Cotran RS, Robbins SL: Basic Pathology, 7th ed. Philadelphia, WB Saunders, 2003.)

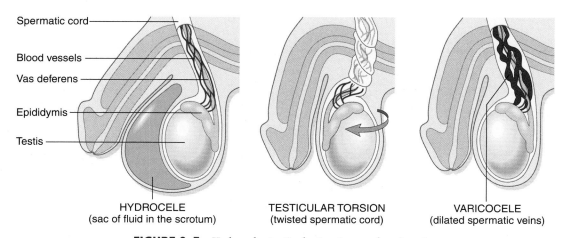

Spermatic cord
Blood vessels
Vas deferens
Epididymis
Testis

HYDROCELE
(sac of fluid in the scrotum)

TESTICULAR TORSION
(twisted spermatic cord)

VARICOCELE
(dilated spermatic veins)

FIGURE 9–7 Hydrocele, testicular torsion, and varicocele.

hydrocele	**Sac of clear fluid in the scrotum.**

Hydroceles may be congenital or occur as a response to infection or tumors. Often idiopathic, they can be differentiated from testicular masses by *transillumination* (shining a light source to the side of a scrotal enlargement). If the hydrocele does not resolve on its own, the sac fluid is aspirated via needle and syringe, or hydrocelectomy may be necessary. In this procedure, the sac is surgically removed through an incision in the scrotum (Fig. 9–7).

testicular torsion	**Twisting of the spermatic cord** (see Fig. 9–7).

The rotation of the spermatic cord cuts off blood supply to the testis. Torsion occurs most frequently in the first year of life and during puberty. Surgical correction within 5 hours of onset of symptoms can save the testis.

varicocele	**Enlarged, dilated veins near the testicle.**

This condition is associated with oligospermia and azoospermia. Oligospermic men with varicocele and scrotal pain should have a varicocelectomy. In this procedure, the internal spermatic vein is ligated (the affected segment is cut out and the ends are tied off), leading to a marked increase in fertility (see Fig. 9–7).

Prostate Gland

carcinoma of the prostate (prostate cancer)	**Malignant tumor of the prostate gland.**

This cancer commonly occurs in men who are older than 50 years of age. **Digital rectal examination** (Fig. 9–8) can detect the tumor at a later stage, but early detection depends on a **prostate-specific antigen (PSA) test**. PSA is a protein that is secreted by tumor cells into the bloodstream. PSA levels are elevated in prostate cancer patients even at an early stage of tumor growth. The normal PSA level is 4.0 ng/mL or less.

Diagnosis requires identification by a pathologist of abnormal prostate tissue in a prostate biopsy. **Transrectal ultrasound (TRUS)** guides the precise placement of the biopsy needle. Multiple needle biopsy specimens are taken through the rectal wall. Computed tomography (CT) detects lymph node metastases.

Treatment consists of surgery (prostatectomy), radiation therapy, and/or hormonal chemotherapy. Because prostatic cells are stimulated to grow in the presence of androgens, antiandrogen hormones slow tumor growth by depriving the cells of testosterone. Prostate cancer also is treated with leupron, a hormone that blocks pituitary stimulation of the testes and reduces the level of androgens in the bloodstream. Radioactive seeds implanted in the prostate also are used to destroy tumor cells.

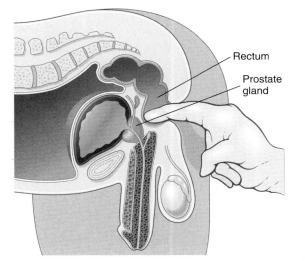

PSA

FIGURE 9–8 Digital rectal examination (DRE) of the prostate gland.

prostatic hyperplasia

Benign growth of cells within the prostate gland; benign prostatic hyperplasia (BPH).

BPH is a common condition in men older than 60 years of age. Urinary obstruction and inability to empty the bladder completely are symptoms. Figure 9–9 shows the prostate gland with BPH and with carcinoma. Surgical treatment by **transurethral resection of the prostate (TURP)** relieves the obstruction, but overgrowth of cells may recur over several years. In this procedure, an endoscope (resectoscope) is inserted into the penis and through the urethra. Prostatic tissue is removed by an electrical hot-loop attached to the resectoscope.

Several drugs to relieve BPH symptoms have been approved by the FDA. Finasteride (Proscar) inhibits production of a potent testosterone that promotes enlargement of the prostate. Other drugs, alpha-blockers such as tamsulosin (Flomax), act by relaxing the smooth muscle of the prostate and the neck of the bladder.

Lasers also may be used to destroy prostatic tissue and relieve obstruction. A **laser TURP** or **GreenLight PVP** procedure employs a green light laser at the end of an endoscope.

FIGURE 9–9 The prostate gland with carcinoma and benign prostatic hyperplasia (BPH). Carcinoma usually arises around the sides of the gland, whereas BPH occurs in the center of the gland. Because prostate cancers are located more peripherally, they can be palpated on digital rectal examination (DRE).

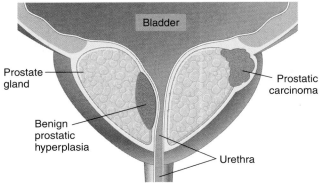
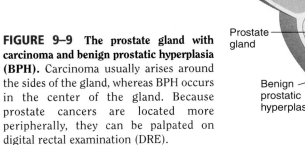

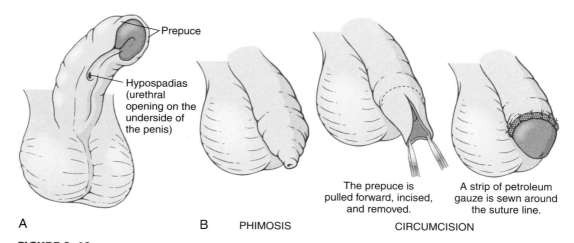

A

B   PHIMOSIS

The prepuce is
pulled forward, incised,
and removed.

A strip of petroleum
gauze is sewn around
the suture line.

CIRCUMCISION

FIGURE 9–10   **A, Hypospadias.** Surgical repair involves excising a portion of the prepuce, wrapping it (to be used as a graft) around a catheter, suturing it to the distal part of the urethra, and bringing it to the exit at the tip of the penis. **B, Phimosis** and **circumcision** to correct the condition.

Penis

hypospadias; hypospadia

Congenital abnormality in which the male urethral opening is on the undersurface of the penis (Fig. 9–10, A), instead of at its tip.

Hypospadias (-spadias means the condition of tearing or cutting) occurs in 1 in every 300 live male births and can be corrected surgically.

phimosis

Narrowing (stricture) of the opening of the prepuce over the glans penis; phim/o means to muzzle.

This condition can interfere with urination and cause secretions to accumulate under the prepuce, leading to infection. Treatment is by circumcision (cutting around the prepuce to remove it) (see Fig. 9–10, B).

SEXUALLY TRANSMITTED DISEASES (STDs)

Sexually transmitted diseases are infections transmitted by sexual or other genital contact. Sexually transmitted infections (STIs) and venereal diseases (from Latin *Venus,* the goddess of love) occur in both men and women and are the most easily communicable diseases in the world.

chlamydial infection

Bacteria *(Chlamydia trachomatis)* invade the urethra and reproductive tract of men and women.

Within 3 weeks after becoming infected, men may experience dysuria and notice a white or clear discharge from the penis.

Infected women may notice a yellowish vaginal discharge (from the endocervix), but often the disease is asymptomatic. Antibiotics cure the infection, but if untreated, this STD can cause salpingitis (pelvic inflammatory disease [PID]) and infertility in women.

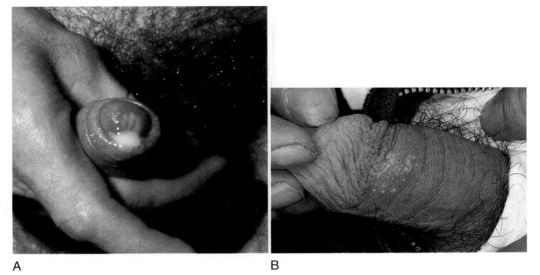

A   B

FIGURE 9–11   **A, Gonorrhea.** Discharge from the penis can be seen. **B, Herpes genitalis.** The classic blisters (vesicles) are evident. (**A** from Morse SA, et al: Atlas of Sexually Transmitted Diseases and AIDS, 2nd ed. London, Gower, 2003. **B** from Swartz MH: Textbook of Physical Diagnosis, History and Examination, 4th ed. Philadelphia, WB Saunders, 2002.)

gonorrhea

Inflammation of the genital tract mucous membranes, caused by infection with gonococci (berry-shaped bacteria).

Other areas of the body, such as the eye, oral mucosa, rectum, and joints, may be affected as well. Signs and symptoms include dysuria and a yellow, mucopurulent (**purulent** means pus-filled) discharge from the male urethra. See Figure 9–11, *A*. The ancient Greeks mistakenly thought that this discharge was a leakage of semen, so they named the condition gonorrhea, meaning discharge of seed (gon/o = seed).

Many women carry the disease asymptomatically, whereas others have pain, vaginal and urethral discharge, and salpingitis (PID). As a result of sexual activity, men and women can acquire anorectal and pharyngeal gonococcal infections as well. Chlamydial infection and gonorrhea often occur together. When treating these infections, doctors give antibiotics for both and treat both partners.

herpes genitalis

Infection of the skin and mucosa of the genitals, caused by the herpes simplex virus (HSV) and marked by blisters.

Most cases of herpes genitalis are caused by HSV type II (although some are caused by HSV type I, which commonly is associated with oral infections such as cold sores or fever blisters). The usual clinical presentation is reddening of skin with formation of small, fluid-filled blisters and ulcers. See Figure 9–11, *B*. Initial episodes also may involve inguinal lymphadenopathy, fever, headache, and malaise. Remissions and relapse periods occur; no drug is known to be effective as a cure. Neonatal herpes is a serious complication that affects infants born to women with active infection near the time of delivery. Gynecologists may deliver infants by cesarean section to prevent infection of these babies by HSV. Studies suggest that women with herpes genitalis have a higher risk of developing vulvar and cervical cancer.

9

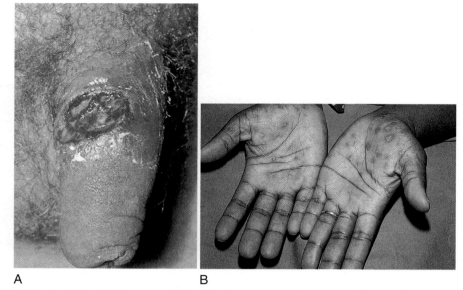

A   B

FIGURE 9–12   **Syphilis. A, Primary syphilis** with **chancre** on penis. **B, Secondary syphilis** showing rash on palms of hands. This stage may last up to 2 years. (**A** from Swartz MH: Textbook of Physical Diagnosis, History and Examination, 4th ed. Philadelphia, WB Saunders, 2002. **B** from Callen JP, et al: Color Atlas of Dermatology, 2nd ed. Philadelphia, WB Saunders, 2000.)

syphilis	**Chronic STD caused by a spirochete (spiral-shaped bacterium).**
	A **chancre** (hard ulcer or sore) usually appears on the external genitalia a few weeks after bacterial infection. See Figure 9–12, *A*. Two to six months after the chancre disappears, secondary syphilis begins (see Fig. 9–12, *B*). Tertiary syphilis includes damage to the brain, spinal cord, and heart, which may appear years after the earlier symptoms disappear. Syphilis (which was so often fatal in early times that it was known as the "great pox"—versus the more familiar smallpox) can be congenital in the fetus if it is transmitted from the mother during pregnancy. Penicillin is effective for treatment in most cases.

LABORATORY TESTS AND CLINICAL PROCEDURES

LABORATORY TESTS

PSA test	**Measures levels of prostate-specific antigen (PSA) in the blood.**
	PSA is produced by cells within the prostate gland. Elevated levels of PSA are associated with enlargement of the prostate gland and may be a sign of prostate cancer.
semen analysis	**Ejaculated fluid is examined microscopically.**
	Sperm cells are counted and examined for motility and shape. The test is part of fertility studies and also is required to establish the effectiveness of vasectomy. Men with sperm counts of less than 20 million/mL of semen usually are sterile (not fertile). Sterility can result in an adult male who becomes ill with mumps, an infectious disease affecting the testes (inflammation and deterioration of spermatozoa).

CLINICAL PROCEDURES

castration

Surgical excision of testicles or ovaries.

Castration may be performed to reduce production and secretion of hormones that stimulate growth of malignant cells (in breast cancer and prostate cancer). When a boy is castrated before puberty, he becomes a **eunuch** (Greek, *eune*, couch; *echein*, to guard). Male secondary sex characteristics fail to develop.

circumcision

Surgical procedure to remove the prepuce of the penis.

See Figure 9–10, *B*.

digital rectal examination (DRE)

Finger palpation through the anal canal and rectum to examine the prostate gland.

See Figure 9–8.

photoselective vaporization of the prostate (GreenLight PVP)

Removal of tissue to treat benign prostatic hyperplasia (BPH) using a green light laser (laser TURP).

This minimally invasive procedure is expected to replace TURP for treatment of BPH. It is quick, with minimal side effects and fast recovery time.

transurethral resection of the prostate (TURP)

Excision of benign prostatic hyperplasia using a resectoscope through the urethra.

This procedure treats benign prostatic hyperplasia (BPH). An electrical hot loop destroys the prostatic tissue, which is removed through the resectoscope (Fig. 9–13).

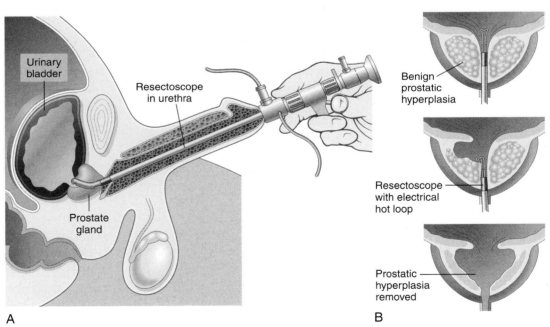

A   B

FIGURE 9–13   Transurethral resection of the prostate (TURP). A, The resectoscope contains a light, valves for controlling irrigating fluid, and an electrical loop that cuts tissue and seals blood vessels. **B,** The urologist uses a wire loop through the resectoscope to remove obstructing tissue one piece at a time. The pieces are carried by the fluid into the bladder and flushed out at the end of the operation.

9

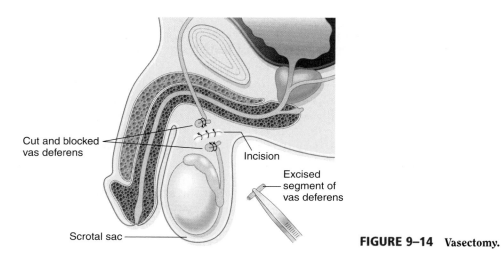

Cut and blocked vas deferens

Incision

Excised segment of vas deferens

Scrotal sac

FIGURE 9–14 Vasectomy.

vasectomy	**Bilateral surgical removal of a part of the vas deferens.**

A urologist cuts the vas deferens on each side, removes a piece, and performs a **ligation** (tying and binding off) of the free ends with sutures (Fig. 9–14). The procedure is performed using local anesthesia and through an incision in the scrotal sac. Because spermatozoa cannot leave the body, the vasectomized male is sterile, but not castrated. Normal hormone secretion, sex drive, and potency (ability to have an erection) are intact. The body reabsorbs unexpelled sperm. In a small number of cases, a vasovasostomy can successfully reverse vasectomy.

ABBREVIATIONS

BPH	benign prostatic hyperplasia (also called benign prostatic hypertrophy)	**TRUS**	transrectal ultrasound [examination]; test to assess the prostate gland and to guide the precise placement of a biopsy needle
DRE	digital rectal examination		
GU	genitourinary		
HSV	herpes simplex virus	**TUIP**	transurethral incision of the prostate; successful in less enlarged prostates and less invasive than TURP
NSU	nonspecific urethritis (not due to gonorrhea or chlamydial infection)		
PID	pelvic inflammatory disease	**TUMT**	transurethral microwave thermotherapy
PSA	prostate-specific antigen	**TUNA**	transurethral needle ablation; radiofrequency energy destroys prostate tissue
PVP	photoselective vaporization of the prostate; GreenLight PVP		
RPR	rapid plasma reagin [test]; a test for syphilis	**TURP**	transurethral resection of the prostate
STD	sexually transmitted diseases		
STI	sexually transmitted infection		

PRACTICAL APPLICATIONS

Reproduced here is a case report from actual medical records. Background data and explanations of more difficult terms are added in brackets. Answers to the questions are on page 325.

CASE REPORT: A MAN WITH POST-TURP COMPLAINTS

The patient is a 70-year-old man who underwent a TURP for BPH 5 years ago and now has severe obstructive urinary symptoms with a large postvoid residual.

On DRE, his prostate was found to be large, bulky, and nodular, with palpable extension to the left seminal vesicle. His PSA level was 120 ng/mL [normal is 0 to 4 ng/mL] and a bone scan was negative. A pelvic sonogram revealed bilateral external iliac adenopathy with lymph nodes measuring 1.5 cm on average [normal lymph node size is less than 1 cm]. A prostatic biopsy revealed a poorly differentiated adenocarcinoma.

This patient most likely has at least stage D1 disease [distant metastases with pelvic lymph node involvement]. Recommendation is hormonal drug treatment to suppress secretion of testosterone, which stimulates prostatic tumor growth.

Questions on the Case Report

1. Five years previously, the patient had which type of surgery?
   a. Removal of testicles
   b. Perineal prostatectomy
   c. Partial prostatectomy (transurethral)

2. What was the reason for the surgery then?
   a. Cryptorchism
   b. Benign overgrowth of the prostate gland
   c. Testicular cancer

3. What symptom does he have now?
   a. Burning pain on urination
   b. Urinary retention
   c. Premature ejaculation

4. What examination allowed the physician to feel the tumor?
   a. Palpation by a finger inserted into the rectum
   b. Pelvic sonogram
   c. Prostate-specific antigen test

5. Where had the tumor spread?
   a. Pelvic lymph nodes
   b. Pelvic lymph nodes and left seminal vesicle
   c. Pelvic bone

6. What is likely to stimulate prostatic adenocarcinoma growth?
   a. Hormonal drug treatment
   b. Prostatic biopsy
   c. Testosterone secretion

7. Stage D1 means that the tumor
   a. Is localized to the hip area
   b. Is confined to the prostate gland
   c. Has spread to lymph nodes and other organs

8. Why is staging of tumors important?
   a. To classify the extent of spread of the tumor and to plan treatment
   b. To make the initial diagnosis
   c. To make an adequate biopsy of the tumor

9

ABOUT ANABOLIC STEROIDS

Anabolic steroids are male hormones (androgens) that increase body weight and muscle size and may be used by doctors to increase growth in boys who do not mature physically as expected for their age. Steroids also may be used by athletes in an effort to increase strength and enhance performance; however, significant detrimental side effects of these drugs have been recognized:

- High levels of anabolic steroids cause acne, hepatic tumors, and sterility (testicular atrophy and oligospermia).
- In women, the androgenic effect of anabolic steroids leads to male hair distribution, deepening of the voice, amenorrhea, and clitoral enlargement.
- Anabolic steroid use also causes hypercholesterolemia, hypertension, jaundice (liver abnormalities), and salt and water retention (edema).

EXERCISES

Remember to check your answers carefully with those given in the Answers to Exercises, page 324.

A. Build medical terms for the following definitions.

1. inflammation of the testes _____

2. inflammation of the tube that carries the spermatozoa to the vas deferens _____

3. resection of the prostate gland _____

4. inflammation of the prostate gland _____

5. the process of producing (the formation of) sperm cells _____

6. fixation of undescended testicle _____

7. inflammation of the glans penis _____

8. condition of scanty sperm _____

9. no sperm or semen are produced _____

10. pertaining to a testicle _____

B. Give the meanings of the following medical terms.

1. hypospadias _____

2. parenchyma _____

3. stroma _____

4. cryogenic _____

5. interstitial cells of the testes _____

6. testosterone _____

7. phimosis _____

8. azoospermia _____

9. androgen _____

10. testicular seminoma _____

11. teratocarcinoma _____

C. Give medical terms for the following descriptions.

1. tube above each testis; carries and stores sperm _____

2. gland surrounding the urethra at the base of the urinary bladder _____

3. parenchymal tissue of the testes; produces spermatozoa _____

4. sperm cell _____

5. foreskin _____

6. male gonad; produces hormone and sperm cells _____

7. pair of sacs; secrete fluid into ejaculatory ducts _____

8. sac on outside of the body enclosing the testes _____

9. tube carrying sperm from the epididymis toward the urethra _____

10. pair of glands near the urethra; secrete fluid into the urethra _____

D. Match the term in Column I with its meaning in Column II. Write the correct letter in the space provided.

Column I

1. castration ___C___

2. semen analysis ___G___

3. ejaculation ___h___

4. purulent ___F___

5. vasectomy ___B___

6. circumcision ___D___

7. ligation ___A___

8. cryosurgery ___E___

Column II

A. To tie off or bind.
B. Removal of a piece of the vas deferens.
C. Orchiectomy.
D. Removal of the prepuce.
E. Destruction of tissue by freezing.
F. Pus-filled.
G. Test of fertility (reproductive ability).
H. Ejection of sperm and fluid from the urethra.

E. Give medical terms for the following abnormal conditions.

1. prostatic enlargement, nonmalignant _____

2. opening of the urethra on the undersurface of the penis _____

3. sexually transmitted infection with herpes virus_____

4. malignant tumor of the prostate gland _____

5. enlarged, swollen veins near the testes _____

6. sexually transmitted infection with primary stage marked by chancre _____

7. malignant tumor of the testes (three types) _____

_____

8. STD caused by berry-shaped bacteria and marked by inflammation of genital mucosa and

mucopurulent discharge_____

9. undescended testicles _____

10. sac of clear fluid in the scrotum_____

F. Spell out the abbreviations in Column I. Then match each abbreviation with its correct meaning from Column II.

Column I

1. PSA _____ ____

2. BPH _____ ____

3. TURP _____ ____

4. TRUS _____ ____

5. DRE _____ ____

6. HSV _____ ____

7. STD _____ ____

Column II

A. Manual diagnostic procedure to examine the prostate gland.

B. Relieves symptoms of prostate gland enlargement.

C. Etiologic agent of a sexually transmitted disease characterized by blister formation.

D. Noncancerous enlargement of the prostate gland.

E. Chlamydial infection, gonorrhea, and syphilis are examples of this general category of infections.

F. Helpful procedure in guiding a prostatic biopsy needle.

G. High serum levels of this protein indicate prostatic carcinoma.

G. *Review exercise:* Give the meanings of the following word parts.

1. -stasis _____

2. -sclerosis _____

3. -stenosis _____

4. -cele _____

5. -rrhagia _____

6. -ptosis _____

7. -plasia _____

8. -phagia _____

9. -rrhaphy _____

10. -pexy ___fixation___

11. -ectasis _____

12. -centesis _____

13. -genesis _____

14. balan/o _____

15. oophor/o _____

16. salping/o _____

17. hyster/o _____

18. metr/o _____

19. colp/o _____

20. mast/o _____

H. Match the following surgical procedures with the reasons they would be performed.

bilateral orchiectomy
circumcision
hydrocelectomy
orchiopexy

radical (complete)
prostatectomy
GreenLight PVP

varicocelectomy
vasectomy
vasovasostomy

1. carcinoma of the prostate gland _____

2. cryptorchism _____

3. sterilization (hormones remain and potency is not impaired) _____

4. benign prostatic hyperplasia _____

5. abnormal collection of fluid in a scrotal sac _____

6. reversal of sterilization procedure _____

7. teratocarcinoma of the testes _____

8. phimosis _____

9. ligation of swollen, twisted veins above the testes _____

I. Use the given definitions to complete the terms. Check your answers carefully.

1. gland at the base of the urinary bladder in males: pro_____ gland

2. coiled tube on top of each testis: epi_____

3. essential cells of an organ: par_____

4. foreskin: pre_____

5. bacterial infection that invades the urethra and reproductive tract of men and women and is the
   major cause of nonspecific urethritis in males and cervicitis in females: ch_____

6. ulcer that forms on genital organs after infection with syphilis: ch_____

7. androgen produced by the interstitial cells of the testis: test_____

8. fluid secreted by male reproductive glands and ejaculated with sperm: se_____

J. Circle the correct term(s) to complete the following sentences.

1. When Fred was a newborn infant, his doctors could feel only one testicle within the scrotum and
   suggested close monitoring of his condition of **(gonorrhea, cryptorchism, prostatic hyperplasia)**.

2. Bob had many sexual partners, one of whom had been diagnosed with **(testosterone, phimosis,
   chlamydial infection)**, a highly communicable STD.

3. At age 65, Mike had some difficulty with urgency and discomfort when urinating. His doctor did a
   digital rectal examination to examine his **(prostate gland, urinary bladder, vas deferens)**.

4. Just after Nick's birth, his parents had a difficult time deciding whether to have their infant son
   undergo **(TURP, castration, circumcision)**.

5. Ted noticed a hard ulcer on his penis and made an appointment with his doctor, a
   (gastroenterologist, gynecologist, urologist). The doctor viewed a specimen of the ulcer under the
   microscope and did a blood test, which revealed that Ted had contracted **(gonorrhea, herpes
   genitalis, syphilis)**, so the ulcer was a **(eunuch, chancre, seminoma)**.

6. After his fifth child was born, Art decided to have a **(vasovasostomy, hydrocelectomy, vasectomy)**
   to prevent conception of another child. A/an **(nephrologist, urologist, abdominal surgeon)**
   performed the procedure to cut and ligate the **(urethra, epididymis, vas deferens)**.

7. Twenty-six-year-old Lance noticed a hard testicular mass. His physician prescribed a brief trial with
   (antibodies, antibiotics, pain killers) to rule out **(epididymitis, testicular cancer, varicocele)**. The
   mass remained and Lance underwent **(epididymectomy, orchiectomy, prostatectomy)** and lymph
   node resection. The mass was a **(seminoma, prostate cancer, hydrocele)**.

8. Sarah and Steve had been trying to conceive a child for 7 years. Steve had a **(digital rectal examination, TURP, semen analysis)**, which revealed 25 percent normal sperm count with 10 percent motility. He was told he had **(anorchism, aspermia, oligospermia)**.

9. To boost his sperm count, Steve was given **(estrogen, testosterone, progesterone)**. As a side effect, this **(androgen, progestin, enzyme)** gave him a case of acne lasting several months.

10. Sarah eventually became pregnant. An ultrasound examination showed two embryos in separate **(peritoneal, scrotal, amniotic)** sacs. Sarah delivered two healthy **(identical, fraternal, perineal)** twin girls.

MEDICAL SCRAMBLE

Unscramble the letters to form suffixes from the clues. Use the letters in squares to complete the bonus term. Answers are found on page 325.

1. *Clue:* Ulcer associated with an STD

___ [ ] ___ ___ ___ ___ ___   RACEHCN

2. *Clue:* Collection of fluid in the scrotal sac (hernia)

___ [ ] ___ ___ ___ ___ [ ] ___   COYLHERED

3. *Clue:* Inflammation of the testes

___ ___ ___ ___ [ ] ___ [ ] [ ]   TCIOSHRI

4. *Clue:* Gland at the base of the bladder that secretes seminal fluid

[ ] ___ ___ [ ] ___ ___ ___ ___   TOSEPART

BONUS TERM: *Clue:* A common sexually transmitted disease caused by a spirochete.

[ ] [ ] [ ] [ ] [ ] [ ] [ ] [ ]

9

ANSWERS TO EXERCISES

A

1. orchitis
2. epididymitis
3. prostatectomy
4. prostatitis
5. spermatogenesis
6. orchiopexy
7. balanitis
8. oligospermia
9. aspermia
10. testicular

B

1. congenital anomaly in which the urethra opens on the underside of the penis
2. distinctive, essential tissue or cells of an organ, as for example, glomeruli and tubules of the kidney, seminiferous tubules of the testis
3. supportive and connective tissue of an organ
4. pertaining to producing cold or low temperatures
5. cells that produce the hormone testosterone; stimulated by luteinizing hormone from the pituitary gland
6. hormone made by the interstitial cells of the testes; responsible for secondary sex characteristics
7. narrowing, or stenosis, of the foreskin on the glans penis
8. lack of spermatozoa in the semen
9. hormone producing male characteristics
10. malignant tumor of the testes composed of germ or embryonic cells
11. malignant tumor of the testes composed of embryonic tissue, forming bone, hair, skin, cartilage

C

1. epididymis
2. prostate gland
3. seminiferous tubules (semin- = semen, fer = to carry)
4. spermatozoon
5. prepuce
6. testis; testicle
7. seminal vesicles
8. scrotum; scrotal sac
9. vas deferens
10. bulbourethral or Cowper glands

D

1. C
2. G
3. H
4. F
5. B
6. D
7. A
8. E

E

1. benign prostatic hyperplasia
2. hypospadias
3. herpes genitalis
4. adenocarcinoma of the prostate
5. varicocele
6. syphilis
7. embryonal carcinoma; seminoma; teratoma or teratocarcinoma
8. gonorrhea
9. cryptorchism
10. hydrocele

F

1. prostate-specific antigen: G
2. benign prostatic hyperplasia: D
3. transurethral resection of the prostate: B
4. transrectal ultrasound: F
5. digital rectal examination: A
6. herpes simplex virus: C
7. sexually transmitted disease: E

G

1. to stop, control; place
2. hardening
3. narrowing
4. hernia, swelling
5. bursting forth (of blood)
6. prolapse
7. formation
8. eating, swallowing
9. suture
10. fixation
11. widening
12. surgical puncture to remove fluid
13. producing
14. glans penis
15. ovary
16. fallopian tube
17. uterus
18. uterus
19. vagina
20. breast

H

1. radical (complete) prostatectomy
2. orchiopexy
3. vasectomy
4. GreenLight PVP
5. hydrocelectomy
6. vasovasostomy
7. bilateral orchiectomy
8. circumcision
9. varicocelectomy

I

1. prostate
2. epididymis
3. parenchyma
4. prepuce
5. chlamydial infection
6. chancre
7. testosterone
8. semen or seminal fluid

J

1. cryptorchism
2. chlamydial infection
3. prostate gland
4. circumcision
5. urologist; syphilis; chancre
6. vasectomy; urologist; vas deferens
7. antibiotics; epididymitis; orchiectomy; seminoma
8. semen analysis; oligospermia
9. testosterone; androgen
10. amniotic; fraternal

ANSWERS TO PRACTICAL APPLICATIONS

1. c
2. b
3. b
4. a
5. b
6. c
7. c
8. a

ANSWERS TO MEDICAL SCRAMBLE

1. CHANCRE   2. HYDROCELE   3. ORCHITIS   4. PROSTATE
BONUS TERM: SYPHILIS

PRONUNCIATION OF TERMS

PRONUNCIATION GUIDE

ā as in āpe	ă as in ăpple
ē as in ēven	ĕ as in ĕvery
ī as in īce	ĭ as in ĭnterest
ō as in ōpen	ŏ as in pŏt
ū as in ūnit	ŭ as in ŭnder

To test your understanding of the terminology in this chapter, write the meaning of each term in the space provided. In addition, you may wish to cover the terms and write them by looking at your definitions. Make sure your spelling is correct. The page number after each term indicates where it is defined or used in the book, so you can easily check your responses. You will find complete definitions for all of these terms and their audio pronunciations on the CD.

Term	Pronunciation	Meaning
androgen (307)	ĂN-drō-jĕn	_____
anorchism (308)	ăn-ŎR-kĭzm	_____
aspermia (308)	ā-SPĔR-mē-ă	_____
azoospermia (308)	ā-zō-ō-SPĔR-mē-ă	_____
balanitis (307)	băl-ă-NĪ-tĭs	_____
bulbourethral gland (305)	bŭl-bō-ū-RĒ-thrăl glănd	_____
castration (315)	kăs-TRĀ-shŭn	_____
chancre (314)	SHĂNG-kĕr	_____
chlamydial infection (312)	klă-MĬD-ē-ăl ĭn-FEK-shŭn	_____
circumcision (315)	sĭr-kŭm-SĬZH-ŭn	_____
Cowper gland (305)	CŎW-pĕr glănd	_____
cryogenic surgery (307)	krī-ō-GĔN-ĭk SŬR-jĕr-ē	_____
cryptorchism (307)	krĭp-TŎR-kĭzm	_____
ejaculation (305)	ē-jăk-ū-LĀ-shŭn	_____
ejaculatory duct (305)	ē-JĂK-ū-lă-tōr-ē dŭkt	_____
embryonal carcinoma (309)	ĕm-brē-ŌN-ăl kăr-sĭ-NŌ-mă	_____
epididymis (305)	ĕp-ĭ-DĬD-ĭ-mĭs	_____
epididymitis (307)	ĕp-ĭ-dĭd-ĭ-MĪ-tĭs	_____
erectile dysfunction (305)	ē-RĔK-tīl dĭs-FŬNK-shŭn	_____
eunuch (315)	Ū-nŭk	_____
flagellum (305)	flă-JĔL-ŭm	_____
fraternal twins (305)	fră-TĔR-năl twĭnz	_____
glans penis (305)	glănz PĒ-nĭs	_____
gonorrhea (307)	gŏn-ō-RĒ-ă	_____
herpes genitalis (313)	HĔR-pēz jĕn-ĭ-TĂL-ĭs	_____
hydrocele (307)	HĪ-drō-sēl	_____

Term	Pronunciation	Meaning
hypospadias (312)	hī-pō-SPĀ-dē-ăs	
identical twins (305)	ī-DĔN-tĭ-kăl twĭnz	
impotence (305)	ĬM-pō-tĕns	
interstitial cells (306)	ĭn-tĕr-STĬSH-ăl sĕlz	
ligation (316)	lī-GĀ-shŭn	
oligospermia (308)	ŏl-ĭ-gō-SPĔR-mē-ă	
orchiectomy (308)	ŏr-kē-ĔK-tō-mē	
orchiopexy (309)	ŏr-kē-ō-PĔK-sē	
orchitis (308)	ŏr-KĪ-tĭs	
parenchyma (306)	pă-RĔNG-kĭ-mă	
perineum (306)	pĕr-ĭ-NĒ-ŭm	
phimosis (312)	fi-MŌ-sĭs	
photoselective vaporization of the prostate (315)	fō-tō-sĕ-LĔK-tĭv vā-pŏr-ĭ-ZĀ-shŭn of the PRŎS-tāt	
prepuce (306)	PRĒ-pŭs	
prostatectomy (308)	prŏs-tă-TĔK-tō-mē	
prostate gland (306)	PRŎS-tāt glănd	
prostatic hyperplasia (311)	prŏs-TĂT-ĭk hī-pĕr-PLĀ-zē-ă	
prostatitis (308)	prŏs-tă-TĪ-tĭs	
purulent (313)	PŪR-ū-lĕnt	
scrotum (306)	SKRŌ-tŭm	
semen (306)	SĒ-mĕn	
seminal vesicle (306)	SĔM-ĭn-ăl VĔS-ĭ-k'l	
seminiferous tubules (306)	sĕ-mĭ-NĬF-ĕr-ŭs TOOB-ūlz	
seminoma (309)	sĕ-mĭ-NŌ-mă	
spermatogenesis (309)	spĕr-mă-tō-JĔN-ĕ-sĭs	
spermatozoa (306)	spĕr-mă-tō-ZŌ-ă	
spermatozoon (306)	spĕr-mă-tō-ZŌ-ĕn	
spermolytic (308)	spĕr-mō-LĬT-ĭk	
sterilization (306)	stĕr-ĭ-lĭ-ZĀ-shŭn	
stroma (306)	STRŌ-mă	
syphilis (314)	SĬF-ĭ-lĭs	
teratoma (308)	tĕr-ă-TŌ-mă	

Term	Pronunciation	Meaning
testicular (308)	tĕs-TĬK-ū-lăr	_____
testicular torsion (310)	tĕs-TĬK-ū-lăr TŎR-shŭn	_____
testis (306)	TĔS-tĭs	_____
testosterone (306)	tĕs-TŎS-tĕ-rōn	_____
varicocele (308)	VĀR-ĭ-kō-sēl	_____
vas deferens (306)	văs DĔF-ĕr-ĕnz	_____
vasectomy (308)	vă-SĔK-tō-mē	_____
vasovasostomy (309)	vă-zō-vă-ZŎS-tō-mē	_____

REVIEW SHEET

Write the meanings of the word parts in the spaces provided. Check your answers with the information in the chapter or in the glossary (Medical Word Parts—English) at the end of the book.

COMBINING FORMS

Combining Form	Meaning	Combining Form	Meaning
andr/o	_____	prostat/o	_____
balan/o	_____	semin/i	_____
cry/o	_____	sperm/o	_____
crypt/o	_____	spermat/o	_____
epididym/o	_____	terat/o	_____
gon/o	_____	test/o	_____
hydr/o	_____	varic/o	_____
orch/o	_____	vas/o	_____
orchi/o	_____	zo/o	_____
orchid/o	_____		

SUFFIXES

Suffix	Meaning	Suffix	Meaning
-cele	_____	-one	_____
-ectomy	_____	-pexy	_____
-gen	_____	-plasia	_____
-genesis	_____	-rrhea	_____
-genic	_____	-stomy	_____
-lysis	_____	-tomy	_____
-lytic	_____	-trophy	_____

 Please refer to the enclosed CD for additional exercises and images related to this chapter.

chapter 10

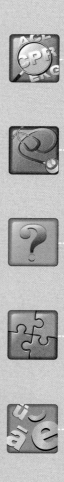

Nervous System

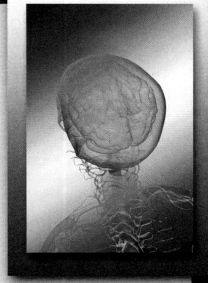

THIS CHAPTER IS DIVIDED INTO THE FOLLOWING SECTIONS

In this chapter you will

- Name, locate, and describe the functions of the major organs and parts of the nervous system.
- Recognize nervous system combining forms and make terms using them with new and familiar suffixes.
- Define several pathologic conditions affecting the nervous system.
- Describe some laboratory tests, clinical procedures, and abbreviations that pertain to the system.
- Apply your new knowledge to understanding medical terms in their proper contexts, such as medical reports and records.

Image Description: Posterior stylized view of the central nervous system within the skeletal torso.

10

INTRODUCTION

The nervous system is one of the most complex of all human body systems. More than 100 billion nerve cells operate constantly all over the body to coordinate the activities we do consciously and voluntarily, as well as those that occur unconsciously or involuntarily. We speak; we move muscles; we hear; we taste; we see; we think; our glands secrete hormones; we respond to danger, pain, temperature, and touch; and we have memory, association, and discrimination. All of these functions compose only a small number of the many activities controlled by our nervous systems.

Microscopic **nerve cells (neurons)** collected into macroscopic bundles called **nerves** carry electrical messages all over the body. External stimuli, as well as internal chemicals such as **acetylcholine,** activate the cell membranes of nerve cells in order to release stored electrical energy within the cells. This energy, when released and passed through the length of the nerve cell, is called the **nervous impulse.** External **receptors** (sense organs) as well as internal receptors in muscles and blood vessels receive these impulses and transmit them to the complex network of nerve cells in the brain and spinal cord. Within this central part of the nervous system, impulses are recognized, interpreted, and finally relayed to other nerve cells that extend out to all parts of the body, such as muscles, glands, and internal organs.

GENERAL STRUCTURE OF THE NERVOUS SYSTEM

The nervous system is classified into two major divisions: the **central nervous system (CNS)** and the **peripheral nervous system.** The central nervous system consists of the **brain** and **spinal cord.** The peripheral nervous system consists of **cranial nerves** and **spinal nerves, plexuses** and peripheral nerves throughout the body. See Figure 10–1. Cranial nerves carry impulses between the brain and the head and neck. The one exception is the 10th cranial nerve, called the vagus nerve. It carries messages to and from the neck, chest, and abdomen. Figure 10–2 shows cranial nerves, their functions, and the parts of the body that they carry messages to and from. Spinal nerves carry messages between the spinal cord and the chest, abdomen, and extremities.

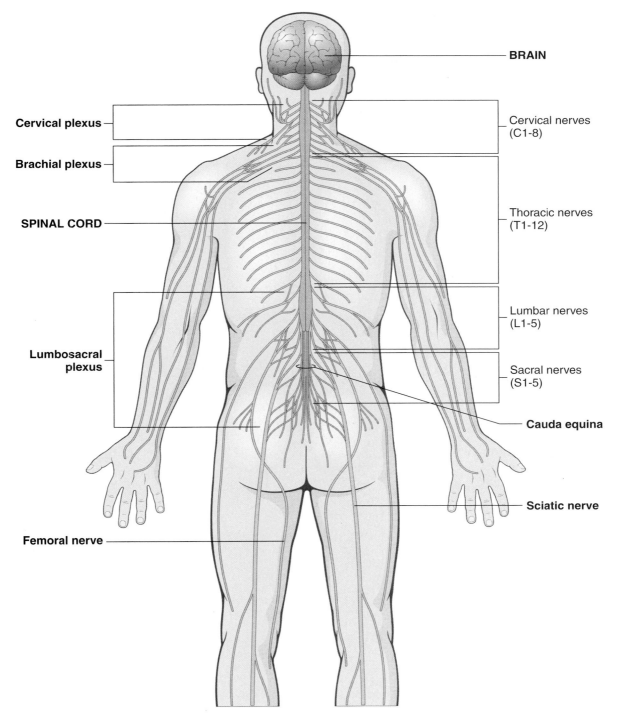

BRAIN

Cervical plexus

Brachial plexus

SPINAL CORD

Lumbosacral
plexus

Femoral nerve

Cervical nerves
(C1-8)

Thoracic nerves
(T1-12)

Lumbar nerves
(L1-5)

Sacral nerves
(S1-5)

Cauda equina

Sciatic nerve

FIGURE 10–1   **The brain and the spinal cord, spinal nerves, and spinal plexuses.** The **femoral nerve** is a lumbar nerve leading to and from the thigh (femur). The **sciatic nerve** is a nerve beginning in a region of the hip. The **cauda equina** (Latin for horse's tail) is a bundle of spinal nerves below the end of the spinal cord.

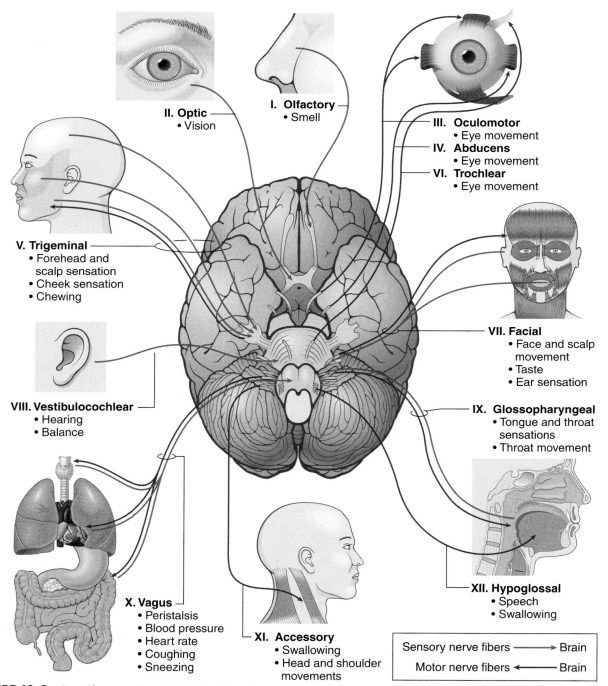

II. Optic
• Vision

I. Olfactory
• Smell

III. Oculomotor
• Eye movement
IV. Abducens
• Eye movement
VI. Trochlear
• Eye movement

V. Trigeminal
• Forehead and scalp sensation
• Cheek sensation
• Chewing

VIII. Vestibulocochlear
• Hearing
• Balance

VII. Facial
• Face and scalp movement
• Taste
• Ear sensation

IX. Glossopharyngeal
• Tongue and throat sensations
• Throat movement

X. Vagus
• Peristalsis
• Blood pressure
• Heart rate
• Coughing
• Sneezing

XI. Accessory
• Swallowing
• Head and shoulder movements

XII. Hypoglossal
• Speech
• Swallowing

Sensory nerve fibers	⟶ Brain
Motor nerve fibers	⟵ Brain

FIGURE 10–2   Cranial nerves (I to XII) leading from the base of the brain and showing the parts of the body they affect. Some are **sensory** or **afferent** nerves (carry messages **toward** the brain), and others are **motor** or **efferent** nerves (carrying messages **from** the brain to muscles and organs). Some nerves (mixed) carry both sensory and motor fibers.

The spinal and cranial nerves are composed of nerves that help the body respond to changes in the outside world. They include **sense receptors** for sight (eye), hearing and balance (ear), smell (olfactory), and **sensory (afferent) nerves** that carry messages related to changes in the environment *toward* the spinal cord and brain. In addition, **motor (efferent) nerves** travel *from* the spinal cord and brain to muscles of the body, telling them how to respond.

In addition to the spinal and cranial nerves (whose functions are mainly voluntary and involved with sensations of smell, taste, sight, hearing, and muscle movements), the peripheral nervous system also contains a large group of nerves that function involuntarily or automatically, without conscious control. These peripheral nerves belong to the **autonomic nervous system.** This system of nerve fibers carries impulses *away from* the central nervous system, to the glands, heart, blood vessels, and involuntary muscles found in the walls of tubes like the intestines and hollow organs like the stomach and urinary bladder. The autonomic nerves generally carry impulses away from the central nervous system.

Some autonomic nerves are **sympathetic** nerves and others are **parasympathetic** nerves. The sympathetic nerves stimulate the body in times of stress and crisis; they increase heart rate and forcefulness, dilate (relax) airways so more oxygen can enter, increase blood pressure, stimulate the adrenal glands to secrete epinephrine (adrenaline), and inhibit intestinal contractions, slowing digestion. The parasympathetic nerves normally act as a balance for the sympathetic nerves. Parasympathetic nerves slow down heart rate, contract the pupils of the eye, lower blood pressure, stimulate peristalsis to clear the rectum, and increase the quantity of secretions like saliva.

A **plexus** is a large network of nerves in the peripheral nervous system. The cervical, brachial (brachi/o means arm), and lumbosacral plexuses are examples. Figure 10–1 illustrates the relationship of the brain and spinal cord to the spinal nerves and plexuses.

Figure 10–3 summarizes the divisions of the central and peripheral nervous systems.

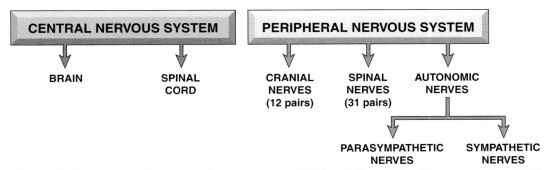

FIGURE 10–3 **Divisions of the central nervous system (CNS) and the peripheral nervous system (PNS).** The autonomic nervous system is a part of the peripheral nervous system.

NEURONS, NERVES, AND GLIA

A **neuron** is an individual nerve cell, a microscopic structure. Impulses pass along the parts of a nerve cell in a definite manner and direction. The parts of a neuron are pictured in Figure 10–4; label it as you study the following.

A **stimulus** begins an impulse in the branching fibers of the neuron, which are called **dendrites** [1]. A change in the electrical charge of the dendrite membranes is thus begun, and the nervous impulse moves along the dendrites like the movement of falling dominoes. The impulse, traveling in only one direction, next reaches the **cell body** [2], which contains the **cell nucleus** [3]. Small collections of nerve cell bodies outside the brain and spinal cord are called **ganglia** (*singular*: **ganglion**). Extending from the cell body is the **axon** [4], which carries the impulse away from the cell body. Axons can be covered with a fatty tissue called a **myelin sheath** [5]. The myelin sheath gives a white appearance to the nerve fiber—hence the term white matter, as in parts of the spinal cord and the white matter of the brain and

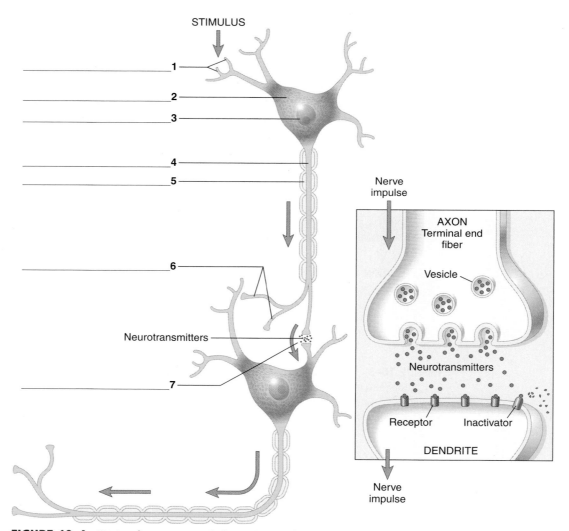

FIGURE 10–4   Parts of a neuron and the pathway of a nervous impulse. Neurons are the **parenchymal** (essential) **cells** of the nervous system. The *boxed drawing* shows what happens in a synapse. Vesicles store neurotransmitters in the terminal end fibers of axons. Receptors on the dendrites pick up the neurotransmitters. Inactivators end the activity of neurotransmitters when they have finished their job.

most peripheral nerves. The gray matter of the brain and spinal cord is composed of the cell bodies of neurons that appear gray because they are not covered by a myelin sheath.

The nervous impulse passes through the axon to leave the cell via the **terminal end fibers** [6] of the neuron. The space where the nervous impulse jumps from one neuron to another is called the **synapse** [7]. The transfer of the impulse across the synapse depends on the release of a chemical substance, called a **neurotransmitter,** by the neuron that brings the impulse to the synapse. See Figure 10–4 (boxed diagram). Tiny sacs (vesicles) containing the neurotransmitter are located at the ends of neurons, and they release the neurotransmitter into the synapse. **Acetylcholine, norepinephrine, epinephrine (adrenaline), dopamine, serotonin** and **endorphins** are examples of neurotransmitters.

Whereas a neuron is a microscopic structure within the nervous system, a **nerve** is macroscopic, able to be seen with the naked eye. A nerve consists of a bundle of dendrites and axons that travel together like strands of rope. Peripheral nerves that carry impulses *to* the brain and spinal cord from stimulus receptors like the skin, eye, ear, and nose are **sensory nerves;** those that carry impulses *from* the CNS to organs that produce responses, such as muscles and glands, are **motor nerves.**

Neurons and nerves are the **parenchymal** tissue of the nervous system; they do the essential work of the system by conducting impulses throughout the body. The **stromal** tissue of the nervous system is called **glia (neuroglia)** and consists of several types of specialized cells. This tissue holds the nervous system together and helps it ward off infection and injury with phagocytosis (engulfing waste products and foreign material). Glial cells do not transmit impulses. They are far more numerous than neurons and can reproduce.

There are four types of supporting or glial (neuroglial) cells. **Astrocytes (astroglial cells)** are star-like (astr/o means star) and transport water and salts between capillaries and neurons. **Microglial cells** are small cells with many branching processes. As phagocytes, they protect neurons in response to inflammation. **Oligodendroglial cells (oligodendrocytes)** have few (olig/o means few or scanty) dendrites. These cells form the myelin sheath. **Ependymal cells** (Greek *ependyma* means upper garment) line membranes within the brain and spinal cord where cerebrospinal fluid (CSF) circulates.

Glial cells, particularly the astrocytes, are associated with blood vessels and regulate the passage of potentially harmful substances from the blood into the nerve cells of the brain. This protective barrier between the blood and brain cells is called the **blood-brain barrier.** Figure 10–5 illustrates glial cells.

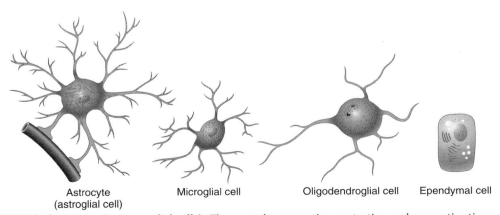

Astrocyte (astroglial cell)   Microglial cell   Oligodendroglial cell   Ependymal cell

FIGURE 10–5   Glial cells (neuroglial cells). These are the supportive, protective, and connective tissue cells of the CNS. Glial cells are **stromal** (framework) **tissue,** whereas neurons carry nervous impulses.

THE BRAIN

The brain controls body activities. In the human adult, it weighs about 3 pounds and has many different parts, all of which control different aspects of body functions.

The largest part of the brain is the "thinking" area or **cerebrum.** On the surface of the cerebrum, nerve cells lie in sheets, called the **cerebral cortex.** These sheets, arranged in folds called **gyri,** are separated from each other by grooves, known as **sulci.** The brain is divided in half, a right side and a left side, which are called **cerebral hemispheres.** Each hemisphere is subdivided into four major lobes named for the cranial (skull) bones that overlie them. Figure 10–6 shows these lobes—frontal, parietal, occipital, and temporal— as well as gyri and sulci.

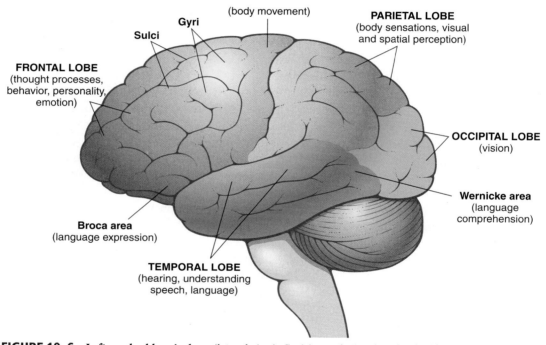

Gyri

Sulci

(body movement)

PARIETAL LOBE
(body sensations, visual
and spatial perception)

FRONTAL LOBE
(thought processes,
behavior, personality,
emotion)

OCCIPITAL LOBE
(vision)

Wernicke area
(language
comprehension)

Broca area
(language expression)

TEMPORAL LOBE
(hearing, understanding
speech, language)

FIGURE 10–6   **Left cerebral hemisphere** (lateral view). **Gyri** (convolutions) and **sulci** (fissures) are indicated. Notice the lobes of the cerebrum and the functional centers that control speech, vision, movement, hearing, thinking, and other processes. Neurologists believe the two hemispheres have different abilities. The **left brain** is more concerned with language, mathematical functioning, reasoning, and analytical thinking. The **right brain** is more active in spatial relationships, art, music, emotions, and intuition.

The cerebrum has many functions. Thought, judgment, memory, association, and discrimination take place within it. In addition, sensory impulses are received through afferent cranial nerves, and when registered in the cortex, they are the basis for perception. Cranial nerves carry motor impulses from the cerebrum to muscles and glands, and these produce movement and activity. Figure 10–6 shows the location of some of the centers in the cerebral cortex that control speech, vision, smell, movement, hearing, and thought processes.

In the middle of the cerebrum, there are spaces, or canals, called **ventricles** (pictured in Fig. 10–7). They contain a watery fluid that flows throughout the brain and around the spinal cord. This fluid is **cerebrospinal fluid (CSF)**, and it protects the brain and spinal cord from shock, by acting like a cushion. CSF usually is clear and colorless and contains lymphocytes, sugar, and proteins. Spinal fluid can be withdrawn for diagnosis or relief of pressure on the brain; this is called a **lumbar puncture (LP).** A hollow needle is inserted in the lumbar region of the spinal column below the region where the nervous tissue of the spinal cord ends, and CSF is withdrawn.

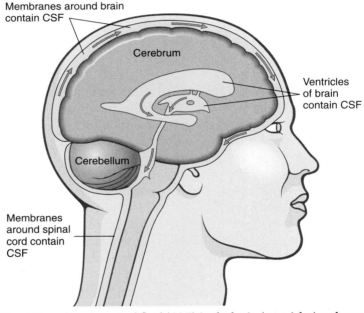

FIGURE 10–7   **Circulation of cerebrospinal fluid (CSF) in the brain (ventricles) and around the spinal cord.** CSF is formed within the ventricles and circulates between the membranes around the brain and within the spinal cord. CSF empties into the bloodstream through the membranes surrounding the brain and spinal cord.

10

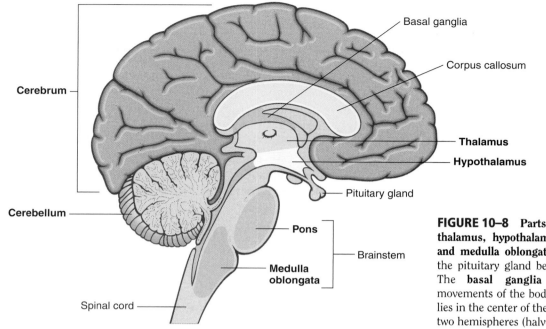

Cerebrum

Cerebellum

Spinal cord

Basal ganglia

Corpus callosum

Thalamus

Hypothalamus

Pituitary gland

Pons

Brainstem

**Medulla
oblongata**

FIGURE 10–8 **Parts of the brain: cerebrum,
thalamus, hypothalamus, cerebellum, pons,
and medulla oblongata.** Note the location of
the pituitary gland below the hypothalamus.
The **basal ganglia** regulate intentional
movements of the body. The **corpus callosum**
lies in the center of the brain and connects the
two hemispheres (halves).

Two other important parts of the brain are the **thalamus** and the **hypothalamus** (Fig.
10–8). The thalamus integrates and monitors sensory impulses from skin, suppressing
some and magnifying others. Perception of pain is controlled by this area of the brain. The
hypothalamus (below the thalamus) contains neurons that control body temperature,
sleep, appetite, sexual desire, and emotions such as fear and pleasure. The hypothalamus
also regulates the release of hormones from the pituitary gland at the base of the brain and
integrates the activities of the sympathetic and parasympathetic nervous systems.

The following structures within the brain lie in the back and below the cerebrum and
connect the cerebrum with the spinal cord: cerebellum, pons, and medulla oblongata. The
pons and medulla are part of the **brainstem.**

The **cerebellum** functions to coordinate voluntary movements and to maintain balance
and posture.

The **pons** is a part of the brainstem that literally means bridge. It contains nerve fiber
tracts that connect the cerebellum and cerebrum with the rest of the brain. Nerves to the
eyes and face lie here.

The **medulla oblongata**, also in the brainstem, connects the spinal cord with the rest
of the brain. Nerve tracts cross from right to left and left to right in the medulla oblongata.
For example, nerve cells that control movement of the left side of the body are found in the
right half of the cerebrum. These cells send out axons that cross over (decussate) to the
opposite side of the brain in the medulla oblongata and then travel down the spinal cord.

In addition, the medulla oblongata contains three important vital centers that regulate
internal activities of the body:

1. **Respiratory center**—controls muscles of respiration in response to chemicals or
other stimuli
2. **Cardiac center**—slows the heart rate when the heart is beating too rapidly
3. **Vasomotor center**—affects (constricts or dilates) the muscles in the walls of blood
vessels, thus influencing blood pressure

Figure 10–8 shows the locations of the thalamus, hypothalamus, cerebellum, pons, and
medulla oblongata. Table 10–1 reviews the functions of these parts of the brain.

Table 10-1

Functions of the Parts of the Brain

Structure	Function(s)
Cerebrum	Thinking, personality, sensations, movements, memory
Thalamus	Relay station for sensory impulses; pain
Hypothalamus	Body temperature, sleep, appetite, emotions, control of the pituitary gland
Cerebellum	Coordination of voluntary movements and balance
Pons	Connection of nerves (to the eyes and face)
Medulla oblongata	Nerve fibers cross over, left to right and right to left; contains centers to regulate heart, blood vessels, and respiratory system

THE SPINAL CORD AND MENINGES

SPINAL CORD

The **spinal cord** is a column of nervous tissue extending from the medulla oblongata to the second lumbar vertebra within the vertebral column. Below the end of the spinal cord is the **cauda equina** (Latin for horse's tail), a fan of nerve fibers (see Fig. 10–1). The spinal cord carries all the nerves to and from the limbs and lower part of the body, and it is the pathway for impulses going to and from the brain. A cross-sectional view of the spinal cord (Fig. 10–9) reveals an inner region of **gray matter** (containing cell bodies and dendrites) and an outer region of **white matter** (containing the nerve fiber tracts with myelin sheaths) conducting impulses to and from the brain.

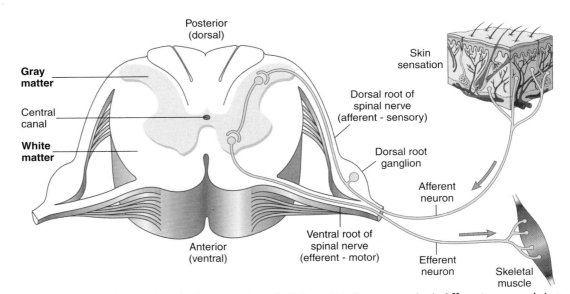

FIGURE 10–9 The spinal cord, showing gray and white matter (transverse view). **Afferent neurons** bring impulses from a sensory receptor (such as the skin) into the spinal cord. **Efferent neurons** carry impulses from the spinal cord to effector organs (such as skeletal muscle). The central canal is the space through which CSF travels.

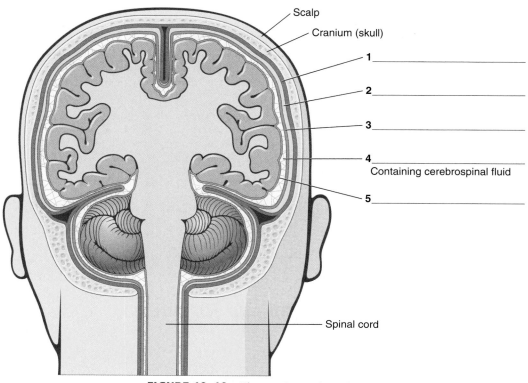

FIGURE 10–10 **The meninges,** frontal view.

MENINGES

The **meninges** are three layers of connective tissue membranes that surround the brain and spinal cord. Label Figure 10–10 as you study the following description of the meninges.

The outermost membrane of the meninges is the **dura mater** [1]. This thick, tough membrane contains channels (dural sinuses) that contain blood. The **subdural space** [2] is below the dural membrane. The second layer surrounding the brain and spinal cord is the **arachnoid membrane** [3]. The arachnoid (spider-like) membrane is loosely attached to the other meninges by web-like fibers, so there is a space for fluid between the fibers and the third membrane. This is the **subarachnoid space** [4], containing CSF. The third layer of the meninges, closest to the brain and spinal cord, is the **pia mater** [5]. It contains delicate (Latin *pia*) connective tissue with a rich supply of blood vessels. Most physicians refer to the pia and arachnoid membranes together as the pia-arachnoid.

VOCABULARY

This list reviews the new terms introduced in the text. Short definitions reinforce your understanding of the terms. Refer to the Pronunciation of Terms section for help with unfamiliar or more difficult words.

acetylcholine	Neurotransmitter chemical released at the ends (synapses) of nerve cells.
afferent nerves	Carry messages *toward* the brain and spinal cord (sensory nerves)
arachnoid membrane	Middle layer of the three membranes (meninges) that surround the brain and spinal cord. The Greek *arachne* means spider.
astrocyte	A type of glial (neurologic) cell that transports water and salts from capillaries.
autonomic nervous system	Nerves that control involuntary body functions of muscles, glands, and internal organs.
axon	Microscopic fiber that carries the nervous impulse along a nerve cell.
blood-brain barrier	Blood vessels (capillaries) that selectively let certain substances enter the brain tissue and keep other substances out.
brainstem	Lower portion of the brain that connects the cerebrum with the spinal cord. The pons and medulla oblongata are part of the brainstem.
cauda equina	Collection of spinal nerves below the end of the spinal cord.
cell body	Part of a nerve cell that contains the nucleus.
central nervous system (CNS)	Brain and the spinal cord.
cerebellum	Posterior part of the brain that coordinates muscle movements and maintains balance.
cerebral cortex	Outer region of the cerebrum; containing sheets of nerve cells; gray matter of the brain.
cerebrospinal fluid (CSF)	Fluid that circulates throughout the brain and spinal cord.
cerebrum	Largest part of the brain; responsible for voluntary muscular activity, vision, speech, taste, hearing, thought, and memory.
cranial nerves	Twelve pairs of nerves that carry messages to and from the brain.
dendrite	Microscopic branching fiber of a nerve cell that is the first part to receive the nervous impulse.
dura mater	Thick, outermost layer of the meninges surrounding and protecting the brain and spinal cord (Latin for hard mother).
efferent nerves	Carry messages *away from* the brain and spinal cord; motor nerves.
ependymal cell	A glial cell that lines membranes within the brain and spinal cord and helps form cerebrospinal fluid.
ganglion (*plural*: **ganglia**)	Collection of nerve cell bodies in the peripheral nervous system.

glial cell (neuroglial cell)	Cell in the nervous system that is supportive and connective in function. Examples are astrocytes, microglial cells, ependymal cells, and oligodendrocytes.
gyrus (*plural:* **gyri**)	Sheet of nerve cells that produces a rounded fold on the surface of the cerebellum; convolution.
hypothalamus	Portion of the brain beneath the thalamus; controls sleep, appetite, body temperature, and secretions from the pituitary gland.
medulla oblongata	Part of the brain just above the spinal cord; controls breathing, heartbeat, and the size of blood vessels; nerve fibers cross over here.
meninges	Three protective membranes that surround the brain and spinal cord.
microglial cell	Phagocytic glial cell that removes waste products from the central nervous system.
motor nerves	Carry messages away from the brain and spinal cord to muscles and organs; efferent (ef [a form of ex] = away) nerves.
myelin sheath	White fatty tissue that surrounds, and insulates the axon of a nerve cell. Myelin speeds impulse conduction along axons.
nerve	Macroscopic cordlike collection of fibers (axons and dendrites) that carry electrical impulses.
neuron	Nerve cell that carries impulses throughout the body.
neurotransmitter	Chemical messenger, released at the end of a nerve cell. It stimulates or inhibits another cell, which can be a nerve cell, muscle cell, or gland cell. Examples of neurotransmitters are acetylcholine, norepinephrine, dopamine, and serotonin.
oligodendroglial cell	Glial cell that forms the myelin sheath covering axons. Also called oligodendrocyte.
parasympathetic nerves	Involuntary, autonomic nerves that regulate normal body functions such as heart rate, breathing, and muscles of the gastrointestinal tract.
parenchyma	Essential, distinguishing tissue of the nervous system; includes the brain and spinal cord. This is to distinguish it from surrounding tissues, such as the meninges. *Pronunciation:* păr-ĔN-kĭ-mă.
peripheral nervous system	Nerves outside the brain and spinal cord; cranial, spinal, and autonomic nerves.
pia mater	Thin, delicate inner membrane of the meninges.
plexus (*plural:* **plexuses**)	Large, interlacing network of nerves. Examples are lumbosacral, cervical, and brachial (brachi/o means arm) plexuses. The term originated from the Indo-European *plek* meaning to weave together.
pons	Part of the brain anterior to the cerebellum and between the medulla and the rest of the midbrain (Latin *pons* means bridge). It is a bridge connecting various parts of the brain.
receptor	Organ that receives a nervous stimulation and passes it on to nerves within the body. The skin, ears, eyes, and taste buds are receptors.
sciatic nerve	Nerve extending from the base of the spine down the thigh, lower leg, and foot. **Sciatica** is pain or inflammation along the course of the nerve.

sensory nerves	Carry messages to the brain and spinal cord from a receptor; afferent (af [a form of ad] = toward) nerves.
spinal nerves	Thirty-one pairs of nerves arising from the spinal cord. Each spinal nerve affects a particular area of the skin.
stimulus (*plural*: **stimuli**)	Agent of change (light, sound, touch) in the internal or external environment that evokes a response.
stroma	Connective and supporting tissue of an organ. Glial cells are the stromal tissue of the brain.
sulcus (*plural*: **sulci**)	Depression or groove in the surface of the cerebral cortex; fissure.
sympathetic nerves	Autonomic nerves that influence bodily functions involuntarily in times of stress.
synapse	Space through which a nervous impulse is transmitted from one neuron to another or from a neuron to another cell, such as a muscle or gland cell. From the Greek *synapsis*, a point of contact.
thalamus	Main relay center of the brain. It conducts impulses between the spinal cord and the cerebrum; incoming sensory messages are relayed through the thalamus to appropriate centers in the cerebrum. Latin *thalamus* means room. The Romans, who named this structure, thought this part of the brain was hollow, like a little room.
vagus nerve	Tenth cranial nerve; its branches reach to the larynx, trachea, bronchi, lungs, aorta, esophagus, and stomach. Latin *vagus* means wandering. Unlike the other cranial nerves, the vagus leaves the head and "wanders" into the abdominal and thoracic cavities.
ventricles of the brain	Canals in the brain that contain cerebrospinal fluid.

COMBINING FORMS AND TERMINOLOGY

This section is divided into terms that describe organs and structures of the nervous system and those that relate to neurologic symptoms. Write the meanings of the medical terms in the spaces provided.

ORGANS AND STRUCTURES

Combining Form	Meaning	Terminology	Meaning
cerebell/o	cerebellum	cerebellar _____	
cerebr/o	cerebrum	cerebrospinal fluid _____	
		cerebral cortex _____ *Cortical means pertaining to the cortex or outer area of an organ.*	

Combining Form	Meaning	Terminology	Meaning
dur/o	dura mater	subdural hematoma _____ *Remember: Hematomas are not tumors of blood, but are collections of blood.*	
		epidural hematoma _____ *Figure 10–11 shows subdural, epidural, and intracerebral hematomas.*	
encephal/o	brain	encephalitis _____	
		encephalopathy _____	
		anencephaly _____ *This is a congenital brain malformation; it is not compatible with life and may be detected with amniocentesis or ultrasonography of the fetus.*	
gli/o	glial cells	glioblastoma _____ *This is a highly malignant tumor (-blast means immature). Gliomas are tumors of glial (neuroglial) cells.*	
lept/o	thin, slender	leptomeningeal _____ *The pia and arachnoid membranes are known as the leptomeninges because of their thin, delicate structure.*	
mening/o, meningi/o	membranes, meninges	meningeal _____	
		meningioma _____ *Slowly growing, benign tumor.*	
		myelomeningocele _____ *Neural tube defect caused by failure of the neural tube to close during embryonic development. This abnormality occurs in infants born with spina bifida. See page 350.*	

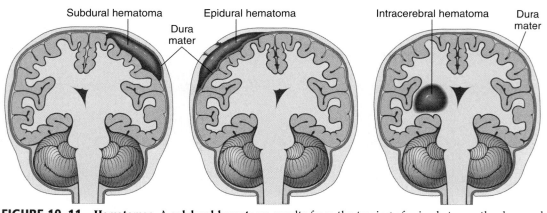

FIGURE 10–11 **Hematomas.** A **subdural hematoma** results from the tearing of veins between the dura and arachnoid membranes. It often is the result of blunt trauma, such as from blows to the head in boxers and in elderly patients who have fallen out of bed. An **epidural hematoma** occurs between the skull and the dura as the result of a ruptured meningeal artery, usually after a fracture of the skull. An **intracerebral hematoma** is caused by bleeding directly into brain tissue, such as can occur in the case of uncontrolled hypertension (high blood pressure).

10

Combining Form	Meaning	Terminology	Meaning
my/o	muscle	myoneural _____	
myel/o	spinal cord (means bone marrow in other contexts)	myelogram _____	
		poliomyelitis _____ _Polio means gray matter. This viral disease affects the gray matter of the spinal cord, leading to paralysis of muscles that rely on the damaged neurons. Effective vaccines developed in the 20th century have made "polio" relatively uncommon._	
neur/o	nerve	neuropathy _____	
		polyneuritis _____	
pont/o	pons	cerebellopontine _____ _-ine means pertaining to._	
radicul/o	nerve root (of spinal nerves)	radiculopathy _____	
		radiculitis _____ _This often results in pain and loss of function._	
thalam/o	thalamus	thalamic _____	
thec/o	sheath (refers to the meninges)	intrathecal injection _____ _Chemicals, such as chemotherapeutic drugs, can be delivered into the subarachnoid space._	
vag/o	vagus nerve (10th cranial nerve)	vagal _____ _This cranial nerve has branches to the head and neck, as well as to the chest._	

SYMPTOMS

Combining Form or Suffix	Meaning	Terminology	Meaning
alges/o **-algesia**	excessive sensitivity to pain	analgesia _____	
		hypalgesia _____ _Diminished sensation to pain. (Notice that the "o" in hypo- is dropped.) Hyperalgesia is increased sensitivity to pain._	
-algia	pain	neuralgia _____ **Trigeminal neuralgia** _involves flashes of pain radiating along the course of the trigeminal nerve (fifth cranial nerve)._	
		cephalgia _____ _Headaches may result from vasodilation (widening) of blood vessels in tissues surrounding the brain or from tension in neck and scalp muscles. A **migraine** is a severe unilateral, vascular headache often accompanied by photophobia (sensitivity to light). Prodromal symptoms sometimes include sensitivity to light and sound and an aura phase of flashes before the eyes and partial blindness._	

10

Combining Form or Suffix	Meaning	Terminology	Meaning
caus/o	burning	causalgia _____	
		Intense burning pain following injury to a sensory nerve.	
comat/o	deep sleep (coma)	comatose _____	
		*A **coma** is a state of unconsciousness from which the patient cannot be aroused. Semicomatose refers to a stupor (unresponsiveness) from which a patient can be aroused. In an irreversible coma (brain death), there is complete unresponsitivity to stimuli, no spontaneous breathing or movement, and a flat EEG.*	
esthesi/o -esthesia	feeling, nervous sensation	anesthesia _____	
		Lack of normal sensation (e.g., absence of sense of touch or pain). Two common types of regional anesthesia are spinal and epidural (caudal) blocks (Fig. 10–12).	
		hyperesthesia _____	
		A light touch with a pin may provoke increased sensation. Diminished sensitivity to pain is called hypesthesia.	
		paresthesia _____	
		Par- (from para-) means abnormal. Paresthesias include burning, prickling, tingling sensations, or numbness. They are the "pins and needless" feeling, numbness and tingling when an extremity "falls asleep."	

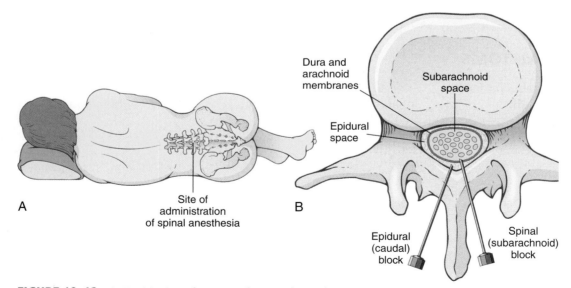

FIGURE 10–12   **A, Positioning of a patient for spinal anesthesia. B,** Cross-sectional view of the spinal cord showing injection sites for **epidural** and **spinal blocks (anesthesia).** Epidural (caudal) anesthesia is achieved by injecting an agent into the epidural space and commonly is used in obstetrics. Spinal anesthesia is achieved by injecting a local anesthetic into the subarachnoid space. Patients may experience loss of sensation and paralysis of feet, legs, and abdomen.

10

Combining Form or Suffix	Meaning	Terminology	Meaning
kines/o, kinesi/o -kinesia -kinesis -kinetic	movement	bradykinesia _____	
		hyperkinesis _____ _Amphetamines (CNS stimulants) are used to treat hyperkinesis in children, but the mechanism of their action is not understood._	
		dyskinesia _____ _Condition marked by involuntary, spasmodic movements._ **Tardive** _(occurring late)_ **dyskinesia** _may develop in people who receive certain antipsychotic drugs for extended periods._	
		akinetic _____	
-lepsy	seizure	epilepsy _____ _See page 352._	
		narcolepsy _____ _Sudden, uncontrollable compulsion to sleep (narc/o = stupor, sleep). Amphetamines and stimulant drugs are prescribed to prevent attacks._	
lex/o	word, phrase	dyslexia _____ _Reading, writing, and learning disorders._	
-paresis	weakness	hemiparesis _____ _Affects either right or left side (half) of the body._ **Paresis** _also is used by itself to mean partial paralysis or weakness of muscles._	
-phasia	speech	aphasia _____ **Motor** _(also called Broca or expressive)_ **aphasia** _is present when the patient knows what he or she wants to say but cannot say it. The patient with_ **sensory aphasia** _articulates (pronounces) words easily but uses them inappropriately. This patient has difficulty understanding written and verbal commands and cannot repeat them._	
-plegia	paralysis (loss or impairment of the ability to move parts of the body)	hemiplegia _____ _Affects right or left half of the body and results from a stroke or other brain injury. The hemiplegia is contralateral to the brain lesion because motor nerve fibers from the right half of the brain cross to the left side of the body (in the medulla oblongata)._	
		paraplegia _____ _Originally, the term paraplegia meant a stroke (paralysis) on one side (para-). Now, however, the term means paralysis of both legs and the lower part of the body caused by injury or disease of the spinal cord or cauda equina._	
		quadriplegia _____ _Quadri- means four. All four extremities are affected. Injury is at the cervical level of the spinal cord._	

-phasia/-phagia
Don't confuse the suffix _-phasia_ with _-phagia,_ meaning to swallow or eat.

10

Combining Form or Suffix	Meaning	Terminology	Meaning
-praxia	action	apraxia _____ *Movements and behavior are not purposeful. A patient with motor apraxia cannot use an object or perform a task. Motor weakness is not the cause.*	
-sthenia	strength	neurasthenia _____ *Nervous exhaustion and fatigue, often following depression.*	
syncop/o	to cut off, cut short	syncopal _____ **Syncope** *(SĬN-kō-pē) means fainting; sudden and temporary loss of consciousness caused by inadequate flow of blood to the brain. The term comes from a Greek word meaning cutting into pieces, thus a fainting spell meant one's strength was "cut off." Remember: syncopal means pertaining to fainting and is an adjective. A patient can experience a syncopal episode.*	
tax/o	order, coordination	ataxia _____ *Persistent unsteadiness on the feet can be caused by a disorder involving the cerebellum.*	

PATHOLOGIC CONDITIONS

The bones of the skull, the vertebral column, and the meninges, containing CSF, provide a hard box with an interior cushion around the brain and spinal cord. In addition, glial cells surrounding neurons form a blood-brain barrier that prevents many potentially harmful substances in the bloodstream from gaining access to neurons. However, these protective factors are counterbalanced by the extreme sensitivity of nerve cells to oxygen deficiency (brain cells die in a few minutes when deprived of oxygen).

Neurologic disorders may be classified in the following categories:

- Congenital
- Degenerative, movement, and seizure
- Infectious (meningitis and encephalitis)

- Neoplastic (tumors)
- Traumatic
- Vascular (stroke)

CONGENITAL DISORDERS

hydrocephalus

Abnormal accumulation of fluid (CSF) in the brain.

If circulation of CSF in the brain or spinal cord is impaired, it accumulates under pressure in the ventricles of the brain. To relieve pressure on the brain, a catheter (shunt) can be placed from the ventricle of the brain into the peritoneal space (ventriculoperitoneal shunt) or right atrium of the heart so that the CSF is continuously drained from the brain.

Hydrocephalus also can occur in adults as a result of tumors and infections.

spina bifida

Congenital defects in the lumbar spinal column caused by imperfect union of vertebral parts (neural tube defect).

In **spina bifida occulta** the vertebral defect is covered over with skin and evident only on x-ray or other imaging examination. **Spina bifida cystica** is a more severe

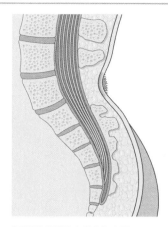
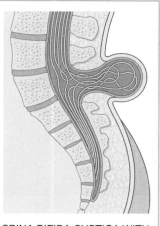

SPINA BIFIDA OCCULTA
Posterior vertebrae have not fused.
No herniation of the spinal cord or
meninges. There may be visible
signs on the skin such as a mole,
dimple, or patch of hair.

SPINA BIFIDA CYSTICA WITH
MENINGOCELE
External protruding sac contains
meninges and CSF.

SPINA BIFIDA CYSTICA WITH
MYELOMENINGOCELE
External sac contains meninges,
CSF, and the spinal cord. Often
associated with hydrocephalus
and paralysis.

A

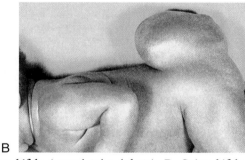

B

FIGURE 10–13 **A, Spina bifida** (neural tube defects). **B, Spina bifida cystica** with myelomeningocele. (**B** from Frazier MS, Drzymkowski JW: Essentials of Human Diseases and Conditions, 3rd ed. Philadelphia, WB Saunders, 2004, p. 51.)

form, with cyst-like protrusions. In **meningocele,** the meninges protrudes to the outside of the body, and in **myelomeningocele** (meningomyelocele), both the spinal cord and meninges protrude. See Figure 10–13, *A* and *B*.

The etiology of neural tube defects is unknown. Defects originate in the early weeks of pregnancy as the spinal cord and vertebrae develop. Prenatal diagnosis is helped by imaging methods and testing maternal blood samples for alpha-fetoprotein.

DEGENERATIVE, MOVEMENT, AND SEIZURE DISORDERS

Alzheimer disease (AD)

Brain disorder marked by gradual and progressive mental deterioration (dementia) with personality changes and impairment of daily functioning.

Characteristics of AD include confusion, memory failure, disorientation, restlessness, and speech disturbances. Anxiety, depression, and emotional disturbances can occur as well. The disease sometimes begins in middle life with slight defects in memory and behavior, but can worsen after the age of 70. On

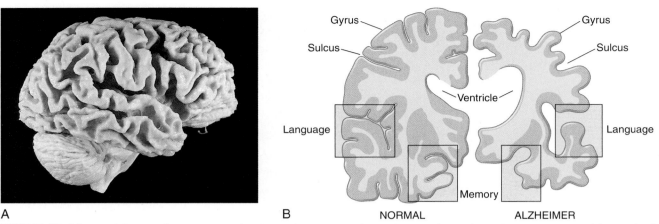

Gyrus Sulcus Ventricle Language Language Memory NORMAL ALZHEIMER

A B

FIGURE 10–14 **A, Alzheimer disease.** Generalized loss of brain parenchyma (neuronal tissue) results in narrowing of the cerebral gyri and widening of the sulci. **B,** Cross-sectional specimens of a normal brain and of a brain from a person with Alzheimer disease. (**A** from Kumar V, Cotran RS, Robbins SL: Robbins Basic Pathology, 7th ed. Philadelphia, WB Saunders, 2003, p. 843.)

autopsy there is atrophy of the cerebral cortex and widening of the cerebral sulci, especially in the frontal and temporal regions (Fig. 10–14, *A* and *B*). Microscopic examination shows **senile plaques** resulting from degeneration of neurons and **neurofibrillary tangles** (bundles of fibrils in the cytoplasm of a neuron) in the cerebral cortex. Deposits of **amyloid** (a protein) occur in neurofibrillary tangles, senile plaques, and blood vessels. The cause of AD remains unknown, although genetic factors may play a role. A mutation on chromosome 14 has been linked to familial cases. There is as yet no effective treatment.

amyotrophic lateral sclerosis (ALS)	**Degenerative disorder of motor neurons in the spinal cord and brainstem.**

ALS presents in adulthood. Symptoms are weakness and atrophy of muscles in the hands, forearms, and legs; difficulty in swallowing and talking and dyspnea develop as the throat and respiratory muscles become affected. Etiology (cause) and cure for ALS both are unknown.

A famous baseball player, Lou Gehrig, became a victim of this disease in the mid-1900s, so the condition was known as Lou Gehrig's disease.

epilepsy	**Chronic brain disorder characterized by recurrent seizure activity.**

A seizure is an abnormal, sudden excessive discharge of electrical activity within the brain. Seizures are often symptoms of underlying brain pathologic conditions, such as brain tumors, meningitis, vascular disease, or scar tissue from a head injury. **Tonic-clonic seizures (grand mal or ictal events)** are characterized by a sudden loss of consciousness, falling down, and then tonic contractions (stiffening of muscles) followed by clonic contractions (twitching and jerking movements of the limbs). These convulsions often are preceded by an **aura,** which is a peculiar sensation experienced by the affected person before onset of a seizure. Dizziness, numbness, and visual or olfactory (sense of smell) disturbances are examples of an aura. **Absence seizures (petit mal seizures)** are a minor form of seizure consisting of momentary clouding of consciousness and loss of awareness of the person's surroundings. Drug therapy (anticonvulsants) is used for control of epileptic seizures.

After seizures, there may be neurologic symptoms such as weakness called **postictal events.**

The term epilepsy comes from the Greek *epilepsis,* meaning a laying hold of. The Greeks thought a victim of a seizure was laid hold of by some mysterious force.

10

Huntington disease	**Hereditary disorder marked by degenerative changes in the cerebrum leading to abrupt involuntary movements and mental deterioration.**

This condition typically begins in adulthood and results in personality changes, along with choreic (meaning dance-like) movements (uncontrollable, irregular, jerking movements of the arms and legs and facial grimacing).

The genetic defect in patients with Huntington disease is located on chromosome 4. Patients can be tested for the gene; however, no cure exists, and management is symptomatic.

multiple sclerosis (MS)	**Destruction of the myelin sheath on neurons in the CNS and its replacement by plaques of sclerotic (hard) tissue.**

One of the leading causes of neurologic disability in persons 20 to 40 years of age, MS is a chronic disease often marked by long periods of stability (remission) and worsening (relapse). **Demyelination** (loss of myelin insulation) prevents the conduction of nerve impulses through the axon and causes paresthesias, muscle weakness, unsteady **gait** (manner of walking), and paralysis. There may be visual (blurred and double vision) and speech disturbances as well. Areas of scarred myelin (plaques) can be seen on MRI scans of the brain. See Figure 10–15. Etiology is unknown but probably involves an autoimmune disease of lymphocytes reacting against myelin. Disease-modifying drugs (DMDs) can slow the progression of MS by preventing the immune system from destroying myelin.

myasthenia gravis (MG)	**Autoimmune neuromuscular disorder characterized by weakness (-asthenia) of voluntary muscles (attached to bones).**

Myasthenia gravis is a chronic autoimmune disorder. Antibodies block the ability of acetylcholine (neurotransmitter) to transmit the nervous impulse from nerve to muscle cell. Onset of symptoms usually is gradual, with ptosis of the upper eyelid, double vision (diplopia), and facial weakness. Therapy to reverse symptoms includes anticholinesterase drugs, which inhibit the enzyme that breaks down acetylcholine. Corticosteroids (prednisone) and immunosuppressive drugs (azathioprine, methotrexate, and cyclophosphamide) are also used in treatment. **Thymectomy** is also a method of treatment and is beneficial to many patients.

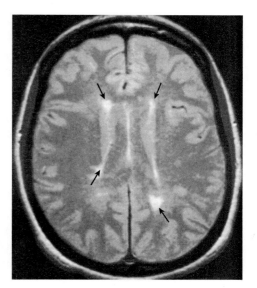

FIGURE 10–15 Multiple sclerosis. This MRI scan shows multiple abnormal white areas that correspond to MS plaques. (From Haaga JR, Lanzieri C, Gilkeson R: CT and MR Imaging of the Whole Body, 4th ed., vol. 1, St. Louis, Mosby, 2003, p. 465.)

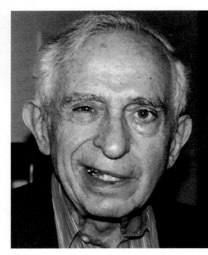

A   B

FIGURE 10–16 **A, Bell palsy.** Notice the paralysis on the left side of this man's face. His eyelid does not close properly, his forehead is not wrinkled as would be expected, and there is clear paralysis of the lower face. **B,** The palsy spontaneously resolved after 6 months.

palsy   **Paralysis (partial or complete loss of motor function).**

Cerebral palsy is partial paralysis and lack of muscular coordination caused by loss of oxygen (hypoxia) or blood flow to the cerebrum during pregnancy or in the perinatal period. **Bell palsy** (or Bell's palsy) (see Fig. 10–16) is paralysis on one side of the face. The likely cause is a viral infection, and therapy is directed against the virus (antiviral drugs) and nerve swelling.

Parkinson disease (parkinsonism)   **Degeneration of neurons in the basal ganglia, occurring in later life and leading to tremors, weakness of muscles, and slowness of movement.**

This slowly progressive condition is caused by a deficiency of **dopamine** (a neurotransmitter) made by cells in the basal ganglia (see Fig. 10–8). Motor disturbances include stooped posture, shuffling gait, muscle stiffness (rigidity), dyskinesias, and often a tremor of the hands.

Therapy with drugs such as levodopa plus carbidopa (Sinemet) to increase dopamine levels in the brain is **palliative** (relieving symptoms but not curative). Implantation of fetal brain tissue containing dopamine-producing cells is an experimental treatment but has produced uncertain results.

Tourette syndrome   **Involuntary, spasmodic, twitching movements; uncontrollable vocal sounds; and inappropriate words.**

These involuntary movements, usually beginning with twitching of the eyelid and muscles of the face with verbal outbursts, are called **tics.** Although the cause of Tourette syndrome is not known, it is associated with either an excess of dopamine or a hypersensitivity to dopamine. Psychological problems do not cause Tourette syndrome, but physicians have had some success in treating it with the antipsychotic drug haloperidol (Haldol), antidepressants, and mood stabilizers.

INFECTIOUS DISORDERS

herpes zoster (shingles)   **Viral infection affecting peripheral nerves.**

Blisters and pain spread along peripheral nerves and are caused by inflammation due to a herpes virus **(herpes zoster),** the same virus that causes chickenpox (varicella). Reactivation of the chickenpox virus (herpes varicella-zoster), which remained in the body after the person had chickenpox, occurs. Painful vesicular skin eruptions (blisters form) follow the underlying route of cranial or spinal nerves. The skin innervation by spinal or cranial nerves is called a **dermatome.**

| meningitis | **Inflammation of the meninges; leptomeningitis.** |

This condition can be caused by bacteria (pyogenic meningitis) or viruses (aseptic or viral meningitis). Signs and symptoms are fever and signs of meningeal irritation, such as headache, photophobia (sensitivity to light), and a stiff neck. Lumbar punctures are performed to examine CSF. Physicians use antibiotics to treat the more serious pyogenic form, and antivirals for the viral form.

human immunodeficiency virus (HIV) encephalopathy

Brain disease and dementia occurring with AIDS.

Many patients with AIDS develop neurologic dysfunction. In addition to encephalitis and dementia (loss of mental functioning), some patients develop brain tumors and other infections.

NEOPLASTIC DISORDERS

brain tumor

Abnormal growth of brain tissue and meninges.

Most primary brain tumors arise from glial cells **(gliomas)** or the meninges **(meningiomas).** Types of gliomas include **astrocytoma** (Fig. 10–17, *A*), **oligodendroglioma,** and **ependymoma.** The most malignant form of astrocytoma is **glioblastoma multiforme** (-blast means immature) (see Fig. 10–17, *B*). Tumors can cause swelling **(cerebral edema)** and hydrocephalus. If CSF pressure is increased, swelling also may occur near the optic nerve (at the back of the eye). Gliomas are removed surgically, and radiotherapy is used for tumors that are not completely resected. Steroids are given to reduce swelling after surgery.

Meningiomas usually are benign and surrounded by a capsule, but they may cause compression and distortion of the brain.

Tumors in the brain may be single or multiple metastatic growths. Most arise from the lung, breast, skin (melanoma), kidney, and gastrointestinal tract and spread to the brain.

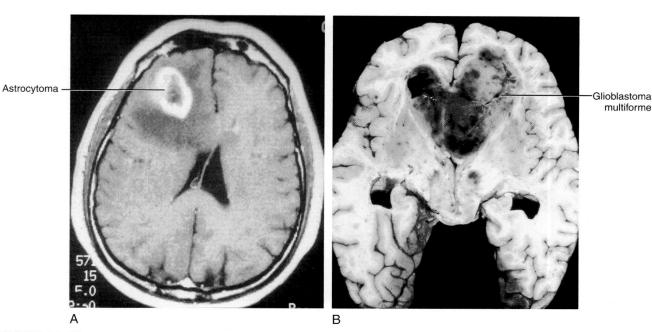

A   B

FIGURE 10–17 **A,** Computed tomographic scan of brain showing a large tumor (an astrocytoma) in the cerebral hemisphere and pronounced peritumoral edema. **B,** Glioblastoma multiforme appearing as a necrotic, hemorrhagic, infiltrating mass. (From Kumar V, Abbas AK, Fausto N: Robbins and Cotran Pathologic Basis of Disease, 7th ed. Philadelphia, WB Saunders, 2005, p. 1402.)

10

TRAUMATIC DISORDERS

cerebral concussion

Temporary brain dysfunction (brief loss of consciousness) after injury, usually clearing within 24 hours.

There is no evidence of structural damage to the brain tissue. Severe concussions may lead to coma.

cerebral contusion

Bruising of brain tissue as a result of direct trauma to the head; neurologic deficits persist longer than 24 hours.

A cerebral contusion usually is associated with a fracture of the skull. Subdural and epidural hematomas occur, leading to permanent brain injury with altered memory or speech or development of epilepsy.

VASCULAR DISORDERS

cerebrovascular accident (CVA)

Disruption in the normal blood supply to the brain; stroke.

This condition, also known as a **cerebral infarction,** is the result of a loss of oxygen to the brain. There are three types of strokes (Fig. 10–18):

1. **Thrombotic**—blood clot **(thrombus)** in the arteries leading to the brain, resulting in occlusion (blocking) of the vessel. Atherosclerosis leads to this common type of stroke as blood vessels become blocked over time. Before total occlusion occurs, a patient may experience symptoms that point to the gradual occlusion of blood vessels. These short episodes of neurologic dysfunction are known as **TIAs (transient ischemic attacks).**
2. **Embolic**—an **embolus** (a dislodged thrombus) travels to cerebral arteries and occludes a small vessel. This type of stroke occurs very suddenly.
3. **Hemorrhagic**—a blood vessel, such as the cerebral artery, breaks and bleeding occurs. This type of stroke can be fatal and results from advancing age, atherosclerosis, or high blood pressure, all of which result in degeneration of cerebral blood vessels. With small hemorrhages, the body reabsorbs the blood and the patient makes good recovery with only

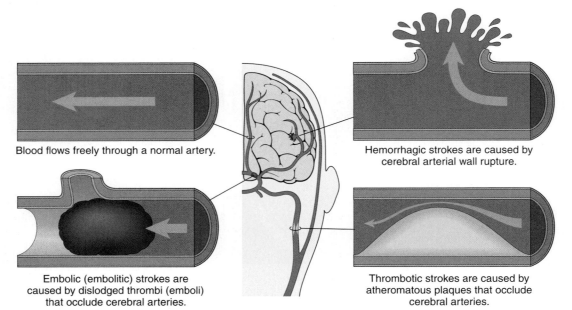

Blood flows freely through a normal artery.

Hemorrhagic strokes are caused by cerebral arterial wall rupture.

Embolic (embolitic) strokes are caused by dislodged thrombi (emboli) that occlude cerebral arteries.

Thrombotic strokes are caused by atheromatous plaques that occlude cerebral arteries.

FIGURE 10–18   Three types of strokes: embolic, hemorrhagic, and thrombotic. (Modified from Ignatavicius DD, Workman ML: Medical-Surgical Nursing: Critical Thinking for Collaborative Care, 4th ed. Philadelphia, WB Saunders, 2002, p. 975.)

10

slight disability. In a younger patient, cerebral hemorrhage is usually caused by mechanical injury associated with skull fracture or rupture of an arterial **aneurysm** (weakened area in the vessel wall that balloons and may eventually burst).

The major risk factors for stroke are hypertension, diabetes, smoking, and heart disease. Other risk factors include obesity, substance abuse (cocaine), and elevated cholesterol levels.

Thrombotic strokes are treated medically with anticoagulant (clot-dissolving) drug therapy. Tissue plasminogen activator (tPA) is started within 3 hours after the onset of a stroke. Surgical intervention with carotid endarterectomy (removal of the atherosclerotic plaque along with the inner lining of the affected carotid artery) is also possible.

STUDY SECTION

The following list reviews the new terms used in the Pathologic Conditions section. Practice spelling each term and know its meaning.

absence seizure	Minor (petit mal) form of seizure, consisting of momentary clouding of consciousness and loss of awareness of surroundings.
aneurysm	Enlarged, weakened area in an arterial wall, which may rupture, leading to hemorrhage and CVA (stroke).
astrocytoma	Malignant tumor of astrocytes (glial brain cells).
aura	Peculiar sensation experienced by some persons with epilepsy before onset of an actual seizure.
blast	Immature cells (as in glio*blast*oma).
dementia	Mental decline and deterioration.
demyelination	Destruction of myelin on axons of nerves (as in multiple sclerosis).
dopamine	CNS neurotransmitter, deficient in patient with Parkinson disease.
embolus	A mass (clot) of material travels through the bloodstream and suddenly blocks a vessel.
gait	Manner of walking.
herpes zoster	Herpes virus that causes shingles—eruption of blisters in a pattern that follows the path of peripheral nerves around the trunk of the body; zoster means "girdle."
ictal event	Pertaining to a sudden, acute onset, as the convulsions of an epileptic seizure.
occlusion	Blockage.
palliative	Relieving symptoms but not curing.
thymectomy	Removal of the thymus gland (a lymphocyte-producing gland in the chest); used as treatment for myasthenia gravis.
TIA	Transient ischemic attack.
tic	Involuntary movement of a small group of muscles, as of the face; characteristic of Tourette syndrome.
tonic-clonic seizure	Major (grand mal) convulsive seizure marked by sudden loss of consciousness, stiffening of muscles, and twitching and jerking movements.

LABORATORY TESTS AND CLINICAL PROCEDURES

LABORATORY TESTS

cerebrospinal fluid analysis

Samples of CSF are examined.

Doctors measure water, glucose, sodium, chloride, and protein as well as the number of red (RBC) and white (WBC) blood cells. CSF analysis can also detect tumor cells (via cytology), bacteria, and viruses. These studies are used to diagnose infection, tumors, or multiple sclerosis.

CLINICAL PROCEDURES

X-Ray Tests

cerebral angiography

X-ray imaging of the arterial blood vessel system in the brain after injection of contrast material.

Contrast is injected into the femoral artery (in thigh), and x-ray motion pictures are taken. These images diagnose vascular disease (aneurysm, occlusion, hemorrhage) in the brain.

computed tomography (CT) of the brain

X-ray technique that generates computerized cross-sectional images of the brain and spinal cord.

Contrast material may be injected intravenously to highlight abnormalities. The contrast leaks through the **blood-brain barrier** from blood vessels into the brain tissue and shows tumors, hemorrhage, and blood clots. Operations are performed using the CT scan as a road map.

myelography

X-ray imaging of the spinal canal after injection of contrast medium into the subarachnoid space.

CT scans and magnetic resonance imaging (MRI) are now replacing myelography, which is a more invasive technique.

Magnetic Resonance Techniques

magnetic resonance imaging (MRI) of the brain

Magnetic and radio waves create an image of the brain in all three planes.

MRI and CT complement each other in diagnosing brain and spinal cord lesions. MRI is excellent for viewing strokes and tumors and changes caused by trauma and Alzheimer disease. **Magnetic resonance angiography (MRA)** produces images of blood vessels using magnetic resonance techniques.

Radionuclide Studies

positron emission tomography (PET) scan

Computerized radiologic technique using radioactive glucose to image the metabolic activity of cells.

PET scans provide valuable information about the function of brain tissue in patients with Alzheimer disease, stroke, schizophrenia, and epilepsy (see Fig. 10–19).

Ultrasound Examination

Doppler/ultrasound studies

Sound waves detect blood flow in the carotid and intracranial arteries.

The carotid artery carries blood to the brain. These studies detect occlusion in blood vessels.

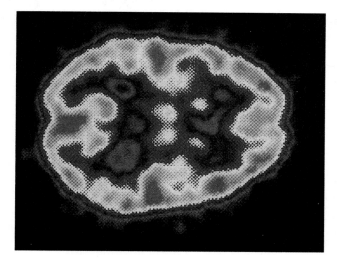

FIGURE 10–19 A **PET scan of the brain** showing decreased metabolic activity after a seizure (noted as green areas on the scan). (From Black JM, Hawks JH, Keene AM: Medical-Surgical Nursing: Clinical Management for Positive Outcomes, 6th ed., Philadelphia, WB Saunders, 2001, p. 197.)

Other Procedures

electroencephalography (EEG)   **Recording of the electrical activity of the brain.**

EEG demonstrates seizure activity resulting from brain tumors, other diseases, and injury to the brain.

lumbar puncture (LP)   **CSF is withdrawn from between two lumbar vertebrae** (Fig. 10–20).

A device to measure the pressure of CSF may be attached to the end of the needle after it has been inserted. Contrast medium for myelography or injection of intrathecal medicines may be administered as well. Some patients experience headache after LP. An informal name for this procedure is "spinal tap."

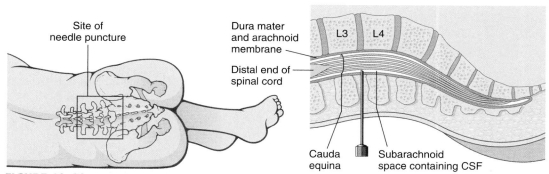

FIGURE 10–20   Lumbar puncture. The patient lies laterally, with the knees drawn up to the abdomen and the chin brought down to the chest. This position increases the spaces between the vertebrae. The lumbar puncture needle is inserted between the third and fourth (or the fourth and fifth) lumbar vertebrae and then is advanced to enter the subarachnoid space.

10

stereotactic radiosurgery

Use of a specialized instrument to locate and treat targets in the brain.

The stereotactic instrument is fixed onto the skull and guides the insertion of a needle by three-dimensional measurement. A **gamma knife** (high-energy radiation beam) treats deep and often inaccessible intracranial brain tumors and abnormal blood vessel masses **(arteriovenous malformations)** without surgical incision. Proton stereotactic radiosurgery (PSRS) delivers a uniform dose of proton radiation to a target and spares surrounding normal tissue. See Figure 10–21, *A* and *B*.

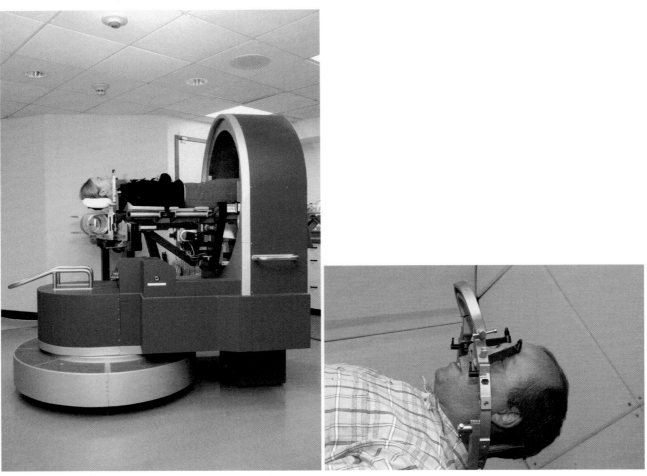

A   B

FIGURE 10–21 **A,** Patient on high-precision robotic bed used for **stereotactic radiosurgery. B, Stereotactic frame** holds the head in place for treatment with proton beam radiosurgery. (Courtesy Department of Radiation Therapy, Massachusetts General Hospital, Boston.)

ABBREVIATIONS

AD	Alzheimer disease		**MAC**	monitored anesthetic care
AFP	alpha-fetoprotein; elevated levels in amniotic fluid and maternal blood are associated with congenital malformations of the nervous system, such as anencephaly and spina bifida		**MG**	myasthenia gravis
			MRA	magnetic resonance angiography
			MRI	magnetic resonance imaging
			MS	multiple sclerosis
			½P	hemiparesis
ALS	amyotrophic lateral sclerosis—Lou Gehrig's disease		**PET**	positron emission tomography
			PSRS	proton stereotactic radiosurgery
AVM	arteriovenous malformation; congenital tangle of arteries and veins in the cerebrum		**Sz**	seizure
			TBI	traumatic brain injury
CNS	central nervous system		**TENS**	transcutaneous electrical nerve stimulation; technique using a battery-powered device to relieve acute and chronic pain
CSF	cerebrospinal fluid			
CT	computed tomography			
CVA	cerebrovascular accident		**TIA**	transient ischemic attack; temporary interference with the blood supply to the brain
EEG	electroencephalography			
GABA	gamma-aminobutyric acid (neurotransmitter)		**tPA**	tissue plasminogen activator; a clot-dissolving drug used as therapy for strokes
ICP	intracranial pressure (normal pressure is 5 to 15 mm Hg)			
LP	lumbar puncture			

PRACTICAL APPLICATIONS

Answers to the following case report are on page 373.

CASE REPORT

This patient was admitted on January 14 with a history of progressive right hemiparesis for the previous 1 to 2 months; fluctuating numbness of the right arm, thorax, and buttocks; jerking of the right leg; periods of speech arrest; diminished comprehension in reading; and recent development of a hemiplegic gait. He is suspected of having a left parietal tumor [the parietal lobes of the cerebrum are on either side under the roof of the skull].

Examinations done before hospitalization included skull films, EEG, and CSF analysis, which were all normal. After admission, an MRI was abnormal in the left parietal region, as was the EEG.

An MRA to assess cerebral blood vessels was attempted, but the patient became progressively more restless and agitated after sedation, so the procedure was stopped. During the recovery phase from the sedation, the patient was alternately somnolent [sleepy] and violent, but it was later apparent that he had developed almost a complete aphasia and right hemiplegia.

In the next few days, he became more alert, although he remained dysarthric [from the Greek *arthroun,* to utter distinctly] and hemiplegic.

MRI and MRA under general anesthesia on January 19 showed complete occlusion of the left internal carotid artery with cross-filling of the left anterior and middle cerebral arteries from the right internal carotid circulation.

Final diagnosis: Left cerebral infarction caused by left internal carotid artery occlusion.

[Fig. 10–22 shows the common carotid arteries and their branches within the head and brain.]

Questions on the Case Report

1. The patient was admitted with a history of
   a. Right-sided paralysis caused by a previous stroke
   b. Paralysis on the left side of his body
   c. Increasing slight paralysis on the right side of his body

2. The patient also has experienced periods of
   a. Aphasia and dyslexia
   b. Dysplastic gait
   c. Apraxia and aphasia

3. After his admission, where did the MRI show an abnormality?
   a. Right posterior region of the brain
   b. Left and right sides of the brain
   c. Left side of the brain

4. What test determined the final diagnosis?
   a. EEG for both sides of the brain
   b. CSF analysis and cerebral angiography
   c. Magnetic resonance imaging and magnetic resonance angiography

5. What was the final diagnosis?
   a. A stroke; necrotic tissue in the left cerebrum caused by blockage of an artery
   b. Cross-filling of blood vessels from the left to the right side of the brain
   c. Cerebral palsy on the left side of the brain with cross-filling of two cerebral arteries

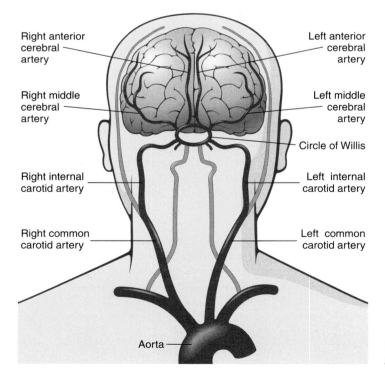

Right anterior cerebral artery

Left anterior cerebral artery

Right middle cerebral artery

Left middle cerebral artery

Circle of Willis

Right internal carotid artery

Left internal carotid artery

Right common carotid artery

Left common carotid artery

Aorta

FIGURE 10–22 Common carotid arteries and their branches.

? EXERCISES

Remember to check your answers carefully with those given in the Answers to Exercises, page 372.

A. Match the following neurologic structures with their meanings as given below.

astrocyte	dendrite	neuron
axon	meninges	oligodendroglial cell
cauda equina	myelin sheath	plexus
cerebral cortex		

1. microscopic fiber leading from the cell body that carries the nervous impulse along a nerve cell

    _____

2. large, interlacing network of nerves _____

3. three protective membranes surrounding the brain and spinal cord _____

4. microscopic branching fiber of a nerve cell that is the first part to receive the nervous impulse

    _____

5. outer region of the largest part of the brain; composed of gray matter

    _____

6. glial cell that transports water and salts between capillaries and nerve cells

    _____

7. glial cell that produces myelin _____

8. a nerve cell that transmits a nerve impulse _____

9. collection of spinal nerves below the end of the spinal cord at the level of the second lumbar

    vertebra _____

10. fatty tissue that surrounds the axon of a nerve cell _____

B. Give the meanings of the following terms.

1. dura mater _____

2. central nervous system _____

3. peripheral nervous system _____

4. arachnoid membrane _____

5. hypothalamus _____

6. synapse _____

7. sympathetic nerves _____

8. medulla oblongata _____

9. pons _____

10. cerebellum _____

11. thalamus _____

12. ventricles of the brain _____

13. brainstem _____

14. cerebrum _____

15. ganglion _____

C. Match the following terms with the meanings or associated terms below.

glia (neuroglia)	neurotransmitter	sensory nerves
gyri	parenchymal cell	subarachnoid space
motor nerves	pia mater	sulci

1. innermost meningeal membrane _____

2. carry messages away from (efferent) the brain and spinal cord to muscles and glands

   _____

3. carry messages toward (afferent) the brain and spinal cord from receptors

   _____

4. grooves in the cerebral cortex _____

5. contains cerebrospinal fluid _____

6. elevations in the cerebral cortex _____

7. chemical that is released at the end of a nerve cell and stimulates or inhibits another cell

   (example: acetylcholine) _____

8. essential cell of the nervous system; a neuron _____

9. connective and supportive (stromal) tissue _____

D. Circle the correct term for the given definition.

1. disease of the brain **(encephalopathy, myelopathy)**

2. part of the brain that controls muscular coordination and balance **(cerebrum, cerebellum)**

3. collection of blood above the dura mater **(subdural hematoma, epidural hematoma)**

4. inflammation of the pia and arachnoid membranes **(leptomeningitis, causalgia)**

5. condition of absence of a brain **(hypalgesia, anencephaly)**

6. inflammation of the gray matter of the spinal cord **(poliomyelitis, polyneuritis)**

7. pertaining to the membranes around the brain and spinal cord **(cerebellopontine, meningeal)**

8. disease of nerve roots (of spinal nerves) **(neuropathy, radiculopathy)**

9. hernia of the spinal cord and meninges **(myelomeningocele, meningioma)**

10. pertaining to the tenth cranial nerve **(thalamic, vagal)**

E. Give the meanings of the following terms.

1. cerebral cortex_____

2. intrathecal _____

3. polyneuritis _____

4. thalamic_____

5. myelogram_____

6. meningioma_____

7. glioma _____

8. subdural hematoma _____

F. Match the following neurologic symptoms with the meanings below.

aphasia	dyslexia	narcolepsy
ataxia	hemiparesis	neurasthenia
bradykinesia	hyperesthesia	paraplegia
causalgia	motor apraxia	syncope

1. reading disorder _____

2. condition of no coordination _____

3. condition of slow movement _____

4. condition of increased sensation _____

5. seizure of sleep; uncontrollable compulsion to sleep _____

6. inability to speak _____

7. inability to perform a task _____

8. slight paralysis in the right or left half of the body _____

9. burning pain _____

10. paralysis in the lower part of the body _____

11. fainting _____

12. nervous exhaustion (lack of strength) and fatigue _____

10

G. Give the meanings of the following terms.

1. analgesia _____

2. motor aphasia _____

3. paresis _____

4. quadriplegia _____

5. asthenia _____

6. comatose _____

7. paresthesia _____

8. hyperkinesis _____

9. anesthesia _____

10. causalgia _____

11. akinetic _____

12. hypalgesia _____

13. dyskinesia _____

14. migraine _____

H. Match the following terms with their descriptions below. The terms in **boldface** are clues!

Alzheimer disease   Huntington disease   myasthenia gravis
amyotrophic lateral sclerosis   hydrocephalus   Parkinson disease
Bell palsy   multiple sclerosis   myelomeningocele
epilepsy

1. Destruction of myelin sheath (demyelination) and its replacement by **hard** plaques

   _____

2. Sudden, transient disturbances of brain function cause **seizures** _____

3. The **spinal** column is imperfectly joined (a **split** in a vertebra occurs), and part of the meninges

   and spinal cord can herniate out of the spinal cavity _____

4. **Atrophy** of muscles and paralysis caused by damage to motor neurons in the spinal cord and

   brainstem _____

5. Patient displays bizarre, abrupt, involuntary, dance-like movements, as well as decline in mental

   functions _____

10

6. Cerebrospinal **fluid** accumulates in the **head** (in the ventricles of the brain)

   _____

7. **Loss of muscle strength** due to the inability of a neurotransmitter (acetylcholine) to transmit

   impulses from nerve cells to muscle cells _____

8. Degeneration of nerves in the basal ganglia occur in later life, leading to tremors, shuffling
   gait, and muscle stiffness; **dopamine** (neurotransmitter) is deficient in the brain

   _____

9. Deterioration of mental capacity **(dementia);** autopsy shows cerebral cortex atrophy, widening of

   cerebral sulci, and microscopic neurofibrillary tangles _____

10. Unilateral facial **paralysis** _____

I. Give the meanings of the following terms for abnormal conditions.

1. astrocytoma _____

2. pyogenic meningitis _____

3. Tourette syndrome _____

4. cerebral contusion _____

5. cerebrovascular accident _____

6. cerebral concussion _____

7. herpes zoster _____

8. cerebral embolus _____

9. cerebral thrombosis _____

10. cerebral hemorrhage _____

11. cerebral aneurysm _____

12. HIV encephalopathy _____

J. Match the term in Column I with the letter of its associated term or meaning in Column II.

Column I		*Column II*
1. ataxia	_____	A. Relieving, but not curing
2. aura	_____	B. Virus that causes chickenpox and shingles
3. transient ischemic attack	_____	C. Uncoordinated gait
4. tonic-clonic seizure	_____	D. Neurotransmitter
5. herpes zoster	_____	E. Peculiar sensation experienced by patient before onset of seizure
6. palliative	_____	F. Malignant brain tumor of immature glial cells
7. dopamine	_____	G. Major epileptic seizure; ictal event
8. occlusion	_____	H. Interruption of blood supply to the cerebrum; mini-stroke
9. absence seizure	_____	I. Minor epileptic seizure
10. glioblastoma multiforme	_____	J. Blockage

K. Describe what happens in the following two procedures.

1. MRI of the brain _____

2. stereotactic radiosurgery with gamma knife

_____

L. Give the meanings of the following abbreviations and then select the letter of the best association for each.

Column I

1. EEG _____ ____
2. PET _____ ____
3. AFP _____ ____
4. MS _____ ____
5. MRI _____ ____
6. LP _____ ____
7. CVA _____ ____
8. AD _____ ____
9. TIA _____ ____
10. CSF _____ ____

Column II

A. Gradually progressive dementia.
B. Stroke; embolus, hemorrhage, or thrombosis are etiological factors.
C. Intrathecal medications can be administered through this procedure.
D. This fluid is analyzed for abnormal blood cells, chemicals, and protein.
E. Procedure to diagnose abnormal electrical activity in the brain.
F. Neurologic symptoms and/or signs due to temporary interference of blood supply to the brain.
G. High levels in amniotic fluid and maternal blood are associated with spina bifida.
H. Diagnostic procedure that allows excellent visualization of soft tissue in the brain.
I. Radioactive materials, such as glucose, are taken up by the brain, and images recorded.
J. Destruction of the myelin sheath in the CNS occurs with plaques of hard scar tissue.

M. Circle the terms that complete the meanings of the sentences.

1. Maria had such severe headaches that she could find relief only with strong analgesics. Her condition of **(spina bifida, migraine, epilepsy)** was debilitating.

2. Paul was in a coma after his high-speed car accident. His physicians were concerned that he had suffered a **(palsy, myelomeningocele, contusion and subdural hematoma)** as a result of the accident.

3. Dick went to the emergency department complaining of dizziness, nausea, and headache. The physician, suspecting increased ICP, prescribed corticosteroids, and Dick's symptoms disappeared. They returned, however, when the steroids were discontinued. A/an **(MRI of the brain, electroencephalogram, CSF analysis)** revealed a large brain lesion. It was removed surgically and determined to be an **(embolus, glioblastoma multiforme, migraine)**.

4. Dorothy felt weakness in her hand and numbness in her arm, and noticed blurred vision, all signs of **(herpes zoster, meningitis, TIA)**. Her physician requested **(myelography, MRA, lumbar puncture)** to assess any damage to cerebral blood vessels and possible stroke.

5. When Bill noticed ptosis and muscle weakness in his face, he reported these symptoms to his doctor. The doctor diagnosed his condition as **(Tourette syndrome, Huntington disease, myasthenia gravis)** and prescribed **(dopamine, anticonvulsants, anticholinesterase drugs)**, which relieved his symptoms.

6. To rule out bacterial **(epilepsy, encephalomalacia, meningitis)**, Dr. Phillips, a pediatrician, requested an **(EEG, PET scan, LP)** be performed on the febrile (feverish) child.

10

7. Eight-year-old Barry reversed his letters and had difficulty learning to read and write words. His family physician diagnosed his problem as **(aphasia, dyslexia, ataxia)**.

8. After his head hit the steering wheel during a recent automobile accident, Clark noticed **(hemiparesis, paraplegia, hyperesthesia)** on the left side of his body. A head CT scan revealed **(narcolepsy, neurasthenia, subdural hematoma)**.

9. For her 35th birthday, Elizabeth's husband threw her a surprise party. She was so startled by the crowd that she experienced a weakness of muscles and loss of consciousness. Friends placed her on her back in a horizontal position with her head low to improve blood flow to her brain. She soon recovered from her **(myoneural, syncopal, hyperkinetic)** episode.

10. Near his 65th birthday, Edward began having difficulty remembering recent events. Over the next five years, he developed age-related **(dyslexia, dementia, seizures)** and was diagnosed with **(multiple sclerosis, myasthenia gravis, Alzheimer disease)**.

11. Elderly Mrs. Smith had been taking an antipsychotic drug for 5 years when she began exhibiting lip smacking and darting movements of her tongue. Her doctor described her condition as **(radiculitis, tardive dyskinesia, hemiparesis)** and discontinued her drug. The condition, acquired after use of the drug, would be considered **(iatrogenic, congenital, ictal)**.

N. Complete the spelling of the following terms based on their meanings.

1. part of the brain that controls sleep, appetite, temperature, and secretions of the pituitary gland:

   hypo_____

2. pertaining to fainting: syn_____

3. abnormal tingling sensations: par_____

4. slight paralysis: par_____

5. inflammation of a spinal nerve root: _____itis

6. inability to speak: a_____

7. movements and behavior that are not purposeful: a_____

8. lack of muscular coordination: a_____

9. reading, writing, and learning disorders: dys_____

10. excessive movement: hyper_____

11. paralysis in one half (right or left) of the body: _____plegia

12. paralysis in the lower half of the body: _____plegia

13. paralysis in all four limbs: _____plegia

14. nervous exhaustion and fatigue: neur_____

MEDICAL SCRAMBLE

Unscramble the letters to form suffixes related to nervous system conditions from the clues. Use the letters in squares to complete the bonus term. Answers are found on page 373.

1. *Clue:* Abnormal electrical activity in the brain

___ ___ ___ ___ ___ [ ] [ ]   EYPIPESL

2. *Clue:* Inflammation of membranes surrounding the brain and spinal cord

___ [ ] ___ ___ ___ ___ ___ ___ ___   SIETMINGNI

3. *Clue:* Paralysis

[ ] ___ ___ [ ] ___   SAYLP

4. *Clue:* Mental decline and deterioration

___ ___ ___ ___ [ ] ___ ___ [ ]   ENETIDAM

BONUS TERM: *Clue:* Space between nerve cells.

[ ] [ ] [ ] [ ] [ ] [ ] [ ]

10

ANSWERS TO EXERCISES

A

1. axon
2. plexus
3. meninges
4. dendrite
5. cerebral cortex
6. astrocyte
7. oligodendroglial cell
8. neuron
9. cauda equina
10. myelin sheath

B

1. outermost meningeal layer surrounding the brain and spinal cord
2. brain and the spinal cord
3. nerves outside the brain and spinal cord; cranial, spinal, and autonomic nerves
4. middle meningeal membrane surrounding the brain and spinal cord
5. part of the brain below the thalamus; controls sleep, appetite, body temperature, and secretions from the pituitary gland
6. space through which a nervous impulse is transmitted from a nerve cell to another nerve cell or to a muscle or gland cell
7. autonomic nerves that influence body functions involuntarily in times of stress
8. part of the brain just above the spinal cord that controls breathing, heartbeat, and the size of blood vessels
9. part of the brain anterior to the cerebellum and between the medulla and the upper parts of the brain; connects these parts of the brain
10. posterior part of the brain that coordinates voluntary muscle movements
11. part of the brain below the cerebrum; relay center that conducts impulses between the spinal cord and the cerebrum
12. canals in the interior of the brain that are filled with CSF
13. lower portion of the brain that connects the cerebrum with the spinal cord (includes the pons and the medulla)
14. largest part of the brain; controls voluntary muscle movement, vision, speech, hearing, thought, memory
15. collection of nerve cell bodies outside the brain and spinal cord

C

1. pia mater
2. motor nerves
3. sensory nerves
4. sulci
5. subarachnoid space
6. gyri
7. neurotransmitter
8. parenchymal cell
9. glia (neuroglia)

D

1. encephalopathy
2. cerebellum
3. epidural hematoma
4. leptomeningitis
5. anencephaly
6. poliomyelitis
7. meningeal
8. radiculopathy
9. myelomeningocele
10. vagal

E

1. outer region of the cerebrum (contains gray matter)
2. pertaining to within a sheath through the meninges and into the subarachnoid space
3. inflammation of many nerves
4. pertaining to the thalamus
5. x-ray study of the spine (after contrast is injected via lumbar puncture)
6. tumor of the meninges
7. tumor of neuroglial cells (a brain tumor)
8. mass of blood below the dura mater (outermost meningeal membrane)

F

1. dyslexia
2. ataxia
3. bradykinesia
4. hyperesthesia
5. narcolepsy
6. aphasia
7. motor apraxia
8. hemiparesis
9. causalgia
10. paraplegia
11. syncope
12. neurasthenia

G

1. lack of sensitivity to pain
2. inability to speak (cannot articulate words, but can understand speech and knows what she or he wants to say)
3. slight paralysis
4. paralysis in all four extremities (damage is to the cervical part of the spinal cord)
5. no strength (weakness)
6. pertaining to coma (loss of consciousness from which the patient cannot be aroused)
7. condition of abnormal sensations (prickling, tingling, numbness, burning) for no apparent reason
8. excessive movement
9. condition of no sensation or nervous feeling
10. intense burning pain
11. pertaining to without movement
12. diminished sensation to pain
13. impairment of the ability to perform voluntary movements
14. recurrent vascular headache with severe pain unilateral onset, and photophobia (sensitivity to light)

H

1. multiple sclerosis
2. epilepsy
3. myelomeningocele
4. amyotrophic lateral sclerosis

5. Huntington disease
6. hydrocephalus
7. myasthenia gravis

8. Parkinson disease
9. Alzheimer disease
10. Bell palsy

I

1. tumor of neuroglial brain cells (astrocytes)
2. inflammation of the meninges (bacterial infection with pus formation)
3. involuntary spasmodic, twitching movements (tics), uncontrollable vocal sounds, and inappropriate words
4. bruising of brain tissue as a result of direct trauma to the head
5. disruption of the normal blood supply to the brain; stroke or cerebral infarction

6. temporary brain dysfunction; loss of consciousness that usually clears within 24 hours
7. neurologic condition caused by infection with herpes zoster virus; blisters form along the course of peripheral nerves
8. blockage of a blood vessel in the cerebrum caused by material from another part of the body that suddenly occludes the vessel

9. blockage of a blood vessel in the cerebrum caused by the formation of a clot within the vessel
10. bursting forth of blood from a cerebral artery (can cause a stroke)
11. widening of a blood vessel (artery) in the cerebrum; the aneurysm can burst and lead to a CVA
12. brain disease (dementia and encephalitis) caused by infection with AIDS virus

J

1. C
2. E
3. H
4. G

5. B
6. A
7. D

8. J
9. I
10. F

K

1. use of magnetic and radio waves to create an image (in frontal, transverse, or sagittal plane) of the brain

2. an instrument (stereotactic) is fixed onto the skull and locates a target by three-dimensional measurement;

gamma radiation beams are used to treat deep brain lesions

L

1. electroencephalography: E
2. positron emission tomography: I
3. alpha-fetoprotein: G
4. multiple sclerosis: J

5. magnetic resonance imaging: H
6. lumbar puncture: C
7. cerebrovascular accident: B

8. Alzheimer disease: A
9. transient ischemic attack: F
10. cerebrospinal fluid: D

M

1. migraine
2. contusion and subdural hematoma
3. MRI of the brain; glioblastoma multiforme
4. TIA; MRA

5. myasthenia gravis; anticholinesterase drugs
6. meningitis; LP
7. dyslexia

8. hemiparesis; subdural hematoma
9. syncopal
10. dementia; Alzheimer disease
11. tardive dyskinesia; iatrogenic

N

1. hypothalamus
2. syncopal
3. paresthesias
4. paresis
5. radiculitis

6. aphasia
7. apraxia
8. ataxia
9. dyslexia
10. hyperkinesis

11. hemiplegia
12. paraplegia
13. quadriplegia
14. neurasthenia

ANSWERS TO PRACTICAL APPLICATIONS

1. c
2. a
3. c

4. c
5. a

ANSWERS TO MEDICAL SCRAMBLE

1. EPILEPSY   2. MENINGITIS   3. PALSY   4. DEMENTIA

BONUS TERM: SYNAPSE

PRONUNCIATION OF TERMS

PRONUNCIATION GUIDE

ā as in āpe   ă as in ăpple
ē as in ēven   ĕ as in ĕvery
ī as in īce   ĭ as in ĭnterest
ō as in ōpen   ŏ as in pŏt
ū as in ūnit   ŭ as in ŭnder

To test your understanding of the terminology in this chapter, write the meaning of each term in the space provided. In addition, you may wish to cover the terms and write them by looking at your definitions. Make sure your spelling is correct. The page number after each term indicates where it is defined or used in the book, so you can easily check your responses. You will find complete definitions for all of these terms and their audio pronunciations on the CD.

VOCABULARY AND COMBINING FORMS AND TERMINOLOGY

Term	Pronunciation	Meaning
acetylcholine (343)	ăs-ĕ-tĭl-KŌ-lēn	
afferent nerves (343)	ĂF-fĕr-ĕnt nĕrvz	
akinetic (349)	ă-kĭ-NĔT-ĭk	
analgesia (347)	ăn-ăl-JĒ-zē-ă	
anencephaly (346)	ăn-ĕn-SĔF-ă-lē	
anesthesia (348)	ăn-ĕs-THĒ-zē-ă	
aphasia (349)	ă-FĀ-zē-ă	
apraxia (350)	ā-PRĂK-sē-ă	
arachnoid membrane (343)	ă-RĂK-noyd MĔM-brān	
astrocyte (343)	ĂS-trō-sīt	
ataxia (350)	ă-TĂK-sē-ă	
autonomic nervous system (343)	ăw-tō-NŌM-ĭk NĔR-vŭs SĬS-tĕm	
axon (343)	ĂK-sŏn	
blood-brain barrier (343)	blŭd-brān BĂ-rē-ĕr	
bradykinesia (349)	brā-dē-kĭ-NĒ-zē-ă	
brainstem (343)	BRĀN-stĕm	
cauda equina (343)	KĂW-dă ĕ-KWĬ-nă	
causalgia (348)	kăw-ZĂL-jă	
cell body (343)	sĕl BŎD-ē	
central nervous system (343)	SĔN-trăl NĔR-vŭs SĬS-tĕm	
cephalgia (347)	sĕ-FĂL-jă	
cerebellar (345)	sĕr-ĕ-BĔL-ăr	
cerebellopontine (347)	sĕr-ĕ-bĕl-ō-PŎN-tēn	

Term	Pronunciation	Meaning
cerebellum (343)	sĕr-ĕ-BĔL-ŭm	_____
cerebral cortex (345)	sĕ-RĒ-brăl (_or_ SĔR-ĕ-brăl) KŎR-tĕks	_____
cerebrospinal fluid (345)	sĕ-rē-brō-SPĪ-năl FLOO-ĭd	_____
cerebrum (343)	sĕ-RĒ-brŭm	_____
coma (348)	KŌ-mă	_____
comatose (348)	KŌ-mă-tōs	_____
cranial nerves (343)	KRĀ-nē-ăl nĕrvz	_____
dendrite (343)	DĔN-drīt	_____
dura mater (343)	DŬR-ă MĂ-tĕr	_____
dyslexia (349)	dĭs-LĔK-sē-ă	_____
dyskinesia (349)	dĭs-kĭ-NĒ-zē-ă	_____
efferent nerve (343)	ĔF-fĕr-ĕnt nĕrvz	_____
encephalitis (346)	ĕn-sĕf-ă-LĪ-tĭs	_____
encephalopathy (346)	ĕn-sĕf-ă-LŎP-ă-thē	_____
ependymal cell (343)	ĕp-ĔN-dĭ-măl sĕl	_____
epidural hematoma (346)	ĕp-ĕ-DŪ-răl hē-mă-TŌ-mă	_____
ganglion (343)	GĂNG-lē-ŏn	_____
glial cell (344)	GLĒ-ăl sĕl	_____
glioblastoma (346)	glē-ō-blă-STŌ-mă	_____
gyrus; gyri (344)	JĪ-rŭs; JĪ-rē	_____
hemiparesis (349)	hĕm-ē-pă-RĒ-sĭs	_____
hemiplegia (349)	hĕm-ē-PLĒ-jă	_____
hypalgesia (347)	hīp-ăl-GĒ-zē-ă	_____
hyperesthesia (348)	hī-pĕr-ĕs-THĒ-zē-ă	_____
hyperkinesis (349)	hī-pĕr-kĭ-NĒ-sĭs	_____
hypothalamus (344)	hī-pō-THĂL-ă-mŭs	_____
intrathecal (347)	ĭn-tră-THĒ-kăl	_____
leptomeningeal (346)	lĕp-tō-mĕn-ĭn-JĒ-ăl	_____
medulla oblongata (344)	mĕ-DŪL-ă (_or_ mĕ-DŬL-ă) ŏb-lŏn-GĂ-tă	_____
meningeal (346)	mĕ-NĬN-jē-ăl _or_ mĕ-nĭn-JĒ-ăl	_____
meninges (344)	mĕ-NĬN-jēz	_____

10

Term	Pronunciation	Meaning
meningioma (346)	mĕ-nĭn-jē-Ō-mă	
microglial cell (344)	mĭ-krō-GLĒ-ăl sĕl	
migraine (347)	MĪ-grān	
motor nerves (344)	MŌ-tĕr nĕrvz	
myelin sheath (344)	MĪ-ĕ-lĭn shēth	
myelogram (347)	MĪ-ĕ-lō-grăm	
myelomeningocele (346)	mī-ĕ-lō-mĕ-NĬN-gō-sēl	
myoneural (347)	mī-ō-NŬR-ăl	
narcolepsy (349)	NĂR-kō-lĕp-sē	
nerve (344)	nĕrv	
neuralgia (347)	nŭr-ĂL-jă	
neurasthenia (350)	nŭr-ăs-THĒ-nē-ă	
neuroglia (347)	nŭr-ō-GLĒ-ă	
neuron (344)	NŪR-ŏn	
neuropathy (347)	nūr-ŎP-ă-thē	
neurotransmitter (344)	nūr-ō-trănz-MĬT-ĕr	
oligodendroglial cell (344)	ŏl-ĭ-gō-dĕn-drō-GLĒ-ăl sĕl	
paraplegia (349)	păr-ă-PLĒ-jă	
parasympathetic nerves (344)	păr-ă-sĭm-pă-THĔT-ĭk nĕrvz	
parenchyma (344)	păr-ĔN-kĭ-mă	
paresis (349)	pă-RĒ-sĭs	
paresthesia (348)	păr-ĕs-THĒ-zē-ă	
peripheral nervous system (344)	pĕ-RĬF-ĕr-ăl NĔR-vŭs SĬS-tĕm	
pia mater (344)	PĒ-ă MĂ-tĕr	
plexus (344)	PLĔK-sŭs	
poliomyelitis (347)	pō-lē-ō-mī-ĕ-LĪ-tĭs	
polyneuritis (347)	pŏl-ē-nŭ-RĪ-tĭs	
pons (344)	pŏnz	
quadriplegia (349)	kwŏd-rĭ-PLĒ-jă	
radiculitis (347)	ră-dĭk-ū-LĪ-tĭs	
radiculopathy (347)	ră-dĭk-ū-LŎP-ă-thē	

Term	Pronunciation	Meaning
receptor (344)	rē-SĚP-tŏr	_____
sciatic nerve (344)	sī-ĂT-ĭk nĕrv	_____
sensory nerves (345)	SĚN-sō-rē nĕrvz	_____
spinal nerves (345)	SPĪ-năl nĕrvz	_____
stimulus (345)	STĬM-ū-lŭs	_____
stroma (345)	STRŌ-mă	_____
subdural hematoma (346)	sŭb-DŪ-răl hē-mă-TŌ-mă	_____
sulcus; sulci (345)	SŬL-kŭs; SŬL-sī	_____
sympathetic nerves (345)	sĭm-pă-THĚT-ĭk nĕrvz	_____
synapse (345)	SĬN-ăps	_____
syncopal (350)	SĬN-kō-păl	_____
syncope (350)	SĬN-kō-pē	_____
thalamic (347)	THĂL-ă-mĭk *or* thă-LĂM-ĭk	_____
thalamus (345)	THĂL-ă-mŭs	_____
trigeminal neuralgia (347)	trī-GĚM-ĭn-ăl nŭr-ĂL-jă	_____
vagal (347)	VĀ-găl	_____
vagus nerve (345)	VĀ-gŭs nĕrv	_____
ventricles of the brain (345)	VĚN-trĭ-k'lz of the brān	_____

PATHOLOGY, LABORATORY TESTS, AND CLINICAL PROCEDURES

Term	Pronunciation	Meaning
absence seizure (357)	ĂB-sĕns SĒ-zhŭr	_____
Alzheimer disease (351)	ĂLZ-hī-mĕr dĭ-ZĒZ	_____
amyotrophic lateral sclerosis (352)	ā-mī-ō-TRŌ-fĭk LĂ-tĕr-ăl sklĕ-RŌ-sĭs	_____
aneurysm (357)	ĂN-ūr-ĭ-zĭm	_____
astrocytoma (355)	ăs-trō-sī-TŌ-mă	_____
aura (352)	ĂW-ră	_____
Bell palsy (354)	bĕl PĂL-zē	_____
cerebral angiography (358)	sĕ-RĒ-brăl ăn-jē-ŌG-ră-fē	_____
cerebral concussion (356)	sĕ-RĒ-brăl kŏn-KŬS-shŭn	_____
cerebral contusion (356)	sĕ-RĒ-brăl kŏn-TOO-shŭn	_____
cerebral hemorrhage (356)	sĕ-RĒ-brăl HĔM-ōr-ĭj	_____

Term	Pronunciation	Meaning
cerebral palsy (354)	sĕ-RĒ-brăl (*or* SĔR-ĕ-brăl) PĂL-zē	_____
cerebrospinal fluid analysis (358)	sĕ-rē-brō-SPĪ-năl FLOO-ĭd ă-NĂL-ĭ-sĭs	_____
cerebrovascular accident (356)	sĕ-rē-brō-VĂS-kū-lăr ĂK-sĭ-dĕnt	_____
computed tomography (358)	kŏm-PŪ-tĕd tō-MŎG-ră-fē	_____
dementia (357)	dĕ-MĔN-shē-ă	_____
demyelination (353)	dē-mī-ĕ-lĭ-NĀ-shun	_____
dopamine (357)	DŌ-pă-mēn	_____
Doppler/ultrasound studies (358)	DŎP-lĕr ŬL-tră-sound STŬ-dēz	_____
electroencephalography (359)	ĕ-lĕk-trō-ĕn-sĕf-ă-LŎG-ră-fē	_____
embolus (357)	ĔM-bō-lŭs	_____
epilepsy (352)	ĔP-ĭ-lĕp-sē	_____
gait (357)	GĀT	_____
glioblastoma multiforme (355)	glē-ō-blăs-TŌ-mă mŭl-tē-FŎR-mă	_____
herpes zoster (354)	HĔR-pēz ZŎS-tĕr	_____
HIV encephalopathy (355)	HIV ĕn-sĕf-ă-LŎP-ă-thē	_____
Huntington disease (353)	HŬN-ting-tŏn dĭ-ZĒZ	_____
hydrocephalus (350)	hī-drō-SĔF-ă-lŭs	_____
ictal event (357)	ĬK-tăl ē-VĔNT	_____
lumbar puncture (359)	LŬM-băr PŬNK-shŭr	_____
magnetic resonance imaging (358)	măg-NĔT-ĭk RĔ-zō-nănce ĬM-ă-jĭng	_____
meningitis (355)	mĕn-ĭn-JĪ-tĭs	_____
meningocele (351)	mĕ-NĬN-gō-sĕl	_____
multiple sclerosis (353)	mūl-tĭ-p'l sklĕ-RŌ-sĭs	_____
myasthenia gravis (353)	mī-ăs-THĒ-nē-ă GRĂ-vĭs	_____
occlusion (357)	ō-KLŪ-zhŭn	_____
palliative (354)	PĂ-lē-ă-tĭv	_____
palsy (354)	PĂWL-zē	_____

Term	Pronunciation	Meaning
Parkinson disease (354)	PĂR-kĭn-sŭn dĭ-ZĒZ	_____
positron emission tomography (358)	PŎS-ĭ-trŏn ē-MĬ-shŭn tō-MŎG-ră-fē	_____
shingles (354)	SHĬNG-ŭlz	_____
spina bifida (350)	SPĪ-nă BĬF-ĭ-dă	_____
stereotactic radiosurgery (360)	stĕ-rē-ō-TĂK-tĭk ră-dē-ō-SŬR-gĕr-ē	_____
thrombosis (356)	thrŏm-BŌ-sĭs	_____
tic (354)	tĭk	_____
tonic-clonic seizure (352)	TŎN-ĭk-KLŌ-nĭk SĒ-zhŭr	_____
Tourette syndrome (354)	tŭ-RĔT SĬN-drōm	_____
transient ischemic attack (356)	TRĂN-zē-ĕnt ĭs-KĒ-mĭk ă-TĂK	_____

10

REVIEW SHEET

10

Write the meanings of the word parts in the spaces provided. Check your answers with the information in the chapter or in the glossary (Medical Word Parts—English) at the end of the book.

COMBINING FORMS

Combining Form	Meaning	Combining Form	Meaning
alges/o		lex/o	
angi/o		mening/o, meningi/o	
caus/o		my/o	
cephal/o		myel/o	
cerebell/o		narc/o	
cerebr/o		neur/o	
comat/o		olig/o	
crani/o		pont/o	
cry/o		radicul/o	
dur/o		spin/o	
encephal/o		syncop/o	
esthesi/o		tax/o	
gli/o		thalam/o	
hydr/o		thec/o	
kines/o, kinesi/o		troph/o	
lept/o		vag/o	

PREFIXES

Prefix	Meaning	Prefix	Meaning
a-, an-		micro-	
dys-		para-	
epi-		polio-	
hemi-		poly-	
hyper-		quadri-	
hypo-		sub-	
intra-			

10

SUFFIXES

Suffix	Meaning	Suffix	Meaning
algesia	_____	-ose	_____
-algia	_____	-paresis	_____
-blast	_____	-pathy	_____
-cele	_____	-phagia	_____
-esthesia	_____	-phasia	_____
-gram	_____	-plegia	_____
-graphy	_____	-praxia	_____
-ine	_____	-ptosis	_____
-itis	_____	-sclerosis	_____
-kinesia, -kinesis	_____	-sthenia	_____
-kinetic	_____	-tomy	_____
-lepsy	_____	-trophy	_____
-oma	_____		

 Please refer to the enclosed CD for additional exercises and images related to this chapter.

chapter 11

Cardiovascular System

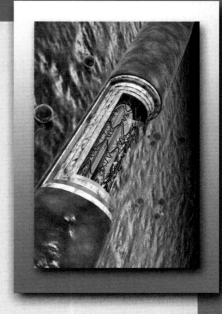

THIS CHAPTER IS DIVIDED INTO THE FOLLOWING SECTIONS

In this chapter you will

- Name the parts of the heart and associated blood vessels and their functions in the circulation of blood.
- Trace the pathway of blood through the heart.
- Identify and describe major pathologic conditions affecting the heart and blood vessels.
- Define combining forms that relate to the cardiovascular system.
- Describe important laboratory tests and clinical procedures pertaining to the cardiovascular system, and recognize relevant abbreviations.
- Apply your new knowledge to understand medical terms in their proper context, such as in medical reports and records.

Image Description: An angioplasty procedure in which a catheter, stent, and balloon are inserted into a blocked part of the coronary artery.

383

INTRODUCTION

Body cells are dependent on a constant supply of nutrients and oxygen. When the supplies are delivered and then chemically combined, they release the energy necessary to do the work of each cell. How does the body ensure that oxygen and food will be delivered to all of its cells? The cardiovascular system, consisting of the heart (a powerful muscular pump) and blood vessels (fuel line and transportation network), performs this important work. This chapter explores terminology related to the heart and blood vessels.

BLOOD VESSELS AND THE CIRCULATION OF BLOOD

BLOOD VESSELS

There are three types of blood vessels in the body: **arteries, veins,** and **capillaries.**

Arteries are large blood vessels that carry blood away from the heart. Their walls are lined with connective tissue, muscle tissue, and elastic fibers, with an innermost layer of epithelial cells called **endothelium.** Endothelial cells, found in all blood vessels, secrete factors that affect the size of blood vessels, reduce blood clotting, and promote the growth

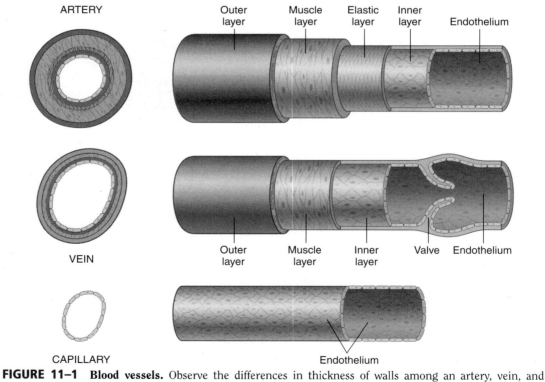

FIGURE 11–1   Blood vessels. Observe the differences in thickness of walls among an artery, vein, and capillary. All three vessels are lined with endothelium. Endothelial cells actively secrete substances that prevent clotting and regulate the tone of blood vessels. Examples of endothelial secretions are endothelium-derived relaxing factor (EDRF) and endothelin (a vasoconstrictor). (Some parts modified from Damjanov I: Pathology for the Health-Related Professions, 3rd ed. Philadelphia, WB Saunders, 2006, p. 139.)

of blood vessels. Because arteries carry blood away from the heart, they must be strong enough to withstand the high pressure of the pumping action of the heart. Their elastic walls allow them to expand as the heartbeat forces blood into the arterial system throughout the body. Smaller branches of arteries are **arterioles.**

Arterioles are thinner than arteries and carry the blood to the tiniest of blood vessels, the capillaries.

Capillaries have walls that are only one endothelial cell in thickness. These delicate, microscopic vessels carry nutrient-rich, oxygenated blood from the arteries and arterioles to the body cells. Their thin walls allow passage of oxygen and nutrients out of the bloodstream and into cells. There, the nutrients are burned in the presence of oxygen (catabolism) to release energy. At the same time, waste products such as carbon dioxide and water pass out of cells and into the thin-walled capillaries. Waste-filled blood then flows back to the heart in small veins or **venules,** which branch to form larger vessels called veins.

Veins have thinner walls compared with arteries. They conduct blood (that has given up most of its oxygen) toward the heart from the tissues. Veins have little elastic tissue and less connective tissue than that typical of arteries, and blood pressure in veins is extremely low compared with pressure in arteries. In order to keep blood moving back toward the heart, veins have **valves** that prevent the backflow of blood and keep the blood moving in one direction. Muscular action also helps the movement of blood in veins. Figure 11–1 illustrates the differences in blood vessels. Figure 11–2 reviews their characteristics and relationship to each other.

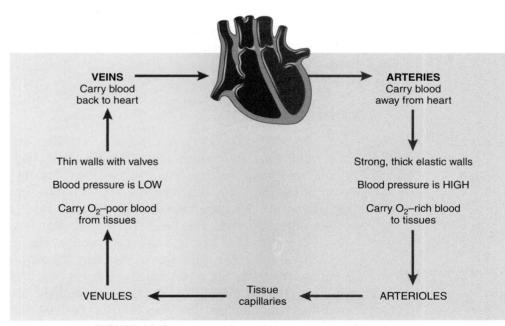

FIGURE 11–2 Relationship and characteristics of blood vessels.

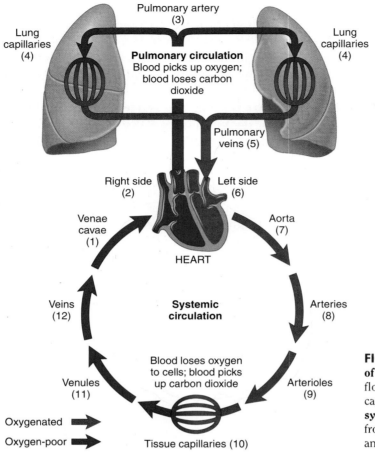

Pulmonary artery
(3)

Lung
capillaries
(4)

Lung
capillaries
(4)

Pulmonary circulation
Blood picks up oxygen;
blood loses carbon
dioxide

Pulmonary
veins (5)

Right side
(2)

Left side
(6)

Venae
cavae
(1)

Aorta
(7)

HEART

Veins
(12)

**Systemic
circulation**

Arteries
(8)

Venules
(11)

Blood loses oxygen
to cells; blood picks
up carbon dioxide

Arterioles
(9)

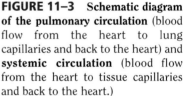

Oxygenated

Oxygen-poor

Tissue capillaries (10)

FIGURE 11–3 Schematic diagram of the pulmonary circulation (blood flow from the heart to lung capillaries and back to the heart) and **systemic circulation** (blood flow from the heart to tissue capillaries and back to the heart.)

CIRCULATION OF BLOOD

Arteries, arterioles, veins, venules, and capillaries, together with the heart, form a circulatory system for the flow of blood. Figure 11–3 is a more detailed representation of the entire circulatory system. Refer to it as you read the following paragraphs. (Note that the numbers in the following paragraphs correspond with those in Fig. 11–3.)

Blood that is deficient in oxygen flows through two large veins, the **venae cavae** [1], on its way from the tissue capillaries to the heart. The blood became oxygen-poor at the tissue capillaries when oxygen left the blood and entered the body cells.

Oxygen-poor blood enters the **right side of the heart** [2] and travels through that side and into the **pulmonary artery** [3], a vessel that divides in two: one branch leading to the left lung, the other to the right lung. The arteries continue dividing and subdividing within the lungs, forming smaller and smaller vessels (arterioles) and finally reaching the **lung capillaries** [4]. The pulmonary artery is unusual in that it is the only artery in the body that carries blood deficient in oxygen.

While passing through the lung (pulmonary) capillaries, blood absorbs the oxygen that entered the body during inhalation. The newly oxygenated blood next returns immediately to the heart through **pulmonary veins** [5]. The pulmonary veins are unusual in that they are the only veins in the body that carry oxygen-rich **(oxygenated)** blood. The circulation of blood through the vessels from the heart to the lungs and then back to the heart again is the **pulmonary circulation.**

Oxygen-rich blood enters the **left side of the heart** [6] from the pulmonary veins. The muscles in the left side of the heart pump the blood out of the heart through the largest single artery in the body, the **aorta** [7]. The aorta moves up at first (ascending aorta) but then arches over dorsally and runs downward (descending aorta) just in front of the vertebral column. The aorta divides into numerous branches called **arteries** [8] that carry the oxygenated blood to all parts of the body. The names of some of these arterial branches will be familiar to you: brachial (brachi/o means arm), axillary, splenic, gastric, and renal arteries. The **carotid** arteries supply blood to the head and neck.

The relatively large arterial vessels branch further to form smaller **arterioles** [9]. The arterioles, still containing oxygenated blood, branch into smaller **tissue capillaries** [10], which are near the body cells. Oxygen leaves the blood and passes through the thin capillary walls to enter the body cells. There, food is broken down, in the presence of oxygen, and energy is released.

This chemical process also releases **carbon dioxide (CO₂)** as a waste product. Carbon dioxide passes out from the cell into the tissue capillaries at the same time that oxygen enters. Thus the blood returning to the heart from tissue capillaries through **venules** [11] and **veins** [12] is filled with carbon dioxide but is depleted of oxygen.

As this oxygen-poor blood enters the heart from the venae cavae, the circuit is complete. The pathway of blood from the heart to the tissue capillaries and back to the heart is the **systemic circulation.**

Figure 11–4 shows the aorta, selected arteries, and pulse points (beat of the heart as felt through the walls of arteries).

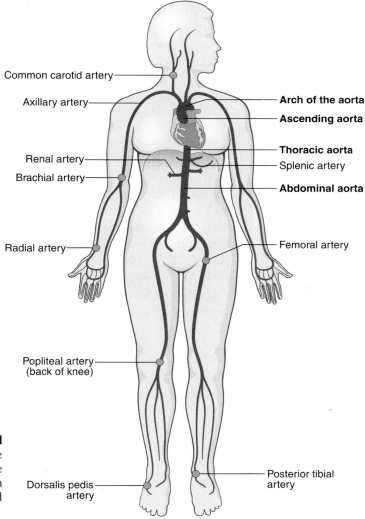

FIGURE 11–4 The aorta and arteries. *Solid gold dots* indicate **pulse points** in arteries. These are areas in which the pulse (expansion and contraction of a superficial artery) can be felt.

ANATOMY OF THE HEART

The human heart weighs less than a pound, is roughly the size of an adult fist, and lies in the thoracic cavity, just behind the breastbone in the mediastinum (between the lungs).

The heart is a pump, consisting of four chambers: two upper chambers called **atria** (*singular:* **atrium**) and two lower chambers called **ventricles.** It is actually a double pump, bound into one organ and synchronized very carefully. Blood passes through each pump in a definite pattern. Pump station number one, on the right side of the heart, sends oxygen-deficient blood to the lungs, where the blood picks up oxygen and releases its carbon dioxide. The newly oxygenated blood returns to the left side of the heart to pump station number two and does not mix with the oxygen-poor blood in pump station number one. Pump station number two then forces the oxygenated blood out to all parts of the body. At the body tissues, the blood loses its oxygen, and on returning to the heart, to pump station number one, blood poor in oxygen (rich in carbon dioxide) is sent out to the lungs to begin the cycle anew.

Label Figure 11–5 as you learn the names of the parts of the heart and the vessels that carry blood to and from it.

Oxygen-poor blood enters the heart through the two largest veins in the body, the **venae cavae.** The **superior vena cava** [1] drains blood from the upper portion of the body, and the **inferior vena cava** [2] carries blood from the lower part of the body.

The venae cavae bring oxygen-poor blood that has passed through all of the body to the **right atrium** [3], the thin-walled upper right chamber of the heart. The right atrium contracts to force blood through the **tricuspid valve** [4] (cusps are the flaps of the valves) into the **right ventricle** [5], the lower right chamber of the heart. The cusps of the tricuspid valve form a one-way passage designed to keep the blood flowing in only one direction. As the right ventricle contracts to pump oxygen-poor blood through the **pulmonary valve** [6] into the **pulmonary artery** [7], the tricuspid valve stays shut, thus preventing blood from pushing back into the right atrium. The pulmonary artery then branches to carry oxygen-deficient blood to each lung.

The blood that enters the lung capillaries from the pulmonary artery soon loses its large quantity of carbon dioxide into the lung tissue, and the carbon dioxide is expelled. At the same time, oxygen enters the capillaries of the lungs and is brought back to the heart via the **pulmonary veins** [8]. The newly oxygenated blood enters the **left atrium** [9] of the heart from the pulmonary veins. The walls of the left atrium contract to force blood through the **mitral valve** [10] into the **left ventricle** [11].

The left ventricle has the thickest walls of all four heart chambers (three times the thickness of the right ventricular wall). It must pump blood with great force so that the blood travels through arteries to all parts of the body. The left ventricle propels the blood through the **aortic valve** [12] into the **aorta** [13], which branches to carry blood all over the body. The aortic valve closes to prevent return of aortic blood to the left ventricle.

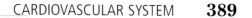

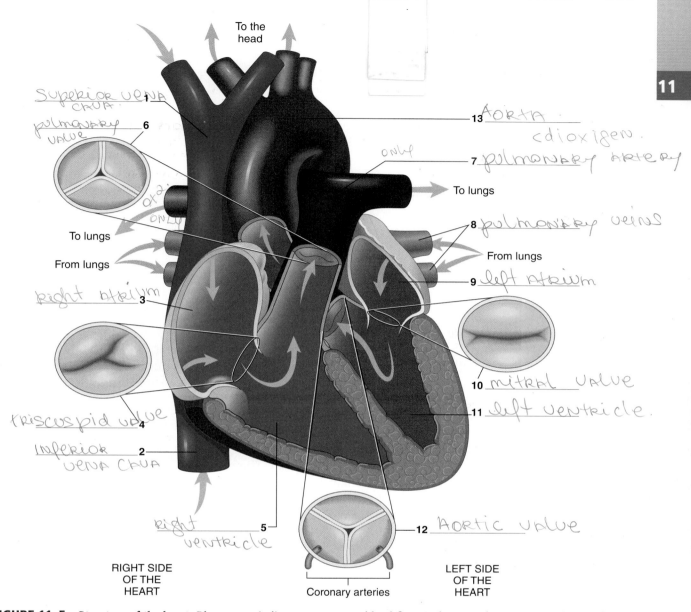

To the
head

SUPERIOR VENA CAVA — 1

pulmonary VALUE — 6

13 — AORTA
cdioxigen.

oxy
only

To lungs

From lungs

right atrium 3 —

7 — pulmonary artery
To lungs

8 — pulmonary veins
From lungs

9 — left Atrium

right — 5
ventricle

triscuspid value 4 —

INFERIOR VENA CAVA — 2

10 — mitral value

11 — left ventricle

12 — AORTIC value

RIGHT SIDE
OF THE
HEART

Coronary arteries

LEFT SIDE
OF THE
HEART

FIGURE 11–5 **Structure of the heart.** *Blue arrows* indicate oxygen-poor blood flow. *Red arrows* show oxygenated blood flow.

septum
(musc. sep/ right/left

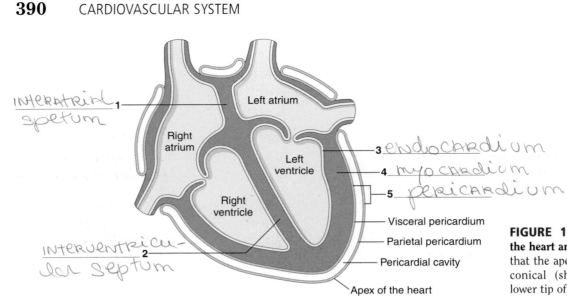

INTERATRIAL
SPETUM 1

INTERVENTRICU-
lar septum 2

3 endocARdium
4 myocHardium
5 periCARdium

FIGURE 11–6 **The walls of the heart and pericardium.** Note that the apex of the heart is the conical (shaped like a cone) lower tip of the heart.

In Figure 11–6 notice that the four chambers of the heart are separated by partitions called **septa** (*singular:* **septum**). (Label Fig. 11–6 as you read these paragraphs.) The **interatrial septum** [1] separates the two upper chambers (atria), and the **interventricular septum** [2], a muscular wall, comes between the two lower chambers (ventricles).

Figure 11–6 shows the three layers of the heart. The **endocardium** [3], a smooth layer of endothelial cells, lines the interior of the heart and heart valves. The **myocardium** [4], the middle, muscular layer of the heart wall, is its thickest layer. The **pericardium** [5], a fibrous and membranous sac, surrounds the heart. It is composed of two layers, the **visceral pericardium,** adhering to the heart, and the **parietal** (parietal means wall) **pericardium,** lining the outer fibrous coat. The **pericardial cavity** (between the visceral and the parietal pericardia) normally contains 10 to 15 mL of pericardial fluid, which lubricates the membranes as the heart beats.

Figure 11–7 reviews the pathway of blood through the heart.

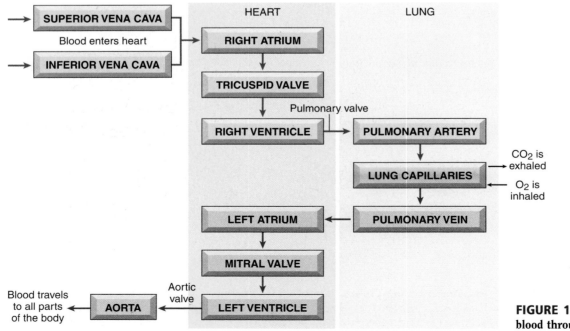

FIGURE 11–7 Pathway of blood through the heart.

PHYSIOLOGY OF THE HEART

HEARTBEAT AND HEART SOUNDS

There are two phases of the heartbeat: **diastole** (relaxation) and **systole** (contraction). Diastole occurs when the ventricle walls relax and blood flows into the heart from the venae cavae and the pulmonary veins. The tricuspid and mitral valves open in diastole, as blood passes from the right and left atria into the ventricles. The pulmonary and aortic valves close during diastole (Fig. 11–8).

Systole occurs next, as the walls of the right and left ventricles contract to pump blood into the pulmonary artery and the aorta. Both the tricuspid and the mitral valves are closed during systole, thus preventing the flow of blood back into the atria (see Fig. 11–8).

This diastole-systole cardiac cycle occurs between 70 and 80 times per minute (100,000 times a day). The heart pumps about 3 ounces of blood with each contraction. This means that about 5 quarts of blood are pumped by the heart in 1 minute (75 gallons an hour and about 2000 gallons a day).

Closure of the heart valves is associated with audible sounds, such as "lubb-dubb," which can be heard on listening to a normal heart with a stethoscope. The "lubb" is associated with closure of the tricuspid and mitral valves at the beginning of systole, and the "dubb" with the closure of the aortic and pulmonary valves at the end of systole. The "lubb" sound is called the first heart sound (S_1) and the "dubb" is the second heart sound (S_2) because the normal cycle of the heartbeat starts with the beginning of systole. An abnormal heart sound is known as a **murmur.**

CONDUCTION SYSTEM OF THE HEART

What keeps the heart at its perfect rhythm? Although the heart has nerves that affect its rate, they are not primarily responsible for its beat. The heart starts beating in the embryo before it is supplied with nerves, and continues to beat in experimental animals even when the nerve supply is cut.

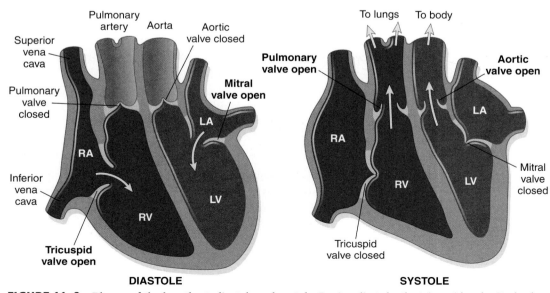

FIGURE 11–8   Phases of the heartbeat: diastole and systole. During diastole, the tricuspid and mitral valves are open as blood enters the ventricles. During systole, the pulmonary and aortic valves are open as blood is pumped to the pulmonary artery and aorta. LA = left atrium; LV = left ventricle; RA = right atrium; RV = right ventricle.

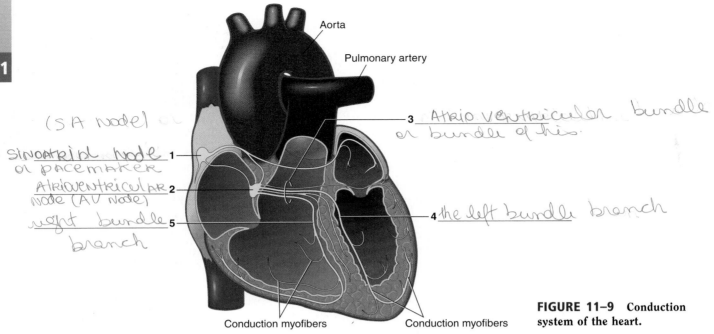

Aorta

Pulmonary artery

3 Atrio ventricular bundle or bundle of his.

(SA node)

sinoatrial node 1 or pacemaker

Atrioventricular 2 node (AV node)

right bundle 5 branch

4 the left bundle branch

Conduction myofibers   Conduction myofibers

FIGURE 11-9 **Conduction system of the heart.**

Label Figure 11–9 as you read the following. Primary responsibility for initiating the heartbeat rests with a small region of specialized muscle tissue in the posterior portion of the right atrium, where an electrical impulse originates. This is the **sinoatrial node (SA node) or pacemaker** [1] of the heart. The current of electricity generated by the pacemaker causes the walls of the atria to contract and force blood into the ventricles.

Almost like ripples in a pond of water when a stone is thrown, the wave of electricity passes from the pacemaker to another region of the myocardium. This region is within the interatrial septum and is the **atrioventricular node (AV node)** [2]. The AV node immediately sends the excitation wave to a bundle of specialized muscle fibers called the **atrioventricular bundle,** or **bundle of His** [3]. Within the interventricular septum, the bundle of His divides into **the left bundle branch** [4] and **right bundle branch** [5], which form the conduction myofibers that extend through the ventricle walls and stimulate them to contract. Thus systole occurs and blood is pumped away from the heart. A short rest period follows, and then the pacemaker begins the wave of excitation across the heart again.

The record used to detect these electrical changes in heart muscle as the heart beats is an **electrocardiogram** (ECG or EKG, from the Greek root *kardia*). The normal ECG shows five waves, or **deflections,** that represent the electrical changes as a wave of excitation spreads through the heart. The deflections are called **P, QRS,** and **T** waves. Figure 11–10 illustrates P, QRS, and T waves in a normal ECG.

Heart rhythm (originating in the SA node and traveling through the heart) is called **normal sinus rhythm (NSR).** Sympathetic nerves speed up the heart rate during conditions of emotional stress or vigorous exercise. Parasympathetic nerves slow the heart rate when there is no need for extra pumping.

BLOOD PRESSURE

Blood pressure is the force that the blood exerts on the arterial walls. This pressure is measured with a **sphygmomanometer.** See Figure 11–11.

The sphygmomanometer consists of a rubber bag inside a cloth cuff that is wrapped around the upper arm, just above the elbow. The rubber bag is inflated with air using a

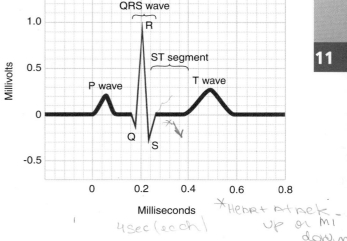

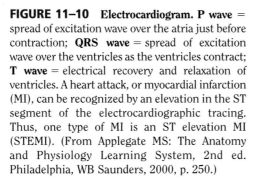

FIGURE 11–10 **Electrocardiogram. P wave** = spread of excitation wave over the atria just before contraction; **QRS wave** = spread of excitation wave over the ventricles as the ventricles contract; **T wave** = electrical recovery and relaxation of ventricles. A heart attack, or myocardial infarction (MI), can be recognized by an elevation in the ST segment of the electrocardiographic tracing. Thus, one type of MI is an ST elevation MI (STEMI). (From Applegate MS: The Anatomy and Physiology Learning System, 2nd ed. Philadelphia, WB Saunders, 2000, p. 250.)

4 sec (each)

Heart Attack - up or MI down

hand bulb pump. As the bag is pumped up, the pressure within it increases and is measured on a recording device attached to the cuff.

The brachial artery in the upper arm is compressed by the air pressure in the bag. When there is sufficient air pressure in the bag to stop the flow of blood, the pulse in the lower arm (where the observer is listening with a stethoscope) drops.

Air is then allowed to escape from the bag and the pressure is lowered slowly, allowing the blood to begin to make its way through the gradually opening artery. At the point when the person listening with the stethoscope first hears the sounds of the pulse beats, the reading on the device attached to the cuff shows the higher, systolic, blood pressure (pressure in the artery when the left ventricle is contracting to force the blood into the aorta and other arteries).

As air continues to escape, the sounds become progressively louder. Finally, when a change in sound from loud to soft occurs, the observer makes note of the pressure on the recording device. This is the diastolic blood pressure (pressure in the artery when the ventricles relax and the heart fills, receiving blood from the venae cavae and pulmonary veins).

Blood pressure is expressed as a fraction; for example, 120/80, in which the upper (120) is the systolic pressure and the lower number (80) is the diastolic pressure.

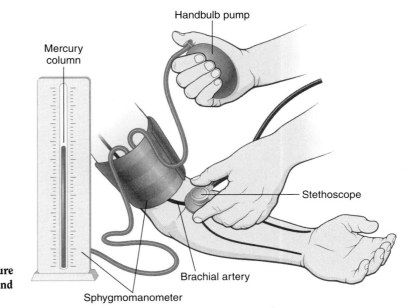

FIGURE 11–11
Measurement of blood pressure with a sphygmomanometer and stethoscope.

VOCABULARY

This list reviews new terms introduced in the text. Short definitions reinforce your understanding of the terms. See page 431 of this chapter for pronunciation of terms.

aorta	Largest artery in the body.
arteriole	Small artery.
artery	Largest type of blood vessel; carries blood away from the heart to all parts of the body. Notice that artery and away begin with an a.
atrioventricular bundle (bundle of His)	Specialized muscle fibers connecting the atria with the ventricles and transmitting electrical impulses between them. His is pronounced as "hiss."
atrioventricular node (AV node)	Specialized tissue in the wall between the atria. Electrical impulses pass from the pacemaker (SA node) through the AV node and the atrioventricular bundle or bundle of His toward the ventricles.
atrium (*plural:* **atria**)	One of two upper chambers of the heart.
capillary	Smallest blood vessel. Materials pass to and from the bloodstream through the thin capillary walls.
carbon dioxide (CO_2)	Gas (waste) released by body cells, transported via veins to the heart, and then to the lungs for exhalation.
coronary arteries	Blood vessels that branch from the aorta and carry oxygen-rich blood to the heart muscle.
deoxygenated blood	Blood that is oxygen-poor.
diastole	Relaxation phase of the heartbeat. From the Greek *diastole*, dilation.
electrocardiogram	Record of the electricity flowing through the heart. The electricity is represented by waves or deflections called P, QRS, or T.
endocardium	Inner lining of the heart.
endothelium	Innermost lining of blood vessels.
mitral valve	Valve between the left atrium and the left ventricle; bicuspid valve.
murmur	Abnormal heart sound caused by improper closure of the heart valves.
myocardium	Muscular, middle layer of the heart.
normal sinus rhythm	Heart rhythm originating in the sinoatrial node with a resting rate of 60 to 100 beats per minute.
oxygen	Gas that enters the blood through the lungs and travels to the heart to be pumped via arteries to all body cells.
pacemaker (sinoatrial node)	Specialized nervous tissue in the right atrium that begins the heartbeat. An artificial cardiac pacemaker is an electronic apparatus implanted in the chest to stimulate heart muscle that is weak and not functioning.
pericardium	Double-layered membrane surrounding the heart.
pulmonary artery	Artery carrying oxygen-poor blood from the heart to the lungs.
pulmonary circulation	Flow of blood from the heart to the lungs and back to the heart.
pulmonary valve	Valve positioned between the right ventricle and the pulmonary artery.

pulmonary vein	One of two pairs of vessels carrying oxygenated blood from the lungs to the left atrium of the heart.
pulse	Beat of the heart as felt through the walls of the arteries.
septum (*plural:* **septa**)	Partition or wall dividing a cavity; such as between the right and left atria (interatrial septum) and right and left ventricles (interventricular septum).
sinoatrial node (SA node)	Pacemaker of the heart.
sphygmomanometer	Instrument to measure blood pressure.
systemic circulation	Flow of blood from body tissue to the heart and then from the heart back to body tissues.
systole	Contraction phase of the heartbeat. From the Greek *systole*, a contracting.
tricuspid valve	Located between the right atrium and the right ventricle; it has three (tri-) leaflets, or cusps.
valve	Structure in veins or in the heart that temporarily closes an opening so that blood flows in only one direction.
vein	Thin-walled vessel that carries blood from body tissues and lungs back to the heart. Veins contain valves to prevent backflow of blood.
vena cava (*plural:* **venae cavae**)	Largest vein in the body. The superior and inferior venae cavae return blood to the right atrium of the heart.
ventricle	One of two lower chambers of the heart.
venule	Small vein.

COMBINING FORMS AND TERMINOLOGY

Write the meaning of the medical term in the space provided.

Combining Form	Meaning	Terminology	Meaning
angi/o	vessel	angiogram	record – vessel *[handwritten]*
		angioplasty	Surgical repairing of vessel *[handwritten]*
aort/o	aorta	aortic stenosis	tightening the aorta. *[handwritten]*
arter/o, arteri/o	artery	arteriosclerosis	hardening of arteries *[handwritten]*
		arterial anastomosis *From the Greek* anastomoien, *to provide a mouth.*	New connection between arteries *[handwritten]*
		arteriography	x-ray imaging of blood after injection of contrast material *[handwritten]*
		endarterectomy *See page 414.*	Surgical removal of plaque from the inner layer of an artery *[handwritten]*

[handwritten bottom note] -graphy – process of recording

11

Combining Form	Meaning	Terminology	Meaning
ather/o	yellowish plaque, fatty substance (Greek *athere* means porridge)	atheroma	*mass of yellowish plaque* (handwritten)
		The suffix -oma means mass or collection. Atheromas are collections of plaque that protrude into the **lumen** (opening) of an artery, weakening the muscle lining.	
		atherosclerosis	
		The major form of arteriosclerosis in which deposits of yellow plaque (atheromas) containing cholesterol and lipids are found within the lining of the artery. See Figure 11–12.	
		atherectomy	
atri/o	atrium, upper heart chamber	atrial	
		atrioventricular	
brachi/o	arm	brachial artery	
cardi/o	heart	cardiomegaly	*enlargement of the heart* (handwritten)
		cardiomyopathy	*disease cond. of heart muscle* (handwritten)
		Toxic or infectious agents may be the cause, but often the etiology is unknown (idiopathic). **Hypertrophic cardiomyopathy** is abnormal thickening of heart walls (septa), which causes narrowing (stenosis) of the aortic valve.	
		bradycardia	*cond. slow heart beat* (handwritten)
		Slower than 60 beats per minute. Normal pulse is about 60 to 80 beats per minute.	
		tachycardia	*cond. of rapid heart beat* (handwritten)
		Faster than 100 beats per minute.	
		cardiogenic shock	
		Results from failure of the heart in its pumping action. **Shock** is circulatory failure associated with inadequate delivery of oxygen and nutrients to body tissues.	

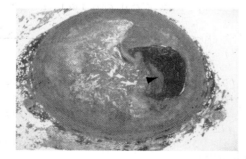

FIGURE 11–12 Atherosclerosis. *Arrow* points to accumulated plaque in lumen of an artery. (From Kumar V, Cotran RS, Robbins SL: Robbins Basic Pathology, 6th ed., Philadelphia, WB Saunders, 1997; courtesy Sid Murphree, MD, Department of Pathology, University of Texas Southwestern Medical School.)

Combining Form	Meaning	Terminology	Meaning
cholesterol/o	cholesterol (a lipid substance)	hypercholesterolemia *High levels of cholesterol in the blood.*	
coron/o	heart	coronary arteries ___ *These arteries come down over the top of the heart like a crown (corona); see Figure 11-22, A, page 411.*	
cyan/o	blue	cyanosis *deficient oxygen in the blood.* *This bluish discoloration of the skin indicates diminished oxygen content of the blood.*	
myx/o	mucus	myxoma ___ *A benign tumor derived from connective tissue, with cells embedded in soft mucoid stromal tissue. These tumors occur most frequently in the left atrium.*	
ox/o	oxygen	hypoxia *deficience of oxygen in tissues* *Inadequate oxygen in tissues.* **Anoxia** *is absence of oxygen in tissues.*	
pericardi/o	pericardium	pericardiocentesis *surgical puncture to remove fluids from the pericardium*	
phleb/o	vein	phlebotomy ___ *A phlebotomist is trained in opening veins for phlebotomy.*	
		thrombophlebitis *clot of veins inflammation* *Also called phlebitis.*	
sphygm/o	pulse	sphygmomanometer *to measure blood pressure* *A manometer measures pressure.*	
steth/o	chest	stethoscope ___ *A misnomer because the examination is by ear, not by eye.* **Auscultation** *means listening to sounds within the body, typically using a stethoscope.*	
thromb/o	clot	thrombolysis *breakdown of the clot vein*	
valvul/o, valv/o	valve	valvuloplasty *surgical repair of the valve* *A balloon-tipped catheter dilates a cardiac valve.*	
		mitral valvulitis *inflammation of mitral valve.* *Most commonly caused by rheumatic fever.*	
		valvotomy *surgical of the vein*	
vas/o	vessel	vasoconstriction *narrowing of the vessel* *Constriction means to tighten or narrow.*	
		vasodilation *dilatation of the vein*	
vascul/o	vessel	vascular *pertaining to the vessel*	

Hypo- below

11

Combining Form	Meaning	Terminology	Meaning
ven/o, ven/i	vein	venous _____	
		A venous cutdown is a small surgical incision to permit access to a collapsed vein. An intravenous infusion is delivery of fluids into a vein.	
		venipuncture _____	
		This procedure is performed for phlebotomy or to start an intravenous infusion.	
ventricul/o	ventricle, lower heart chamber	interventricular septum _____	

PATHOLOGY: THE HEART AND BLOOD VESSELS

HEART   *problem*

arrhythmias
same

Abnormal heart rhythms (dysrhythmias).

Arrhythmias are problems with the conduction or electrical system of the heart. More than 4 million Americans have recurrent cardiac arrhythmias.

Examples of cardiac arrhythmias are:

1. **bradycardia and heart block (atrioventricular block)**

sino atrial

Failure of proper conduction of impulses from the SA node through the AV node to the atrioventricular bundle (bundle of His).

AtriumoENtriculAR

Damage to the SA node may cause its impulses to be too weak to activate the AV node and impulses fail to reach the ventricles. The heart beats slowly and bradycardia results. If the failure occurs only occasionally, the heart misses a beat in a rhythm at regular intervals (partial heart block). If no impulses reach the AV node from the SA node, the ventricles contract slower than the atria and are not coordinated. This is complete heart block.

Right and left bundle branch block (RBBB and LBBB) are common types of heart block. They involve delay or failure of impulses traveling through the right and left bundle branches to the ventricles.

Implantation of an artificial **cardiac pacemaker** overcomes arrhythmias and keeps the heart beating at the proper rate. The pacemaker power source is a generator that contains a computer and lithium battery. It is implanted under the skin just below the collarbone, with wires or leads to both chambers, usually on the right side of the heart. A newer type of pacemaker, called a **biventricular pacemaker,** treats delays and abnormalities in ventricular contractions (as in LBBB) and also can improve symptoms of congestive heart failure. See Figure 11–13.

2. **flutter**

Rapid but regular contractions, usually of the atria.

Heart rhythm may reach up to 300 beats per minute. Atrial flutter is often symptomatic of heart disease and frequently requires treatment such as medication, electrical cardioversion or catheter ablation (see below under fibrillation).

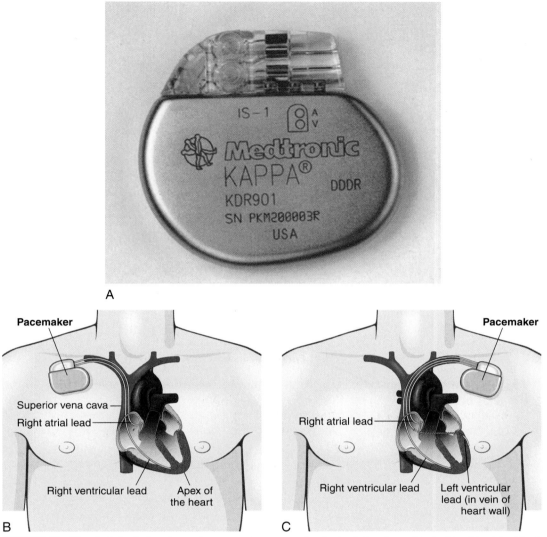

FIGURE 11–13 **A,** A dual-chamber, rate-responsive **pacemaker** (actual size shown) is designed to detect body movement and automatically increase or decrease paced heart rates based on levels of physical activity. **B, Cardiac pacemaker** with leads in both the right atrium and the right ventricle enable it to sense and pace in both heart chambers. **C, Biventricular pacemaker** with leads in the right atrium and the right ventricle and left ventricle to synchronize ventricular contractions. (**A** from Lewis SM, Heitkemper MM, Dirksen SR: Medical-Surgical Nursing, 6th ed., St. Louis, Mosby, 2004, p. 877.)

3. fibrillation	Rapid, random, inefficient, and irregular contractions of the artria and ventricles (350 beats or more per minute).

In **atrial fibrillation** (AF), the most common type of cardiac arrhythmia, electrical impulses move randomly throughout the atria. This causes the atria to quiver instead of contracting in a coordinated rhythm. Common symptoms are **palpitations** (uncomfortable sensations in the chest from missed heartbeats), fatigue, and shortness of breath. Patients with chronic or intermittent AF

Palpitation/Palpation
Don't confuse *palpitations* with *palpation,* which means to touch, feel, or examine with the hands and fingers.

are at risk for stroke because ineffective atrial contractions can lead to the formation of blood clots that may travel to the brain.

In **ventricular fibrillation** (VF), electrical impulses move randomly throughout the ventricles. This life-threatening situation may result in sudden cardiac death or cardiac arrest (sudden stoppage of heart movement) unless help is provided immediately. If treatment is immediate, VF can be interrupted with cardioversion (application of an electrical shock). Cardioversion stops electrical activity in the heart for a brief moment so that normal rhythm takes over. Medications such as **digoxin** can slow the heart rate to treat atrial fibrillation. Other drugs can convert fibrillation to normal sinus rhythm.

An **implantable cardioverter-defibrillator (ICD)** is a small electrical device that is implanted inside the chest (near the collarbone) to sense arrhythmias and terminate them with an electric shock. Candidates for ICDs are people who have had or are at high risk for having ventricular tachycardia, fibrillation, and cardiac arrest. **Automatic external defibrillators (AEDs)** may be found in airports and public places and are used in an emergency situation to reverse ventricular fibrillation.

Radiofrequency catheter ablation (RFA) is a minimally invasive treatment to treat cardiac arrhythmias. The technique, using radiofrequency energy delivered from the tip of a catheter inserted through a blood vessel and into the heart, destroys tissue that causes arrhythmias. This is a relatively low-risk procedure that provides a permanent cure in most situations.

congenital heart disease   **Abnormalities in the heart at birth.**

The following conditions are congenital anomalies resulting from some failure in the development of the fetal heart.

1. coarctation of the aorta (CoA)   **Narrowing (coarctation) of the aorta.**

Figure 11–14, *A*, shows coarctation of the aorta. Surgical treatment consists of removal of the constricted region and end-to-end anastomosis of the aortic segments.

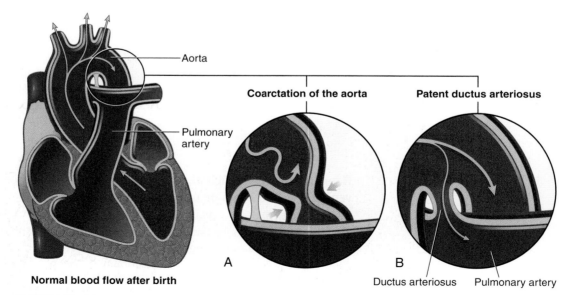

FIGURE 11–14   A, Coarctation of the aorta. Localized narrowing of the aorta reduces the supply of blood to the lower part of the body. **B, Patent ductus arteriosus.** The ductus arteriosus fails to close after birth, and blood from the aorta flows through it into the pulmonary artery.

2. patent ductus arteriosus (PDA)

A duct (ductus arteriosus) between the aorta and the pulmonary artery, which normally closes soon after birth, remains open (patent).

This condition, illustrated in Figure 11–14, *B*, results in the flow of oxygenated blood from the aorta into the pulmonary artery. PDA occurs in premature infants, causing cyanosis, fatigue, and rapid breathing. Although the defect often closes on its own within months after birth, treatment may be necessary if patency continues. Treatments include use of a drug (indomethacin) to promote closure; surgery via catheterization (with coil embolization to "plug" the ductus); and ligation (tying off) via a small incision between the ribs.

3. septal defects

Small holes in the septa between the atria (atrial septal defects) or the ventricles (ventricular septal defects). Figure 11–15, *A*, shows a ventricular septal defect.

Although many septal defects close spontaneously, others require open heart surgery to close the hole between heart chambers. Septal defects are closed while maintaining a general circulation by means of a **heart-lung machine.** This machine, connected to the patient's circulatory system, relieves the heart and lungs of pumping and oxygenation functions during heart surgery.

Alternatively, septal defects may be repaired with a less invasive catheter technique using a device (Amplatzer device) in the defect to close it.

4. tetralogy of Fallot (fă-LŌ)

A congenital malformation of the heart involving four (tetra-) distinct defects.

The condition, named for Etienne Fallot, the French physician who described it in 1888, is illustrated in Figure 11–15, *B*. The four defects are:

1. **Pulmonary artery stenosis.** Pulmonary artery is narrow or obstructed.
2. **Ventricular septal defect.** Large hole between two ventricles lets venous blood pass from the right to the left ventricle and out to the aorta without oxygenation.
3. **Shift of the aorta to the right.** Aorta overrides the interventricular septum. Oxygen-poor blood passes from the right ventricle to the aorta.
4. **Hypertrophy of the right ventricle.** Myocardium works harder to pump blood through a narrowed pulmonary artery.

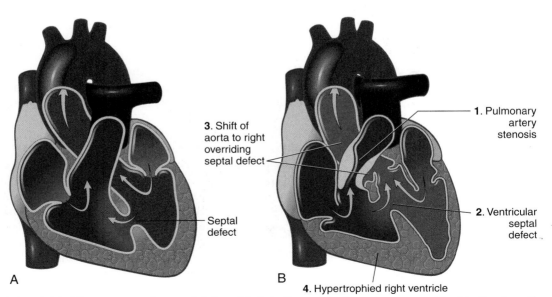

3. Shift of aorta to right overriding septal defect

Septal defect

A

1. Pulmonary artery stenosis

2. Ventricular septal defect

4. Hypertrophied right ventricle

B

FIGURE 11–15 **A, Ventricular septal defect.** A hole in the ventricular septum causes blood to flow from the left ventricle to the right and into the lungs via the pulmonary artery. **B, Tetralogy of Fallot** showing the four defects. The flow of blood is indicated by the *arrows*.

An infant with this condition is described as a "blue baby" because of the extreme degree of **cyanosis** present at birth. Surgery for tetralogy of Fallot includes a patch closure of the ventricular septal defect and removing obstruction to the outflow at the pulmonary artery.

Other congenital conditions such as **transposition of the great arteries (TGA)** (pulmonary artery arises from the left ventricle and the aorta from the right ventricle) cause cyanosis and hypoxia as well. Surgical correction of TGA involves an arterial switch procedure (pulmonary artery and aorta are reconnected in their proper positions).

congestive heart failure (CHF)   **The heart is unable to pump its required amount of blood (more blood enters the heart from the veins than leaves through the arteries).**

Blood accumulates in the lungs (left-sided heart failure) causing **pulmonary edema** (fluid seeps out of capillaries into the tiny air sacs of the lungs). Damming back of blood resulting from right-sided heart failure results in accumulation of fluid in the abdominal organs (liver and spleen) and subcutaneous tissue of the legs.

Symptoms of CHF include shortness of breath (SOB), fatigue, and exercise intolerance. The most common causes of CHF in the United States are high blood pressure and coronary artery disease. Therapy includes lowering dietary intake of sodium and diuretics to promote loss of fluids.

Digoxin and other drugs such as **angiotensin-converting enzyme (ACE) inhibitors** and **beta-blockers** improve the performance of the heart and its pumping activity. ACE inhibitors, beta-blockers, and newer angiotensin receptor blockers (ARBs) decrease pressure inside blood vessels to treat hypertension (high blood pressure).

If drug therapy and lifestyle changes fail to control congestive heart failure, heart transplantation may be the only treatment option. While waiting for a transplant, patients may need a device to assist the heart's pumping. A **left ventricular assist device (LVAD)** is a booster pump implanted in the abdomen, with a cannula (tube) inserted into the left ventricle. It pumps blood out of the heart to all parts of the body. LVAD may be used either as a "bridge to transplant" or as a "destination" therapy when heart transplantation is not possible. Because of the severe shortage of donor hearts, research efforts are directed at developing total artificial hearts.

coronary artery disease (CAD)   **Disease of the arteries surrounding the heart.**

The coronary arteries are a pair of blood vessels that arise from the aorta and supply oxygenated blood to the heart. After blood leaves the heart via the aorta, a portion is at once led back over the surface of the heart through the coronary arteries.

CAD usually is the result of **atherosclerosis.** This is the deposition of fatty compounds on the inner lining of the coronary arteries (any other artery can be similarly affected). The ordinarily smooth lining of the artery becomes roughened as the atherosclerotic plaque collects in the artery.

The plaque first causes plugging of the coronary artery. Next, the roughened lining of the artery may rupture or cause abnormal clotting of blood, leading to a **thrombotic occlusion** (blocking of the coronary artery by a clot). Blood flow is decreased **(ischemia)** or stopped entirely, leading to death **(necrosis)** of a part of the myocardium. This sequence of events constitutes a **myocardial infarction,** or heart attack, and the area of dead myocardial tissue is known as an infarct. The infarcted area is eventually replaced by scar tissue. Figure 11–16, *A,* shows coronary arteries branching from the aorta and illustrates coronary artery occlusion leading to ischemia and infarction of heart muscle. Figure 11–17 is a photograph of myocardium after an acute myocardial infarction.

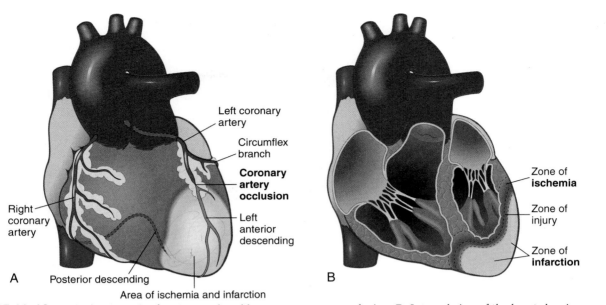

FIGURE 11–16 A, **Ischemia** and **infarction** produced by coronary artery occlusion. **B,** Internal view of the heart showing an area damaged by **myocardial infarction.**

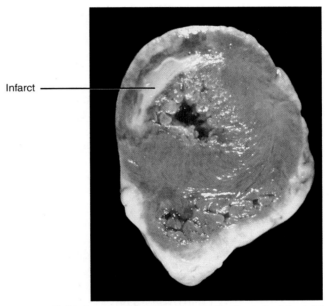

FIGURE 11–17 Acute **myocardial infarction (MI),** 5 to 7 days old. The infarct is visible as a well-demarcated, pale yellow lesion in the posterolateral region of the left ventricle. The border of the infarct is surrounded by a dark red zone of acute inflammation. (From Kumar V, Cotran RS, Robbins SL: Robbins Basic Pathology, 7th ed. Philadelphia, WB Saunders, 2003, p. 369.)

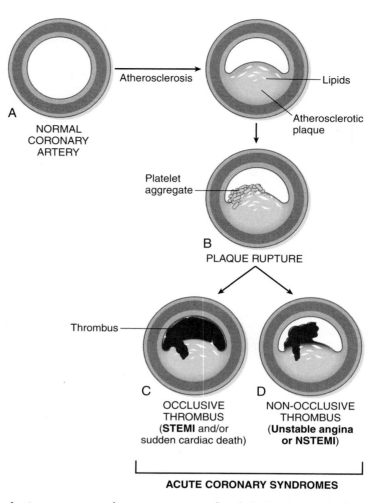

FIGURE 11–18 **Acute coronary syndromes: sequence of pathologic changes leading to cardiac event.** **A,** Plaque formation from lipid collection. **B,** Rupture or erosion of the plaque, causing platelet aggregation on the plaque. **C,** Formation of a thrombus that is occlusive, totally blocks the artery, and produces a **myocardial infarction** (MI) or **ST** segment (on ECG) **E**levation **M**I (STEMI). **D,** Alternatively, a nonocclusive thrombus may form, which causes **unstable angina** (chest pain at rest or with increasing frequency) or NSTEMI (**N**on-**ST E**levation **M**yocardial **I**nfarction).

Acute coronary syndromes (ACSs) are conditions caused by myocardial ischemia. These conditions are **unstable angina** (chest pain at rest or chest pain of increasing frequency) and **myocardial infarction** (see Fig. 11–18).

Patients with ACSs benefit from early angiography (x-ray imaging of coronary arteries) and angioplasty to improve blood flow to the heart muscle (revascularization). Drugs used to treat ACSs are anticoagulants (low-molecular-weight heparin) and antiplatelet agents such as aspirin and clopidogrel (Plavix).

For acute attacks of angina, **nitroglycerin** is given sublingually (under the tongue). This drug, one of several called **nitrates,** is a powerful vasodilator that increases coronary blood flow and lowers blood pressure to decrease the work of the heart.

Physicians advise patients to avoid risk factors such as smoking, obesity, and lack of exercise, and they prescribe effective drugs to prevent CAD and ACSs. These drugs include **aspirin** (to prevent clumping of platelets), **beta-blockers** (to reduce the force and speed of the heartbeat and to lower blood pressure), **ACE inhibitors** (to reduce high blood pressure and the risk of future heart attack even if the patient is not hypertensive), **calcium channel blockers** (to relax muscles in blood vessels), and **statins** (to lower cholesterol levels).

Cardiac surgeons perform an open heart operation called **coronary artery bypass grafting (CABG)** to treat CAD by replacing clogged vessels. Interventional cardiologists perform **percutaneous coronary intervention (PCI),** in which catheterization with balloons and stents opens clogged coronary arteries.

endocarditis	**Inflammation of the inner lining of the heart caused by bacteria (bacterial endocarditis).**

Damage to the heart valves from infection or trauma produces lesions called **vegetations** (resembling cauliflower) that break off into the bloodstream as **emboli** (material that travels through the blood). The emboli lodge in other vessels, leading to a transient ischemic attack (TIA), or stroke, or in small vessels of the skin, where multiple pinpoint hemorrhages known as **petechiae** (from the Italian *petechio*, a fleabite) form. Antibiotics can cure bacterial endocarditis.

hypertensive heart disease	**High blood pressure affecting the heart.**

This condition results from narrowing of arterioles, which leads to increased pressure in arteries. The heart is affected (left ventricular hypertrophy) because it pumps more vigorously to overcome the increased resistance in the arteries.

mitral valve prolapse (MVP)	**Improper closure of the mitral valve.**

This condition occurs because the mitral valve enlarges and prolapses into the left atrium during systole. The physician hears a midsystolic click on **auscultation** (listening with a stethoscope). Most people with MVP live normal lives, but because prolapsed valves can on rare occasions become infected, persons with MVP are advised to have preventive antibiotics at the time of dental procedures if the murmur is present.

murmur	**An extra heart sound, heard between normal beats.**

Murmurs are heard with the aid of a stethoscope and usually are caused by a valvular defect or disease that disrupts the smooth flow of blood in the heart. They also are heard in cases of interseptal defects, in which blood flows abnormally between chambers through holes in the septa. Functional murmurs are not caused by valve or septal defects and do not seriously endanger a person's health.

A **bruit** (brū-Ē) is an abnormal sound or murmur heard on auscultation. A **thrill,** which is a vibration felt on palpation of the chest, often accompanies a murmur.

pericarditis	**Inflammation of the membrane (pericardium) surrounding the heart.**

In most instances, pericarditis results from disease elsewhere in the body (such as pulmonary infection). Bacteria and viruses cause the condition, or the etiology may be idiopathic. Malaise, fever, and chest pain occur, and auscultation with a stethoscope often reveals a pericardial friction rub (heard as a scraping or grating sound). Compression of the heart caused by collection of fluid in the pericardial cavity is **cardiac tamponade** (tăm-pō-NŎD). Treatment includes anti-inflammatory drugs and other agents to manage pain. If the pericarditis is infective, antibiotics or antifungals are prescribed, depending on the microorganisms detected in specimens obtained by pericardiocentesis.

11

rheumatic heart disease	**Heart disease caused by rheumatic fever.**

Rheumatic fever is a childhood disease that follows after a streptococcal infection. The heart valves can be damaged by inflammation and scarred (with **vegetations**), so that they do not open and close normally (see Fig. 11–19, *A*). **Mitral stenosis,** atrial fibrillation, and congestive heart failure, caused by weakening of the myocardium, also can result from rheumatic heart disease. Treatment consists of reduced activity, drugs to control arrhythmia, surgery to repair a damaged valve, and anticoagulant therapy to prevent emboli from forming. Artificial and porcine (pig) valve implants can replace deteriorated heart valves (Figure 11–19, *B* and *C*).

BLOOD VESSELS

aneurysm	**Local widening (dilation) of an arterial wall.**

An aneurysm (Greek, *aneurysma*, widening) usually is caused by atherosclerosis and hypertension or a congenital weakness in the vessel wall. Aneurysms are common in the aorta but may occur in peripheral vessels as well. The danger of an aneurysm is rupture and hemorrhage. Treatment depends on the vessel involved, the site, and the health of the patient. In aneurysms of small vessels in the brain **(berry aneurysms),** treatment is occlusion of the vessel with small clips. For larger arteries, such as the aorta, the aneurysm is resected and a synthetic graft is sewn within the affected vessel. Figure 11–20, *A*, shows an abdominal aortic aneurysm, and Figure 11–20, *B*, illustrates a synthetic graft in place. Stent grafts also may be placed less invasively as an alternative to surgery in some patients.

deep vein thrombosis (DVT)	**A blood clot (thrombus) forms in a large vein, usually in a lower limb.**

This condition may result in a **pulmonary embolism** (clot travels to the lung) if not treated effectively. Anticoagulants (blood-thinning drugs) such as heparin are used to prevent pulmonary emboli.

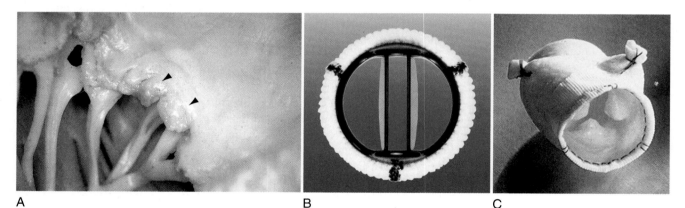

A   B   C

FIGURE 11–19 **A, Acute rheumatic mitral valvulitis with chronic rheumatic heart disease.** Small vegetations are visible along the line of closure of the mitral valve leaflet *(arrows)*. Previous episodes of rheumatic valvulitis have caused fibrous thickening and fusion of the chordae tendineae of the valves. **B, Artificial heart valve. C, Porcine xenograft valve.** A xenograft valve (Greek *xen/o* means stranger) is tissue that is transferred from an animal of one species (pig) to one of another species (human). (**A** from Kumar V, Cotran RS, Robbins SL: Basic Pathology, 7th ed. Philadelphia, WB Saunders, 2003, p. 377. **B** and **C** from Lewis SM, Heitkemper MM, Dirksen SR: Medical-Surgical Nursing: Assessment and Management of Clinical Problems, 6th ed. St. Louis, Mosby, 2004, p. 906.)

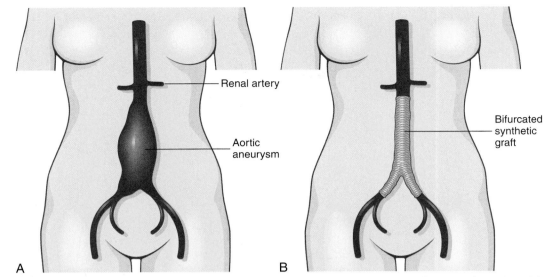

FIGURE 11–20 **A, Abdominal aortic aneurysm.** A dissecting aortic aneurysm is splitting or dissection of the wall of the aorta by blood entering a tear or hemorrhage within the walls of the vessel. **B, Bifurcated synthetic graft** in place.

hypertension (HTN)

High blood pressure.

Most high blood pressure is **essential hypertension,** with no identifiable cause. In adults, a blood pressure of 140/90 mm Hg or greater is considered high. Diuretics, beta-blockers, ACE inhibitors, and calcium channel blockers are used to treat essential hypertension. Losing weight, limiting sodium (salt) intake, stopping smoking, and reducing fat in the diet also can reduce blood pressure.

In **secondary hypertension,** the increase in pressure is caused by another associated lesion, such as glomerulonephritis, pyelonephritis, or disease of the adrenal glands.

peripheral vascular disease (PVD)

Blockage of blood vessels outside the heart.

Any artery can be affected, such as the carotid (neck), **femoral** (thigh), and **popliteal** (back of the knee). A sign of PVD in the lower extremities is **intermittent claudication** (absence of pain or discomfort in a leg at rest, but pain, tension, and weakness after walking has begun). Treatment is exercise, avoidance of nicotine (which causes vessel constriction), and control of risk factors such as hypertension, hyperlipidemia, and diabetes. Surgical treatment includes endarterectomy and bypass grafting (from the normal proximal vessel around the diseased area to a normal vessel distally).

Percutaneous treatments include balloon angioplasty, atherectomy, and stenting. **Embolic protection devices** are parachute-like filters used to capture embolic debris during stenting.

Raynaud (rā-NŌ) disease

Recurrent episodes of pallor and cyanosis primarily in fingers and toes.

Of uncertain cause, this disorder is marked by intense constriction and vasospasm of arterioles often of young, otherwise healthy women and may be secondary to some other, more serious problem. Episodes can be triggered by cold temperatures, emotional stress, or cigarette smoking. Protecting the body from cold and use of vasodilators are effective treatments.

Raynaud's phenomenon is a similar condition of arterial insufficiency but secondary to arterial narrowing from other conditions, such as atherosclerosis, systemic lupus erythematosus, or scleroderma.

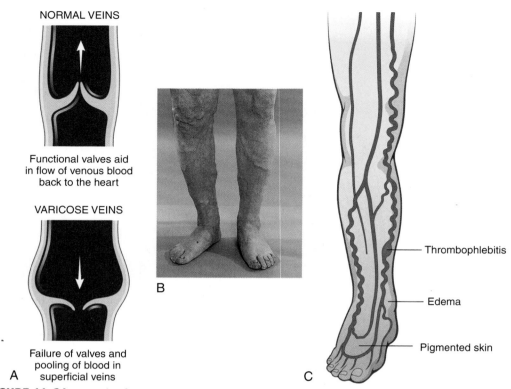

NORMAL VEINS

Functional valves aid
in flow of venous blood
back to the heart

VARICOSE VEINS

Failure of valves and
pooling of blood in
A   superficial veins

B

C

Thrombophlebitis

Edema

Pigmented skin

FIGURE 11–21   A, Valve function in normal vein and varicose vein. **B,** Varicose veins. **C,** The slow flow in veins increases susceptibility to clot formation (**thrombophlebitis**), **edema,** and **pigmented skin** (blood pools in the lower parts of the leg and fluid leaks from distended small capillaries). If a thrombus becomes loosened from its place in the vein, it can travel to the lungs **(pulmonary embolism)** and block a blood vessel there. (**B** from Forbes CD, Jackson WF: Color Atlas and Text of Clinical Medicine, 3rd ed. London, Mosby, 2003.)

varicose veins

Abnormally swollen and twisted veins, usually occurring in the legs.

This condition is caused by damaged valves that fail to prevent the backflow of blood (Fig. 11–21, *A* to *C*). The blood then collects in the veins, which distend to many times their normal size. Because of the slow flow of blood in the varicose veins and frequent injury to the vein, thrombosis may occur as well. **Hemorrhoids** (piles) are varicose veins near the anus.

Physicians now treat varicose veins with sclerotherapy (injections with sclerosing solution) or laser and pulsed-light treatments to seal off veins. Surgical interventions such as vein stripping and ligation are used less frequently.

STUDY SECTION

Practice spelling each term and know its meaning.

acute coronary syndromes	Consequences of plaque rupture in coronary arteries: unstable angina and myocardial infarction.
angina (pectoris)	Chest pain resulting from myocardial ischemia. Stable angina occurs predictably with exertion; unstable angina is chest pain that occurs more often and with less exertion.

angiotensin-converting enzyme (ACE) inhibitor	Antihypertensive drug that blocks the conversion of angiotensin I to angiotensin II and thus dilates blood vessels. It prevents heart attacks, CHF, stroke, and death. See page 864 for names of ACE inhibitors and other cardiovascular drugs.
auscultation	Listening for sounds in blood vessels or other body structures, typically using a stethoscope.
beta-blockers	Drugs used to treat angina, hypertension, and arrhythmias. They block the action of epinephrine (adrenaline) at receptor sites on cells, slowing the heartbeat and reducing the workload on the heart.
biventricular pacemaker	Device enabling ventricles to beat together (in synchrony) so that more blood is pumped out of the heart.
bruit	An abnormal blowing or swishing sound heard during auscultation of an artery or organ.
calcium channel blockers	Drugs used to treat angina and hypertension. They dilate blood vessels by blocking the influx of calcium into muscle cells lining vessels.
cardiac arrest	Sudden, unexpected stopping of heart action; sudden cardiac death.
cardiac tamponade	Pressure on the heart caused by fluid in the pericardial space.
claudication	Pain, tension, and weakness in a leg after walking has begun, but absence of pain at rest.
digoxin	A drug that treats arrhythmias and strengthens the heartbeat.
embolus (pl. **emboli**)	A clot or other substance that travels to a distant location and suddenly blocks a blood vessel.
infarction	Area of dead tissue.
nitrates	Drugs used in the treatment of angina. They dilate blood vessels, increasing blood flow and oxygen to myocardial tissue.
nitroglycerin	A nitrate drug used in the treatment of angina.
occlusion	Closure of a blood vessel.
palpitations	Uncomfortable sensations in the chest related to cardiac arrhythmias, such as premature ventricular contractions (PVCs).
patent	Open.
pericardial friction rub	Scraping or grating noise heard on auscultation of the heart; suggestive of pericarditis.
petechiae	Small, pinpoint hemorrhages.
statins	Drugs used to lower cholesterol in the bloodstream.
thrill	Vibration felt on touching the body over an area of turmoil in blood flow (as a blocked artery).
vegetations	Clumps of platelets, clotting proteins, microorganisms, and red blood cells on the endocardium in conditions such as bacterial endocarditis and rheumatic heart disease.

LABORATORY TESTS AND CLINICAL PROCEDURES

LABORATORY TESTS

11

BNP test	**Measurement of BNP (brain natriuretic peptide) in blood.**
	This test identifies patients at risk for major complications after MI and with CHF. BNP is elevated in CHF. It is secreted when the heart becomes overloaded. It acts like a diuretic to help heart function return to normal.
lipid tests (lipid profile)	**Measurement of cholesterol and triglycerides (fats) in a blood sample.**
	High levels of lipids are associated with atherosclerosis. The National Guideline for total cholesterol in the blood is less than 200 mg/dL. **Saturated fats** (animal origin, such as milk, butter, and meats) increase cholesterol in the blood, whereas **polyunsaturated fats** (of vegetable origin, such as corn and safflower oil) decrease blood cholesterol.
	Treatment of hyperlipidemia includes proper diet (low fat, high fiber intake) and exercise. Niacin (a vitamin) also helps reduce lipids. Drug therapy includes **statins,** which reduce the risk of heart attack, stroke, and cardiovascular death. Statins lower cholesterol by reducing its production in the liver. Examples are simvastatin (Zocor), atorvastatin (Lipitor), and pravastatin (Pravachol).
lipoprotein electrophoresis	**Lipoproteins (combinations of fat and protein) are physically separated in a blood sample.**
	Examples of lipoproteins are **low-density lipoprotein (LDL)** and **high-density lipoprotein (HDL).** High levels of LDL are associated with atherosclerosis. The National Guideline for LDL is less than 130 mg/dL in normal persons and less than 70 mg/dL in patients with CAD, PVD, and diabetes mellitus. High levels of HDL protect adults from atherosclerosis. Factors that increase HDL are estrogen, exercise, and alcohol in moderation.
serum enzyme tests	**Chemicals measured in the blood as evidence of a heart attack.**
	Damaged heart muscle releases enzymes into the bloodstream. The substances tested for are **creatine kinase (CK), troponin-I (cTnI),** and **troponin-T (cTnT).** Troponin is a protein released into circulation after myocardial injury.

CLINICAL PROCEDURES: DIAGNOSTIC

X-Ray and Electron Beam Tests

angiography	**X-ray imaging of blood vessels after injection of contrast material.**
	Arteriography is x-ray imaging of arteries after injection of contrast via a catheter into the aorta or an artery.
computerized tomography angiography (CTA)	**Three-dimensional x-ray images of the heart and coronary arteries using computed tomography (CT) (64-slice CT scanner).**
	This new technique takes 192 images of the heart per second. Cross-sectional images are assembled by computer into a three-dimensional picture. It is less invasive than angioplasty (contrast material is injected into a small peripheral vein with a small needle) and provides spectacular views of the coronary arteries for diagnosis and use in stenting and angioplasty. See Figure 11-22, *A.*
digital subtraction angiography (DSA)	**Video equipment and a computer produce x-ray images of blood vessels.**
	After taking an initial x-ray picture and storing it in a computer, physicians inject contrast material and take a second image of that area. The computer compares

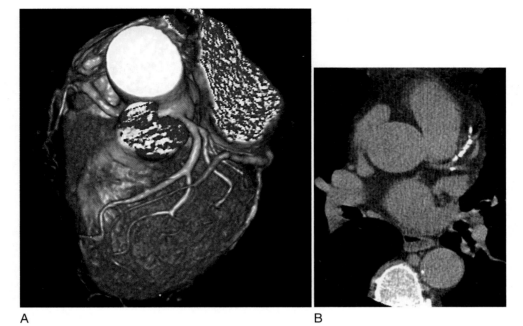

A   B

FIGURE 11–22 A, Computed tomography angiography showing coronary arteries. **B, Electron beam computed tomography** showing significant calcification in the coronary arteries, indicating advanced coronary artery disease. (**A** courtesy Massachusetts General Hospital, Boston; **B** from Crawford MH, DiMarco JP, Paulus WJ: Cardiology, 2nd ed., St. Louis, Mosby, 2004, p. 224.)

the two images and subtracts digital data for the first from the second, leaving an image of vessels with contrast.

electron beam computed tomography (EBCT *or* EBT)	**Electron beams and CT identify calcium deposits in and around coronary arteries to diagnose early CAD.** This new test is faster (called ultrafast CT) than a standard CT scan and takes a clear picture of coronary arteries while the heart is beating. See Figure 11–22, *B*.

Ultrasound Examination

Doppler ultrasound studies	**Sound waves measure movement of blood flow.** An instrument focuses sound waves on blood vessels and echoes bounce off red blood cells. The examiner can hear various alterations in blood flow caused by vessel obstruction. **Duplex ultrasound** combines Doppler and conventional ultrasound to allow physicians to image the structure of blood vessels and measure the speed of blood flow. Carotid artery occlusion, aneurysms, varicose veins, and other vessel disorders can be diagnosed with Duplex ultrasound.
echocardiography (ECHO)	**Echoes generated by high-frequency sound waves produce images of the heart.** ECHOs show the structure and movement of the heart. In **transesophageal echocardiography (TEE),** a transducer placed in the esophagus provides ultrasound and Doppler information. This technique detects cardiac masses, prosthetic valve function, aneurysms, and pericardial fluid.

Nuclear Cardiology

positron emission tomography (PET) scan	**Images show blood flow and myocardial function following uptake of radioactive substances.** PET scanning can detect CAD, myocardial function, and differences between ischemic heart disease and cardiomyopathy.

11

technetium Tc 99m sestamibi scan	**Technetium Tc 99m sestamibi injected intravenously is taken up in cardiac tissue, where it is detected by scanning.**
	This scan is used in persons who have had an MI, to assess the amount of damaged heart muscle. It also is used with an exercise tolerance test **(ETT-MIBI)**. Sestamibi is a radioactive tracer compound used to define areas of poor blood flow in heart muscle.
thallium 201 scan	**Concentration of a radioactive substance is measured in the myocardium.**
	Thallium studies show the viability of heart muscle. Infarcted or scarred myocardium shows up as "cold spots."

Magnetic Resonance Imaging (MRI)

cardiac MRI	**Images of the heart are produced with magnetic waves.**
	These images in multiple planes give information about aneurysms, cardiac output, and patency of peripheral and coronary arteries. The magnetic waves emitted during MRI could interfere with implanted pacemakers because of their metal content, so it is currently contraindicated for a patient with a pacemaker to undergo cardiac MRI. **Magnetic resonance angiography (MRA)** is a type of MRI that gives highly detailed images of blood vessels. Physicians use MRA to view arteries and blockage inside arteries.

Other Diagnostic Procedures

cardiac catheterization	**A thin, flexible tube is guided into the heart via a vein or an artery.**
	This procedure detects pressures and patterns of blood flow in the heart. Contrast may be injected and x-ray images taken of the heart and blood vessels (see Fig. 11–23).
electrocardiography (ECG)	**Recording of electricity flowing through the heart.**
	Continuous monitoring of a patient's heart rhythm in hospitals is performed via **telemetry** (electronic transmission of data—tele/o means distant). Normal sinus rhythm begins in the SA node and is between 60 to 100 beats per minute. Figure 11–24 shows ECG (EKG) strips for normal sinus rhythm and several types of dysrhythmias (abnormal rhythms).

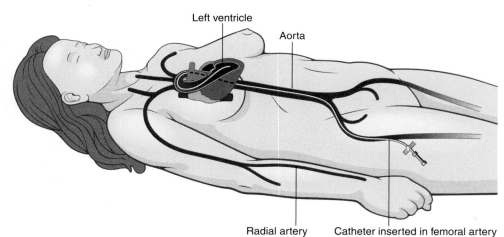

Left ventricle

Aorta

Radial artery   Catheter inserted in femoral artery

FIGURE 11–23 Left-sided cardiac catheterization. The catheter is passed retrograde (backward) from the femoral artery into the aorta and then into the left ventricle. Catheterization also is performed via the radial artery by an increasing number of interventional cardiologists. For right-sided cardiac catheterization, the cardiologist inserts a catheter through the femoral vein and advances it to the right atrium and right ventricle and into the pulmonary artery. Catheterization through the radial artery is also performed.

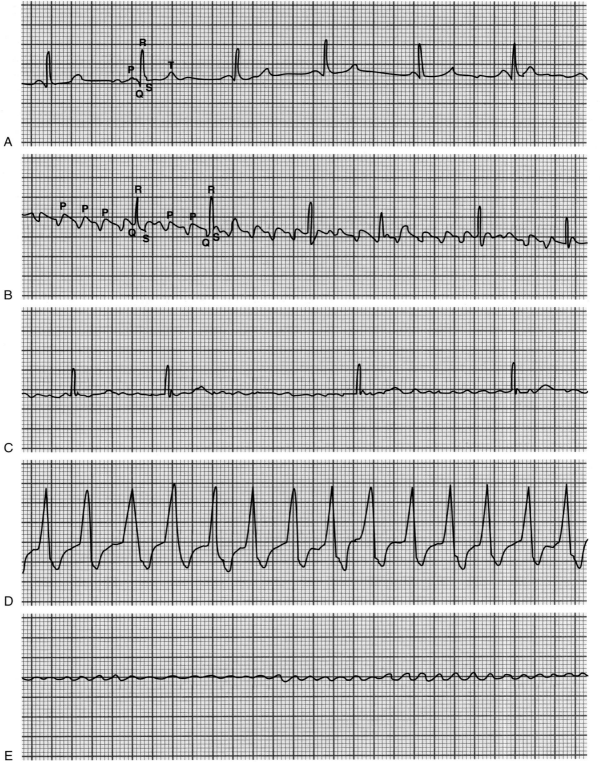

FIGURE 11–24 **ECG rhythm strips showing normal sinus rhythm and dysrhythmias (arrhythmias).** (From Hicks GH: Cardiopulmonary Anatomy and Physiology, Philadelphia, WB Saunders, 2000.)

  A, Normal sinus rhythm. Notice the regularity of the P, QRS, and T waves.

  B, Atrial flutter. Notice the rapid atrial rate (P wave) compared with the slower ventricular rate (ARS).

  C, Atrial fibrillation. P waves are replaced by irregular and rapid fluctuations. There are no effective atrial contractions.

  D, Ventricular tachycardia. Ventricular rate may be as high as 250 beats per minute. The rhythm is regular, but the atria are not contributing to ventricular filling and blood output is poor.

  E, Ventricular fibrillation. Notice the abnormal, irregular waves. Ventricles in fibrillation cannot pump blood effectively. Circulation stops and sudden cardiac death follows if fibrillation is not reversed.

11

Holter monitoring	**An ECG device is worn during a 24-hour period to detect cardiac arrhythmias.** Rhythm changes are correlated with symptoms recorded in a diary.
stress test	**Exercise tolerance test (ETT) determines the heart's response to physical exertion (stress).** A common protocol uses 3-minute stages at set speeds and elevations of a treadmill. Continual monitoring of vital signs and ECG rhythms is important in the diagnosis of CAD and left ventricular function.

CLINICAL PROCEDURES: TREATMENT

cardioversion (defibrillation)	**Very brief discharges of electricity, applied across the chest to stop arrhythmias.** For patients at high risk of sudden cardiac death from ventricular dysrhythmias, an implantable cardioverter-defibrillator (ICD) or automatic implantable cardioverter-defibrillator (AICD) is placed in the upper chest.
coronary artery bypass grafting (CABG)	**Arteries and veins are anastomosed to coronary arteries to detour around blockages.** Internal mammary (breast) and radial (arm) arteries and saphenous (leg) vein grafts are used to keep the myocardium supplied with oxygenated blood (see Fig. 11–25). Cardiac surgeons perform minimally invasive CABG surgery with smaller incisions instead of the traditional sternotomy to open the chest. Vein and artery grafts are removed endoscopically with small incisions as well. Although most operations are performed with a heart-lung machine ("on-pump"), an increasing number are performed "off pump" with a beating heart.
endarterectomy	**Surgical removal of plaque from the inner layer of an artery.** Fatty deposits (atheromas) and thromboses are removed to open clogged arteries. **Carotid endarterectomy** is a procedure to remove plaque buildup in the carotid artery to reduce risk of stroke.

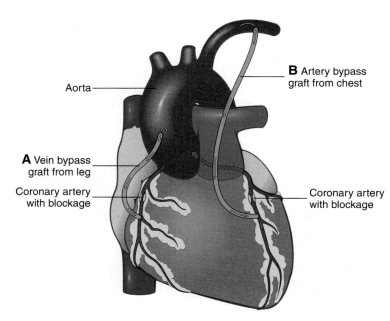

Aorta

B Artery bypass graft from chest

A Vein bypass graft from leg

Coronary artery with blockage

Coronary artery with blockage

FIGURE 11–25 Coronary artery bypass graft (CABG) surgery with anastomosis of vein and arterial grafts. **A,** Section of a vein is removed from the leg and anastomosed (upside down because of its directional valves) to a coronary artery to bypass an area of arteriosclerotic blockage. **B,** An internal mammary artery is grafted to a coronary artery to bypass a blockage.

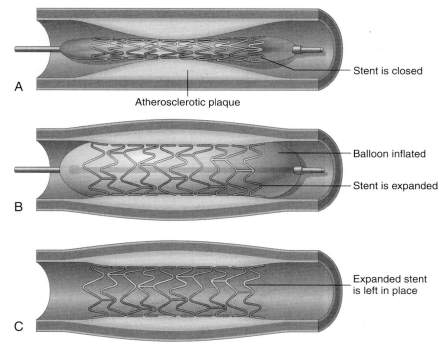

Stent is closed

Atherosclerotic plaque

Balloon inflated

Stent is expanded

Expanded stent is left in place

FIGURE 11–26 Placement of an intra-coronary artery drug-eluting stent. **A,** The stent is positioned at the site of the lesion. **B,** The balloon is inflated, expanding the stent and compressing the plaque. **C,** When the balloon is withdrawn, the stent supports the artery and releases a drug to reduce the risk of restenosis. Stents are stainless steel scaffolding devices that help to hold open arteries, such as the coronary, renal, and carotid arteries.

extracorporeal circulation	**A heart-lung machine diverts blood from the heart and lungs while the heart is repaired.** Blood leaves the body, enters the heart-lung machine, where it is oxygenated, and then returns to a blood vessel (artery) to circulate through the bloodstream. The machine uses the technique of **extracorporeal membrane oxygenation (ECMO).**
heart transplantation	**A donor heart is transferred to a recipient.** While waiting for a transplant, a patient may need a **left ventricular assist device (LVAD),** which is a booster pump implanted in the abdomen with a cannula (flexible tube) to the left ventricle.
percutaneous coronary intervention (PCI)	**A balloon-tipped catheter is inserted into a coronary artery to open the artery; stents are put in place.** An interventional cardiologist places the catheter in the femoral or radial artery and then threads it up the aorta into the coronary artery. **Stents** (expandable slotted tubes that serve as permanent scaffolding devices) create wide lumens and make restenosis less likely. New **drug-eluting stents (DESs)** are coated with polymers that elute (release) antiproliferative drugs to prevent scar tissue formation leading to restenosis (see Fig. 11–26). Stents also are placed in carotid, renal, and other peripheral arteries. PCI techniques include percutaneous transluminal coronary angioplasty (PTCA), stent placement, laser angioplasty (a small laser on the tip of a catheter vaporizes plaque), and atherectomy.
thrombolytic therapy	**Drugs to dissolve clots are injected into the bloodstream of patients with coronary thrombosis.** Tissue plasminogen activator **(tPA)** and **streptokinase** restore blood flow to the heart and limit irreversible damage to heart muscle. The drugs are given within 12 hours after the onset of a heart attack. Thrombolytic agents reduce mortality in patients with myocardial infarction by 25 percent.

ABBREVIATIONS

AAA	abdominal aortic aneurysm
ACE inhibitor	angiotensin-converting enzyme inhibitor
ACLS	advanced cardiac life support; CPR plus drugs and defibrillation
ACS	acute coronary syndrome
ADP	adenosine diphosphate; ADP blockers are used to prevent cardiovascular-related death, heart attack, and strokes and after all stent procedures
AED	automatic external defibrillator
AF, a-fib	atrial fibrillation
AICD	automatic implantable cardioverter-defibrillator
AMI	acute myocardial infarction
ARVD	arrhythmogenic right ventricular dysplasia
AS	aortic stenosis
ASD	atrial septal defect
AV, A-V	atrioventricular
AVR	aortic valve replacement
BBB	bundle branch block
BNP	brain natriuretic peptide; elevated in congestive heart failure
BP	blood pressure
CABG	coronary artery bypass grafting
CAD	coronary artery disease
CCU	coronary care unit
Cath	catheterization
CHF	congestive heart failure
CK	creatine kinase; released into the bloodstream after injury to heart or skeletal muscles
CoA	coarctation of the aorta
CPR	cardiopulmonary resuscitation
CRT	cardiac resynchronization therapy; biventricular pacing
CTNI *or* **cTnI**	cardiac troponin I; troponin is a protein released into the bloodstream after myocardial injury
CTNT *or* **cTnT**	cardiac troponin T
CV	cardiovascular
DES	drug-eluting stent
DSA	digital subtraction angiography
DVT	deep vein thrombosis
ECMO	extracorporeal membrane oxygenation
ECG	electrocardiography
ECHO	echocardiography
EF	ejection fraction; measure of the amount of blood that pumps out of the heart with each beat
EPS	electrophysiology study; electrode catheters are inserted into veins and threaded into the heart and electrical conduction is measured (tachycardias are provoked and analyzed)
ETT	exercise tolerance test
ETT-MIBI	exercise tolerance test combined with a radioactive tracer (sestamibi) scan
HDL	high-density lipoprotein; high blood levels are associated with lower incidence of coronary artery disease
HTN	hypertension (high blood pressure)
IABP	intra-aortic balloon pump; used to support patients in cardiogenic shock
ICD	implantable cardioverter-defibrillator
LAD	left anterior descending (coronary artery)
LDL	low-density lipoprotein
LMWH	low-molecular-weight heparin
LV	left ventricle
LVAD	left ventricular assist device
LVH	left ventricular hypertrophy
MI	myocardial infarction
MR	mitral regurgitation
MUGA	multiple-gated acquisition scan; a radioactive test of heart function
MVP	mitral valve prolapse
NSR	normal sinus rhythm
NSTEMI	non–ST elevation myocardial infarction
PAC	premature atrial contraction
PCI	percutaneous coronary intervention
PDA	patent ductus arteriosus; posterior descending artery
PVC	premature ventricular contraction
RFA	radiofrequency catheter ablation
SA, S-A	sinoatrial

SCD	sudden cardiac death	TEE	transesophageal echocardiography
SOB	shortness of breath	TGA	transposition of the great arteries
SPECT	single photon emission computed tomography; used for myocardial imaging with sestamibi scans	tPA	tissue-type plasminogen activator; a drug used to prevent thrombosis
		UA	unstable angina
SSCP	substernal chest pain	VF	ventricular fibrillation
STEMI	ST elevation myocardial infarction	VSD	ventricular septal defect
SVT	supraventricular tachycardia; rapid heart beats arising from the atria and causing palpitations, SOB, and dizziness	VT	ventricular tachycardia
		WPW	Wolff-Parkinson-White syndrome; an abnormal ECG pattern often associated with paroxysmal tachycardia
Tc	technetium		

PRACTICAL APPLICATIONS

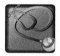

OPERATING ROOM SCHEDULE: GENERAL HOSPITAL

Match the operative treatment in Column I with the appropriate surgical indication (diagnosis) in Column II. Answers are found on page 431.

Column I

1. Coronary artery bypass graft   _E_
2. Left carotid endarterectomy   _C_
3. Sclerosing injections and laser treatment   _H_
4. LV aneurysmectomy   _I_
5. Atrial septal defect repair   _D_
6. Left ventricular assist device   _A_
7. Pericardiocentesis   _B_
8. Aortic valve replacement   _J_
9. Pacemaker implantation   _G_
10. Femoral-popliteal bypass graft   _F_

Column II

A. Congestive heart failure
B. Cardiac tamponade (fluid in the space surrounding the heart)
C. Atherosclerotic occlusion of a main artery leading to the head
D. Congenital hole in the wall of the upper chamber of the heart
E. Disabling angina and extensive coronary atherosclerosis despite medical therapy
F. Peripheral vascular disease
G. Heart block
H. Varicose veins
I. Protrusion of the wall of a lower heart chamber
J. Aortic stenosis

CASES

Case 1: A 24-year-old woman with a history of palpitations [heartbeat is unusually strong, rapid, or irregular, so that patient is aware of it] and vague chest pains enters the hospital. With the patient supine, you hear a midsystolic click that is followed by a grade 3/6 [moderately loud—6/6 is loud and 1/6 is quiet] honking murmur.

1. Your diagnosis is:
   a. Tetralogy of Fallot
   b. Mitral valve prolapse
   c. Raynaud phenomenon
   d. Congestive heart failure

Case 2: Mr. Smith was admitted to the telemetry unit for cardiac monitoring following an episode of chest pain. His cardiac enzymes (CK, troponin-T, and troponin-I) were slightly elevated and the ECG showed elevation in the ST segment. An angiogram reveals plaque blocking the LAD. PCI with DES is recommended.

2. What did the ECG reveal?
   a. NSTEMI and unstable angina
   b. Aortic aneurysm
   c. CHF
   d. STEMI   *St elevation myocardial Infarction*

3. Your diagnosis for this patient is:
   a. Heart attack
   b. Rheumatic heart disease
   c. Unstable angina
   d. Patent ductus arteriosus

4. What treatment is recommended?
   a. Coronary artery bypass grafting
   b. Catheterization with drug-eluting stent placement
   c. Defibrillation and cardioversion
   d. Thrombolytic drugs

coronary artery disease

Case 3: Charles Jones, a 72-year-old politician, has had CAD for nearly 25 years, resulting in four MIs. Recently, he has been aware of palpitations and slight dizziness. Results of Holter monitoring revealed four episodes of ventricular tachycardia and PVCs. Since ventricular tachycardia can lead to VF, a potentially fatal dysrhythmia, his cardiologist recommended electrophysiologic studies. These studies showed the need for ICD to reverse potential arrhythmias and SCD.   *ventricular fibrillation*   *implantable cardioverter defibrillator*

5. What were Mr. Jones' physicians most concerned about preventing?
   a. Hypercholesterolemia and coronary artery disease
   b. Shortness of breath and substernal chest pain
   c. Ventricular fibrillation and cardiac arrest
   d. Stroke and blood clots to the brain

6. What treatment is recommended?
   a. Pacemaker implantation
   b. Cardioverter-defibrillator implantation
   c. Resynchronization therapy (biventricular pacing)
   d. Reversing myocardial ischemia

Case 4: A 42-year-old female runner recovering from an upper respiratory infection comes to the ED complaining of chest pain that is sharp, constant, worse when she is lying down and improved with sitting up and leaning forward. Serum CK and troponin I levels rule out an acute MI. The ED physician auscultates a pericardial friction rub and orders a STAT bedside echocardiogram to assess for pericardial effusion.

7. What's your diagnosis for this patient?
   a. Myocardial ischemia   *non-St elevation myocardial infarction*
   b. Unstable angina and NSTEMI
   c. Endocarditis
   d. Pericarditis

8. The danger of this condition is the risk for progression to:
   a. Cardiac tamponade
   b. Aneurysm
   c. Pulmonary embolism
   d. Claudication

? EXERCISES

Remember to check your answers carefully with those given in the Answers to Exercises, page 428.

A. Match the following terms with their meanings below.

aorta	inferior vena cava	superior vena cava
arteriole	mitral valve	tricuspid valve
atrium	pulmonary artery	ventricle
capillary	pulmonary vein	venule

1. valve that lies between the right atrium and the right ventricle _triscupid valve_

2. smallest blood vessel _capillary_

3. carries oxygenated blood from the lungs to the heart _pulmonary vein_

4. largest artery in the body _AORTA_

5. brings oxygen-poor blood into the heart from the upper parts of the body _Superior vena cava_

6. upper chamber of the heart _Atrium_

7. carries oxygen-poor blood to the lungs from the heart _pulmonary artery_

8. small artery _Arteriole_

9. valve that lies between the left atrium and the left ventricle _mitral valve_

10. brings blood from the lower half of the body to the heart _infi. vena cava_

11. a small vein _venule_

12. lower chamber of the heart _ventricle_

B. Trace the path of blood through the heart. Begin as the blood enters the right atrium from the venae cavae (and include the valves within the heart).

1. _right atrium_

2. _triscupid valve_

3. _right ventricle_

4. _pulmonary valve_

5. _pulmonary artery_

6. capillaries of the lung

7. _pulmonary vein_

8. _left atrium_

9. _mitral valve_

10. _left ventricle_

11. _aortic valve_

12. aorta

C. Complete the following sentences.

1. The pacemaker of the heart is the _Sinotrial node_.

2. The sac-like membrane surrounding the heart is the _pericardium_.

11

3. The wall of the heart between the right and the left atria is the _interatrial spetum_.

4. The relaxation phase of the heartbeat is called _diastole_.

5. Specialized conductive tissue in the wall between the ventricles is the _Atrioventricular bundle_.

6. The inner lining of the heart is the _endocardium_.

7. The contractive phase of the heartbeat is called _systole_.

8. A gas released as a metabolic product of catabolism is _carbon dioxide (CO_2)_.

9. Specialized conductive tissue at the base of the wall between the two upper heart chambers is the _atrioventricular (AV) Node_.

10. The inner lining of the pericardium, adhering to the outside of the heart, is the _visceral pericardium_.

11. An abnormal heart sound due to improper closure of heart valves is a _murmur_.

12. The beat of the heart as felt through the walls of arteries is called the _pulse_.

D. Complete the following terms using the given definitions.

1. hardening of arteries: **arterio** _sclerosis_

2. disease condition of heart muscle: **cardio** _myopathy_

3. enlargement of the heart: **cardio** _megaly_

4. inflammation of a vein: **phleb** _itis_

5. condition of rapid heartbeat: _tachy_ **cardia**

6. condition of slow heartbeat: _brady_ **cardia**

7. high levels of cholesterol in the blood: **hyper** _cholesterolemie_

8. surgical repair of a valve: **valvulo** _plasty_

9. condition of deficient oxygen: **hyp** _oxia_

10. pertaining to an upper heart chamber: _atri_ **al**

11. narrowing of the mitral valve: **mitral** _stenosis_

12. breakdown of a clot: **thrombo** _lysis_

E. Give the meanings of the following terms.

1. cyanosis _discoloration of the skin owing to deficient oxygen in the blood_

2. phlebotomy _incision of a vein_

3. arterial anastomosis _new connection between arteries_

4. cardiogenic shock _circulatory failure due poor heart function_

5. atheroma _mass of yellowish plaque (fatty substance)_

6. arrhythmia _Abnormal heart rhythm_

7. sphygmomanometer _Instrument to mesure blood pressure_

8. stethoscope _inst. to listen to the sounds within the chest_

9. mitral valvulitis _inflammation of the mitral valve_

10. atherosclerosis _hardening of arteries with yellowish (fatty substance) plaque_

11. vasoconstriction _narrowing of a vessel_

12. vasodilation _widening of a vessel_

F. Match the following pathologic conditions of the heart with their meanings below.

atrial septal defect

coarctation of the aorta

congestive heart failure

coronary artery disease

endocarditis

fibrillation

flutter

hypertensive heart disease

mitral valve prolapse

patent ductus arteriosus

pericarditis

tetralogy of Fallot

1. inflammation of the inner lining of the heart _endocarditis_

2. rapid but regular atrial or ventricular contractions _flutter_

3. small hole between the upper heart chambers; congenital anomaly _atrial septal defect_

4. improper closure of the valve between the left atrium and ventricle during systole
   mitral valve prolapse

5. blockage of the arteries surrounding the heart leading to ischemia _coronary artery disease_

6. high blood pressure affecting the heart _hypertensive heart disease_

7. rapid, random, ineffectual, and irregular contractions of the heart _fibrillation_

8. inflammation of the sac surrounding the heart _pericarditis_

9. inability of the heart to pump its required amount of blood _congestive heart failure_

10. congenital malformation involving four separate heart defects _tetralogy of fallot_

11. congenital narrowing of the large artery leading from the heart _coarctation of the aorta_

12. a duct between the aorta and the pulmonary artery, which normally closes soon after birth,
    remains open _patent ductus arteriosus_

G. Give the meanings of the following terms.

1. heart block _failure of proper conduction of impulses through the AV node_

2. cardiac arrest _unexpected stoppage of heart action_

3. palpitations _uncomfortable sensations in the chest associated with arrhythmias_

4. artificial cardiac pacemaker _battery-operated placed in the chest to send electrical current to the heart to establish normal rhythm._

5. thrombotic occlusion _blockage of a vessel by a clot._

6. angina _chest pain result for insufficient oxygen to the heart muscle_

7. myocardial infarction _heart attack (and the necrosis)_

8. necrosis _abnormal condition of the death (dead tissue)_

9. infarction _damage or death of tissue due to deprivation of oxygen_

10. ischemia _blood is held back from an area of the body_

11. nitroglycerin _arithetic drug used in the treatment of angine_

12. digoxin _drug that treats arrhythmias and strengthens heart beat_

13. bruit _abnormal sound (murmur)_

14. thrill _vibration felt a palpitation of the chest_

15. acute coronary syndromes _consequences of plaque rupture in coronary arteries_

16. pericardial friction rub _scraping or gratining noise on auscultation, indicate pericarditis_

17. deep vein thrombosis _clot formation in a large vein, usually in lower limb_

18. biventricular pacemaker _device enabling ventricles to heat in synchrony._

H. Match the following terms with their descriptions.

aneurysm
auscultation
claudication
emboli

essential hypertension
murmur
peripheral vascular disease
petechiae

Raynaud disease
rheumatic heart disease
secondary hypertension
vegetations

1. lesions that form on heart valves after damage by infection _vegetations_

2. clots that travel to and suddenly block a blood vessel _emboli_

3. small, pinpoint hemorrhages _petechiae_

4. an extra heart sound, heard between normal beats and caused by a valvular defect or condition that disrupts the smooth flow of blood through the heart _murmur_

5. listening with a stethoscope _auscultation_

6. heart disease caused by rheumatic fever _rheumatic heart disease_

7. high blood pressure in arteries when the etiology is idiopathic _essential hypertension_

8. high blood pressure related to kidney disease _secondary hypertension_

9. episodes of ischemia with pallor and numbness in fingers and toes caused by a temporary constriction of arterioles in the skin _Raynaud disease_

10. local widening of an artery _peripheral vascular disease_

11. pain, tension, and weakness in a limb after walking has begun _claudication_

12. blockage of arteries in the lower extremities; etiology is atherosclerosis _peripheral vascular disease_

I. Give short answers for the following.

1. Types of drugs used to treat acute coronary syndromes include _beta blockers, statins, aspirin, calcium channel blockers_.

2. When damaged valves in veins fail to prevent the backflow of blood, a condition (swollen, twisted vein) that results is _varicose veins_.

3. Swollen, twisted veins in the rectal region are called _hemorrhoids_.

4. Name the four defects in tetralogy of Fallot from their descriptions:

   a. narrowing of the artery leading to the lungs from the heart: _pulmonary artery stenosis_

   b. gap in the wall between the ventricles: _ventricular septal defect_

   c. the large vessel leading from the left ventricle moves over the interventricular septum: _shift of the aorta to the right_

   d. excessive development of the wall of the right lower heart chamber: _hypertrophy of the right ventricle._

J. Select from the list of cardiac tests and procedures to complete the definitions below.

angiography	echocardiography	lipoprotein electrophoresis
cardiac MRI	electrocardiography	serum enzyme test
cardioversion	endarterectomy	stress test
coronary artery bypass graft	lipid tests (profile)	thallium 201 scan

1. surgical removal of plaque from the inner lining of an artery _endarterectomy_

2. application of brief electrical discharges across the chest to stop a cardiac arrhythmia; defibrillation _cardioversion_

3. measurement of levels of fatty substances (cholesterol and triglycerides) in the bloodstream _lipid tests (profile)_

4. measurement of the heart's response to physical exertion (patient monitored while jogging on a treadmill) _stress test_

5. measurement of serum creatine kinase (CK) and troponin-T and troponin-I after myocardial infarction _serum enzyme test_

6. injection of contrast into vessels and x-ray imaging _angiography_

7. recording of the electricity in the heart _electrocardiography._

8. intravenous injection of a radioactive substance and measurement of its accumulation in heart muscle _thallium 201 scan_

9. use of echoes from high-frequency sound waves to produce images of the heart

echocardiography

10. separation of HDL and LDL from a blood sample _lipoprotein electrophoresis_

11. anastomosis of vessel grafts to existing coronary arteries to maintain blood supply to the myocardium _coronary artery bypass graft._

12. beaming of magnetic waves at the heart to produce images of its structure _cardiac MRI_

K. Give the meanings for the following terms.

1. digital subtraction angiography _____

2. heart transplantation_____

3. ETT-MIBI _____

4. Doppler ultrasound _____

5. Holter monitoring_____

6. thrombolytic therapy_____

7. extracorporeal circulation_____

8. cardiac catheterization _____

9. percutaneous coronary intervention _____

10. drug-eluting stent _____

11. electron beam computed tomography _____

12. computerized tomography angiography _____

L. Identify the following cardiac dysrhythmias from their abbreviations.

1. AF_____

2. VT_____

3. VF_____

4. PVC_____

5. PAC_____

M. Identify the following abnormal cardiac conditions from their abbreviations.

1. CHF _____

2. VSD _____

3. MI_____

4. PDA _____

5. MVP _____

6. AS _____

7. CAD _____

8. ASD _____

N. Match the following abbreviations for cardiac tests and procedures with their explanations below.

BNP	ECMO	LDL
CRT	ETT	LVAD
cTnI or cTnT	ETT-MIBI	RFA
ECHO	ICD	TEE

1. serum enzyme test for myocardial infarction _____

2. booster pump implanted in the abdomen with a cannula leading to the heart as a "bridge to transplant" _____

3. ultrasound imaging of the heart using transducer within the esophagus _____

4. device implanted in the chest that senses and corrects arrhythmias by shocking the heart _____

5. catheter delivery of a high-frequency current to damage a small portion of the heart muscle and reverse an abnormal heart rhythm _____

6. procedure to determine the heart's response to physical exertion (stress) _____

7. cardiac imaging using high-frequency sound waves pulsed through the chest wall and bounced off heart structures _____

8. radioactive test of heart function with stress test _____

9. technique using heart-lung machine to divert blood from the heart and lungs while the heart is being repaired _____

10. biventricular pacing to correct serious abnormal ventricular rhythms _____

11. lipoprotein sample is measured _____

12. brain chemical measured to identify patients at risk for complications after MI and with CHF _____

11

O. Spell the term correctly from its definition.

belong

1. pertaining to the heart: _____ CORO N _____ ary

2. not a normal heart rhythm: arr _y th miA_____

3. abnormal condition of blueness: _____ CYAN osis

4. relaxation phase of the heartbeat: _____ diAS ___ tole

5. chest pain: _____ ANGINA _____ pectoris

6. inflammation of a vein: _____ phe b _____ itis

enlargment

7. widening of a vessel: vaso ___ dilAtion _____

8. enlargement of the heart: cardio ___ megaly _____

9. hardening of arteries with fatty plaque: _____ ARthe RO sclerosis

10. swollen veins in the rectal region: _____ Hemo RRh oids

P. Match the following terms with their meanings below.

aneurysmorrhaphy	endarterectomy	STEMI
atherectomy	PCI	thrombolytic therapy
CABG	pericardiocentesis	valvotomy
embolectomy		

1. incision of a heart valve ___ VAL votomy _____

2. removal of a clot that has traveled into a blood vessel and suddenly caused occlusion
   ___ embolectomy _____

3. coronary artery bypass graft (to relieve ischemia) ___ CABG _____

4. surgical puncture to remove fluid from the pericardial space ___ pericardiocentesis

5. insertion of a balloon-tipped catheter and stents into a coronary artery ___ PCI _____

6. removal of the inner lining of an artery to make it wider ___ endarterectomy ___

7. suture (repair) of a ballooned-out portion of an artery ___ aneurysmorrhaphy ___

8. removal of plaque from an artery ___ Atherectomy ___

9. type of acute coronary syndrome ___ STEMI - ___

10. use of streptokinase and tPA to dissolve clots ___ thrombolytic therapy ___

Q. Select the boldface term that best completes each sentence.

1. Bill was having pain in his chest that radiated up his neck and down his arm. He called his family physician, who thought Bill should report to the local hospital's emergency department (ED) immediately. The first test performed in the ED was a/an **(stress test, ECG, CABG)**.

2. Dr. Kelly explained to the family that their observation of the bluish color of baby Charles' skin helped her make the diagnosis of a/an **(thrombotic, aneurysmal, septal)** defect in the baby's heart, which needed immediate attention.

3. Mr. Duggan had a fever of unknown origin. When the doctors completed an echocardiogram and saw vegetations on his mitral valve, they suspected **(bacterial endocarditis, hypertensive heart disease, angina)**.

4. Claudia's hands turned red, almost purple, whenever she went out into the cold or became stressed. Her physician thought it might be wise to evaluate her for **(varicose veins, Raynaud disease, intermittent claudication)**.

5. Daisy's heart felt like it was skipping beats every time she drank coffee. Her physician suggested that she wear a/an **(Holter monitor, LVAD, CABG)** for 24 hours to assess the nature of the arrhythmia.

6. Paola's father and grandfather died of heart attacks. Her physician tells her that she has inherited a tendency to accumulate fats in her bloodstream. Blood tests reveal high levels of **(enzymes, lipids, nitroglycerin)**. Discussing her family history with her **(gynecologist, hematologist, cardiologist)**, she understands that she has familial **(hypocholesterolemia, hypercholesterolemia, cardiomyopathy)**.

7. While exercising, Bernard experienced a pain (cramp) in his calf muscle. The pain disappeared when he was resting. After performing **(Holter monitoring, Doppler ultrasound, echocardiography)** on his leg to assess blood flow, Dr. Shaw found **(stenosis, fibrillation, endocarditis)**, indicating poor circulation. She recommended a daily exercise program, low-fat diet, careful foot care, and antiplatelet drug therapy to treat Bernard's intermittent **(palpitations, hypertension, claudication)**.

8. Carol noticed that her 6-week-old son Louis had a slightly bluish or **(jaundiced, cyanotic, diastolic)** coloration to his skin. She consulted a pediatric **(dermatologist, hematologist, cardiologist)**, who performed **(echocardiography, PET scan, endarterectomy)** and diagnosed Louis' condition as **(endocarditis, congestive heart disease, tetralogy of Fallot)**.

9. Seventy-eight-year-old John Smith had coronary artery disease and high blood pressure for the past 10 years. His history included an acute heart attack, or **(MI, PDA, CABG)**. He often was tired and complained of **(dyspnea, nausea, migraine headaches)** and swelling in his ankles. His physician diagnosed his condition as **(aortic aneurysm, congestive heart failure, congenital heart disease)** and recommended restricted salt intake, diuretics, and an **(ACE inhibitor, antibiotic, analgesic)**.

10. Sarah had a routine checkup that included **(auscultation, vasoconstriction, vasodilation)** of her chest with a **(catheter, stent, stethoscope)** to listen to her heart. Her physician noticed a midsystolic murmur characteristic of **(DVT, MVP, LDL)**. An echocardiogram confirmed the diagnosis.

MEDICAL SCRAMBLE

Unscramble the letters to form cardiovascular terms from the clues. Use the letters in squares to complete the bonus term. Answers are found on page 431.

1. *Clue:* Localized widening of an arterial wall

   ☐ __ __ __ ☐ ☐ __ __   R M E Y U A S N

2. *Clue:* Contraction phase of the heart beat

   __ __ __ ☐ __ __ __   E O S L S T Y

3. *Clue:* Swollen, dilated veins in the rectal region

   ☐ __ ☐ __ ☐ __ ☐ __ ☐ __ __   R I H E O D R S H M O

4. *Clue:* Blue discoloration of skin due to hypoxia

   __ __ ☐ __ __ __ __ __   O C N S Y S A I

BONUS TERM: *Clue:* Flutter and fibrillation are examples

   ☐ ☐ ☐ ☐ ☐ ☐ ☐ ☐ ☐ ☐

ANSWERS TO EXERCISES

A

1. tricuspid valve
2. capillary
3. pulmonary vein
4. aorta
5. superior vena cava
6. atrium
7. pulmonary artery
8. arteriole
9. mitral valve
10. inferior vena cava
11. venule
12. ventricle

B

1. right atrium
2. tricuspid valve
3. right ventricle
4. pulmonary valve
5. pulmonary artery
6. capillaries of the lung
7. pulmonary veins
8. left atrium
9. mitral valve
10. left ventricle
11. aortic valve
12. aorta

C

1. sinoatrial (SA) node
2. pericardium
3. interatrial septum
4. diastole
5. atrioventricular bundle or bundle of His
6. endocardium
7. systole
8. carbon dioxide (CO_2)
9. atrioventricular (AV) node
10. visceral pericardium (the outer lining is the parietal pericardium)
11. murmur
12. pulse

11

D

1. arteriosclerosis
2. cardiomyopathy
3. cardiomegaly
4. phlebitis
5. tachycardia
6. bradycardia
7. hypercholesterolemia
8. valvuloplasty
9. hypoxia
10. atrial
11. mitral stenosis
12. thrombolysis

E

1. bluish discoloration of the skin owing to deficient oxygen in the blood
2. incision of a vein
3. new connection between arteries
4. circulatory failure due to poor heart function
5. mass of yellowish plaque (fatty substance)
6. abnormal heart rhythm
7. instrument to measure blood pressure
8. instrument to listen to sounds within the chest
9. inflammation of the mitral valve
10. hardening of arteries with a yellowish, fatty substance (plaque)
11. narrowing of a vessel
12. widening of a vessel

F

1. endocarditis
2. flutter
3. atrial septal defect
4. mitral valve prolapse
5. coronary artery disease
6. hypertensive heart disease
7. fibrillation
8. pericarditis
9. congestive heart failure
10. tetralogy of Fallot
11. coarctation of the aorta
12. patent ductus arteriosus

G

1. failure of proper conduction of impulses through the AV node to the atrioventricular bundle (bundle of His)
2. sudden unexpected stoppage of heart action
3. uncomfortable sensations in the chest associated with arrhythmias
4. battery-operated device that is placed in the chest and wired to send electrical current to the heart to establish a normal sinus rhythm
5. blockage of a vessel by a clot
6. chest pain resulting from insufficient oxygen being supplied to the heart muscle (ischemia)
7. area of necrosis (tissue death in the heart muscle; heart attack)
8. abnormal condition of death (dead tissue)
9. damage or death of tissue due to deprivation of oxygen
10. blood is held back from an area of the body
11. nitrate drug used in the treatment of angina
12. drug that treats arrhythmias and strengthens the heartbeat
13. abnormal sound (murmur) heard on auscultation
14. vibration felt on palpation of the chest
15. consequences of plaque rupture in coronary arteries; MI and unstable angina
16. scraping or grating noise on auscultation of heart; indicates pericarditis
17. clot formation in a large vein, usually in lower limb
18. device enabling ventricles to heat in synchrony; cardiac resynchronization therapy.

H

1. vegetations
2. emboli
3. petechiae
4. murmur
5. auscultation
6. rheumatic heart disease
7. essential hypertension
8. secondary hypertension
9. Raynaud disease
10. aneurysm
11. claudication
12. peripheral vascular disease

I

1. beta-blockers, ACE inhibitors, statins, aspirin, calcium channel blockers
2. varicose veins
3. hemorrhoids
4. a. pulmonary artery stenosis
   b. ventricular septal defect
   c. shift of the aorta to the right
   d. hypertrophy of the right ventricle

J

1. endarterectomy
2. cardioversion
3. lipid tests (profile)
4. stress test
5. serum enzyme test (-ase means enzyme)
6. angiography (arteriography)
7. electrocardiography
8. thallium 201 scan
9. echocardiography
10. lipoprotein electrophoresis
11. coronary artery bypass graft
12. cardiac MRI

11

K

1. Video equipment and a computer produce x-ray pictures of blood vessels by taking two pictures (without and with contrast) and subtracting the first image (without contrast) from the second.
2. A donor heart is transferred to a recipient.
3. Exercise tolerance test combined with a radioactive tracer scan.
4. An instrument that focuses sound waves on a blood vessel to measure blood flow.
5. A compact version of an electrocardiograph is worn during a 24-hour period to detect cardiac arrhythmias.

6. Treatment with drugs (streptokinase and tPA) to dissolve clots after a heart attack.
7. A heart-lung machine is used to divert blood from the heart and lungs during surgery. The machine oxygenates the blood and sends it back into the bloodstream.
8. A catheter (tube) is inserted into an artery or vein and threaded into the heart chambers. Contrast can be injected to take x-ray pictures, patterns of blood flow can be detected, and blood pressures can be measured.

9. A balloon-tipped catheter is inserted into a coronary artery to open the artery; stents are put in place.
10. Stents are expandable slotted tubes that are placed in arteries during PCI. They release polymers that prevent plaque from reforming.
11. Electron beams and CT identify calcium deposits in and around coronary arteries to diagnose CAD.
12. X-ray images of the heart and coronary arteries using CT technology.

L

1. atrial fibrillation
2. ventricular tachycardia
3. ventricular fibrillation

4. premature ventricular contraction
5. premature atrial contraction

M

1. congestive heart failure
2. ventricular septal defect
3. myocardial infarction

4. patent ductus arteriosus
5. mitral valve prolapse
6. aortic stenosis

7. coronary artery disease
8. atrial septal defect

N

1. cTnI: troponin I and troponin T
2. LVAD: left ventricular assist device
3. TEE: transesophageal echocardiography
4. ICD: implantable cardioverter/defibrillator
5. RFA: radiofrequency catheter ablation

6. ETT: exercise tolerance test
7. ECHO: echocardiography
8. ETT-MIBI: exercise tolerance test with sestamibi scan
9. ECMO: extracorporeal membrane oxygenation

10. CRT: cardiac resynchronization therapy
11. LDL: low-density lipoprotein; high levels indicate risk for CAD
12. BNP: brain natriuretic peptide

O

1. coronary
2. arrhythmia
3. cyanosis
4. diastole

5. angina pectoris
6. phlebitis
7. vasodilation

8. cardiomegaly
9. atherosclerosis
10. hemorrhoids

P

1. valvotomy
2. embolectomy
3. CABG
4. pericardiocentesis

5. PCI
6. endarterectomy
7. aneurysmorrhaphy
8. atherectomy

9. STEMI (ST segment elevation myocardial infarction)
10. thrombolytic therapy

Q

1. ECG
2. septal
3. bacterial endocarditis
4. Raynaud disease
5. Holter monitor

6. lipids; cardiologist; hypercholesterolemia
7. Doppler ultrasound; stenosis; claudication

8. cyanotic; cardiologist; echocardiography; tetralogy of Fallot
9. MI; dyspnea; congestive heart failure; ACE inhibitor
10. auscultation; stethoscope; MVP

ANSWERS TO PRACTICAL APPLICATIONS

Operating Room Schedule

1. E	5. D	8. J
2. C	6. A	9. G
3. H	7. B	10. F
4. I		

Cases

Case 1	*Case 3*	*Case 4*
1. b	5. c	7. d
Case 2	6. b	8. a
2. d		
3. a		
4. b		

ANSWERS TO MEDICAL SCRAMBLE

1. ANEURYSM   2. SYSTOLE   3. HEMORRHOIDS   4. CYANOSIS
BONUS TERM: ARRHYTHMIA

PRONUNCIATION OF TERMS

PRONUNCIATION GUIDE

ā as in āpe	ă as in ăpple
ē as in ēven	ĕ as in ĕvery
ī as in īce	ĭ as in ĭnterest
ō as in ōpen	ŏ as in pŏt
ū as in ūnit	ŭ as in ŭnder

To test your understanding of the terminology in this chapter, write the meaning of each term in the space provided. In addition, you may wish to cover the terms and write them by looking at your definitions. Make sure your spelling is correct. The page number after each term indicates where it is defined or used in the book, so you can easily check your responses. You will find complete definitions for all of these terms and their audio pronunciations on the CD.

Term	Pronunciation	Meaning
angiogram (395)	ĂN-jē-ō-grăm	_____
angioplasty (395)	ĂN-jē-ō-plăs-tē	_____
anoxia (397)	ă-NŎK-sē-ă	_____
aorta (394)	ā-ŌR-tă	_____
aortic stenosis (395)	ā-ŌR-tĭk stĕ-NŌ-sĭs	_____
arrhythmia (398)	ā-RĬTH-mē-ă	_____
arterial anastomosis (395)	ăr-TĒ-rē-ăl ă-năs-tō-MŌ-sĭs	_____
arteriography (395)	ăr-tē-rē-ŎG-ră-fē	_____
arteriole (394)	ăr-TĒ-rē-ōl	_____
arteriosclerosis (395)	ăr-tē-rē-ō-sklĕ-RŌ-sĭs	_____
artery (394)	ĂR-tĕ-rē	_____
atherectomy (396)	ă-thĕ-RĔK-tō-mē	_____
atheroma (396)	ăth-ĕr-Ō-mă	_____
atherosclerosis (396)	ăth-ĕr-ō-sklĕ-RŌ-sĭs	_____

11

Term	Pronunciation	Meaning
atrial (396)	Ā-trē-ăl	
atrioventricular bundle (394)	ā-trē-ō-věn-TRĬK-ū-lăr BŬN-dl	
atrioventricular node (394)	ā-trē-ō-věn-TRĬK-ū-lăr nōd	
atrium; atria (394)	Ā-trē-ŭm; Ā-trē-ă	
brachial artery (396)	BRĀ-kē-ăl ĂR-tě-rē	
bradycardia (396)	brād-ē-KĂR-dē-ă	
bundle of His (394)	BŬN-dl of Hĭss	
capillary (394)	KĂP-ĭ-lăr-ē	
carbon dioxide (394)	KĂR-bŏn dī-ŎK-sīd	
cardiogenic shock (396)	kăr-dē-ō-JĔN-ĭk shŏk	
cardiomegaly (396)	kăr-dē-ō-MĔG-ă-lē	
cardiomyopathy (396)	kăr-dē-ō-mī-ŎP-ă-thē	
coronary arteries (394)	KŎR-ō-năr-ē ĂR-tě-rēz	
cyanosis (397)	sī-ă-NŌ-sĭs	
deoxygenated blood (394)	dē-ŎK-sĭ-jě-NĀ-těd blŭd	
diastole (394)	dī-ĂS-tō-lē	
electrocardiogram (394)	ě-lěk-trō-KĂR-dē-ō-grăm	
endocardium (394)	ěn-dō-KĂR-dē-ŭm	
endothelium (394)	ěn-dō-THĒ-lē-um	
hypercholesterolemia (397)	hī-pěr-kō-lěs-těr-ŏl-Ē-mē-ă	
hypoxia (397)	hī-PŎK-sē-ă	
interventricular septum (398)	ĭn-těr-věn-TRĬK-ū-lăr SĔP-tŭm	
mitral valve (394)	MĪ-trăl vălv	
mitral valvulitis (397)	MĪ-trăl văl-vū-LĪ-tĭs	
myocardium (394)	mī-ō-KĂR-dē-ŭm	
myxoma (397)	mĭk-SŌ-mă	
normal sinus rhythm (394)	NŎR-măl SĪ-nus RĬ-thěm	
oxygen (394)	ŎK-sĭ-jěn	
pacemaker (394)	PĀS-mā-kěr	
pericardiocentesis (397)	pěr-ĭ-kăr-dē-ō-sěn-TĒ-sĭs	
pericardium (394)	pěr-ĭ-KĂR-dē-ŭm	
phlebotomy (397)	flě-BŎT-ō-mē	
pulmonary artery (394)	PŬL-mō-něr-ē ĂR-těr-ē	
pulmonary circulation (394)	PŬL-mō-něr-ē sěr-kū-LĀ-shŭn	

Term	Pronunciation	Meaning
pulmonary valve (394)	PŬL-mō-nĕr-ē vălv	_____
pulmonary vein (395)	PŬL-mō-nĕr-ē vān	_____
pulse (395)	pŭls	_____
septum; septa (395)	SĔP-tŭm; SĔP-tă	_____
sinoatrial node (395)	sī-nō-Ā-trē-ăl nōd	_____
sphygmomanometer (395)	sfĭg-mō-mă-NŎM-ĕ-tĕr	_____
stethoscope (397)	STĔTH-ō-skōp	_____
systemic circulation (395)	sĭs-TĔM-ĭk sĕr-kū-LĀ-shŭn	_____
systole (395)	SĬS-tō-lē	_____
tachycardia (396)	tăk-ē-KĂR-dē-ă	_____
thrombolysis (397)	thrŏm-BŎL-ĭ-sĭs	_____
thrombophlebitis (397)	thrŏm-bō-flĕ-BĪ-tĭs	_____
tricuspid valve (395)	trī-KŬS-pĭd vălv	_____
valve (395)	vălv	_____
valvotomy (397)	văl-VŎT-ō-mē	_____
valvuloplasty (397)	văl-vū-lō-PLĂS-tē	_____
vascular (397)	VĂS-kū-lăr	_____
vasoconstriction (397)	văz-ō-kŏn-STRĬK-shŭn	_____
vasodilation (397)	văz-ō-dī-LĀ-shŭn	_____
vein (395)	vān	_____
vena cava; venae cavae (395)	VĒ-nă KĀ-vă; VĒ-nē KĀ-vē	_____
venipuncture (398)	vĕ-nĭ-PŬNK-chŭr	_____
venous (398)	VĒ-nŭs	_____
ventricle (395)	VĔN-trĭ-k'l	_____
venule (395)	VĔN-ū'l	_____

PATHOLOGY, LABORATORY TESTS, AND CLINICAL PROCEDURES

Term	Pronunciation	Meaning
ACE inhibitor (405)	ĀCE ĭn-HĬB-ĭ-tŏr	_____
acute coronary syndromes (404)	ă-KŪT kŏr-ō-NĂR-ē SĬN-drōmz	_____
aneurysm (406)	ĂN-ū-rĭzm	_____
angina (408)	ăn-JĪ-nă _or_ ĂN-jĭ-nă	_____
angiography (410)	ăn-jē-ŎG-ră-fē	_____

11

Term	Pronunciation	Meaning
atrioventricular block (398)	ā-trē-ō-věn-TRĬK-ū-lăr blŏk	
atrial fibrillation (399)	Ā-trē-ăl fĭb-rĭ-LĀ-shŭn	
auscultation (409)	ăw-skŭl-TĀ-shŭn	
beta-blocker (409)	BĀ-tă-BLŎK-ĕr	
bruit (409)	BRŪ-ē	
calcium channel blocker (409)	KĂL-sē-ŭm CHĂ-něl BLŎK-ĕr	
cardiac arrest (409)	KĂR-dē-ăk ā-RĔST	
cardiac catheterization (412)	KĂR-dē-ăk kăth-ě-těr-ĭ-ZĀ-shŭn	
cardiac MRI (412)	KĂR-dē-ăk MRI	
cardiac tamponade (409)	KĂR-dē-ăk tăm-pō-NŎD	
cardioversion (414)	kăr-dē-ō-VĚR-zhŭn	
claudication (409)	klăw-dě-KĀ-shŭn	
coarctation of the aorta (400)	kō-ărk-TĀ-shŭn of the ā-ŎR-tă	
computed tomography angiography (410)	kŏm-PŪ-těd tō-MŎG-ră-fē ăn-jē-ŎG-ră-fē	
congenital heart disease (400)	kŏn-GĔN-ĭ-tăl hărt dĭ-ZĒZ	
congestive heart failure (402)	kŏn-GĔS-tĭv hărt FĀL-ŭr	
coronary artery disease (402)	kŏr-ō-NĂR-ē ĂR-tě-rē dĭ-ZĒZ	
coronary artery bypass grafting (414)	kŏr-ō-NĂR-ē ĂR-tě-rē BĪ-păs GRĂFT-ĭng	
deep vein thrombosis (406)	dēp vān thrŏm-BŌ-sĭs	
digoxin (409)	dĭj-ŎK-sĭn	
digital subtraction angiography (410)	DĬJ-ĭ-tăl sŭb-TRĂK-shŭn ăn-jē-ŎG-ră-fē	
Doppler ultrasound (411)	DŎP-lěr ŬL-tră-sŏnd	
echocardiography (411)	ěk-ō-kăr-dē-ŌG-ră-fē	
electrocardiography (412)	ē-lěk-trō-kăr-dē-ŌG-ră-fē	
electron beam computed tomography (411)	ē-LĔK-trŏn bēm kŏm-PŪ-tě-rīzd tō-MŎG-ră-fē	
embolus; emboli (409)	ĔM-bō-lŭs; ĔM-bō-lī	
endarterectomy (414)	ěnd-ăr-těr-ĔK-tō-mē	
endocarditis (405)	ěn-dō-kăr-DĪ-tĭs	
extracorporeal circulation (415)	ěks-tră-kŏr-PŎR-ē-ăl sěr-kū-LĀ-shŭn	
fibrillation (399)	fĭb-rĭ-LĀ-shŭn	

Term	Pronunciation	Meaning
flutter (398)	FLŬ-tĕr	
heart transplantation (415)	hărt trănz-plăn-TĀ-shŭn	
hemorrhoids (408)	HĔM-ō-roydz	
Holter monitoring (414)	HŎL-tĕr MŎN-ĭ-tĕ-rĭng	
hypertension (407)	hī-pĕr-TĔN-shŭn	
implantable cardioverter defibrillator (400)	ĭm-PLĂNT-ăbl kăr-dē-ō-VĔR-tĕr dē-FĬB-rĭ-lā-tŏr	
infarction (409)	ĭn-FĂRK-shŭn	
ischemia (402)	ĭs-KĒ-mē-ă	
left ventricular assist device (415)	lĕft vĕn-TRĬ-kū-lăr ă-SĬST dĕ-VĪS	
lipid tests (410)	LĬ-pĭd tĕsts	
lipoprotein electrophoresis (410)	lī-pō-PRŌ-tēn ē-lĕk-trō-fŏr-Ē-sĭs	
mitral stenosis (406)	MĬ-trăl stĕ-NŌ-sĭs	
mitral valve prolapse (405)	MĬ-trăl vălv PRŌ-laps	
murmur (405)	MŬR-mĕr	
myocardial infarction (402)	mī-ō-KĂR-dē-ăl ĭn-FĂRK-shŭn	
nitroglycerin (409)	nī-trō-GLĬS-ĕr-ĭn	
occlusion (409)	ŏ-KLŪ-zhĕn	
palpitations (409)	păl-pĭ-TĀ-shŭnz	
patent ductus arteriosus (401)	PĀ-tĕnt DŬK-tŭs ăr-tēr-ē-Ō-sŭs	
percutaneous coronary intervention (415)	pĕr-kū-TĀ-nē-ŭs KŎR-ō-năr-ē ĭn-tĕr-VĔN-shŭn	
pericardial friction rub (409)	pĕr-ĭ-KĂR-dē-ăl FRĬK-shŭn rŭb	
pericarditis (405)	pĕr-ĭ-kăr-DĬ-tĭs	
peripheral vascular disease (407)	pĕ-RĬ-fĕr-ăl VĂS-kū-lăr dĭ-ZĒZ	
petechiae (409)	pĕ-TĒ-kē-ē	
positron emission tomography (411)	pŏs-ĭ-tron ē-MĬSH-un tō-MŎG-ră-fē	
radiofrequency catheter ablation (400)	rā-dē-ō-FRĒ-qwĕn-sē KĂTH-ĕ-tĕr ăb-LĀ-shŭn	
Raynaud disease (407)	rā-NŌ dĭ-ZĒZ	
rheumatic heart disease (406)	roo-MĂT-ik hărt dĭ-ZĒZ	
septal defects (401)	SĔP-tăl DĒ-fĕkts	

11

Term	Pronunciation	Meaning
serum enzyme tests (410)	SĔ-rum ĔN-zīm tĕsts	_____
statins (409)	STĂ-tĭnz	_____
stress test (414)	STRĔS tĕst	_____
telemetry (412)	tĕl-ĔM-ĕ-trē	_____
tetralogy of Fallot (401)	tĕ-TRĂL-ō-jē of fă-LŌ	_____
technetium 99m sestamibi scan (412)	tĕk-NĒ-shē-ŭm 99m sĕs-tă-MĬ-bē skăn	_____
thallium 201 scan (412)	THĂL-ē-um 201 skăn	_____
thrill (409)	thrĭl	_____
thrombolytic therapy (415)	thrŏm-bō-LĬ-tĭk THĔ-ră-pē	_____
thrombotic occlusion (402)	thrŏm-BŎT-ĭk ō-KLŪ-zhŭn	_____
varicose veins (408)	VĂR-ĭ-kōs vānz	_____
vegetations (409)	vĕj-ĕ-TĀ-shŭnz	_____

REVIEW SHEET

Write the meanings of each word part in the space provided. Check your answers with the information in the chapter or in the Glossary (Medical Word Parts—English) at the end of the book.

COMBINING FORMS

Combining Form	Meaning	Combining Form	Meaning
aneurysm/o	aneurysm- *widened blood vessel*	myx/o	*mucus*
angi/o	*vessel*	ox/o	*oxygen*
aort/o	*aorta*	pericardi/o	*surrounding heart*
arter/o, arteri/o	*artery*	phleb/o	*vein*
ather/o	*plaque*	pulmon/o	*lung*
atri/o	*atrium*	sphygm/o	*pulse*
axill/o	*armpit*	steth/o	*chest*
brachi/o	*arm*	thromb/o	*clot*
cardi/o	*heart*	valv/o	*valve*
cholesterol/o	*cholesterol*	valvul/o	*valve*
coron/o	*heart*	vas/o	*vessel*
cyan/o	*blue*	vascul/o	*vessel*
isch/o	*ischium (part of hip bone)*	ven/o, ven/i	*vein*
my/o	*muscle*	ventricul/o	*ventricle*

SUFFIXES

Suffix	Meaning	Suffix	Meaning
-constriction	narrowing	-oma	tumor
-dilation	expanding	-osis	condition usually
-emia	blood condition	-plasty	surgical repair
-graphy	process of recording	-sclerosis	hardening
-lysis	breakdown / separate	-stenosis	tightening
-megaly	enlargement	-tomy	process of cutting
-meter	measure		

PREFIXES

Prefix	Meaning	Prefix	Meaning
a-, an-	not / without	hypo-	deficient / below
brady-	slow	inter-	between
de-	down, less, removed	peri-	surrounding
dys-	bad, bb normal	tachy-	fast
endo-	in, within	tetra-	four
hyper-	excessive	tri-	three

 Please refer to the enclosed CD for additional exercises and images related to this chapter.

chapter 12

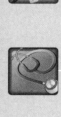

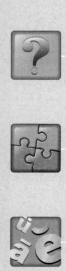

Combining Form	Meaning	Terminology	Meaning
lob/o	lobe of the lung	lobectomy _____ *Figure 12–5 shows four different types of pulmonary resections.*	
mediastin/o	mediastinum	mediastinoscopy _____ *An endoscope is inserted through an incision in the chest.*	
nas/o	nose	paranasal sinuses _____ *Para- means near in this term.*	
		nasogastric intubation _____	
orth/o	straight, upright	orthopnea _____ *An abnormal condition in which breathing (-pnea) is easier in the upright position. A major cause of orthopnea is congestive heart failure (the lungs fill with fluid when the patient is lying flat). Physicians assess the degree of orthopnea by the number of pillows a patient requires to sleep comfortably (e.g., two-pillow orthopnea).*	

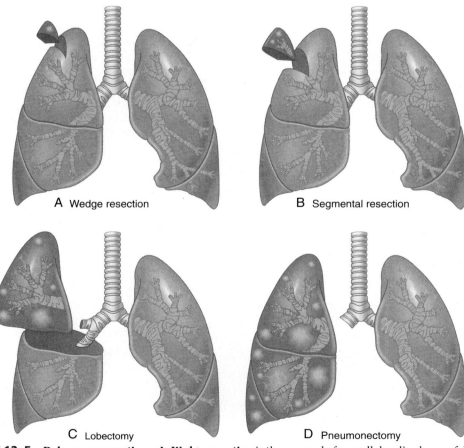

A Wedge resection

B Segmental resection

C Lobectomy

D Pneumonectomy

FIGURE 12–5   Pulmonary resections. A, Wedge resection is the removal of a small, localized area of diseased tissue near the surface of the lung. Pulmonary function and structure are relatively unchanged after healing. **B, Segmental resection** is the removal of a bronchiole and its alveoli (one or more lung segments). The remaining lung tissue expands to fill the previously occupied space. **C, Lobectomy** is the removal of an entire lobe of the lung. After lobectomy, the remaining lung increases in size to fill the space in the thoracic cavity. **D, Pneumonectomy** is the removal of an entire lung. Techniques such as removal of ribs and elevation of the diaphragm are used to reduce the size of the empty thoracic space.

12

Combining Form	Meaning	Terminology	Meaning
ox/o	oxygen	hypoxia _____ *Tissues have a decreased amount of oxygen, and cyanosis can result.*	
pector/o	chest	expectoration _____ *Expectorated sputum can contain mucus, blood, cellular debris, pus, and microorganisms.*	
pharyng/o	pharynx, throat	pharyngeal _____	
phon/o	voice	dysphonia _____ *Hoarseness or other voice impairment.*	
phren/o	diaphragm	phrenic nerve _____ *The motor nerve to the diaphragm.*	
pleur/o	pleura	pleurodynia _____ *The suffix -dynia means pain. The intercostal muscles are inflamed.*	
		pleural effusion _____ *An **effusion** is the escape of fluid from blood vessels or lymphatics into a cavity or into tissue spaces.*	
pneum/o, pneumon/o	air, lung	pneumothorax _____ *The suffix -thorax means chest. Air accumulates in the pleural cavity, between the layers of the pleura (Fig. 12–6).*	
		pneumonectomy _____	
pulmon/o	lung	pulmonary _____	
rhin/o	nose	rhinorrhea _____	
		rhinoplasty _____	

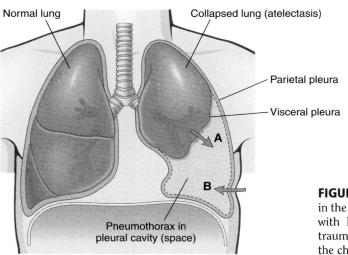

FIGURE 12–6 Pneumothorax. Air gathers in the pleural cavity. This condition can occur with lung disease, as in **A,** or can follow trauma to and perforation of (a hole through) the chest wall, as in **B.**

12

Combining Form	Meaning	Terminology	Meaning
sinus/o	sinus, cavity	sinusitis _____	
spir/o	breathing	spirometer _____	
		expiration _____	
		Note that the s is omitted (when it's preceded by an x).	
		respiration _____	
		Cheyne-Stokes respirations *are marked by rhythmic changes in the depth of breathing. The pattern occurs every 45 seconds to 3 minutes. The cause may be heart failure or brain damage, both of which affect the respiratory center in the brain.*	
tel/o	complete	atelectasis _____	
		Collapsed lung; incomplete expansion (-ectasis) of a lung (Fig. 12–7). Atelectasis may occur after surgery when a patient experiences pain and does not take deep breaths, preventing full expansion of the lungs.	
thorac/o	chest	thoracotomy _____	
		thoracic _____	
tonsill/o	tonsils	tonsillectomy *Removal of the Tonsils*	
		The oropharyngeal (palatine) tonsils are removed.	
trache/o	trachea, windpipe	tracheotomy _____	
		tracheal stenosis _____	
		Having an endotracheal tube in place for a prolonged period may lead to tracheal trauma or the formation of scar tissue.	

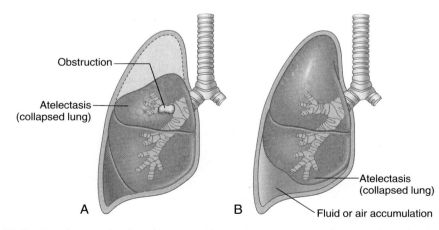

FIGURE 12–7   Two forms of atelectasis. A, An obstruction prevents air from reaching distal airways, and alveoli collapse. The most frequent cause is blockage of a bronchus by a mucous or mucopurulent (pus-filled) plug, as might occur postoperatively. **B,** Accumulations of fluid, blood, or air within the pleural cavity collapse the lung. This can occur with congestive heart failure (poor circulation leads to fluid buildup in the pleural cavity) or because of leakage of air caused by a pneumothorax.

SUFFIXES

12

Suffix	Meaning	Terminology	Meaning
-ema	condition	empyema _____	
		Em- at the beginning of this term means in. Empyema (pyothorax) is a collection of pus in the pleural cavity.	
-osmia	smell	anosmia _____	
-pnea	breathing	apnea _____	
		Sleep apnea *is sudden cessation of breathing during sleep. It can result in hypoxia, leading to cognitive impairment, hypertension, and arrhythmias. Obstructive sleep apnea (OSA) involves narrowing or occlusion in the upper airway.* ***Continuous positive airway pressure (CPAP)*** *is gentle ventilatory support used to keep the airways open. See Figure 12–8.*	
		dyspnea _____	
		Dys- means abnormal here and is associated with shortness of breath (SOB). ***Paroxysmal*** *(sudden)* ***nocturnal*** *(at night)* ***dyspnea*** *may be experienced by patients with congestive heart failure when they recline in bed. Patients often describe the sensation as "air hunger."*	
		hyperpnea _____	
		An increase in the depth of breathing, occurring normally with exercise and abnormally with any condition in which the supply of oxygen is inadequate.	
		tachypnea _____	
		Excessively rapid and shallow breathing; hyperventilation.	
-ptysis	spitting	hemoptysis _____	
-sphyxia	pulse	asphyxia _____	
		Blockage of breathing and severe hypoxia leads to hypoxemia, hypercapnia, loss of consciousness, and death (lack of pulse).	
-thorax	pleural cavity, chest	hemothorax _____	
		pyothorax _____	
		Empyema of the chest.	

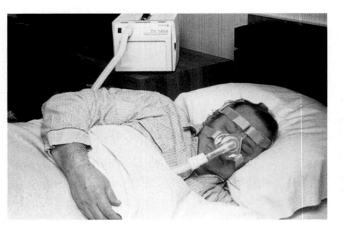

FIGURE 12–8 This man is sleeping with a **nasal CPAP** (continuous positive airway pressure) mask in place. The pressure supplied by air coming from the compressor opens the oropharynx and nasopharynx. (From Lewis SM, Heitkemper MM, Dirksen SR: Medical-Surgical Nursing: Assessment and Management of Clinical Problems, 6th ed. St. Louis, Mosby, 2004, p. 575.)

DIAGNOSTIC AND PATHOLOGIC TERMS

DIAGNOSTIC TERMS

auscultation

Listening to sounds within the body.

This procedure, performed with a stethoscope, is used chiefly for diagnosing conditions of the lungs, pleura, heart, and abdomen, as well as to determine the condition of the fetus during pregnancy.

percussion

Tapping on a surface to determine the difference in the density of the underlying structure.

Tapping over a solid organ produces a dull sound without resonance. Percussion over an air-filled structure, such as the lung, produces a resonant, hollow note. When the lungs or the pleural space are filled with fluid and become more dense, as in pneumonia, resonance is replaced by dullness.

pleural rub

Scratchy sound produced by the motion of inflamed or irritated pleural surfaces rubbing against each other; also called a friction rub.

Pleural rub occurs when the pleura are thickened by inflammation, scarring, or neoplastic cells. It is heard by auscultation and can be felt by placing the fingers on the chest wall.

rale (crackle)

Fine crackling sound heard on auscultation (during inspiration) when there is fluid in the alveoli.

rhonchus (*plural:* **rhonchi**)

Loud rumbling sound heard on auscultation of bronchi obstructed by sputum.

Rhonchi indicate congestion and inflammation in larger bronchial tubes.

sputum

Material expelled from the chest by coughing or clearing the throat.

Purulent (containing pus) sputum often is green or brown. It results from infection and also may be seen with asthma. Blood-tinged sputum is suggestive of tuberculosis or malignancy. A **sputum culture** is growing sputum in a nutrient medium to detect the presence of a pathogen. **Culture and sensitivity (C&S)** studies identify the sputum pathogen and determine which antibiotic will be effective in destroying or reducing its growth.

stridor

Strained, high-pitched, relatively loud sound made on inspiration; associated with obstruction of the larynx or trachea.

wheeze

Continuous high-pitched whistling sound heard when air is forced through a narrow space during inspiration or expiration.

Usually caused by tightening of the bronchi in patients with asthma.

PATHOLOGIC TERMS

Upper Respiratory Disorders

croup

Acute viral infection in infants and children; characterized by obstruction of the larynx, barking cough, and stridor.

The most common causative agents are influenza viruses or **respiratory syncytial virus (RSV)**.

12

diphtheria	**Acute infection of the throat and upper respiratory tract caused by the diphtheria bacterium (*Corynebacterium*).**

Inflammation occurs, and a leathery, opaque membrane (Greek *diphthera*, leather membrane) forms in the pharynx and respiratory tract.

Immunity to diphtheria (by production of antibodies) is induced by the administration of weakened toxins (antigens) beginning between the sixth and eighth weeks of life. These injections usually are given as combination vaccines with pertussis and tetanus toxins and so are called **DPT** injections.

epistaxis	**Nosebleed.**

Epistaxis is a Greek word meaning a dropping. It commonly results from irritation of nasal mucous membranes, trauma, vitamin K deficiency, clotting abnormalities, or hypertension.

pertussis	**Highly contagious bacterial infection of the pharynx, larynx, and trachea caused by *Bordetella pertussis*. Also known as whooping cough.**

Pertussis is characterized by **paroxysmal** (sudden) coughing that ends in a loud "whooping" inspiration.

Bronchial Disorders

asthma	**Chronic inflammatory disorder with airway obstruction caused by bronchial edema, bronchoconstriction, and increased mucus production.**

Associated signs and symptoms of asthma are dyspnea, wheezing, and cough. Etiology can involve allergy or infection. Triggers to asthmatic attacks include exercise, strong odors, cold air, stress, allergens (e.g., dust, molds, pollens, foods) and medications (aspirin, beta-blockers). Asthma treatments are inhaled anti-inflammatory agents (long-term control with glucocorticoids), bronchodilators (quick-relief control with albuterol and theophylline), and trigger avoidance by patient education. Other conditions, such as gastroesophageal reflux disease (GERD), sinusitis, or allergic rhinitis, or certain medications can impede asthma control.

bronchiectasis	**Chronic dilation of a bronchus secondary to infection in the lower lobes of the lung.**

This condition is caused by chronic infection with loss of elasticity of the bronchi. Secretions puddle and do not drain normally. Signs and symptoms are cough, fever, and expectoration of foul-smelling, **purulent** (pus-containing) sputum. Treatment is **palliative** (noncurative) and includes antibiotics, mucolytics, bronchodilators, respiratory therapy, and surgical resection if other treatment is not effective.

chronic bronchitis	**Inflammation of the bronchi persisting over a long time.**

Infection and cigarette smoking are etiologic factors. Signs and symptoms include excessive secretion of mucus, a productive cough, and obstruction of respiratory passages. Chronic bronchitis, asthma, and emphysema (lung disease in which air exchange at the alveoli is severely impaired) all are components of chronic obstructive pulmonary disease (COPD).

cystic fibrosis	**Inherited disorder of exocrine glands resulting in thick, mucous secretions that do not drain normally.**

The exocrine glands affected are the pancreas (insufficient secretion of enzymes), sweat glands (abnormal salt production), and epithelium (lining cells) of the respiratory tract. Chronic airway obstruction, infection, bronchiectasis, and respiratory failure are the end result. Therapy includes replacement of pancreatic enzymes and treatment of pulmonary obstruction and infection.

The gene responsible for cystic fibrosis is known, and persons carrying the gene may be identified. There is no known cure, although lung transplantation can extend life and restore lung function.

Lung Disorders

atelectasis

Incomplete (atel/o) expansion (-ectasis) of alveoli; collapsed, functionless, airless lung or portion of a lung. Caused by tumor or other obstruction of the bronchus, or poor respiratory effort.

In atelectasis, the bronchioles and alveoli (pulmonary parenchyma) resemble a collapsed balloon. Common causes of atelectasis include poor inspiratory effort after surgery, blockage of a bronchus or smaller bronchial tube by secretions, tumor, and chest wounds that permit air, fluid, or blood to accumulate in the pleural cavity. Acute atelectasis requires removal of the underlying cause (tumor, foreign body, mucous plug) and therapy to open airways. Respiration also can be limited by pain.

emphysema

Hyperinflation of air sacs with destruction of alveolar walls. (See Figure 12–9, *A* and *B*).

Loss of elasticity and the breakdown of alveolar walls result in expiratory flow limitation. There is a strong association between cigarette smoking and emphysema. As a result of the destruction of lung parenchyma, including blood vessels, pulmonary artery pressure rises and the right side of the heart must work harder to pump blood. This leads to right ventricular hypertrophy and heart failure **(cor pulmonale).**

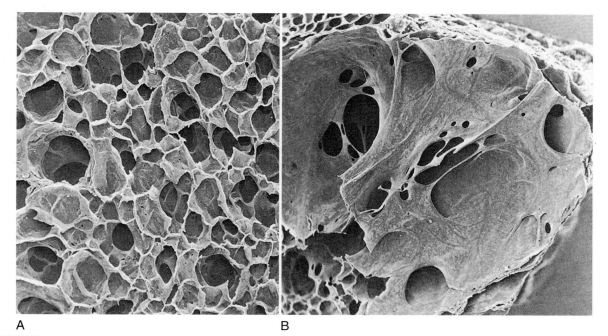

A   B

FIGURE 12–9   **A,** Normal lung tissue. **B, Emphysema.** Notice the overinflation of air sacs with destruction of alveolar walls. (From Thibodeau GA, Patton KT: Anatomy & Physiology, 6th ed., St. Louis, Mosby, 2007, p. 868.)

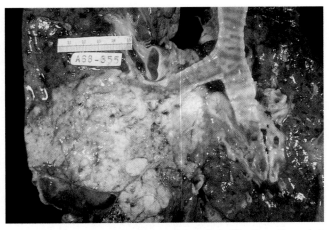

FIGURE 12–10 **Lung cancer.** The gray-white tumor tissue is infiltrating the substance of the lung. This tumor was identified as a squamous cell carcinoma. Squamous cell carcinomas arise in major bronchi and spread to local hilar lymph nodes. (From Kumar V, Cotran RS, Robbins SL: Robbins Basic Pathology, 7th ed. Philadelphia, WB Saunders, 2003, p. 501.)

lung cancer

Malignant tumor arising from the lungs and bronchi (see Fig. 12–10).

This group of cancers, often associated with cigarette smoking, is the most frequent fatal malignancy. Lung cancers are divided into two general categories: **non–small cell lung cancer (NSCLC)** and **small cell lung cancer (SCLC).**

NSCLC accounts for 90 percent of lung cancers and comprises two main types: adenocarcinoma (derived from mucus-secreting cells), and squamous cell carcinoma (derived from the lining cells of the upper airway). When lung cancer is diagnosed, physicians assess the *stage* of the tumor (determined by its size and location, including any distant areas of spread) to prepare a protocol for treatment.

For localized tumors, surgery may be curative. When disease is locally advanced (with spread to involve lymph nodes or mediastinum), chemotherapy and radiation therapy are options. Doctors treat metastatic disease (to liver, brain, and bones) with chemotherapy and radiation therapy (irradiation).

SCLC derives from small, round to oval secretory cells found in pulmonary epithelium. It grows rapidly early in its course and quickly spreads outside the lung. Palliative treatment includes surgery, radiation therapy, and chemotherapy.

pneumoconiosis

Abnormal condition caused by dust in the lungs, with chronic inflammation, infection, and brochitis (see Figure 12–11, *A*).

Various forms are named according to the type of dust particle inhaled: **anthracosis**—coal (anthrac/o) dust (black lung disease); **asbestosis**—asbestos (asbest/o) particles (in shipbuilding and construction trades); **silicosis**—silica (silic/o = rocks) or glass (grinder's disease).

pneumonia

Acute inflammation and infection of alveoli, which fill with pus or products of the inflammatory reaction. See Figure 12–11, *B*.

Etiologic agents are pneumococci, staphylococci, and other bacteria, fungi, or viruses. Infection damages alveolar membranes so that an **exudate** (fluid, blood cells, and debris) consolidates the alveoli (sacs become "glued" together, making air exchange less effective). **Lobar pneumonia** (see Figure 12–11, *B*) involves an entire lobe of a lung. **Bronchopneumonia,** common in infants and the elderly, involves patchy consolidation (abscesses) in the lung parenchyma. Treatment includes appropriate antibiotics and, if necessary, oxygen and mechanical ventilation.

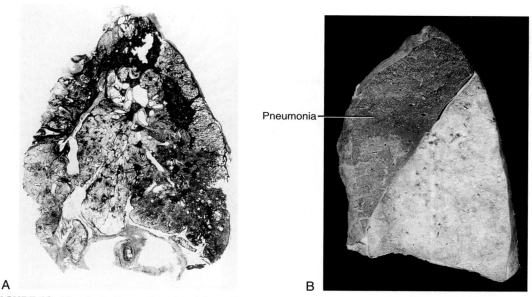

A

B

FIGURE 12–11 **A, Anthracosis** or black lung disease. Notice the dark black deposits of coal dust throughout the lung. **B, Lobar pneumonia** (at autopsy). Notice that the condition affects a lobe of the lung. The patient's signs and symptoms included fever, chills, cough, dark sputum, rapid shallow breathing, and cyanosis. If diagnosis is made early, antibiotic therapy is successful. (**A** from Cotran RS, Kumar V, Collins T: Robbins Pathologic Basis of Disease, 6th ed., Philadelphia, WB Saunders, 1999, p. 731; **B** from Kumar V, Cotran RS, Robbins SL: Robbins Basic Pathology, 7th ed. Philadelphia, WB Saunders, 2003.)

Community-acquired pneumonia results from a contagious respiratory infection, caused by a variety of viruses and bacteria (especially *Mycoplasma* bacteria). It usually is treated at home with oral antibiotics.

Hospital-acquired pneumonia or **nosocomial pneumonia** is acquired during hospitalization (Greek *nosokomeion* means hospital). For example, patients may contract pneumonia while on mechanical ventilation or as a hospital-acquired infection.

Aspiration pneumonia is caused by material, such as food or vomit lodging in bronchi or lungs. It is a danger to the elderly, Alzheimer disease patients, stroke victims, and people with dysphagia.

pulmonary abscess **A large collection of pus (bacterial infection) in the lungs.**

pulmonary edema **Swelling and fluid in the air sacs and bronchioles.**

This condition most commonly is caused by the inability of the heart to pump blood (congestive heart failure). Blood backs up in the pulmonary blood vessels, and fluid seeps out into the alveoli and bronchioles. Acute pulmonary edema requires immediate medical attention, including drugs (diuretics, vasodilators), oxygen in high concentrations, and keeping the patient in a sitting position (to decrease venous return to the heart).

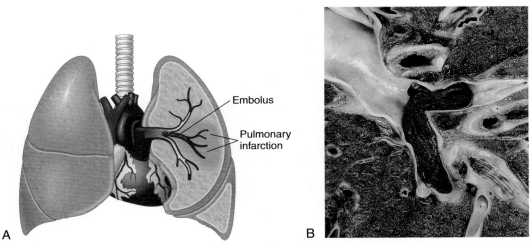

FIGURE 12–12 **Pulmonary embolism** (**A** and **B**). (**B** from Kumar V, Cotran RS, Robbins SL: Robbins Basic Pathology, 7th ed. Philadelphia, WB Saunders, 2003.)

pulmonary embolism (PE)	**Clot (thrombus) or other material lodges in vessels of the lung.** See Figure 12–12, *A* and *B*. The clot travels from distant veins, usually in the legs. Occlusion can produce an area of dead (necrotic) tissue; this condition is called **pulmonary infarction.** PE often causes acute pleuritic chest pain (pain on inspiration) and may be associated with blood in the sputum, fever, and respiratory insufficiency. It is diagnosed by ventilation-perfusion scans that reveal areas of lung that lack adequate blood supply (perfusion). Other useful tests include computed tomography (CT) scans, which will reveal obstruction of pulmonary vessels.
pulmonary fibrosis	**Formation of scar tissue in the connective tissue of the lungs.** This condition may be the result of any inflammation or irritation caused by tuberculosis, pneumonia, or pneumoconiosis.
sarcoidosis	**Chronic inflammatory disease of unknown cause in which small nodules or tubercles develop in lungs, lymph nodes, and other organs.** Bilateral hilar lymphadenopathy or lung involvement is visible on chest x-ray in 90 percent of cases. Many patients are asymptomatic and retain adequate pulmonary function. Others have more active disease and impaired pulmonary function. Corticosteroid drugs are used to prevent progression in these patients.
tuberculosis (TB)	**Infectious disease caused by *Mycobacterium tuberculosis*; lungs usually are involved, but any organ in the body may be affected.** Rod-shaped bacteria called **bacilli** invade the lungs, producing small tubercles (from Latin *tuber*, a swelling) of infection. Early TB usually is asymptomatic and detected on routine chest x-ray. Signs and symptoms of advanced disease are cough, weight loss, night sweats, hemoptysis, and pleuritic pain. Antituberculous chemotherapy (isoniazid, rifampin) is effective in most cases. Immuno-compromised patients are particularly susceptible to antibiotic-resistant TB. It is important and often necessary to treat TB with several drugs at the same time to prevent drug resistance. The PPD skin test (see page 462) is given to most hospital and medical employees because TB is highly contagious.

Pleural Disorders

mesothelioma

Rare malignant tumor arising in the pleura; associated with asbestos exposure.

Mesotheliomas are composed of mesothelium, which forms the lining of the pleural surface.

pleural effusion

Abnormal accumulation of fluid in the pleural space (cavity).

Two types of pleural effusions are exudates (fluid from tumors, infections, trauma, and other diseases) and transudates (fluid from congestive heart failure, pulmonary embolism, or cirrhosis).

pleurisy (pleuritis)

Inflammation of the pleura.

This condition causes pleurodynia and dyspnea and, in chronic cases, pleural effusion.

pneumothorax

Collection of air in the pleural space.

Pneumothorax may occur in the course of a pulmonary disease (emphysema, carcinoma, tuberculosis, or lung abscess) when rupture of any pulmonary lesions near the pleural surface allows communication between an alveolus or bronchus and the pleural cavity. It may also follow trauma and perforation of the chest wall or prolonged high-flow oxygen delivered by a respirator in an intensive care unit (ICU).

  Pleurodesis (-desis means to bind) is the artificial production of adhesions between the parietal and visceral pleura for treatment of persistent pneumothorax and severe pleural effusion. This is accomplished by using talc powder or drugs, such as antibiotics.

STUDY SECTION

Practice spelling each term and know its meaning.

anthracosis	Coal dust accumulation in the lungs.
asbestosis	Asbestos particles accumulate in the lungs.
bacilli (*singular:* **bacillus**)	Rod-shaped bacteria (cause of tuberculosis).
chronic obstructive pulmonary disease (COPD)	Chronic condition of persistent obstruction of air flow through bronchial tubes and lungs. COPD is caused by smoking, chronic infection, and, in a minority of cases, asthma. Patients with predominant **chronic bronchitis** COPD are referred to as "blue bloaters" (cyanotic, stocky build), whereas those with predominant **emphysema** are called "pink puffers" (short of breath, but with near-normal blood oxygen levels, and no change in skin color).
cor pulmonale	Failure of the right side of the heart to pump a sufficient amount of blood to the lungs because of underlying lung disease.
exudate	Fluid, cells, or other substances (pus) that slowly leave cells or capillaries through pores or small breaks in cell membranes.
hydrothorax	Collection of fluid in the pleural cavity.
palliative	Relieving symptoms, but not curing the disease.
paroxysmal	Pertaining to a sudden occurrence, such as a spasm or seizure; oxysm/o means sudden.
pulmonary infarction	Occurrence of necrotic (dead) tissue in the lung.
purulent	Containing pus.
silicosis	Disease due to silica or glass dust in the lungs; occurs in mining occupations.

CLINICAL PROCEDURES

X-RAY TESTS

12

chest x-ray (CXR)

Radiographic image of the thoracic cavity (chest film).

Chest x-rays are taken in the frontal (coronal) plane (see Fig. 12–13, *A*) as posteroanterior (PA) or anteroposterior (AP) views and in the sagittal plane as lateral views. **Chest tomograms** are a series of x-ray images each showing a "slice" of the chest at different depths. Tomograms detect small masses not seen on regular films.

computed tomography (CT) scan of the chest

Computer-generated x-ray images show thoracic structures in cross section.

This test is for diagnosis of lesions difficult to assess by conventional x-ray studies, such as those in the hilum, mediastinum, and pleura.

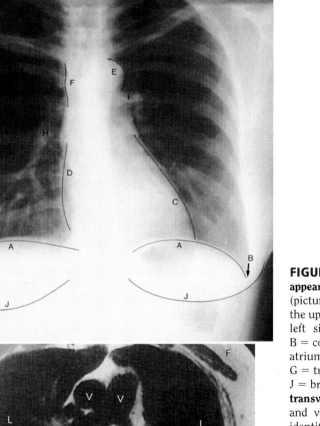

FIGURE 12–13 A, A normal chest x-ray appearance. The image is a posteroanterior (PA) view (picture was taken back to front). The backwards L in the upper corner is placed on the film to indicate the left side of the patient's chest. A = diaphragm; B = costophrenic angle; C = left ventricle; D = right atrium; E = aortic arch; F = superior vena cava; G = trachea; H = right bronchus; I = left bronchus; J = breast shadows. **B, MRI of the upper chest, transverse (axial) view.** Notice the lungs (L), fat (F), and vessels (V). A hilar tumor *(arrow)* is easily identified at the region where bronchial tubes and blood vessels enter the lung. (**A** from Black JM, Hawks JH, Keene AM: Medical-Surgical Nursing: Clinical Management for Positive Outcomes, 6th ed. Philadelphia, WB Saunders, 2001, p. 1644. **B** from Ballinger PW, Frank ED: Merrill's Atlas of Radiographic Positions and Radiologic Procedures, 10th ed. vol. 3. St. Louis, Mosby, 2003, p. 388.)

pulmonary angiography or arteriography	**X-ray images are obtained after radiopaque contrast is injected into the pulmonary artery.**
	The pulmonary angiogram (PA gram) is a study that visualizes the pulmonary circulation to locate obstructions or pathologic conditions such as pulmonary embolism.

MAGNETIC IMAGING

magnetic resonance imaging (MRI) of the chest	**Magnetic waves create detailed images of the chest in frontal, lateral, and cross-sectional (axial) planes.**
	This test is helpful in locating lesions difficult to assess by CT scan (see Fig. 12–13, *B*).

RADIOACTIVE TESTS

positron emission tomography (PET) scan of the lung	**Radioactive substance is injected and images reveal metabolic activity in the lung.**
	This scanning technique can identify malignant tumors, which have higher metabolic activity.
ventilation-perfusion (V/Q) scan	**Detection device records radioactivity in the lung after injection of a radioisotope or inhalation of small amount of radioactive gas (xenon).**
	This test can identify areas of the lung not receiving adequate air flow (ventilation) or blood flow (perfusion). Q is the symbol for blood volume or rate of blood flow.

OTHER PROCEDURES

bronchoscopy	**Fiberoptic or rigid endoscope inserted into the bronchial tubes for diagnosis, biopsy, or collection of specimens.**
	A physician places the bronchoscope through the throat, larynx, and trachea into the bronchi. In **bronchioalveolar lavage (bronchial washing),** fluid is injected and withdrawn. In transbronchial biopsies, a forceps is used to grasp tissue or a brush **(bronchial brushing)** is inserted through the bronchoscope (see Fig. 12–14).

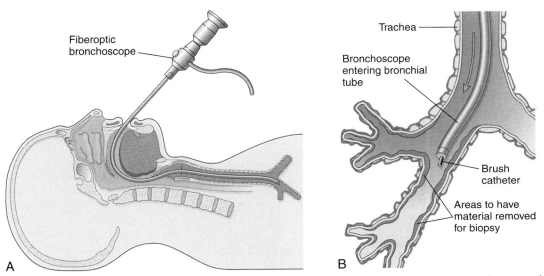

FIGURE 12–14   A, Fiberoptic bronchoscopy. A bronchoscope is passed through the nose, throat, larynx, and trachea into a bronchus. **B, A bronchoscope,** with brush catheter, in place in a bronchial tube.

12

endotracheal intubation	**Placement of a tube through the mouth into the pharynx, larynx, and trachea to establish an airway** (see Fig. 12–15).

This procedure also allows a person to be placed on a **ventilator** (an apparatus that moves air into and out of the lungs).

laryngoscopy	**Visual examination of the voice box.**

A lighted, flexible endoscope is passed through the mouth or nose into the larynx.

lung biopsy	**Removal of lung tissue followed by microscopic examination.**

Specimens may be obtained by bronchoscopy or thoracotomy (open-lung biopsy).

mediastinoscopy	**Endoscopic visual examination of the mediastinum.**

An incision is made above the breastbone (suprasternal) for inspection and biopsy of lymph nodes.

pulmonary function tests (PFTs)	**Tests that measure the ventilation mechanics of the lung (airway function, lung volume, and capacity of the lungs to exchange oxygen and carbon dioxide efficiently).**

PFTs are used for many reasons: (1) to evaluate patients with shortness of breath (SOB); (2) to monitor lung function in patients with known respiratory disease; (3) to evaluate disability; and (4) to assess lung function before surgery or therapy (chemotherapy). A **spirometer** measures the volume and rate of air passing in and out of the lung.

PFTs determine if lung disease is obstructive, restrictive, or both. In **obstructive lung disease** airways are narrowed, which results in resistance to air flow during breathing. A hallmark PFT value in obstructive disease is decreased expiratory flow rate or **FEV_1** (forced expiratory volume in the first second of expiration). Examples of obstructive lung diseases are asthma, COPD, bronchiectasis, cystic fibrosis, and bronchiolitis.

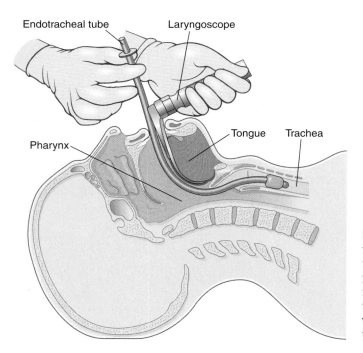

Endotracheal tube   Laryngoscope

Pharynx

Tongue   Trachea

FIGURE 12–15 Endotracheal intubation. The patient is in a supine position; the head is hyperextended, the lower portion of the neck is flexed, and the mouth is opened. A **laryngoscope** is used to hold the airway open, to expose the vocal cords, and as a guide for placing the tube into the trachea.

In **restrictive lung disease** expansion of the lung is limited by disease that affects the chest wall, pleura, or lung tissue itself. A hallmark PFT abnormality in restrictive disease is decreased **total lung capacity (TLC).** Examples of lung conditions that stiffen and scar the lung are pulmonary fibrosis, radiation damage to the lung, and pneumoconiosis. Other causes of restrictive lung disease are neuromuscular conditions that affect the lung, such as myasthenia gravis, muscular dystrophy, and diaphragmatic weakness and paralysis.

The ability of gas to diffuse across the alveolar-capillary membrane is assessed by the diffusion capacity of the lung for carbon monoxide (DL_{co}). A patient breathes in a small amount of carbon monoxide (CO), and the length of time it takes the gas to enter the bloodstream is measured.

thoracentesis	**Surgical puncture to remove fluid from the pleural space.**

This procedure is used to obtain pleural fluid for diagnosis or to drain a pleural effusion. A chest tube may be inserted to allow further drainage of fluid (see Fig. 12–16). New pleural catheters are available for home management of pleural effusions.

thoracotomy	**Major surgical incision of the chest.**

The incision is large, cutting into bone, muscle, and cartilage. It is necessary for lung biopsies and resections (lobectomy and pneumonectomy).

thoracoscopy (thorascopy)	**Visual examination of the chest via small incisions and use of an endoscope.**

Video-assisted thoracic surgery (VATS) allows the surgeon to view the chest from a video monitor. The thorascope (thoracoscope) is equipped with a camera that magnifies the image on the monitor. Thoracoscopy can diagnose and treat conditions of the lung, pleura, and mediastinum.

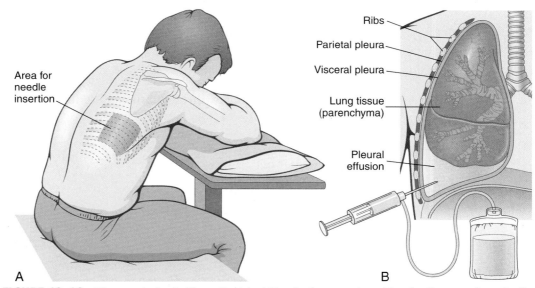

FIGURE 12–16   **Thoracentesis. A,** The patient is sitting in the correct position for the procedure; it allows the chest wall to be pulled outward in an expanded position. **B,** The needle is inserted close to the base of the effusion so that gravity can help with drainage, but it is kept as far away from the diaphragm as possible.

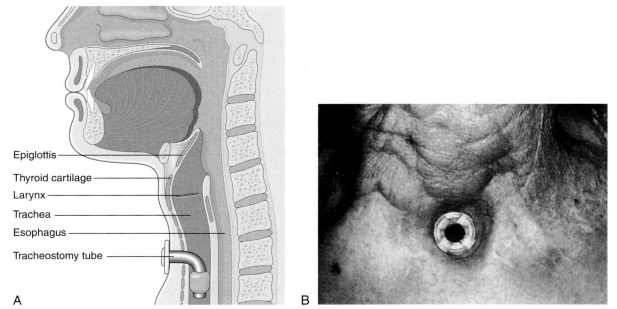

Epiglottis
Thyroid cartilage
Larynx
Trachea
Esophagus
Tracheostomy tube

A   B

FIGURE 12–17 **A, Tracheostomy** with tube in place. **B, Healed tracheostomy** after laryngectomy. (**B** from Black JM, Hawks JH, Keene AM: Medical-Surgical Nursing: Clinical Management for Positive Outcomes, 6th ed. Philadelphia, WB Saunders, 2001, p. 1672.)

tracheostomy	**Surgical creation of an opening into the trachea through the neck.** A tube is inserted to create an airway. The tracheostomy tube may be permanent as well as an emergency device (see Fig. 12–17). A **tracheotomy** is the incision necessary to create a tracheostomy.
tuberculin test	**Determines past or present tuberculous infection based on a positive skin reaction.** Examples are the **Heaf and tine tests**, using purified protein derivative **(PPD)** applied with multiple punctures of the skin, and the **Mantoux test,** using PPD given by intradermal injection.
tube thoracostomy	**Chest tube is passed through an opening in the skin of the chest to continuously drain a pleural effusion.**

ABBREVIATIONS

ABGs	arterial blood gases
AFB	acid-fast bacillus—the type of organism causing tuberculosis
ARDS	acute (formerly adult) respiratory distress syndrome—a group of signs and symptoms including tachypnea, dyspnea, tachycardia, hypoxemia, and cyanosis associated with acute respiratory failure
BAL	bronchioalveolar lavage
Bronch	bronchoscopy
CO₂	carbon dioxide
COPD	chronic obstructive pulmonary disease—airway obstruction associated with emphysema and chronic bronchitis
CPAP	continuous positive airway pressure
CPR	cardiopulmonary resuscitation—three basic steps: A, *a*irway opened by tilting the head; B, *b*reathing restored by mouth-to-mouth breathing; C, *c*irculation restored by external cardiac compression
C&S	culture and sensitivity
CTA	clear to auscultation
CXR	chest x-ray [film]
DL$_{CO}$	diffusion capacity of the lung for carbon monoxide
DOE	dyspnea on exertion
DPI	dry powder inhaler
DPT	diphtheria, pertussis, tetanus—toxoids for vaccination of infants, to provide immunity to these diseases
ERV	expiratory reserve—maximal volume of gas that can be exhaled after resting volume exhalation
FEV$_1$	forced expiratory volume in 1 second
FVC	forced vital capacity—amount of gas that can be forcibly and rapidly exhaled after a full inspiration
HHN	hand-held nebulizer—device for administering aerosolized drug (in fine spray)

HCO₃⁻	bicarbonate—measured in blood to determine acidity or alkalinity
ICU	intensive care unit
IRV	inspiratory reserve volume—maximum volume of gas that can be inhaled beyond normal resting inspiration
LLL	left lower lobe (of lung)
LUL	left upper lobe (of lung)
MDI	metered-dose inhaler—used to deliver aerosolized medications to patients with respiratory disease
NC	nasal cannula
NIV	noninvasive ventilation
NSCLC	non–small cell lung cancer
O₂	oxygen
OSA	obstructive sleep apnea
Paco₂	carbon dioxide partial pressure—a measure of the amount of carbon dioxide in arterial blood
Pao₂	oxygen partial pressure—a measure of the amount of oxygen in arterial blood
PA gram	pulmonary angiogram
PCP	*Pneumocystis* pneumonia—a type of pneumonia seen in patients with AIDS or other immunosuppression
PE	pulmonary embolism
PEP	positive expiratory pressure—mechanical ventilator strategy in which patient takes a deep breath and then exhales through a device that resists air flow (helps refill underventilated areas of the lung)
PEEP	positive end-expiratory pressure—a common mechanical ventilator setting in which airway pressure is maintained above atmospheric pressure
PFTs	pulmonary function tests
PND	paroxysmal nocturnal dyspnea
PPD	purified protein derivative—substance used in a tuberculosis test

12

RDS	respiratory distress syndrome—in the newborn infant, condition marked by dyspnea and cyanosis and related to absence of surfactant, a substance that permits normal expansion of lungs; also called hyaline membrane disease
RLL	right lower lobe (of lung)
RSV	respiratory syncytial virus—a common cause of bronchiolitis, bronchopneumonia, and the common cold, especially in children (in tissue culture, forms syncytia or giant cells, so that cytoplasm flows together).
RUL	right upper lobe (of lung)
RV	residual volume—amount of air remaining in lungs at the end of maximal expiration
SCLC	small cell lung cancer
SIMV	synchronized intermittent mandatory ventilation
SOA	shortness of air
SOB	shortness of breath

TB	tuberculosis
TBNA	transbronchial needle aspiration (for biopsy of lesions)
TLC	total lung capacity—volume of gas in the lungs at the end of maximal inspiration; equals VC plus RV
URI	upper respiratory infection
V_T	tidal volume—amount of air inhaled and exhaled during a normal ventilation
VAP	ventilator-associated pneumonia—bacterial pneumonia in a patient who has been on mechanical ventilation for 48 hours or more
VATS	video-assisted thoracic surgery (thoracoscopy or thorascopy)
VC	vital capacity—equals inspiratory reserve volume plus expiratory reserve volume plus tidal volume
V/Q scan	ventilation-perfusion scan—radioactive test of lung ventilation and blood perfusion throughout the lung capillaries (lung scan)

PRACTICAL APPLICATIONS

Reproduced here are actual medical reports using terms that you have studied in this and previous chapters. Explanations of more difficult terms are added in brackets. Answers to the questions for the autopsy report are on page 475.

CASE REPORT

A 22-year-old known heroin abuser was admitted to an emergency room comatose with shallow respirations. Routine laboratory studies and chest x-rays were done after the patient was aroused. He was then transferred to the ICU. He complained of left-sided chest pain. Examination of the chest x-ray showed three fractured ribs on the right and a large right pleural effusion. Further questioning of a friend revealed that he had fallen and struck the corner of a table after injecting heroin.

The diagnosis was traumatic hemothorax secondary to fractured ribs, and a chest tube was inserted into the right pleural space. No blood could be obtained despite maneuvering of the tube. Another chest x-ray showed that the tube was correctly placed in the right pleural space, but the fractured ribs and pleural effusion were on the left. The radiologist then realized that he had reversed the first film. A second tube was inserted into the left pleural space, and 1500 mL [6 to 7 cups] of blood was evacuated.

AUTOPSY REPORT

Adenocarcinoma, bronchogenic, left lung, with extensive mediastinal, pleural, and pericardial involvement. Metastasis to tracheobronchial lymph nodes, liver, lumbar vertebrae. Pulmonary emboli, multiple, recent, with recent infarct of left lower lobe. The tumor apparently originated at the left main bronchus and extends peripherally. Parenchyma (alveoli) is particularly atelectatic with a centrally located area of hemorrhage in the lower lobe.

Questions about the Autopsy Report

1. What was the patient's primary disease?
   a. Blood clots in the lung
   b. Mediastinal, pleural, and pericardial inflammation
   c. Lung cancer

2. Which was *not* an area of metastasis?
   a. Backbones
   b. Bone marrow
   c. Hepatocytes

3. What event probably was the cause of death?
   a. Infarction of lung tissue caused by pulmonary emboli
   b. COPD
   c. Myocardial infarction

4. What best describes the pulmonary parenchyma in the lower left lobe?
   a. Alveoli are filled with tumor.
   b. Alveoli are collapsed, with central area of bleeding.
   c. Alveoli are filled with pus and blood.

X-RAY AND BRONCHOSCOPY REPORTS

1. CXR: Complete opacification of left hemithorax with deviation of mediastinal structures of right side. Massive pleural effusion.

2. Chest tomograms: Mass most compatible with LUL bronchogenic carcinoma. Possible left paratracheal adenopathy or direct involvement of mediastinum.

3. Bronchoscopy: Larynx, trachea, **carina** [area of bifurcation or forking of the trachea], and left lung all within normal limits. On the right side there was irregularity and roughening of the bronchial mucosa on the lateral aspect of the bronchial wall. This irregularity extended into the RUL, and the apical and posterior segments [divisions of lobes of the lung] each contained inflamed irregular mucosa. Conclusion: Suspicious for infiltrating tumor, but may be nonspecific inflammation. Bronchial washings, brushings, and bxs [biopsies] taken. Bronchial biopsy diagnosis: squamous cell carcinoma. Washings and brushings showed no malignant cells.

EXERCISES

12

Remember to check your answers carefully with those given in the Answers to Exercises, page 473.

A. Match the following anatomic structures with their descriptions below.

adenoids	epiglottis	paranasal sinuses
alveoli	hilum	parietal pleura
bronchi	larynx	pharynx
bronchioles	mediastinum	trachea
cilia	palatine tonsils	visceral pleura

1. Outer fold of pleura lying closer to the ribs_____

2. Collections of lymph tissue in the nasopharynx _____

3. Windpipe _____

4. Lid-like piece of cartilage that covers the voice box _____

5. Branches of the windpipe that lead into the lungs _____

6. Region between the lungs in the chest cavity _____

7. Air-containing cavities in the bones around the nose_____

8. Thin hairs attached to the mucous membrane lining the respiratory tract _____

9. Inner fold of pleura closer to lung tissue_____

10. Throat _____

11. Air sacs of the lung _____

12. Voice box _____

13. Smallest branches of bronchi_____

14. Collections of lymph tissue in the oropharynx _____

15. Midline region of the lungs where bronchi, blood vessels, and nerves enter and exit the lungs

_____

B. Complete the following sentences.

1. The apical part of the lung is the _____.

2. The gas that passes into the bloodstream at the lungs is _____.

3. Breathing in air is called _____.

4. Divisions of the lungs are known as _____.

5. The gas produced by cells and exhaled through the lungs is _____.

6. The space between the visceral and the parietal pleura is the _____.

7. Breathing out air is called _____.

8. The essential tissues of the lung that perform its main function are pulmonary

_____.

9. The exchange of gases in the lung is _____ respiration.

10. The exchange of gases at the tissue cells is _____ respiration.

C. Give meanings for the following terms relating to respiratory disorders and structures.

1. bronchiectasis _____

2. pleuritis _____

3. pneumothorax _____

4. anosmia _____

5. laryngectomy _____

6. nasopharyngitis _____

7. phrenic _____

8. alveolar _____

9. glottis _____

10. tracheal stenosis _____

D. Complete the medical terms for the following respiratory symptoms.

1. excessive carbon dioxide in the blood: hyper_____

2. breathing is easiest or possible only in an upright position: _____pnea

3. difficult breathing: _____pnea

4. condition of blueness of skin: _____osis

5. spitting up blood: hemo_____

6. deficiency of oxygen: hyp_____

7. condition of pus in the pleural cavity: pyo_____ *or* em_____

8. hoarseness; voice impairment: dys_____

9. blood in the pleural cavity: hemo_____

10. nosebleed: epi_____

12

E. Give the meanings of the following medical terms.

1. rales (crackles)_____

2. auscultation _____

3. sputum_____

4. percussion _____

5. rhonchi _____

6. pleural rub_____

7. purulent_____

8. paroxysmal nocturnal dyspnea _____

9. hydrothorax _____

10. pulmonary infarction _____

11. stridor _____

12. wheeze _____

F. Match the following terms with their descriptions below.

asbestosis   croup   lung cancer
asthma   cystic fibrosis   pertussis
atelectasis   diphtheria   sarcoidosis
chronic bronchitis   emphysema

1. acute infectious disease of the throat caused by *Corynebacterium* _____

2. acute respiratory syndrome in children and infants that is marked by obstruction of the larynx

   and stridor _____

3. hyperinflation of air sacs with destruction of alveolar walls _____

4. inflammation of tubes that lead from the trachea; over a long period of time _____

5. chronic inflammatory disorder characterized by airway obstruction _____

6. lung or a portion of a lung is collapsed _____

7. malignant neoplasm originating in a lung or bronchus _____

8. whooping cough _____

9. inherited disease of exocrine glands; mucous secretions lead to airway obstruction

   _____

10. type of pneumoconiosis; dust particles are inhaled _____

11. inflammatory disease in which small nodules form in lungs and lymph nodes _____

G. **Use the following terms and abbreviations to complete the sentences below:**

CPAP	fibrosis	Pao$_2$
DL$_{CO}$	obstructive lung disease	palliative
exudate	OSA	restrictive lung disease
FEV$_1$	Paco$_2$	rhonchi

1. Sarah had a pulmonary function test in which she inhaled as much air as she could and the air that

   she expelled in the first second was measured. This PFT is a/an _____.

2. Dr. Smith heard loud _____ when he auscultated Kate's chest. Her
   bronchial tubes were obstructed with thick mucous secretions.

3. Karl was asked to breathe in a small amount of carbon monoxide and then blood samples were
   taken to detect the gas in his bloodstream. This is a PFT to assess how well gases can diffuse across

   the alveolar membrane, and it is called _____.

4. Formation of scar tissue in the connective tissue of the lungs is pulmonary _____.

5. A purulent _____ consists of white blood cells, microorganisms (dead
   and alive), and other debris.

6. Myasthenia gravis and muscular dystrophy are examples of neuromuscular conditions that produce

   _____.

7. Chronic bronchitis and asthma are examples of _____.

8. Patients with a small pharyngeal airway that closes during sleep may experience

   _____.

9. With nasal _____, positive pressure (air coming from a compressor)
   opens the oropharynx and nasopharynx, preventing obstructive sleep apnea.

10. Doctors realized that they could not cure Jean's adenocarcinoma of the lung. They used

    _____ measures to relieve her uncomfortable symptoms.

11. During an apneic period, a patient experiences severe hypoxemia (decreased

    _____) and hypercapnia (increased _____).

H. **Give the meanings of the following medical terms.**

1. pulmonary abscess_____

2. pulmonary edema _____

3. pneumoconiosis_____

4. pneumonia_____

5. pulmonary embolism _____

6. tuberculosis _____

7. pleural effusion _____

8. pleurisy _____

9. anthracosis_____

10. mesothelioma _____

11. adenoid hypertrophy _____

12. pleurodynia _____

13. expectoration _____

14. tachypnea_____

I. Match the clinical procedure or abbreviation with its description.

bronchial alveolar lavage	mediastinoscopy	tracheostomy
bronchoscopy	pulmonary angiography	tube thoracostomy
endotracheal intubation	pulmonary function tests	tuberculin tests
laryngoscopy	thoracentesis	V/Q scan

1. placement of a tube through the mouth into the trachea to establish an airway _____

2. injection or inhalation of radioactive material and recording images of its distribution in the

   lungs _____

3. PPD, tine, and Mantoux tests _____

4. puncture of the chest wall to obtain fluid from the pleural cavity _____

5. tests that measure the ventilation mechanics of the lung _____

6. creation of an opening into the trachea through the neck to establish an airway _____

7. visual examination of the bronchi _____

8. injection of fluid into the bronchi, followed by withdrawal of the fluid for examination

   _____

9. insertion of an endoscope into the larynx to view the voice box _____

10. x-ray images taken after injection of contrast material into the pulmonary artery

    _____

11. visual examination of the area between the lungs _____

12. continuous drainage of the pleural spaces from a chest tube placed through a small skin

    incision _____

J. Give the meanings of the following abbreviations and then select the letter of the sentences that follow that is the best association for each.

Column I

1. DOE _____ ____

2. PND _____ ____

3. VATS _____ ____

4. CPR _____ ____

5. NSCLC _____ ____

6. ARDS _____ ____

7. COPD _____ ____

8. PFTs _____ ____

9. PPD _____ ____

10. DPT _____ ____

Column II

A. Patients with congestive heart failure and pulmonary edema experience this symptom when they recline in bed.
B. Chronic bronchitis and emphysema are examples.
C. Substance used in the test for tuberculosis.
D. Adenocarcinoma and squamous cell carcinoma are types.
E. Visual examination of the chest via endoscope and a video monitor.
F. Injection in an infant to provide immunity.
G. A spirometer is used for these respiratory tests.
H. This symptom means that a patient has difficulty breathing and becomes short of breath when exercising.
I. Three basic steps: A, airway opened by tilting the head; B, breathing restored by mouth-to-mouth breathing; C, circulation restored by external cardiac compression.
J. A group of symptoms resulting in acute respiratory failure.

K. Match the respiratory system procedures with their meanings.

laryngectomy
lobectomy
pneumonectomy

rhinoplasty
thoracentesis
thoracoscopy (thorascopy)

thoracotomy
tonsillectomy

1. removal of lymph tissue in the oropharynx _____

2. surgical puncture of the chest to remove fluid from the pleural space _____

3. surgical repair of the nose _____

4. incision of the chest _____

5. removal of the voice box _____

6. removal of a region of a lung _____

7. endoscopic examination of the chest _____

8. pulmonary resection _____

12

L. Circle the **boldface** term that best completes the meaning of each sentence.

1. Ruth was having difficulty taking a deep breath, and her chest x-ray showed accumulation of fluid in her pleural spaces. Dr. Smith ordered **(PPD, tracheotomy, thoracentesis)** to relieve the pressure on her lungs.

2. Dr. Wong used her stethoscope to perform **(percussion, auscultation, thoracentesis)** on the patient's chest.

3. Before making a decision to perform surgery on Mrs. Hope, an 80-year-old woman with lung cancer, her physicians ordered **(COPD, bronchoscopy, PFTs)** to determine the functioning of her lungs.

4. Sylvia produced yellow-colored sputum and had a high fever. Her physician told her that she probably had **(pneumonia, pulmonary embolism, pneumothorax)** and needed antibiotics.

5. The night before her thoracotomy for lung biopsy, Mrs. White was told by her anesthesiologist that he would place a/an **(thoracostomy tube, mediastinoscope, endotracheal tube)** down her throat to keep her airways open during surgery.

6. Early in her pregnancy, Sonya had a routine **(PET scan, CXR, MRI)**, which revealed a/an **(epiglottic, alveolar, mediastinal)** mass in the area between her lungs. After delivery of her child, the mass was removed, and biopsy revealed a malignant thymoma (tumor of the thymus gland).

7. Five-year-old Seth was allergic to cats and experienced wheezing, coughing, and difficult breathing at night when he was trying to sleep. After careful evaluation by a **(cardiologist, pulmonologist, neurologist)**, his parents were told that Seth had **(pleurisy, sarcoidosis, asthma)** involving inflammation of his **(nasal passages, pharynx, bronchial tubes)**.

8. Six-year-old Daisy had a habit of picking her nose. During the winter months, heat in her family's house caused drying of her nasal **(mucus, mucous, pleural)** membranes. She had frequent bouts of **(epistaxis, croup, stridor)**.

9. Seventy-five-year-old Beatrice had been a pack-a-day smoker all of her adult life. Over the previous 3 months she noticed a persistent cough, weight loss, blood in her sputum **(hemoptysis, hematemesis, asbestosis)**, and dyspnea. A chest CT scan revealed a mass. Biopsy confirmed the diagnosis of **(tuberculosis, pneumoconiosis, adenocarcinoma)**, which is a type of **(small cell, non–small cell, lymph node)** lung cancer.

10. Carrie's lungs were normal at birth, but thick bronchial secretions soon blocked her **(arterioles, venules, bronchioles)**, which became inflamed. She was losing weight, and tests revealed inadequate amounts of pancreatic enzymes necessary for digestion of fats and proteins. Her pediatrician diagnosed her hereditary condition as **(chronic bronchitis, asthma, cystic fibrosis)**.

MEDICAL SCRAMBLE

Unscramble the letters to form respiratory system–related terms from the clues. Use the letters in squares to complete the bonus term. Answers are found on page 475.

1. *Clue:* Flap of cartilage above the trachea

   ☐ __ __ __ __ ☐ __ __ ☐   I O P T L G E T S I

2. *Clue:* Bacteria causing tuberculosis

   __ __ ☐ ☐ __ ☐ __   L A L C B I I

3. *Clue:* Small airway leading to air sacs

   __ __ __ __ __ __ __ __ __ ☐   O N E B H L R I C O

4. *Clue:* Chronic allergic condition marked by airway obstruction

   ☐ ☐ ☐ __ __ ☐   S M T A H A

BONUS TERM: *Clue:* Collapsed lung

   ☐ ☐ ☐ ☐ ☐ ☐ ☐ ☐ ☐ ☐

ANSWERS TO EXERCISES

A

1. parietal pleura
2. adenoids
3. trachea
4. epiglottis
5. bronchi

6. mediastinum
7. paranasal sinuses
8. cilia
9. visceral pleura
10. pharynx

11. alveoli
12. larynx
13. bronchioles
14. palatine tonsils
15. hilum

B

1. uppermost part
2. oxygen
3. inspiration; inhalation
4. lobes

5. carbon dioxide
6. pleural cavity
7. expiration; exhalation

8. parenchyma
9. external
10. internal

C

1. chronic dilation of a bronchus
2. inflammation of pleura
3. air in the chest (pleural cavity)
4. lack of sense of smell

5. removal of the voice box
6. inflammation of the nose and throat
7. pertaining to the diaphragm

8. pertaining to an air sac
9. opening to the larynx
10. narrowing of the windpipe

12

D

1. hypercapnia
2. orthopnea
3. dyspnea
4. cyanosis
5. hemoptysis
6. hypoxia
7. pyothorax; empyema
8. dysphonia
9. hemothorax
10. epistaxis

E

1. fine crackling sounds heard during inspiration when there is fluid in the alveoli
2. listening to sounds within the body
3. material expelled from the chest by coughing or clearing the throat
4. tapping on the surface to determine the underlying structure
5. loud rumbling sounds on auscultation of chest; bronchi obstructed by sputum
6. abnormal grating sound produced by the motion of pleural surfaces rubbing against each other (caused by inflammation or tumor cells)
7. pus-filled
8. sudden attack of difficult breathing associated with lying down at night (caused by congestive heart failure and pulmonary edema as the lungs fill with fluid)
9. fluid in the pleural cavity
10. area of dead tissue in the lung
11. strained, high-pitched inspirational sound
12. continuous high-pitched whistling sound heard when air is forced through a narrow space; seen in asthma

F

1. diphtheria
2. croup
3. emphysema
4. chronic bronchitis
5. asthma
6. atelectasis
7. lung cancer
8. pertussis
9. cystic fibrosis
10. asbestosis
11. sarcoidosis

G

1. FEV_1 (forced expiratory volume in first second)
2. rhonchi
3. DL_{CO} (diffusion capacity of the lung for carbon monoxide)
4. fibrosis
5. exudate
6. restrictive lung disease
7. obstructive lung disease
8. OSA: obstructive sleep apnea
9. CPAP: continuous positive airway pressure
10. palliative
11. Pao_2, $Paco_2$

H

1. collection of pus in the lungs
2. swelling, fluid collection in the air sacs and bronchioles
3. abnormal condition of dust in the lungs
4. acute inflammation and infection of alveoli; they become filled with fluid and blood cells
5. floating clot or other material blocking the blood vessels of the lung
6. an infectious disease caused by rod-shaped bacilli and producing tubercles (nodes) of infection
7. collection of fluid in the pleural cavity
8. inflammation of pleura
9. abnormal condition of coal dust in the lungs (black-lung disease)
10. malignant tumor arising in the pleura; composed of mesothelium (epithelium that covers the surfaces of membranes such as pleura and peritoneum)
11. excessive growth of cells in the adenoids (lymph tissue in the nasopharynx)
12. pain of the pleura (irritation of pleural surfaces leads to intercostal pain)
13. coughing up of material from the chest
14. rapid breathing; hyperventilation

I

1. endotracheal intubation
2. lung scan
3. tuberculin tests
4. thoracentesis
5. pulmonary function tests
6. tracheostomy
7. bronchoscopy
8. bronchial alveolar lavage
9. laryngoscopy
10. pulmonary angiography
11. mediastinoscopy
12. tube thoracostomy

J

1. dyspnea on exertion: H
2. paroxysmal nocturnal dyspnea: A
3. video-assisted thoracic surgery: E
4. cardiopulmonary resuscitation: I
5. non–small cell lung cancer: D
6. acute (adult) respiratory distress syndrome: J
7. chronic obstructive pulmonary disease: B
8. pulmonary function tests: G
9. purified protein derivative: C
10. diphtheria, pertussis, and tetanus: F

K

1. tonsillectomy
2. thoracentesis
3. rhinoplasty
4. thoracotomy
5. laryngectomy
6. lobectomy
7. thoracoscopy (thorascopy)
8. pneumonectomy

L

1. thoracentesis
2. auscultation
3. PFTs
4. pneumonia
5. endotracheal tube
6. CXR; mediastinal
7. pulmonologist; asthma; bronchial tubes
8. mucous; epistaxis
9. hemoptysis; adenocarcinoma; non–small cell
10. bronchioles; cystic fibrosis

ANSWERS TO PRACTICAL APPLICATIONS

1. c
2. b
3. a
4. b

ANSWERS TO MEDICAL SCRAMBLE

1. EPIGLOTTIS   2. BACILLI   3. BRONCHIOLE   4. ASTHMA
BONUS TERM: ATELECTASIS

PRONUNCIATION OF TERMS

PRONUNCIATION GUIDE

ā as in āpe   ă as in ăpple
ē as in ēven   ĕ as in ĕvery
ī as in īce   ĭ as in ĭnterest
ō as in ōpen   ŏ as in pŏt
ū as in ūnit   ŭ as in ŭnder

To test your understanding of the terminology in this chapter, write the meaning of each term in the space provided. In addition, you may wish to cover the terms and write them by looking at your definitions. Make sure your spelling is correct. The page number after each term indicates where it is defined or used in the book, so you can easily check your responses. You will find complete definitions for all of these terms and their audio pronunciations on the CD.

VOCABULARY AND TERMINOLOGY

Term	Pronunciation	Meaning
adenoidectomy (446)	ăd-ĕ-noyd-ĔK-tō-mē	_____
adenoid hypertrophy (446)	ĂD-ĕ-noyd hī-PĔR-trō-fē	_____
adenoids (444)	ĂD-ĕ-noydz	_____
alveolar (446)	ăl-VĒ-ō-lăr	_____
alveolus; alveoli (444)	ăl-VĒ-ō-lŭs; ăl-VĒ-ō-lī	_____
anosmia (450)	ăn-ŎS-mē-ă	_____
apex of the lung (444)	Ā-pĕkz of the lŭng	_____
apical (444)	Ā-pĭ-kăl	_____
apnea (450)	ăp-NĒ-ă	_____
asphyxia (450)	ăs-FĬK-sē-ă	_____
atelectasis (449)	ă-tĕ-LĔK-tă-sĭs	_____
base of the lung (444)	bās of the lŭng	_____

12

Term	Pronunciation	Meaning
bronchiectasis (446)	brŏng-kē-ĔK-tă-sĭs	_____
bronchiole (444)	BRŎNG-kē-ŏl	_____
bronchiolitis (446)	brŏng-kē-ō-LĪ-tĭs	_____
bronchodilator (446)	brŏng-kō-DĪ-lā-tĕr	_____
bronchospasm (446)	BRŎNG-kō-spăzm	_____
bronchus; bronchi (444)	BRŎNG-kŭs; BRŎNG-kī	_____
carbon dioxide (444)	KĂR-bŏn dī-ŎK-sīd	_____
cilia (445)	SĬL-ē-ă	_____
cyanosis (446)	sī-ă-NŌ-sĭs	_____
diaphragm (445)	DĪ-ă-frăm	_____
dysphonia (448)	dĭs-FŌ-nē-ă	_____
dyspnea (450)	DĬSP-nē-ă	_____
empyema (450)	ĕm-pī-Ē-mă	_____
epiglottis (445)	ĕp-ĭ-GLŎT-ĭs	_____
epiglottitis (446)	ĕp-ĭ-glŏ-TĪ-tĭs	_____
expectoration (448)	ĕk-spĕk-tō-RĀ-shŭn	_____
expiration (445)	ĕks-pĭr-RĀ-shŭn	_____
glottis (445)	GLŎ-tĭs	_____
hemoptysis (450)	hē-MŎP-tĭ-sĭs	_____
hemothorax (450)	hē-mō-THŌ-răks	_____
hilum of the lung (445)	HĪ-lŭm of the lŭng	_____
hilar (445)	HĪ-lăr	_____
hypercapnia (446)	hī-pĕr-KĂP-nē-ă	_____
hyperpnea (450)	hī-PĔRP-nē-ă	_____
hypoxia (448)	hī-PŎK-sē-ă	_____
inspiration (445)	ĭn-spĭ-RĀ-shŭn	_____
laryngeal (446)	lă-RĬN-jē-ăl _or_ lăr-ĭn-JĒ-ăl	_____
laryngospasm (446)	lă-RĬNG-gō-spăzm	_____
laryngitis (446)	lă-rĭn-JĪ-tĭs	_____
larynx (445)	LĂR-ĭnks	_____
lobectomy (447)	lō-BĔK-tō-mē	_____
mediastinoscopy (447)	mē-dē-ă-stī-NŎS-kō-pē	_____
mediastinum (445)	mē-dē-ă-STĪ-nŭm	_____

Term	Pronunciation	Meaning
nasogastric intubation (447)	nā-zō-GĂS-trĭk ĭn-too-BĀ-shŭn	
orthopnea (447)	ŏr-thŏp-NĒ-ă	
oxygen (445)	ŎKS-ĭ-jĕn	
palatine tonsil (445)	PĂL-ĭ-tīn TŎN-sĭl	
paranasal sinus (445)	pă-ră-NĀ-zăl SĪ-nĭs	
parietal pleura (445)	pă-RĪ-ĕ-tăl PLOO-răh	
pharyngeal (448)	fă-RĬN-jē-ăl *or* făr-ĭn-JĒ-ăl	
pharynx (445)	FĂR-ĭnkz	
phrenic nerve (448)	FRĔN-ĭk nĕrv	
pleura (445)	PLOOR-ă	
pleural cavity (445)	PLOOR-ăl KĂ-vĭ-tē	
pleurodynia (448)	ploor-ō-DĬN-ē-ă	
pneumoconiosis (446)	nū-mō-kō-nē-Ō-sĭs	
pneumonectomy (448)	nū-mō-NĔK-tō-mē	
pneumothorax (448)	nū-mō-THŌ-răks	
pulmonary (448)	PŬL-mō-năr-ē	
pulmonary parenchyma (445)	pŭl-mō-NĂR-ē pă-RĔN-kă-mă	
pyothorax (450)	pī-ō-THŌ-răks	
respiration (445)	rĕs-pĕ-RĀ-shĕn	
rhinoplasty (448)	RĪ-nō-plăs-tē	
rhinorrhea (448)	rī-nō-RĒ-ăh	
sinusitis (449)	sī-nū-SĪ-tĭs	
spirometer (449)	spī-RŎM-ĕ-tĕr	
tachypnea (450)	tăk-ĭp-NĒ-ă	
thoracic (449)	thōr-RĂ-sĭk	
thoracoscopy (461)	thōr-ră-KŎS-kō-pē	
thoracotomy (449)	thōr-ră-KŎT-ō-mē	
tonsillectomy (449)	tŏn-sĭ-LĔK-tō-mē	
trachea (445)	TRĀ-kē-ă	
tracheal stenosis (449)	TRĀ-kē-ăl stĕ-NŌ-sĭs	
tracheotomy (449)	trā-kē-ŎT-ō-mē	
visceral pleura (445)	VĬ-sĕr-ăl PLOO-ră	

12

PATHOLOGIC CONDITIONS, LABORATORY TESTS, AND CLINICAL PROCEDURES

Term	Pronunciation	Meaning
anthracosis (457)	ăn-thră-KŌ-sĭs	_____
asbestosis (457)	ăs-bĕs-TŌ-sĭs	_____
asthma (452)	ĂZ-mă	_____
atelectasis (453)	ă-tĕ-LĔK-tă-sĭs	_____
auscultation (451)	ăw-skŭl-TĀ-shŭn	_____
bacilli (457)	bă-SĬL-ī	_____
bronchioalveolar lavage (459)	BRŎNG-kē-ăl ăl-vē-Ō-lar lă-VĂJ	_____
bronchiectasis (452)	brŏng-kē-ĔK-tă-sĭs	_____
bronchoscopy (459)	brŏng-KŎS-kō-pē	_____
chest tomograms (458)	chĕst TŌ-mō-grămz	_____
chronic bronchitis (452)	KRŎ-nĭk brŏng-KĪ-tĭs	_____
chronic obstructive pulmonary disease (457)	KRŎ-nĭk ŏb-STRŬK-tĭv PŬL-mō-nă-rē dĭ-ZĒZ	_____
computed tomography (458)	kŏm-PŪ-tĭd tō-MŎG-ră-fē	_____
cor pulmonale (453)	kŏr pŭl-mō-NĂ-lē	_____
croup (451)	kroop	_____
cystic fibrosis (452)	SĬS-tĭk fī-BRŌ-sĭs	_____
diphtheria (452)	dĭf-THĔR-ē-ă	_____
emphysema (453)	ĕm-fĭ-ZĒ-mă	_____
endotracheal intubation (460)	ĕn-dō-TRĀ-kē-ăl ĭn-tū-BĀ-shŭn	_____
epistaxis (452)	ĕp-ĭ-STĂK-sĭs	_____
exudate (457)	ĔK-sū-dāt	_____
hydrothorax (457)	hī-drō-THŎR-ăks	_____
laryngoscopy (460)	lăr-ĭng-GŎS-kō-pē	_____
lung biopsy (460)	lŭng BĪ-ŏp-sē	_____
lung cancer (454)	lŭng KĂN-sĕr	_____
magnetic resonance imaging of the chest (459)	măg-NĔ-tĭk RĔ-zō-năns ĬM-ă-gĭng of the chest	_____
mediastinoscopy (460)	mē-dē-ă-stī-NŎS-kō-pē	_____
mesothelioma (457)	mĕz-ō-thē-lē-Ō-mă	_____
obstructive lung disease (460)	ŏb-STRŬK-tĭv lŭng dĭ-ZĒZ	_____

Term	Pronunciation	Meaning
palliative (457)	PĂL-ē-ă-tĭv	_____
paroxysmal (452)	păr-ŏk-SĬZ-măl	_____
percussion (451)	pĕr-KŬSH-ŭn	_____
pertussis (452)	pĕr-TŬS-ĭs	_____
pleural effusion (457)	PLOOR-ăl ĕ-FŪ-zhŭn	_____
pleural rub (451)	PLOOR-ăl rŭb	_____
pleurisy (457)	PLOOR-ĭ-sē	_____
pneumonia (454)	nū-MŌ-nē-ă	_____
pneumothorax (457)	nū-mō-THŎR-ăks	_____
positron emission tomography (459)	PŎS-ĭ-trŏn ē-MĬ-shŭn tō-MŎG-ră-fē	_____
pulmonary abscess (455)	PŬL-mō-nă-rē ĂB-sĕs	_____
pulmonary angiography (459)	PŬL-mō-nă-rē ăn-jē-ŎG-ră-fē	_____
pulmonary edema (455)	PŬL-mō-nă-rē ĕ-DĒ-mă	_____
pulmonary embolism (456)	PŬL-mō-nă-rē ĔM-bō-lĭzm	_____
pulmonary fibrosis (456)	PŬL-mō-nă-rē fī-BRŌ-sĭs	_____
pulmonary function tests (460)	PŬL-mō-nă-rē FŬNK-shŭn tĕsts	_____
pulmonary infarction (455)	PŬL-mō-nă-rē ĭn-FĂRK-shŭn	_____
purulent (457)	PŪ-rū-lĕnt	_____
rale (451)	răhl	_____
restrictive lung disease (461)	rē-STRĬK-tĭv lŭng dĭ-ZĒZ	_____
rhonchus (451)	RŎNG-kŭs	_____
sarcoidosis (456)	săr-koy-DŌ-sĭs	_____
silicosis (457)	sĭ-lĭ-KŌ-sĭs	_____
sputum (451)	SPŪ-tŭm	_____
sputum culture (451)	SPŪ-tŭm KŬL-tŭr	_____
stridor (451)	STRĪ-dŏr	_____
thoracentesis (460)	thō-ră-sĕn-TĒ-sĭs	_____
thoracotomy (461)	thō-ră-KŎ-tō-mē	_____
thorascopy (thoracoscopy) (461)	thō-RĂS-kō-pē (thō-ră-KŎS-kō-pē)	_____
tracheostomy (462)	trā-kē-ŎS-tō-mē	_____
tuberculin test (462)	too-BĔR-kū-lĭn tĕst	_____

12

Term	Pronunciation	Meaning
tuberculosis (456)	too-bĕr-kū-LŌ-sĭs	_____
tube thoracostomy (462)	toob thŏr-ă-KŎS-tō-mē	_____
ventilation-perfusion scan (459)	vĕn-tĭ-LĀ-shŭn-pĕr-FŪ-zhŭn scăn	_____
wheeze (451)	wēz	_____

REVIEW SHEET

Write the meanings of the word parts in the spaces provided. Check your answers with the information in the chapter or in the glossary (Medical Word Parts—English) at the end of the book.

COMBINING FORMS

Combining Form	Meaning	Combining Form	Meaning
adenoid/o	_____	pector/o	_____
alveol/o	_____	pharyng/o	_____
bronch/o	_____	phon/o	_____
bronchi/o	_____	phren/o	_____
bronchiol/o	_____	pleur/o	_____
capn/o	_____	pneum/o	_____
coni/o	_____	pneumon/o	_____
cyan/o	_____	pulmon/o	_____
epiglott/o	_____	py/o	_____
hydr/o	_____	rhin/o	_____
laryng/o	_____	sinus/o	_____
lob/o	_____	spir/o	_____
mediastin/o	_____	tel/o	_____
nas/o	_____	thorac/o	_____
or/o	_____	tonsill/o	_____
orth/o	_____	trache/o	_____
ox/o	_____		

SUFFIXES

Suffix	Meaning	Suffix	Meaning
-algia	_____	-plasty	_____
-capnia	_____	-pnea	_____
-centesis	_____	-ptysis	_____
-dynia	_____	-rrhea	_____
-ectasis	_____	-scopy	_____
-ectomy	_____	-sphyxia	_____
-ema	_____	-stenosis	_____
-lysis	_____	-stomy	_____
-osmia	_____	-thorax	_____
-oxia	_____	-tomy	_____
-phonia	_____	-trophy	_____

PREFIXES

Prefix	Meaning	Prefix	Meaning
a-, an-	_____	hyper-	_____
brady-	_____	hypo-	_____
dys-	_____	para-	_____
em-	_____	per-	_____
eu-	_____	re-	_____
ex-	_____	tachy-	_____

 Please refer to the enclosed CD for additional exercises and images related to this chapter.

chapter 13

Blood System

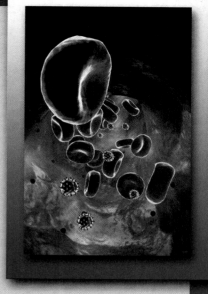

THIS CHAPTER IS DIVIDED INTO THE FOLLOWING SECTIONS

In this chapter you will

- Identify terms relating to the composition, formation, and function of blood.
- Differentiate among the four major blood types.
- Identify terms related to blood clotting.
- Build words and recognize combining forms used in blood system terminology.
- Identify various pathologic conditions affecting blood.
- Describe various laboratory tests and clinical procedures used with hematologic disorders, and recognize relevant abbreviations.
- Apply your new knowledge to understanding medical terms in their proper contexts, such as medical reports and records.

Image Description: Stylized view of blood cells flowing within an artery, seen as if through a fiber-optic camera.

13

INTRODUCTION

The primary function of blood is to maintain a constant environment for the other living tissues of the body. Blood transports nutrients, gases, and wastes to and from the cells of the body. Nutrients from food, digested in the stomach and small intestine, pass into the bloodstream through the lining cells of the small intestine. Blood then carries these nutrients to all body cells. Oxygen enters the body through the air sacs of the lungs. Blood cells then transport the oxygen to cells throughout the body. Blood also helps remove the waste products released by cells. It carries gaseous waste (such as carbon dioxide) to the lungs to be exhaled. It carries chemical waste, such as urea, to the kidneys to be expelled in the urine.

Blood transports chemical messengers called hormones from their sites of secretion in glands, such as the thyroid or pituitary, to distant sites where they regulate growth, reproduction, and energy production. These hormones are discussed later in the endocrine chapter.

Finally, blood contains proteins, white blood cells and antibodies that fight infection, and platelets (thrombocytes) that help the blood to clot.

COMPOSITION AND FORMATION OF BLOOD

Blood is composed of **cells,** or formed elements, suspended in a clear, straw-colored liquid called **plasma.** The cells constitute 45 percent of the blood volume and include **erythrocytes** (red blood cells), **leukocytes** (white blood cells), and **platelets** or **thrombocytes** (clotting cells). The remaining 55 percent of blood is plasma, a solution of water, proteins, sugar, salts, hormones, and vitamins.

CELLS

Beginning at birth, all blood cells originate in the marrow cavity of bones. Both the red blood cells that carry oxygen and the white blood cells that fight infection arise from the same blood-forming or **hematopoietic stem cells.** Under the influence of proteins in the bloodstream and bone marrow, stem cells change their size and shape to become specialized, or **differentiated.** In this process, the cells change in size from large (immature cells) to small (mature forms), and the cell nucleus shrinks (in red cells, the nucleus actually disappears). Figure 13–1 illustrates these changes in the formation of blood cells. Use Figure 13–1 as a reference as you learn the names of mature blood cells and their earlier forms.

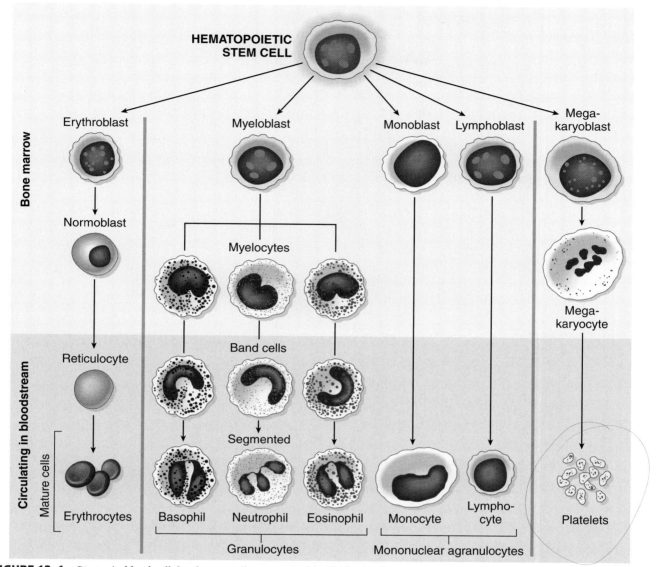

FIGURE 13–1 **Stages in blood cell development (hematopoiesis).** All blood cells originate from **hematopoietic stem cells.** Notice that the suffix **-blast** indicates immature forms of all cells. Band cells are identical to segmented granulocytes except that the nucleus is U-shaped and its lobes are connected by a band rather than by a thin thread, as in segmented forms.

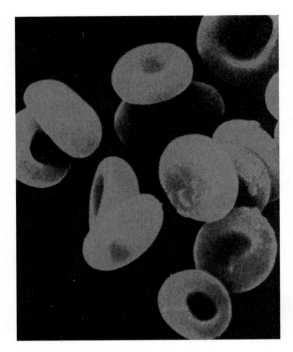

FIGURE 13–2 Normal **erythrocytes** (red blood cells). (From Thibodeau GA, Patton KT: Anatomy & Physiology, 6th ed. St. Louis, Mosby, 2007, p. 650.)

ERYTHROCYTES

As a red blood cell matures (from erythroblast to erythrocyte), it loses its nucleus and assumes the shape of a biconcave disk. This shape (a depressed or hollow surface on each side of the cell, resembling a cough drop with a thin central portion) allows for a large surface area so that absorption and release of gases (oxygen and carbon dioxide) can take place (see Fig. 13–2). Red cells contain the unique protein **hemoglobin,** composed of **heme** (iron-containing pigment) and **globin** (protein). Hemoglobin enables the erythrocyte to carry oxygen. The combination of oxygen and hemoglobin (oxyhemoglobin) produces the bright red color of blood.

Erythrocytes originate in the bone marrow. The hormone called **erythropoietin** (secreted by the kidney) stimulates their production (**-poiesis** means formation). Erythrocytes live and fulfill their role of transporting gases for about 120 days in the bloodstream. After this time, **macrophages** (in the spleen, liver, and bone marrow) destroy the worn-out erythrocytes. This is **hemolysis.** From 2 million to 10 million red cells are destroyed each second, but because they are constantly replaced, the number of circulating cells remains constant (4 to 6 million per μL).

Macrophages break down erythrocytes and hemoglobin into heme and globin (protein) portions. The heme releases iron and decomposes into a yellow/orange pigment called

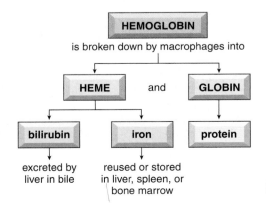

FIGURE 13–3   The breakdown of hemoglobin.

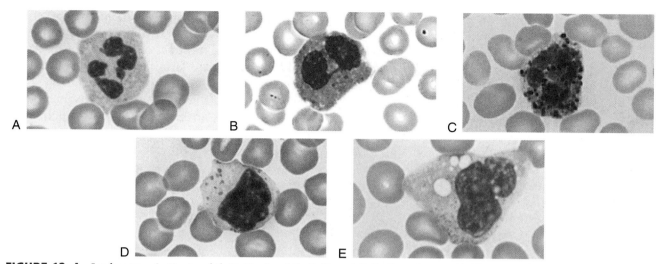

FIGURE 13–4   Leukocytes. A, Neutrophil. B, Eosinophil. C, Basophil. D, Lymphocyte. E, Monocyte. (From Carr JH, Rodak BF: Clinical Hematology Atlas, 2nd ed., St. Louis, Mosby, 2004.)

bilirubin. The iron in hemoglobin is reutilized to form new red cells or is stored in the spleen, liver, or bone marrow. Bilirubin is excreted into bile by the liver, and from bile it enters the small intestine. Finally it is excreted in the stool, where its color changes to brown. Figure 13–3 reviews the sequence of events in hemoglobin breakdown.

LEUKOCYTES

White blood cells (7000 to 9000 cells per μL) are less numerous than erythrocytes, but there are five different types of mature leukocytes, shown in Figure 13-4. These are three polymorphonuclear granulocytic leukocytes (basophil, neutrophil, and eosinophil) and two mononuclear agranulocytic leukocytes (monocyte and lymphocyte).

The **granulocytes,** or **polymorphonuclear leukocytes (PMNs),** are the most numerous (about 60 percent). **Basophils** contain dark-staining granules that stain with a basic (alkaline) dye. The granules contain heparin (an anticlotting substance) and histamine (a chemical released in allergic responses). **Eosinophils** contain granules that stain with eosin, a red acidic dye. They increase in allergic responses and engulf substances that trigger the allergies. **Neutrophils** contain granules that are neutral; they do not stain intensely with either acidic or basic dye. Neutrophils are **phagocytes (phag/o** means to eat or swallow) that accumulate at sites of infection, where they ingest and destroy bacteria. Figure 13–5 shows phagocytosis by a neutrophil.

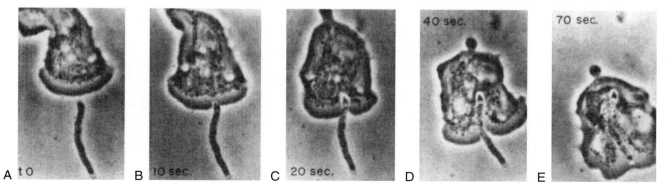

FIGURE 13–5   Phagocytosis (ingestion) of a bacterium by a neutrophil. (From Hirsch JG: Cinemicrophotographic observations of granule lysis in polymorphonuclear leucocytes during phagocytosis. J Exp Med 1962;116:827, by copyright permission of Rockefeller University Press.)

13

Specific proteins called **colony-stimulating factors** (CSFs) promote the growth of granulocytes in bone marrow. **G-CSF** (granulocyte CSF) and **GM-CSF** (granulocyte-macrophage CSF) are given to restore granulocyte production in cancer patients. **Erythropoietin,** like CSFs, can be produced by recombinant DNA techniques. It stimulates red blood cell production (erythropoiesis).

Although all granulocytes are **polymorphonuclear** (they have multilobed nuclei), the term **polymorphonuclear leukocyte ("poly")** often describes the **neutrophil,** which is the most numerous of the granulocytes.

Mononuclear (containing one large nucleus) leukocytes do not have large numbers of granules in their cytoplasm, but they may have a few granules. These are **lymphocytes** and **monocytes** (see Fig. 13–1). Lymphocytes are made in bone marrow and lymph nodes and circulate both in the bloodstream and in the parallel circulating system, the lymphatic system.

Lymphocytes play an important role in the **immune response** that protects the body against infection. They can directly attack foreign matter and, in addition, make **antibodies,** which neutralize and can lead to the destruction of foreign **antigens** (bacteria and viruses). Monocytes are phagocytic cells that also fight disease. They move from the bloodstream into tissues (as **macrophages**) and dispose of dead and dying cells and other tissue debris by phagocytosis.

Table 13–1 reviews the different types of leukocytes, their numbers in the blood, and their functions.

PLATELETS (THROMBOCYTES)

Platelets, or thrombocytes, are formed in red bone marrow from giant cells with multilobed nuclei called **megakaryocytes** (see Fig. 13–6, *A* and *B*). Tiny fragments of a megakaryocyte break off to form platelets. The main function of platelets is to help blood to clot. Specific terms related to blood clotting are discussed later in this chapter.

Table 13–1

Leukocytes

Leukocyte	Percentage of Leukocytes in Blood	Function
GRANULOCYTES		
Basophil	0–1	Contains heparin (prevents clotting) and histamine (involved in allergic responses)
Eosinophil	1–4	Phagocytic cell involved in allergic reactions
Neutrophil	50–70	Phagocytic cell that accumulates at sites of infection
MONONUCLEARS		
Lymphocyte	20–40	Controls the immune response; makes antibodies to antigens
Monocyte	3–8	Phagocytic cell that becomes a macrophage and digests bacteria and tissue debris

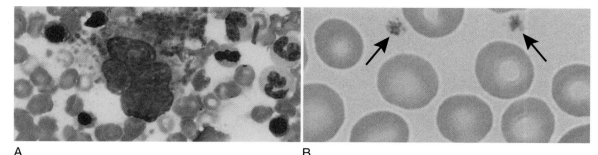

FIGURE 13–6   A, Megakaryocyte. B, Platelets. (From Carr JH, Rodak BF: Clinical Hematology Atlas, 2nd ed., St. Louis, Mosby, 2004.)

PLASMA

Plasma, the liquid part of the blood, consists of water, dissolved proteins, sugar, wastes, salts, hormones, and other substances. The four major plasma proteins are **albumin, globulins, fibrinogen,** and **prothrombin** (the last two are clotting proteins).

Albumin maintains the proper proportion (and concentration) of water in the blood. Because albumin cannot pass easily through capillary walls, it remains in the blood and carries smaller molecules bound to its surface. It attracts water from the tissues back into the bloodstream and thus opposes the water's tendency to leave the blood and leak out into tissue spaces. **Edema** (swelling) results when too much fluid from blood "leaks" out into tissues. This happens in a mild form when a person ingests too much salt (water is retained in the blood and seeps out into tissues) and in a severe form when a person is burned in a fire. In this situation albumin escapes from capillaries as a result of the burn injury. Then water cannot be held in the blood; it escapes through the skin, and blood volume drops.

Globulins are another component of blood and one of the plasma proteins. There are alpha, beta, and gamma globulins. The gamma globulins are **immunoglobulins,** which are antibodies that bind to and sometimes destroy antigens (foreign substances). Examples of immunoglobulin antibodies are **IgG** (found in high concentration in plasma) and **IgA** (found in breast milk, saliva, tears, and respiratory mucus). Other immunoglobulins are **IgM, IgD,** and **IgE.** Immunoglobulins are separated from other plasma proteins by **electrophoresis.** In this process, an electrical current passes through a solution of plasma. The different proteins in plasma separate as they migrate at different speeds to the source of the electricity.

Plasmapheresis (-apheresis means to remove) is the process of separating plasma from cells and then removing the plasma from the patient. In plasmapheresis, the entire blood sample is spun in a centrifuge machine, and the plasma, being lighter in weight than the cells, moves to the top of the sample.

Figure 13–7 reviews the composition of blood.

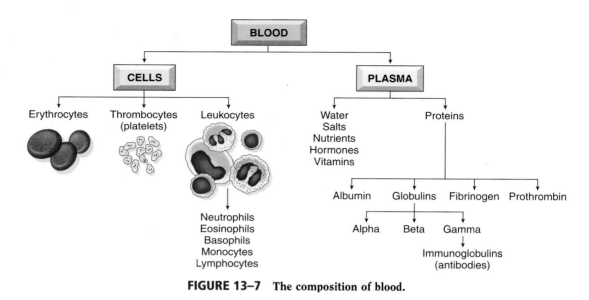

FIGURE 13–7 The composition of blood.

BLOOD TYPES

Transfusions of "whole blood" (cells and plasma) are used to replace blood lost after injury, during surgery, or in severe shock. A patient who is severely anemic and needs only red blood cells will receive a transfusion of **packed red cells** (whole blood with most of the plasma removed). Human blood falls into four main types: A, B, AB, and O. There are harmful effects of transfusing blood from a donor of one blood type into a recipient who has blood of another blood type. Therefore, before blood is transfused, both the blood donor and the blood recipient are tested to be certain that the transfused blood will be compatible with the recipient.

Each of the blood types has a specific combination of factors called **antigens** and **antibodies.** Blood type antigens are inherited, and blood type antibodies are acquired by 6 months of age after exposure to antigens. The antigen and antibody factors of blood types are:

> **Type A,** containing **A antigen** and **anti-B antibody**
> **Type B,** containing **B antigen** and **anti-A antibody**
> **Type AB,** containing **A and B antigens** and **no anti-A or anti-B antibodies**
> **Type O,** containing **no A or B antigens** and **both anti-A and anti-B antibodies**

The problem in transfusing blood from a type A donor into a type B recipient is that A antigens (from the A donor) will react adversely with the anti-A antibodies in the recipient's type B bloodstream. The accidental adverse reaction is **hemolysis,** or breakdown of red blood cells. Intravascular hemolysis may lead to **disseminated intravascular coagulation (DIC),** a coagulation and bleeding disorder. Similar problems can occur in other transfusions if the donor's antigens are incompatible with the recipient's antibodies.

People with type O blood are known as universal donors because their blood contains neither A nor B antigens. The anti-A and anti-B antibodies in O blood do not have an effect in the recipient because the antibodies are diluted in the recipient's bloodstream. Those with type AB blood are known as universal recipients because their blood contains neither anti-A nor anti-B antibodies, so that neither the A nor the B group antigens will cause hemolysis in their blood.

Besides A and B antigens, many other antigens are located on the surface of red blood cells. One of these is called the **Rh factor** (named because it was first found in the blood of a rhesus monkey). The term Rh-positive refers to a person who is born with the Rh antigen on her or his red blood cells. An Rh-negative person does not have the Rh antigen. There are no anti-Rh antibodies normally present in the blood of an Rh-positive or an Rh-negative person. However, if Rh-positive blood is transfused into an Rh-negative person, the recipient may, but not always, begin to develop antibodies that would cause hemolysis of Rh-positive blood if another transfusion were to occur subsequently.

The same reactions occur during pregnancy if the fetus of an Rh-negative woman happens to be Rh-positive. This situation is described in Chapter 4 as an example of an antigen–antibody reaction.

Table 13-2 shows the blood types, their frequency of occurrence in the population, and their antigens and antibodies.

Table 13–2

Blood Types

Type	Percentage in Population	Red Cell Antigens	Plasma Antibodies
A	41	A	Anti-B
B	10	B	Anti-A
AB	4	A and B	Neither anti-A nor anti-B
O	45	Neither A nor B	Anti-A and anti-B
Rh positive	85	Rh factor	No anti-Rh
Rh negative	15	No Rh factor	Anti-Rh (occurs if an Rh-negative person is given Rh-positive blood)

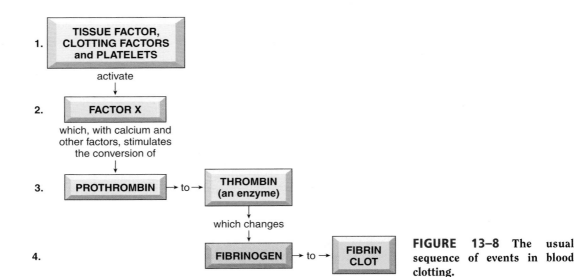

FIGURE 13–8 The usual sequence of events in blood clotting.

BLOOD CLOTTING

Blood clotting, or **coagulation,** is a complicated process involving many different substances and chemical reactions. The final result (usually taking less than 15 minutes) is the formation of a **fibrin clot** from the plasma protein **fibrinogen.** Platelets are important in beginning the process following injury to tissues or blood vessels. The platelets clump, or aggregate, at the site of injury. Then in combination with a protein tissue factor, other clotting factors and calcium promote the formation of a fibrin clot. One of the clotting factors is clotting factor VIII. It is missing in some people who are born with hemophilia. Other hemophiliacs are missing factor IX. Figure 13–8 reviews the basic sequence of events in the clotting process.

The fibrin threads form the clot by trapping red blood cells (Fig. 13–9 shows a red blood cell trapped by fibrin threads). Then the clot retracts into a tight ball, leaving behind a clear fluid called **serum.** Normally, clots (thrombi) do not form in blood vessels unless the vessel is damaged or the flow of blood is impeded. Anticoagulant substances in the bloodstream inhibit blood clotting, so thrombi and emboli (floating clots) do not form. **Heparin,** produced by tissue cells (especially in the liver), is an example of an anticoagulant. Other drugs such as **warfarin (Coumadin)** are given to patients with thromboembolic diseases to prevent the formation of clots and emboli.

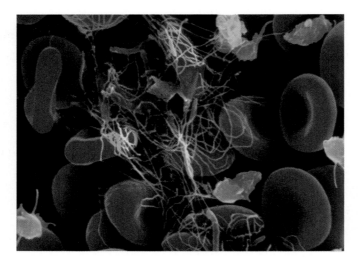

FIGURE 13–9 A red blood cell enmeshed in threads of fibrin. (From Thibodeau GA, Patton KT: Anatomy & Physiology, 6th ed. St. Louis, Mosby, 2007, p. 663.)

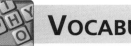

VOCABULARY

This list reviews many of the new terms introduced in the text. Short definitions reinforce your understanding of the terms. Refer to the Pronunciation of Terms section for help with difficult or unfamiliar words.

albumin	Protein in blood; maintains the proper amount of water in the blood.
antibody	Protein (immunoglobulin) produced by lymphocytes in response to bacteria, viruses, or other antigens. An antibody is specific to an antigen and inactivates it.
antigen	Substance (usually foreign) that stimulates the production of an antibody.
basophil	Granulocytic white blood cell with granules that stain blue when exposed to a basic dye.
bilirubin	Orange-yellow pigment in bile. It is formed by the breakdown of hemoglobin when red blood cells die.
coagulation	Blood clotting.
colony-stimulating factor (CSF)	Protein that stimulates the growth and proliferation of white blood cells (granulocytes).
differentiation	Change in structure and function of a cell as it matures; specialization.
electrophoresis	Method of separating serum proteins by electrical charge.
eosinophil	Granulocytic white blood cell with granules that stain red with the acidic dye eosin; associated with allergic reactions.
erythrocyte	Red blood cell. There are about 5 million per microliter (μL) or cubic millimeter (mm^3) of blood.
erythropoietin (EPO)	Hormone secreted by the kidneys that stimulates formation of red blood cells.
fibrin	Protein threads that form the basis of a blood clot.
fibrinogen	Plasma protein that is converted to fibrin in the clotting process.
globulins	Part of blood containing different plasma proteins. Immunoglobulins and alpha and beta globulins are examples.
granulocyte	White blood cell with numerous dark-staining granules: eosinophil, neutrophil, and basophil.
heme	Iron-containing nonprotein portion of the hemoglobin molecule.
hemoglobin	Blood protein containing iron; carries oxygen in red blood cells.
hemolysis	Destruction or breakdown of blood (red blood cells).
heparin	Anticoagulant found in blood and tissue cells.
immune reaction	Response of the immune system to foreign invasion.
immunoglobulin	Protein (globulin) with antibody activity; examples are IgG, IgM, IgA, IgE, IgD. Immun/o means protection.
leukocyte	White blood cell.
lymphocyte	Mononuclear leukocyte that produces antibodies.

13

macrophage	Monocyte that migrates from the blood to tissue spaces. It is a large phagocyte.
megakaryocyte	Large platelet precursor cell found in the bone marrow.
monocyte	Large mononuclear phagocytic leukocyte formed in bone marrow. Monocytes become macrophages as they leave the blood and enter body tissues.
mononuclear	Pertaining to a cell (leukocyte) with a single round nucleus; lymphocytes and monocytes are mononuclear leukocytes.
neutrophil	Granulocytic leukocyte formed in bone marrow; a phagocyte with neutral-staining granules; also called a **polymorphonuclear leukocyte,** or "poly."
plasma	Liquid portion of blood; contains water, proteins, salts, nutrients, hormones, and vitamins.
plasmapheresis	Removal of plasma from withdrawn blood by centrifuge. Collected cells are retransfused back into the donor. Fresh-frozen plasma or salt solution is used to replace withdrawn plasma.
platelet	Smallest blood cell (thrombocyte); these cells clump at sites of injury to prevent bleeding and facilitate clotting.
prothrombin	Plasma protein; converted to thrombin in the clotting process.
reticulocyte	Immature erythrocyte with a network of strands (reticulin) that are seen after staining the cell with special dyes.
Rh factor	Antigen on red blood cells of Rh-positive individuals. The factor was first identified in the blood of a <u>rh</u>esus monkey.
serum	Plasma minus clotting proteins and cells. Clear, yellowish fluid that separates from blood when it is allowed to clot. It is formed from plasma, but does not contain protein-coagulation factors.
stem cell	Unspecialized cell that gives rise to mature, specialized forms. A **hematopoietic stem cell** is the progenitor for all different types of blood cells.
thrombin	Enzyme that converts fibrinogen to fibrin during coagulation.
thrombocyte	Platelet.

COMBINING FORMS, SUFFIXES, AND TERMINOLOGY

Write the meanings of the medical terms in the spaces provided.

COMBINING FORMS

Combining Form	Meaning	Terminology	Meaning
bas/o	base (*alkaline*, the opposite of acid)	<u>bas</u>ophil _____ *The suffix -phil means attraction to.*	

Combining Form	Meaning	Terminology	Meaning
chrom/o	color	hypochromic _____ *Pertaining to a type of anemia with decreased hemoglobin in erythrocytes.*	
coagul/o	clotting	anticoagulant _____	
		coagulopathy _____	
cyt/o	cell	cytology _____	
eosin/o	red, dawn, rosy	eosinophil _____	
erythr/o	red	erythrocytopenia _____ *The suffix -penia means deficiency.*	
granul/o	granules	granulocyte _____	
hem/o	blood	hemolysis _____ *Destruction or breakdown of red blood cells. See hemolytic anemia, page 498.*	
hemat/o	blood	hematocrit _____ *The suffix -crit means to separate. The hematocrit gives the percentage of red blood cells in a volume of blood. See page 503.*	
hemoglobin/o	hemoglobin	hemoglobinopathy _____	
is/o	same, equal	anisocytosis _____ *An abnormality of red blood cells; they are of unequal (anis/o) size; -cytosis means an increase in the number of cells.*	
kary/o	nucleus	megakaryocyte _____	
leuk/o	white	leukocytopenia _____ *Usually is shortened to leukopenia.*	
mon/o	one, single	monocyte _____ *The cell has a single, rather than a multilobed, nucleus.*	
morph/o	shape, form	morphology _____	
myel/o	bone marrow	myeloblast _____ *The suffix -blast indicates an immature cell.*	
		myelogenous _____ *The suffix -genous means pertaining to or produced in.*	
neutr/o	neutral (neither base nor acid)	neutropenia _____ *This term refers to neutrophils.*	
nucle/o	nucleus	mononuclear _____	
		polymorphonuclear _____	

13

Combining Form	Meaning	Terminology	Meaning
phag/o	eat, swallow	phagocyte _____	
poikil/o	varied, irregular	poikilocytosis _____ *Irregularity in the shape of red blood cells. Poikilocytosis occurs in certain types of anemia.*	
sider/o	iron	sideropenia _____	
spher/o	globe, round	spherocytosis _____ *In this condition, the erythrocyte has a round shape, making the cell fragile and easily able to be destroyed.*	
thromb/o	clot	thrombocytopenia _____	

SUFFIXES

Suffix	Meaning	Terminology	Meaning
-apheresis	removal, a carrying away	plasmapheresis _____ *A centrifuge spins blood to remove plasma from the other parts of blood.*	
		leukapheresis _____	
		plateletpheresis _____ *Note that the a of apheresis is dropped in this term. Platelets are removed from the donor's blood (and used in a patient), and the remainder of the blood is reinfused into the donor.*	
-blast	immature cell, embryonic	monoblast _____	
		erythroblast _____	
-cytosis	abnormal condition of cells (increase in cells)	macrocytosis _____ *Macrocytes are erythrocytes that are larger (macro-) than normal size.*	
		microcytosis _____ *These are erythrocytes that are smaller (micro-) than normal size. Table 13–3 reviews terms related to abnormalities of red blood cell morphology.*	
-emia	blood condition	leukemia _____ *See page 501.*	
-globin	protein	hemoglobin _____	
-globulin	protein	immunoglobulin _____	
-lytic	pertaining to destruction	thrombolytic therapy _____ *Used to dissolve clots.*	

Table 13–3

Abnormalities of Red Blood Cell Morphology

Abnormality	Description
Anisocytosis	Cells are **unequal** in size
Hypo**chromia**	Cells have reduced **color** (less hemoglobin)
Macrocytosis	Cells are **large**
Microcytosis	Cells are **small**
Poikilocytosis	Cells are **irregularly shaped**
Spherocytosis	Cells are **rounded**

Suffix	Meaning	Terminology	Meaning
-oid	derived from	myeloid	
-osis	abnormal condition	thrombosis	
-penia	deficiency	granulocytopenia	
		pancytopenia	
-phage	eat, swallow	macrophage	
		A large phagocyte that destroys worn-out red blood cells and foreign material.	
-philia	attraction for (an increase in cell numbers)	eosinophilia	
		neutrophilia	
-phoresis	carrying, transmission	electrophoresis	
-poiesis	formation	hematopoiesis	
		erythropoiesis	
		Erythropoietin is produced by the kidneys to stimulate erythrocyte formation.	
		myelopoiesis	
-stasis	stop, control	hemostasis	

PATHOLOGIC CONDITIONS

Any abnormal or pathologic condition of the blood generally is referred to as a blood **dyscrasia** (disease). The blood dyscrasias discussed in this section are organized in the following manner: diseases of red blood cells, disorders of blood clotting, diseases of white blood cells, and disease of the bone marrow.

DISEASES OF RED BLOOD CELLS

anemia	**Deficiency in erythrocytes or hemoglobin.**

The most common type of anemia is **iron deficiency anemia**; it is caused by a lack of iron, which is required for hemoglobin production (see Fig. 13–10).

Other types of anemia include:

1. aplastic anemia	**Failure of blood cell production due to aplasia (absence of development, formation) of bone marrow cells.**

The cause of most cases of aplastic anemia is unknown (idiopathic), but some cases have been linked to benzene exposure and to antibiotics such as chloramphenicol. **Pancytopenia** occurs when stem cells fail to produce leukocytes, platelets, and erythrocytes. Blood transfusions prolong life, allowing the marrow time to resume its normal functioning, and antibiotics control infections. Bone marrow transplantation and treatment with drugs that inhibit the immune system have been successful as therapy in cases where spontaneous recovery is unlikely.

2. hemolytic anemia	**Reduction in red cells due to excessive destruction.**

One example of hemolytic anemia is **congenital spherocytic anemia** (also called **hereditary spherocytosis**). Instead of their normal biconcave shape, erythrocytes are spheroidal. This shape makes them fragile and easily destroyed (hemolysis). Shortened red cell survival results in increased reticulocytes in blood as the bone marrow compensates for hemolysis of mature erythrocytes. Because the spleen destroys red cells, removing the spleen usually improves this anemia. Figure 13–11 shows the altered shape of erythrocytes in hereditary spherocytosis.

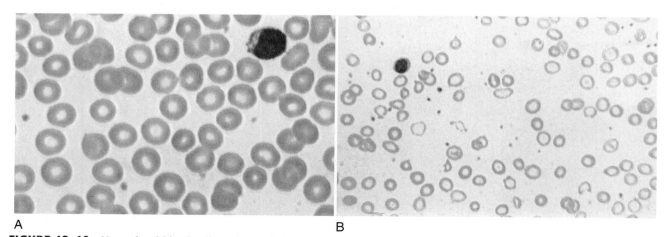

A   B

FIGURE 13–10 **Normal red blood cells and iron deficiency anemia. A, Normal red cells.** Erythrocytes are fairly uniform in size and shape. The red cells are normal in hemoglobin content (normochromic) and size (normocytic). **B, Iron deficiency anemia.** Many erythrocytes are small (microcytic) and have increased central pallor (hypochromic). Red cells in this slide show variation in size (anisocytosis) and shape (poikilocytosis). (From Tkachuk DC, Hirschmann JV, McArthur JR: Atlas of Clinical Hematology. Philadelphia, WB Saunders, 2002, p. 4.)

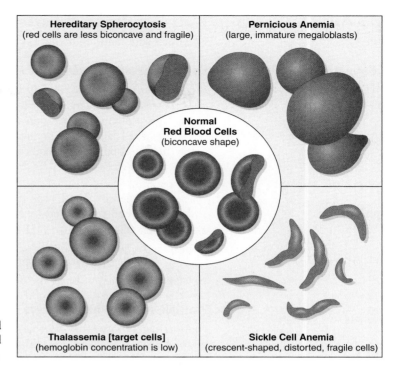

FIGURE 13–11 Normal red blood cells and the abnormal cells in several types of anemia.

3. pernicious anemia	**Lack of mature erythrocytes caused by inability to absorb vitamin B_{12} into the body. (Pernicious means ruinous or hurtful.)**

Vitamin B_{12} is necessary for the proper development and maturation of erythrocytes. Although vitamin B_{12} is a common constituent of food (liver, kidney, sardines, egg yolks, oysters), it cannot be absorbed into the bloodstream without the aid of a special substance called **intrinsic factor** that is normally found in gastric juice. People with pernicious anemia lack this factor in their gastric juice, and the result is unsuccessful maturation of red blood cells, with an excess of large, immature, and poorly functioning cells in the bone marrow and large, often oval red cells (macrocytes) in the circulation. Treatment is administration of vitamin B_{12} for life. Figure 13–11 illustrates cells in pernicious anemia.

4. sickle cell anemia

A hereditary condition characterized by abnormal sickle shape of erythrocytes and by hemolysis.

The crescent, or sickle, shape of the erythrocyte is caused by an abnormal type of hemoglobin (hemoglobin S) in the red cell (see Fig. 13–11). The distorted, fragile erythrocytes cannot pass through small blood vessels normally, leading to thrombosis and infarction (local tissue death from ischemia). Signs and symptoms include arthralgias, acute attacks of abdominal pain, and ulcerations of the extremities. The genetic defect (presence of the hemoglobin S gene) is particularly prevalent in black persons of African or African American ancestry and appears with different degrees of severity. Individuals who inherit just one gene for the trait usually do not have symptoms.

5. thalassemia

An inherited defect in the ability to produce hemoglobin, usually seen in persons of Mediterranean background.

This condition manifests in varying forms and degrees of severity and usually leads to hypochromic anemia with diminished hemoglobin content in red cells (see Fig. 13–11). *Thalassa* is a Greek word meaning sea.

13

hemochromatosis	**Excess iron deposits throughout the body.**
	Hepatomegaly, skin pigmentation, diabetes, and cardiac failure may occur.
polycythemia vera	**General increase in red blood cells (erythremia).**
	Blood consistency is viscous (thick) because of greatly increased numbers of erythrocytes. The bone marrow is hyperplastic, and leukocytosis and thrombocytosis commonly accompany the increase in red blood cells. Treatment consists of reduction of red cell volume to normal levels by phlebotomy (removal of blood from a vein) and by suppressing blood cell production with myelotoxic drugs.

DISORDERS OF BLOOD CLOTTING

hemophilia	**Excessive bleeding caused by hereditary lack of one of the protein substances (either factor VIII or factor IX) necessary for blood clotting.**
	Although the platelet count of a hemophiliac patient is normal, deficiency in clotting factors (VIII or IX) results in a prolonged coagulation time. Treatment consists of administration of the deficient factor.
purpura	**Multiple pinpoint hemorrhages and accumulation of blood under the skin.**
	Hemorrhages into the skin and mucous membranes produce red-purple discoloration of the skin. **Petechiae** are tiny purple or red flat spots appearing on the skin as a result of hemorrhages. **Ecchymoses** are larger blue or purplish patches on the skin (bruises). See Figure 13-12. Purpura can be caused by having too few platelets (thrombocytopenia). The cause may be immunologic, meaning the body produces an antiplatelet factor that harms its own platelets. **Autoimmune thrombocytopenic purpura** (previously idiopathic thrombocytopenia purpura) is a condition in which a patient makes an antibody that destroys platelets. Bleeding time is prolonged; splenectomy (the spleen is the site of platelet destruction) and drug therapy with corticosteroids are common treatments.

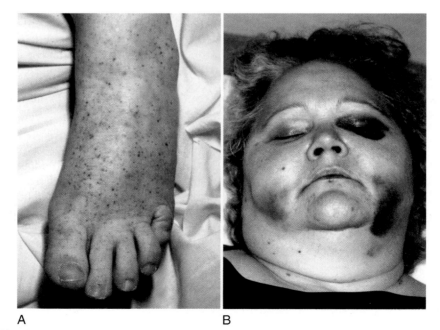

A   B

FIGURE 13–12   **A, Petechiae** result from bleeding from capillaries or small arterioles. **B, Ecchymoses** are larger and more extensive than petechiae. (From Gould BE: Pathophysiology for the Health Professions, 3rd ed. Philadelphia, WB Saunders, 2006, p. 250.)

DISEASES OF WHITE BLOOD CELLS

leukemia

13

Increase in cancerous white blood cells.

Malignant leukocytes fill the marrow and bloodstream. The terms **acute** and **chronic** discriminate between leukemias of primarily immature (acute) or mature (chronic) leukocytes.

Acute leukemias have common clinical characteristics: abrupt, stormy onset of symptoms, fatigue, fever, bleeding, bone pain and tenderness, lymphadenopathy, splenomegaly, hepatomegaly, and CNS abnormalities, such as headache, vomiting, and paralysis. Four types of leukemia are:

1. **Acute myelogenous (myelocytic) leukemia (AML).** Immature granulocytes (myeloblasts) predominate. Platelets and erythrocytes are diminished because of infiltration and replacement of the bone marrow by large numbers of myeloblasts (see Fig. 13–13, *A*).
2. **Acute lymphocytic leukemia (ALL).** Immature lymphocytes (lymphoblasts) predominate. This form is seen most often in children and adolescents; onset is sudden (Fig. 13–13, *B*).
3. **Chronic myelogenous (myelocytic) leukemia (CML).** Both mature and immature granulocytes are present in the marrow and bloodstream. This is a slowly progressive illness with which patients (often adults older than 55) may live for many years without encountering life-threatening problems. New therapies (such as the drug Gleevec) target abnormal proteins responsible for malignancy.
4. **Chronic lymphocytic leukemia (CLL).** Abnormal numbers of relatively mature lymphocytes predominate in the marrow, lymph nodes, and spleen. This most common form of leukemia usually occurs in the elderly and follows a slowly progressive course.

All forms of leukemia are treated with chemotherapy, using drugs that prevent cell division and selectively injure rapidly dividing cells. Effective treatment can lead to a **remission** (disappearance of signs of disease). **Relapse** occurs when leukemia cells reappear in the blood and bone marrow, necessitating further treatment.

Transplantation of normal bone marrow from donors of similar tissue type is successful in restoring normal bone marrow function in some patients with acute

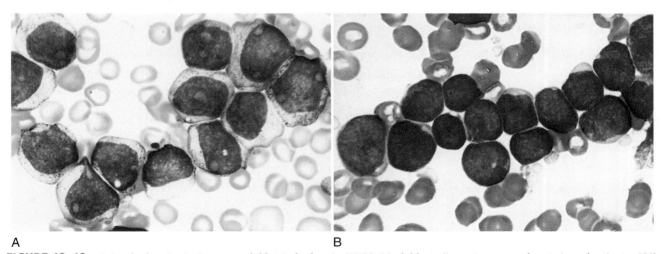

A   B

FIGURE 13–13   **Acute leukemia. A, Acute myeloblastic leukemia** (AML). Myeloblasts (immature granulocytes) predominate. AML affects primarily adults. A majority of patients achieve remission with intensive chemotherapy, but relapse is common. Hematopoietic stem cell transplantation may be a curative therapy. **B, Acute lymphoblastic leukemia** (ALL). Lymphoblasts (immature lymphocytes) predominate. ALL is a disease of children and young adults. Most children are cured with chemotherapy. (Courtesy of Dr. Robert W. McKenna, Department of Pathology, University of Texas Southwestern Medical School, Dallas, TX. From Kumar V, Cotran RS, Robbins SL: Robbins Basic Pathology, 7th ed. Philadelphia, WB Saunders, 2003, p. 424.)

leukemia. This procedure is performed after high-dose chemotherapy, which is administered to eliminate the leukemic cells.

granulocytosis — **Abnormal increase in granulocytes in the blood.**

An increase in neutrophils in the blood may occur in response to infection or inflammation of any type. **Eosinophilia** is an increase in eosinophilic granulocytes, seen in certain allergic conditions, such as asthma, or in parasitic infections (tapeworm, pinworm). **Basophilia** is an increase in basophilic granulocytes seen in certain types of leukemia.

mononucleosis — **An infectious disease marked by increased numbers of leukocytes and enlarged cervical lymph nodes.**

This disease is caused by the Epstein-Barr virus (EBV). Lymphadenitis is present, with fever, fatigue, asthenia (weakness), and pharyngitis. Atypical lymphocytes are present in the blood, liver (hepatomegaly), and spleen (splenomegaly).

Mononucleosis usually is transmitted by direct oral contact (salivary exchange during kissing) and affects primarily young adults. No treatment is necessary for EBV infections. Antibiotics are not effective for self-limited viral illnesses. Rest during the period of acute symptoms and slow return to normal activities are advised.

DISEASES OF BONE MARROW CELLS

multiple myeloma — **Malignant neoplasm of bone marrow.**

The malignant cells (lymphocytes that produce antibodies) destroy bone tissue and cause overproduction of immunoglobulins, including **Bence Jones protein,** an immunoglobulin fragment found in urine. The condition leads to osteolytic lesions, hypercalcemia, anemia, renal damage, and increased susceptibility to infection. Treatment is with analgesics, radiotherapy, **palliative** (relieving, not curing) doses of chemotherapy, and special orthopedic supports. **Autologous bone marrow transplantation (ABMT),** in which the patient serves as his or her own donor for stem cells, may lead to prolonged remission and possible cure.

LABORATORY TESTS AND CLINICAL PROCEDURES

LABORATORY TESTS

antiglobulin test — **Test for the presence of antibodies that coat and damage erythrocytes.**

This test determines the presence of antibodies in infants of Rh-negative women or in patients with autoimmune hemolytic anemia.

bleeding time — **Time required for blood to stop flowing from a tiny puncture wound.**

Normal time is 8 minutes or less. The Simplate or Ivy method is used. Platelet disorders and the use of aspirin prolong bleeding time.

coagulation time — **Time required for venous blood to clot in a test tube.**

Normal time is less than 15 minutes.

complete blood count (CBC) — **Determination of the number of red and white cells and platelets, hemoglobin level and hematocrit, and red cell indices—MCH, MCV, MCHC (see Abbreviations).**

erythrocyte sedimentation rate (ESR)	**Speed at which erythrocytes settle out of plasma.** Venous blood is collected into an anticoagulant, and the blood is placed in a tube in a vertical position. The distance that the erythrocytes sink in a given period of time is the sedimentation rate. The rate increases with infections, joint inflammation, and tumor, which increase the fibrinogen content of the blood. (Also called sed rate for short.)
hematocrit (Hct)	**Percentage of erythrocytes in a volume of blood.** A sample of blood is spun in a centrifuge so that the erythrocytes fall to the bottom of the sample.
hemoglobin test (H, Hg, HGB)	**Total amount of hemoglobin in a sample of peripheral blood.**
partial thromboplastin time (PTT)	**Measures the presence of plasma factors that act in a portion of the coagulation pathway.** This test is used to follow patients taking anticoagulants, such as heparin.
platelet count	**Number of platelets per cubic millimeter (mm³) or microliter (μL) of blood.** Platelets normally average between 150,000 and 350,000 per mm³ (cu mm) or μL.
prothrombin time (PT)	**Test of the ability of blood to clot.** The test measures the time elapsed between the addition of calcium and tissue factor (thromboplastin) to a plasma sample and the appearance of a visible clot. It is used to monitor patients taking the anticoagulant drug warfarin (Coumadin).
red blood cell count (RBC)	**Number of erythrocytes per cubic millimeter (mm³) or microliter (μL) of blood.** The normal number is 4 to 6 million per mm³ (or μL).
red blood cell morphology	**Microscopic examination of a stained blood smear to determine the shape of individual red cells.** Abnormal morphology includes anisocytosis, poikilocytosis, and sickle cells.
white blood cell count (WBC)	**Number of leukocytes per cubic millimeter (mm³) or microliter (μL) of blood.** Automated counting devices record numbers within seconds. Normal number of leukocytes average between 5000 and 10,000 per mm³ (or μL).
white blood cell differential	**Percentage of the total WBC made up by different types of leukocytes.** Some instruments can produce automated differentials, but otherwise the cells are stained and counted under a microscope by a technician. Percentages of neutrophils, eosinophils, basophils, monocytes, lymphocytes, and immature cells are determined. 　　The term **"shift to the left"** describes an increase in immature neutrophils in the blood.

Shift to the Left

The phrase "shift to the left" derives from the early practice of reporting percentages of each WBC type across the top of a page, starting with blasts (immature cells) on the left and more mature cell on the right. An increase in immature neutrophils (as seen with severe infection) would be noted on the left-hand column of a form. Thus a "shift to the left" indicates an infection and the body's effort to fight it by making more neutrophils.

CLINICAL PROCEDURES

apheresis	**Separation of blood into component parts and removal of a select part from the blood.**

This procedure can remove toxic substances or autoantibodies from the blood and can collect blood cells. Leukapheresis, plateletpheresis, and plasmapheresis are examples (see Fig. 13–14). If plasma is removed from the patient and fresh plasma is given, the procedure is termed **plasma exchange.**

blood transfusion

Whole blood or cells are taken from a donor and infused into a patient.

Appropriate testing to ensure a match of red blood cell type (A, B, AB, or O) is essential. Tests also are performed to detect the presence of hepatitis and the acquired immunodeficiency syndrome (AIDS) virus (HIV). **Autologous transfusion** is the collection and later reinfusion of a patient's own blood or blood components. **Packed cells** are a preparation of red blood cells separated from liquid plasma and administered in severe anemia to restore levels of hemoglobin and red cells without overdiluting the blood with excess fluid.

bone marrow biopsy

Microscopic examination of a core of bone marrow removed with a needle.

This procedure is helpful in the diagnosis of blood disorders such as anemia, cell deficiencies, and leukemia. Bone marrow may also be removed by brief suction produced by a syringe, which is termed a **bone marrow aspirate.**

hematopoietic stem cell transplantation

Peripheral stem cells from a compatible donor are administered into a recipient's vein.

Patients with malignant hematologic disease, such as AML, ALL, CLL, CML, and multiple myeloma, are candidates for this treatment. First the donor is treated with a drug that mobilizes stem cells into the blood. Then stem cells are removed from the donor, a process like leukapheresis in Figure 13–14. Meanwhile, the patient undergoes a conditioning process in which radiation and chemotherapy are administered to kill malignant marrow cells and inactivate the patient's immune system so that subsequent stem cells will not be rejected. A cell suspension containing the donor's stem cells, which will repopulate the bone marrow, is then given through a vein to the recipient. **Bone marrow transplantation** follows the same procedure, except bone marrow cells are removed and used rather than peripheral stem cells (see Fig. 13–15). Problems

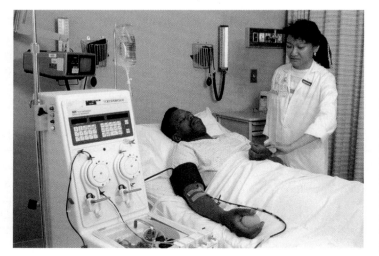

FIGURE 13–14 Leukapheresis. This machine is an automated blood cell separator that removes large numbers of white blood cells and returns red cells, platelets, and plasma to the patient. (From Black JM, Hawks JH, Keene AM: Medical-Surgical Nursing: Clinical Management for Positive Outcomes, 6th ed. Philadelphia, WB Saunders, 2001, p. 2170.)

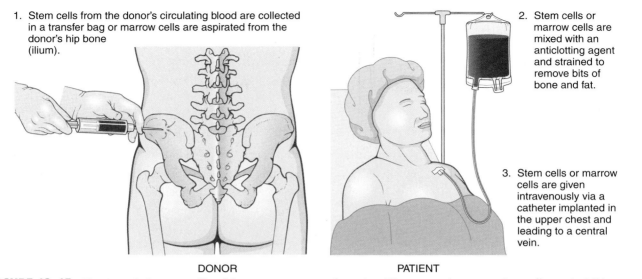

1. Stem cells from the donor's circulating blood are collected in a transfer bag or marrow cells are aspirated from the donor's hip bone (ilium).

2. Stem cells or marrow cells are mixed with an anticlotting agent and strained to remove bits of bone and fat.

3. Stem cells or marrow cells are given intravenously via a catheter implanted in the upper chest and leading to a central vein.

DONOR   PATIENT

FIGURE 13–15 **Hematopoietic stem cell and bone marrow transplantation.** These procedures constitute **allogeneic** (all/o means other, different) **transplantation,** in which a relative or unrelated person having a close or identical HLA (human leukocyte antigen) type is the donor. It carries a high rate of morbidity (disease) and mortality (death) because of complications of incompatibility such as GVHD (graft versus host disease). In **autologous transplantation,** stem cells or bone marrow cells are removed from the patient during a remission phase and given back to the patient after intensive chemotherapy (drug treatment).

encountered subsequently may be serious infection, **graft versus host disease (GVHD),** and relapse of the original disease despite the treatment.

In GVHD, the immunocompetent cells in the donor's tissue recognize the recipient's tissues as foreign and attack them. Because the recipient is totally immunosuppressed, his or her immune system cannot defend against the attack.

ABBREVIATIONS

ABMT	autologous bone marrow transplantation—patient serves as his or her own donor for stem cells	**diff.**	differential count (white blood cells)
ABO	four main blood types—A, B, AB, and O	**EBV**	Epstein-Barr virus, the cause of mononucleosis
ALL	acute lymphocytic leukemia	**eos**	eosinophils
AML	acute myelogenous leukemia	**EPO**	erythropoietin
ASCT	autologous stem cell transplantation	**ESR**	erythrocyte sedimentation rate
baso	basophils	**Fe**	iron
BMT	bone marrow transplantation	**G-CSF**	granulocyte colony-stimulating factor
CBC	complete blood count	**GM-CSF**	granulocyte-macrophage colony-stimulating factor
CLL	chronic lymphocytic leukemia	**g/dL**	gram per deciliter (1 deciliter = one tenth of a liter)
CML	chronic myelogenous leukemia	**GVHD**	graft versus host disease—immune reaction of donor's cells to recipient's tissue
DIC	disseminated intravascular coagulation—bleeding disorder marked by reduction in blood clotting factors due to their use and depletion for intravascular coagulation	**HCL**	hairy cell leukemia—abnormal lymphocytes accumulate in bone marrow, leading to anemia, thrombocytopenia, neutropenia, and infection

Hct	hematocrit	**mm³**	cubic millimeter—one millionth of a liter
Hgb, HGB	hemoglobin		
H and H	hemoglobin and hematocrit	**mono**	monocyte
HLA	human leukocyte antigen	**polys, PMNs, PMNLs**	polymorphonuclear leukocytes; neutrophils
IgA, IgD, IgE, IgG, IgM	immunoglobulins		
		PT	prothrombin time
lymphs	lymphocytes	**PTT**	partial thromboplastin time
MCH	mean corpuscular hemoglobin—average amount of hemoglobin per cell	**RBC**	red blood cell; red blood cell count
		sed rate	erythrocyte sedimentation rate
		segs	segmented, mature white blood cells
MCHC	mean corpuscular hemoglobin concentration—average concentration of hemoglobin in a single red cell; when MCHC is low, the cell is hypochromic	**SMAC**	Sequential Multiple Analyzer Computer—an automated chemistry system that determines substances in serum
		µL	microliter—one millionth of a liter; 1 liter = 1.057 quarts
MCV	mean corpuscular volume—average volume or size of a single red blood cell; when MCV is high, the cells are macrocytic, and when low, the cells are microcytic	**WBC**	white blood cell; white blood cell count
		WNL	within normal limits

PRACTICAL APPLICATIONS

The cases presented here are based on data from actual medical records. Use the table of normal values to help you decide on a probable diagnosis in each case. Answers to the questions are on page 517.

Normal Laboratory Values

WBC 4,500–11,000/mm³ or µL			RBC	M:	4.5–6.0 million per mm³ or µL
Differential:				F:	4.0–5.5 million per mm³ or µL
Segs (polys)	54%–62%		Hct	M:	40–50%
Lymphs	20%–40%			F:	37–47%
Eos	1%–3%		Hgb	M:	14–16 g/dL
Baso	0%–1%			F:	12–14 g/dL
Mono	3%–7%		Platelets 150,000–350,000/mm³ or µL		

THREE SHORT CASES

1. A 65-year-old woman visits her physician complaining of shortness of breath and swollen ankles. Lab tests reveal that her hematocrit is 18.0 and her hemoglobin 5.8. Her blood smear shows macrocytes and her blood level of vitamin B_{12} is very low. What is a likely diagnosis?
   a. Aplastic anemia
   b. Hemochromatosis
   c. Pernicious anemia

2. A 22-year-old college student visits the clinic with a fever and complaining of a sore throat. Blood tests show a WBC of 28,000 per mm^3 with 95% myeloblasts (polys are 5%). Platelet count is 15,000 per mm^3, hemoglobin is 10 g/dL, and the hematocrit is 22.5. What is your diagnosis?
   a. Chronic lymphocytic leukemia
   b. Acute myelogenous leukemia
   c. Thalassemia

3. A 35-year-old woman goes to her physician complaining of spots on her legs and bleeding gums. On examination, she has tiny purple spots covering her legs and evidence of dried blood in her mouth. Her CBC shows hemoglobin 14 g/dL, hematocrit 42%, WBC 5000 per mm^3 with normal differential, and platelet count 4000/mm^3 (with megakaryocytes in bone marrow). What is your diagnosis?
   a. Sickle cell anemia
   b. Hemolytic anemia
   c. Autoimmune thrombocytopenic purpura

CASE REPORT

Four-year-old Sally has been running a low-grade fever for several weeks, with recurrent sore throat and cough. Her mother takes her to the family physician, who diagnoses her condition as otitis. Sally continues to be fatigued and anorexic. Her mother notices bruising on her legs and arms. The family physician finally orders blood tests and an antibiotic drug. Peripheral blood tests reveal Hgb 7.4, platelet count 40,000, and WBC count 85,000 with 90 percent lymphoblasts. A bone marrow biopsy is ordered.

1. What's the likely diagnosis for this patient?
   a. AML
   b. CLL
   c. ALL
   d. CML

2. The probable cause of Sally's ecchymoses is:
   a. Neutropenia
   b. Thrombocytopenia
   c. Anorexia
   d. Otitis

3. The likely explanation for Sally's fatigue is:
   a. Anemia
   b. Sore throat and cough
   c. Thrombocytopenia
   d. Neutropenia

4. Treatment for Sally's condition is likely to be:
   a. Prolonged antibiotic therapy
   b. IV feeding
   c. Surgery to repair the bone marrow
   d. Chemotherapy

? EXERCISES

Remember to check your answers carefully with those given in the Answers to Exercises, page 516.

A. Match the following cells with their meanings as given below.

basophil   hematopoietic stem cell   neutrophil
eosinophil   lymphocyte   platelet
erythrocyte   monocyte

1. mononuclear white blood cell (agranulocyte) formed in lymph tissue; it is a phagocyte and the

   precursor of a macrophage _____

2. thrombocyte or cell that helps blood clot _____

3. cell in the bone marrow that gives rise to different types of blood cells _____

4. mononuclear leukocyte formed in lymph tissue; produces antibodies _____

5. leukocyte with dense, reddish granules having an affinity for red acidic dye; associated with allergic

   reactions _____

6. red blood cell _____

7. leukocyte (polymorphonuclear granulocyte) formed in the bone marrow and having neutral-staining

   granules _____

8. leukocyte (granulocyte) whose granules have an affinity for basic dye; releases histamine and

   heparin _____

B. Give the meanings of the following terms.

1. coagulation _____

2. granulocyte _____

3. mononuclear _____

4. polymorphonuclear _____

5. globulins _____

6. erythroblast _____

7. megakaryocyte _____

8. macrophage _____

9. hemoglobin _____

10. plasma _____

13

11. reticulocyte _____

12. myeloblast _____

C. Give the medical terms for the following descriptions.

1. liquid portion of blood _____

2. orange-yellow pigment produced from hemoglobin when red blood cells are destroyed

_____

3. iron-containing nonprotein part of hemoglobin _____

4. proteins in plasma; separated into alpha, beta, and gamma types _____

5. hormone secreted by the kidneys to stimulate bone marrow to produce red blood cells

_____

6. foreign material that stimulates the production of an antibody _____

7. plasma protein that maintains the proper amount of water in the blood _____

8. proteins made by lymphocytes in response to antigens in the blood _____

D. Give short answers for the following.

1. Name four types of plasma proteins. _____

_____

2. What is the Rh factor? _____

3. What is hemolysis? _____

4. A person with type A blood has _____ antigens and _____ antibodies in his or her blood.

5. A person with type B blood has _____ antigens and _____ antibodies in his or her blood.

6. A person with type O blood has _____ antigens and _____ antibodies in his or her blood.

7. A person with type AB blood has _____ antigens and _____ antibodies in his or her blood.

8. Can you transfuse blood from a type A donor into a type B recipient? _____ Why?

_____

9. Can you transfuse blood from a type AB donor into a type O recipient? _____ Why?

_____

10. What is electrophoresis? _____

11. What is immunoglobulin? _____

12. What is differentiation? _____

13. What is plasmapheresis? _____

E. Match the following terms related to clotting with their meanings as given below.

coagulation	heparin	thrombin
fibrin	prothrombin	warfarin (Coumadin)
fibrinogen	serum	

1. anticoagulant substance found in liver cells, bloodstream, and tissues _____

2. protein threads that form the basis of a blood clot _____

3. plasma protein that is converted to thrombin in the clotting process _____

4. plasma minus clotting proteins and cells _____

5. drug given to patients to prevent formation of clots _____

6. plasma protein that is converted to fibrin in the clotting process _____

7. process of clotting _____

8. enzyme that helps convert fibrinogen to fibrin _____

F. Divide the following terms into component parts and give meanings of the complete terms.

1. anticoagulant _____

2. hemoglobinopathy _____

3. cytology _____

4. leukocytopenia _____

5. morphology _____

6. megakaryocyte _____

7. sideropenia _____

8. phagocyte _____

9. myeloblast _____

10. plateletpheresis _____

11. monoblast _____

12. myelopoiesis _____

13. hemostasis _____

14. thrombolytic _____

15. hematopoiesis _____

G. Match the following terms concerning red blood cells with their meanings as given below.

anisocytosis   hemoglobin   microcytosis
erythrocytopenia   hemolysis   poikilocytosis
erythropoiesis   hypochromic   polycythemia vera
hematocrit   macrocytosis   spherocytosis

1. any irregularity in the shape of red blood cells _____

2. oxygen-containing protein in red blood cells _____

3. formation of red blood cells _____

4. deficiency in numbers of red blood cells _____

5. destruction of red blood cells _____

6. pertaining to reduction of hemoglobin in red blood cells _____

7. variation in size of red blood cells _____

8. abnormal numbers of round, rather than normally biconcave-shaped, red blood cells

 _____

9. increase in number of small red blood cells _____

10. general increase in numbers of red blood cells; erythremia _____

11. increase in numbers of large red blood cells _____

12. separation of blood so that the percentage of red blood cells in relation to the volume of a blood

 sample is measured _____

H. Describe the problem in each of the following forms of anemia.

1. iron deficiency anemia _____

2. pernicious anemia _____

3. sickle cell anemia _____

4. aplastic anemia _____

5. thalassemia _____

I. Give the meanings of the following terms for blood dyscrasias.

1. autoimmune thrombocytopenic purpura _____

2. granulocytosis _____

3. hemophilia _____

4. hemochromatosis _____

5. multiple myeloma _____

6. mononucleosis _____

J. Match the term in Column I with its meaning in Column II. Write the letter of the meaning in the space provided.

Column I

1. relapse   _____

2. remission   _____

3. palliative   _____

4. Bence Jones protein   _____

5. ecchymoses   _____

6. pancytopenia   _____

7. apheresis   _____

8. eosinophilia   _____

9. petechiae   _____

10. packed cells   _____

Column II

A. Deficiency of all blood cells.

B. Immunoglobulin fragment found in the urine of patients with multiple myeloma.

C. Increase in numbers of granulocytes; seen in allergic conditions.

D. Large blue or purplish patches on skin (bruises).

E. Symptoms of the disease return.

F. Tiny purple or flat red spots on skin as a result of small hemorrhages.

G. Symptoms of the disease disappear.

H. Separation of blood into its parts.

I. Preparation of erythrocytes separated from plasma.

J. Relieving but not curing.

K. Match the following laboratory test or clinical procedure with its description.

antiglobulin Coombs test
autologous transfusion
bleeding time
bone marrow biopsy
coagulation time

erythrocyte sedimentation rate
hematocrit
hematopoietic stem cell
  transplantation

platelet count
red blood cell count
red blood cell morphology
white blood cell differential

1. microscopic examination of a stained blood smear to determine the shape of individual red blood

   cells _____

2. percentage of red blood cells in a volume of blood _____

3. determines the number of clotting cells per mm³ or μL of blood _____

4. time required for venous blood to clot in a test tube _____

5. speed at which erythrocytes settle out of plasma _____

6. percentage of the total WBCs made up by different types of white blood cells (immature and

   mature forms) _____

7. test for the presence of antibodies that coat and damage erythrocytes _____

8. peripheral stem cells from a compatible donor are infused into a recipient's vein to repopulate the

   bone marrow _____

9. time required for blood to stop flowing from a small puncture wound _____

10. microscopic examination of a core of bone marrow removed with a needle _____

11. number of erythrocytes per mm^3 or μL of blood _____

12. blood is collected from and later reinfused into the same patient _____

L. Give the meanings of the following abbreviations in Column I and then select from the sentences in Column II the best association for each.

Column I

1. Hgb _____ _____

2. GVHD _____ _____

3. ALL _____ _____

4. PTT _____ _____

5. CML _____ _____

6. G-CSFs _____ _____

7. IgA, IgE, IgD _____ _____

8. CLL _____ _____

9. Hct _____ _____

10. AML _____ _____

Column II

A. Blood protein that helps transport oxygen to body tissues.

B. Malignant condition of white blood cells in which immature granulocytes predominate; normal bone marrow is replaced by myeloblasts.

C. Malignant condition of white blood cells in which immature lymphocytes predominate; children are affected and onset is sudden.

D. Test used to follow patients who are taking certain anticoagulants.

E. Percentage of erythrocytes in a volume of blood.

F. Malignant condition of white blood cells in which both mature and immature granulocytes are present; a slowly progressive illness.

G. Immune reaction of donor's cells/tissue to recipient's cells/tissue; a possible outcome of hematopoietic stem cell or bone marrow transplantation.

H. Proteins containing antibodies.

I. Malignant condition of white blood cells in which relatively mature lymphocytes predominate in lymph nodes, spleen, and bone marrow; usually seen in elderly patients.

J. Proteins that stimulate the formation and proliferation of white blood cells.

M. Circle the boldface terms that best complete the meanings of the sentences.

1. Gary, a 1-year-old African American child, was failing to gain weight normally. He seemed pale and without energy. His blood tests showed a decreased hemoglobin (5.0 g/dL) and decreased hematocrit (16.5%). After a blood smear revealed abnormally shaped red cells, the physician told Gary's mother that her son had **(iron deficiency anemia, hemophilia, sickle cell anemia)**.

2. While in the hospital, Mr. Klein was told he had an elevated **(red blood cell, white blood cell, platelet)** count with a "shift to the left." This was information that confirmed his diagnosis of a systemic infection.

3. While taking warfarin (Coumadin), a blood thinner, Mr. Smith's physician made sure to check his **(prothrombin time, hematocrit, sed rate)**.

13

4. When they checked Babette's blood type during her prenatal examination, she was AB⁻. Her physician told her that she and her baby might have the condition of **(Rh incompatibility, multiple myeloma, pernicious anemia)**.

5. Bobby was diagnosed at a very early age with a bleeding disorder called **(hemophilia, thalassemia, eosinophilia)**. He needed factor VIII regularly, especially after even the slightest traumatic injury.

6. Bill was a 9-year-old boy who suddenly noticed many black and blue marks all over his legs. He had a fever and was tired all the time. The physician did a blood test that revealed pancytopenia. A bone marrow biopsy confirmed the diagnosis of **(acute lymphocytic leukemia, polycythemia vera, aplastic anemia)**.

7. Alice and her friends had been staying up late for weeks, cramming for exams. She developed a sore throat and swollen lymph nodes in her neck and felt fatigued all the time. Dr. Smith did a blood test, and the results showed lymphocytosis and antibodies to EBV in the bloodstream. His diagnosis was **(leukapheresis, lymphocytopenia, mononucleosis)**.

8. Susan was experiencing heavy menstrual periods **(menorrhea, menorrhagia, hemoptysis)**. Because of the bleeding, she frequently felt tired and weak and probably was sideropenic. Her physician performed blood tests that revealed her problem as **(thrombocytopenia, pernicious anemia, iron deficiency anemia)**.

9. Dr. Harris examined a highly allergic patient and sent a blood sample to a **(pulmonary, cardiovascular, hematologic)** pathologist. The physician stained the blood smear and found an abundance of leukocytes with dense, reddish granules. She made the diagnosis of **(basophilia, eosinophilia, neutrophilia)**.

10. George's blood cell counts had been falling in recent weeks. His scheduled laparotomy was canceled because blood tests revealed **(pancytopenia, plasmapheresis, myelopoiesis)**. Bone marrow biopsy determined that the cause was **(hyperplasia, hypoplasia, differentiation)** of all cellular elements.

MEDICAL SCRAMBLE

Unscramble the letters to form blood system terms from the clues. Use the letters in squares to complete the bonus term. Answers are found on page 517.

1. *Clue:* Blood protein

☐ ☐ ___ ☐ ___ ___ ___ MLUINAB

2. *Clue:* Percentage of red blood cells in a volume of blood

___ ___ ___ ☐ ___ ☐ ☐ ___ ___ ☐ CAHOTRETMI

3. *Clue:* Blood protein in erythrocytes

___ ___ ___ ☐ ☐ ___ ___ ___ ___ ☐ GIMOHONEBL

4. *Clue:* Threads of a clot

___ ___ ___ ___ ☐ ___ BIFNIR

BONUS TERM: *Clue:* Process of blood clotting

☐ ☐ ☐ ☐ ☐ ☐ ☐ ☐ ☐ ☐ ☐

ANSWERS TO EXERCISES

A

1. monocyte
2. platelet
3. hematopoietic stem cell
4. lymphocyte
5. eosinophil
6. erythrocyte
7. neutrophil
8. basophil

B

1. blood clotting
2. white blood cell with dense, dark-staining granules (neutrophil, basophil, and eosinophil)
3. pertaining to (having) one (prominent) nucleus (monocytes and lymphocytes are mononuclear leukocytes)
4. pertaining to (having) a many-shaped nucleus (neutrophils are polymorphonuclear leukocytes)
5. plasma proteins in blood; immunoglobulins are examples
6. immature red blood cell
7. forerunner (precursor) of platelets (formed in the bone marrow)
8. large phagocytes formed from monocytes and found in tissues; they destroy worn-out red blood cells and engulf foreign material
9. blood protein found in red blood cells; enables the erythrocyte to carry oxygen
10. liquid portion of blood
11. immature, developing red blood cell with a network of granules in its cytoplasm
12. immature bone marrow cell that is the forerunner of granulocytes

C

1. plasma
2. bilirubin
3. heme
4. globulins
5. erythropoietin
6. antigen
7. albumin
8. antibodies

D

1. albumin, globulins, fibrinogen, and prothrombin
2. an antigen normally found on red blood cells of Rh-positive individuals
3. destruction of red blood cells when incompatible bloods are mixed
4. A; anti-B
5. B; anti-A
6. no A or B; anti-A and anti-B
7. A and B; no anti-A and no anti-B
8. no; the A antigens will agglutinate with the anti-A antibodies in the B person's bloodstream
9. no; the A and B antigens will agglutinate with the anti-A and anti-B antibodies in the O person's bloodstream
10. a method of separating substances (such as proteins) by electrical charge
11. a type of gamma globulin (blood protein) that contains antibodies
12. change in the structure and function (specialization) of a cell as it matures
13. the process of using a centrifuge to separate or remove blood cells from plasma.

E

1. heparin
2. fibrin
3. prothrombin
4. serum
5. warfarin (Coumadin)
6. fibrinogen
7. coagulation
8. thrombin

F

1. anti/coagul/ant—a substance that prevents clotting
2. hemoglobin/o/pathy—disease (abnormality) of hemoglobin
3. cyt/o/logy—study of cells
4. leuk/o/cyt/o/penia—deficiency of white (blood) cells
5. morph/o/logy—study of the shape or form (of cells)
6. mega/kary/o/cyte—cell with a large (mega-) nucleus (kary); platelet precursor
7. sider/o/penia—deficiency of iron
8. phag/o/cyte—cell that eats or swallows other cells
9. myel/o/blast—immature bone marrow cell (gives rise to granulocytes)
10. platelet/pheresis—separation of platelets from the rest of the blood
11. mon/o/blast—immature monocyte
12. myel/o/poiesis—formation of bone marrow cells
13. hem/o/stasis—controlling or stopping the flow of blood
14. thromb/o/lytic—pertaining to destruction of clots
15. hemat/o/poiesis—formation of blood

G

1. poikilocytosis
2. hemoglobin
3. erythropoiesis
4. erythrocytopenia
5. hemolysis
6. hypochromic
7. anisocytosis
8. spherocytosis
9. microcytosis
10. polycythemia vera
11. macrocytosis
12. hematocrit

H

1. lack of iron leading to insufficient hemoglobin production
2. lack of mature erythrocytes due to inability to absorb vitamin B_{12} into the bloodstream (gastric juice lacks a factor that helps absorb B_{12})
3. abnormal shape (crescent shape) of erythrocytes caused by an abnormal type of hemoglobin (hereditary disorder)
4. lack of all types of blood cells due to lack of development of bone marrow cells
5. defect in the ability to produce hemoglobin, leading to hypochromia

I

1. multiple pinpoint hemorrhages due to a deficiency of platelets (patient makes an antibody that destroys her or his own platelets)
2. abnormal condition of excess numbers of granulocytes (eosinophilia and basophilia)
3. excessive bleeding caused by a hereditary lack of factor VIII or factor IX necessary for clotting
4. excessive deposits of iron in tissues of the body
5. malignant neoplasm of bone marrow
6. infectious disease marked by increased numbers of mononuclear leukocytes

J

1. E
2. G
3. J
4. B
5. D
6. A
7. H
8. C
9. F
10. I

K

1. red blood cell morphology
2. hematocrit
3. platelet count
4. coagulation time
5. erythrocyte sedimentation rate
6. white blood cell differential
7. antiglobulin (Coombs) test
8. hematopoietic stem cell transplantation
9. bleeding time
10. bone marrow biopsy
11. red blood cell count
12. autologous transfusion

L

1. hemoglobin: A
2. graft versus host disease: G
3. acute lymphocytic leukemia: C
4. partial thromboplastin time: D
5. chronic myelogenous (myelocytic) leukemia: F
6. granulocyte colony-stimulating factors: J
7. immunoglobulins: H
8. chronic lymphocytic leukemia: I
9. hematocrit: E
10. acute myelogenous (myelocytic) leukemia: B

M

1. sickle cell anemia
2. white blood cell
3. prothrombin time
4. Rh incompatibility
5. hemophilia
6. aplastic anemia
7. mononucleosis
8. menorrhagia; iron deficiency anemia
9. hematologic; eosinophilia
10. pancytopenia; hypoplasia

ANSWERS TO PRACTICAL APPLICATIONS

Three Short Cases
1. c
2. b
3. c

Case Report
1. b   3. a
2. b   4. d

ANSWERS TO MEDICAL SCRAMBLE

1. ALBUMIN   2. HEMATOCRIT   3. HEMOGLOBIN   4. FIBRIN
BONUS TERM: COAGULATION

PRONUNCIATION OF TERMS

PRONUNCIATION GUIDE	
ā as in āpe	ă as in ăpple
ē as in ēven	ĕ as in ĕvery
ī as in īce	ĭ as in ĭnterest
ō as in ōpen	ŏ as in pŏt
ū as in ūnit	ŭ as in ŭnder

To test your understanding of the terminology in this chapter, write the meaning of each term in the space provided. In addition, you may wish to cover the terms and write them by looking at your definitions. Make sure your spelling is correct. The page number after each term indicates where it is defined or used in the book, so you can easily check your responses. You will find complete definitions for all of these terms and their audio pronunciations on the CD.

VOCABULARY AND TERMINOLOGY

Term	Pronunciation	Meaning
albumin (493)	ăl-BŪ-mĭn	_____
anisocytosis (497)	ăn-ī-sō-sī-TŌ-sĭs	_____
antibody (493)	ĂN-tĭ-bŏd-ē	_____
anticoagulant (495)	ăn-tĭ-cō-ĂG-ū-lănt	_____
antigen (493)	ĂN-tĭ-jĕn	_____
basophil (493)	BĀ-sō-fĭl	_____
bilirubin (493)	bĭl-ĭ-ROO-bĭn	_____
coagulation (493)	kō-ăg-ū-LĀ-shŭn	_____
coagulopathy (495)	kō-ăg-ū-LŎP-ă-thē	_____
colony-stimulating factor (493)	KŎL-ō-nē STĬM-ū-lā-tĭng FĂK-tŏr	_____
cytology (495)	sī-TŎL-ō-jē	_____
differentiation (493)	dĭf-ĕr-ĕn-shē-Ā-shŭn	_____
electrophoresis (493)	ē-lĕk-trō-fō-RĒ-sis	_____
eosinophil (493)	ē-ō-SĬN-ō-fĭl	_____
eosinophilia (497)	ē-ō-sĭn-ō-FĬL-ē-ă	_____
erythroblast (496)	ĕ-RĬTH-rō-blăst	_____
erythrocytopenia (495)	ĕ-rĭth-rō-sī-tō-PĒ-nē-ă	_____
erythropoiesis (497)	ĕ-rĭth-rō-poy-Ē-sĭs	_____
erythropoietin (493)	ĕ-rĭth-rō-POY-ĕ-tĭn	_____
fibrin (493)	FĬ-brĭn	_____
fibrinogen (493)	fĭ-BRĬN-ō-jĕn	_____
globulins (493)	GLŎB-ū-lĭnz	_____
granulocyte (493)	GRĂN-ū-lō-sīt	_____

13

Term	Pronunciation	Meaning
granulocytopenia (497)	grăn-ū-lō-sī-tō-PĒ-nē-ă	
hematopoiesis (497)	hē-mă-tō-poy-Ē-sĭs	
hemoglobin (493)	HĒ-mō-glō-bĭn	
hemoglobinopathy (495)	hē-mō-glō-bĭn-ŎP-ă-thē	
hemolysis (493)	hē-MŎL-ĭ-sĭs	
hemostasis (497)	hē-mō-STĀ-sĭs	
heparin (493)	HĔP-ă-rĭn	
hypochromic (495)	hī-pō-KRŌ-mĭk	
immune reaction (493)	ĭm-MŪN rē-ĂK-shŭn	
immunoglobulin (493)	ĭm-ū-nō-GLŎB-ū-lĭn	
leukapheresis (496)	loo-kă-fĕ-RĒ-sĭs	
leukocytopenia (495)	loo-kō-sī-tō-PĒ-nē-ă	
lymphocyte (493)	LĬM-fō-sīt	
macrocytosis (496)	măk-rō-sī-TŌ-sĭs	
macrophage (494)	MĂK-rō-făj	
megakaryocyte (494)	mĕg-ă-KĀR-ē-ō-sīt	
microcytosis (496)	mī-krō-sī-TŌ-sĭs	
monoblast (496)	MŎN-ō-blăst	
monocyte (494)	MŎN-ō-sīt	
mononuclear (494)	mŏn-ō-NŪ-klē-ăr	
morphology (495)	mŏr-FŎL-ō-jē	
myeloblast (495)	MĪ-ĕ-lō-blăst	
myeloid (497)	MĪ-ĕ-loyd	
myelogenous (495)	mī-ĕ-LŎJ-ĕn-ŭs	
myelopoiesis (497)	mī-ĕ-lō-poy-Ē-sĭs	
neutropenia (495)	noo-trō-PĒ-nē-ă	
neutrophil (494)	NOO-trō-fĭl	
neutrophilia (497)	noo-trō-FĬL-ē-ă	
pancytopenia (497)	păn-sī-tō-PĒ-nē-ă	
phagocyte (496)	FĂG-ō-sīt	
plasma (494)	PLĂZ-mă	
plasmapheresis (494)	plăz-mă-fĕ-RĒ-sĭs	
platelet (494)	PLĀT-lĕt	

13

Term	Pronunciation	Meaning
plateletpheresis (496)	plāt-lĕt-fĕ-RĒ-sĭs	_____
poikilocytosis (496)	poy-kĭ-lō-sī-TŌ-sĭs	_____
polymorphonuclear (495)	pŏl-ē-mŏr-fō-NŪ-klē-ăr	_____
prothrombin (494)	prō-THRŎM-bĭn	_____
reticulocyte (494)	rĕ-TĬK-ū-lō-sīt	_____
Rh factor (494)	R-h FĂK-tŏr	_____
serum (494)	SĔ-rŭm	_____
sideropenia (496)	sĭd-ĕr-ō-PĒ-nē-ă	_____
spherocytosis (496)	sfĕr-ō-sī-TŌ-sĭs	_____
stem cell (494)	stĕm sĕl	_____
thrombin (494)	THRŎM-bĭn	_____
thrombocyte (494)	THRŎM-bō-sīt	_____
thrombocytopenia (496)	thrŏm-bō-sī-tō-PĒ-nē-ă	_____
thrombolytic therapy (496)	thrŏm-bō-LĬ-tĭk THĔR-ă-pē	_____
thrombosis (497)	thrŏm-BŌ-sĭs	_____

PATHOLOGIC CONDITIONS, LABORATORY TESTS, AND CLINICAL PROCEDURES

Term	Pronunciation	Meaning
acute lymphocytic leukemia (501)	ă-KŪT lĭm-fō-SĬ-tĭk loo-KĒ-mē-ă	_____
acute myelogenous leukemia (501)	ă-KŪT mī-ĕ-LŎJ-ĕ-nŭs loo-KĒ-mē-ă	_____
antiglobulin test (502)	ăn-tē-GLŎB-ū-lĭn tĕst	_____
apheresis (504)	ă-fĕ-RĒ-sĭs	_____
aplastic anemia (498)	ā-PLĂS-tĭk ă-NĒ-mē-ă	_____
autologous transfusion (504)	ăw-TŎL-ō-gŭs trăns-FŪ-zhŭn	_____
bleeding time (502)	BLĒ-dĭng tīm	_____
blood transfusion (504)	blŭd trăns-FŪ-zhŭn	_____
bone marrow biopsy (504)	bōn MĂ-rō BĪ-ŏp-sē	_____
chronic lymphocytic leukemia (501)	KRŎ-nĭk lĭm-fō-SĬ-tĭk loo-KĒ-mē-ă	_____
chronic myelogenous leukemia (501)	KRŎ-nĭk mī-ĕ-LŎJ-ĕ-nŭs loo-KĒ-mē-ă	_____
coagulation time (502)	kō-ăg-ū-LĀ-shŭn tīm	_____

Term	Pronunciation	Meaning
complete blood count (502)	kŏm-PLĒT blŭd kount	_____
dyscrasia (498)	dĭs-KRĀ-zē-ă	_____
ecchymoses (500)	ĕk-kĭ-MŌ-sēs	_____
erythrocyte sedimentation rate (503)	ĕ-RĬTH-rō-sīt sĕd-ĭ-mĕn-TĀ-shŭn rāt	_____
granulocytosis (502)	grăn-ū-lō-sī-TŌ-sis	_____
hematocrit (503)	hē-MĂT-ō-krĭt	_____
hematopoietic stem cell transplant (504)	hē-mă-tō-poy-Ē-tĭk stĕm sĕl TRĂNS-plănt	_____
hemochromatosis (500)	hē-mō-krō-mă-TŌ-sĭs	_____
hemoglobin test (503)	HĒ-mō-glō-bĭn tĕst	_____
hemolytic anemia (498)	hē-mō-LĬ-tĭk ă-NĒ-mē-ă	_____
hemophilia (500)	hē-mō-FĬL-ē-ă	_____
intrinsic factor (499)	ĭn-TRĬN-sĭk FĂK-tŏr	_____
mononucleosis (502)	mŏ-nō-nū-klē-Ō-sĭs	_____
multiple myeloma (502)	MŬL-tĭ-p'l mī-ĕ-LŌ-mă	_____
palliative (502)	PĂL-ē-ă-tĭv	_____
partial thromboplastin time (503)	PĂR-shŭl thrŏm-bō-PLĂS-tĭn tīm	_____
pernicious anemia (499)	pĕr-NĬSH-ŭs ă-NĒ-mē-ă	_____
petechiae (500)	pĕ-TĒ-kē-ā	_____
platelet count (503)	PLĀT-lĕt kount	_____
polycythemia vera (500)	pŏl-ē-sī-THĒ-mē-ă VĔR-ă	_____
prothrombin time (503)	prō-THRŎM-bĭn tīm	_____
purpura (500)	PŬR-pū-ră	_____
red blood cell count (503)	rĕd blŭd sĕl kount	_____
red blood cell morphology (503)	rĕd blŭd sĕl mŏr-FŎL-ō-jē	_____
relapse (501)	RĒ-lăps	_____
remission (501)	rē-MĬSH-ŭn	_____
sickle cell anemia (499)	SĬK'l sĕl ă-NĒ-mē-ă	_____
thalassemia (499)	thāl-ă-SĒ-mē-ă	_____
white blood cell count (503)	wīt blŭd sĕl kount	_____
white blood cell differential (503)	wīt blŭd sĕl dĭ-fĕr-ĔN-shŭl	_____

REVIEW SHEET

13

Write the meanings of the word parts in the spaces provided. Check your answers with the information in the chapter or in the glossary (Medical Word Parts—English) at the end of the book.

COMBINING FORMS

Combining Form	Meaning	Combining Form	Meaning
bas/o	_____	leuk/o	_____
chrom/o	_____	mon/o	_____
coagul/o	_____	morph/o	_____
cyt/o	_____	myel/o	_____
eosin/o	_____	neutr/o	_____
erythr/o	_____	nucle/o	_____
granul/o	_____	phag/o	_____
hem/o	_____	poikil/o	_____
hemat/o	_____	sider/o	_____
hemoglobin/o	_____	spher/o	_____
is/o	_____	thromb/o	_____
kary/o	_____		

SUFFIXES

Suffix	Meaning	Suffix	Meaning
-apheresis	_____	-osis	_____
-blast	_____	-penia	_____
-cytosis	_____	-phage	_____
-emia	_____	-philia	_____
-globin	_____	-phoresis	_____
-globulin	_____	-plasia	_____
-lytic	_____	-poiesis	_____
-oid	_____	-stasis	_____

PREFIXES

Prefix	Meaning	Prefix	Meaning
a-, an-	_____	micro-	_____
anti-	_____	mono-	_____
hypo-	_____	pan-	_____
macro-	_____	poly-	_____
mega-	_____		

 Please refer to the enclosed CD for additional exercises and images related to this chapter.

chapter 14

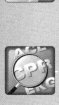

Lymphatic and Immune Systems

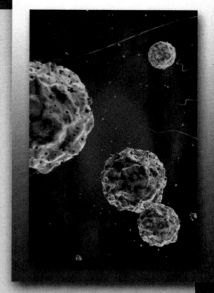

In this chapter you will

- Identify the structures and analyze terms related to the lymphatic and immune systems.
- Recognize terms that describe various pathologic conditions affecting the lymphatic and immune systems.
- Identify laboratory tests, clinical procedures, and abbreviations that are pertinent to the lymphatic and immune systems.
- Apply your new knowledge to understanding medical terms in their proper contexts, such as medical reports and records.

Image Description: Conceptual image of large
lymphocytes.

INTRODUCTION

Lymph is a clear, watery fluid (the term *lymph* comes from the Latin for "clear spring water") that surrounds body cells and flows in a system of lymph vessels that extends throughout the body.

Lymph differs from blood, but it has a close relationship to the blood system. Lymph fluid does not contain erythrocytes or platelets, but it is rich in two types of white blood cells (leukocytes): **lymphocytes** and **monocytes.** The liquid part of lymph is similar to blood plasma in that it contains water, salts, sugar, and wastes of metabolism such as urea and creatinine, but it differs in that it contains less protein. Lymph actually originates from the blood. It is the fluid that filters out of tiny blood capillaries into the spaces between cells. This fluid that surrounds body cells is called **interstitial fluid.** Interstitial fluid passes continuously into specialized thin-walled vessels called **lymph capillaries,** which are found coursing through tissue spaces (Fig. 14–1). The fluid in the lymph capillaries, now called **lymph** instead of interstitial fluid, passes through larger lymphatic vessels and through clusters of lymph tissues **(lymph nodes),** finally reaching large lymph vessels in the upper chest. Lymph enters these large lymphatic vessels, which then empty into the bloodstream. Figure 14–2 illustrates the relationship between the blood and the lymphatic systems.

The lymphatic system has several functions. First, it is a drainage system to transport needed proteins and fluid that have leaked out of the blood capillaries (and into the interstitial fluid) back to the bloodstream via the veins. Second, the lymphatic vessels in the intestines absorb lipids (fats) from the small intestine and transport them to the bloodstream.

A third function of the lymphatic system relates to the **immune system:** the defense of the body against foreign organisms such as bacteria and viruses. Lymphocytes and monocytes, originating in bone marrow, lymph nodes, and organs such as the spleen and thymus gland, protect the body by producing antibodies and by mounting a cellular attack on foreign cells and organisms.

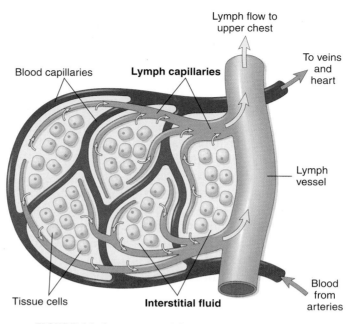

FIGURE 14–1 Interstitial fluid and lymph capillaries.

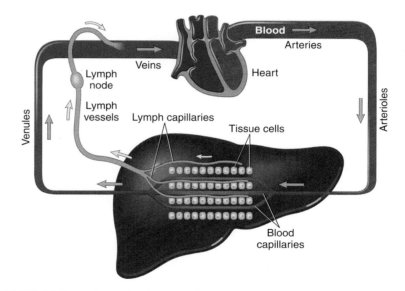

FIGURE 14–2 Relationship between the circulatory systems of blood and lymph.

14

LYMPHATIC SYSTEM

ANATOMY

Label Figure 14–3, *A*, as you read the following paragraphs.

Lymph capillaries [1] begin at the spaces around cells throughout the body. Like blood capillaries, they are thin-walled tubes. Lymph capillaries carry lymph from the tissue spaces to larger **lymph vessels** [2]. Lymph vessels have thicker walls than those of lymph capillaries and, like veins, contain valves so that lymph flows in only one direction, toward the thoracic cavity. Collections of stationary lymph tissue, called **lymph nodes** [3], are located along the path of the lymph vessels. Each lymph node is a mass of lymph cells and vessels, surrounded by a fibrous, connective tissue capsule (Fig. 14–4).

Lymph nodes not only produce lymphocytes but also filter lymph and trap substances from inflammatory and cancerous lesions. Special cells, called **macrophages,** located in lymph nodes (as well as in the spleen, liver, and lungs), phagocytose foreign substances. When bacteria are present in lymph nodes that drain a particular area of the body, the nodes become swollen with collections of cells and their engulfed debris and become tender. Lymph nodes also fight disease when specialized lymphocytes called **B lymphocytes (B cells),** present in the nodes, produce antibodies. Other lymphocytes, the **T lymphocytes (T cells),** attack bacteria and foreign cells by accurately recognizing a cell surface protein as foreign, attaching to the foreign or cancerous cells, poking holes in them, and injecting them with toxic chemicals.

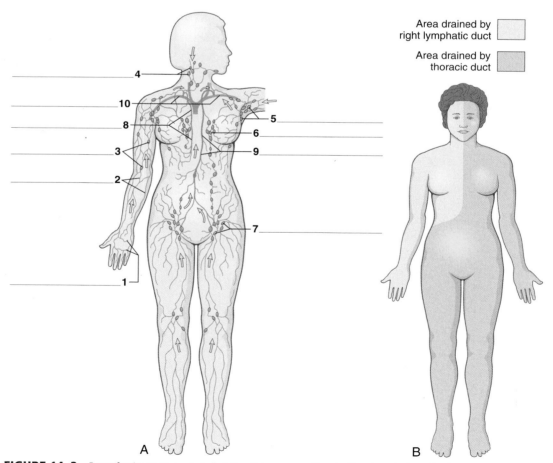

FIGURE 14–3 **Lymphatic system. A,** Label the figure according to the descriptions in the text. **B,** Note the different regions of the body drained by the right lymphatic duct and the thoracic duct.

Label the major sites of lymph node concentration on Figure 14–3, *A*. These are the **cervical** [4], **axillary** (armpit) [5], **mediastinal** [6], and **inguinal** (groin) [7] regions of the body. Remember that **tonsils** are masses of lymph tissue in the throat near the back of the mouth (oropharynx), and **adenoids** are enlarged lymph tissue in the part of the throat near the nasal passages (nasopharynx).

Lymph vessels all lead toward the thoracic cavity and empty into two large ducts in the upper chest. These are the **right lymphatic duct** [8] and the **thoracic duct** [9]. The thoracic duct drains the lower body and the left side of the head, whereas the right lymphatic duct drains the right side of the head and the chest (a much smaller area) (Fig. 14–3, *B*). Both ducts carry the lymph into **large veins** [10] in the neck, where the lymph then enters the bloodstream.

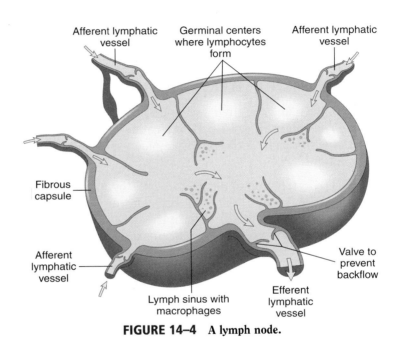

FIGURE 14–4 **A lymph node.**

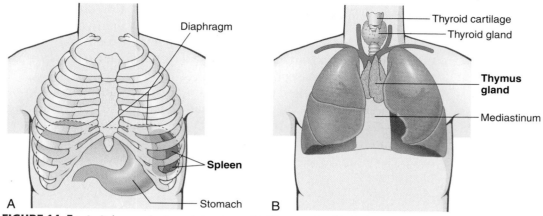

FIGURE 14–5 **A, Spleen** and adjacent structures. **B, Thymus gland** in its location in the mediastinum between the lungs.

SPLEEN AND THYMUS GLAND

The spleen and the thymus gland are organs composed of lymph tissue.

The **spleen** (Fig. 14–5, *A*) is located in the left upper quadrant of the abdomen, adjacent to the stomach. Although the spleen is not essential to life, it has several important functions:

1. Destruction of old erythrocytes by macrophages. In the slow-moving circulation of the spleen, red cell breakdown (hemolysis) liberates hemoglobin, which is converted to bilirubin in the liver and then is added to the bloodstream.
2. Filtration of microorganisms and other foreign material from the blood.
3. Activation of lymphocytes by antigens filtered from the blood. Activated B cell lymphocytes produce antibodies.
4. Storage of blood, especially erythrocytes and platelets. A large number of platelets collect in the splenic blood pool.

The spleen is susceptible to injury. A sharp blow to the upper abdomen (as from the impact of a car's steering wheel) may cause rupture of the spleen. Massive hemorrhage can occur when the spleen is ruptured, and immediate surgical removal (splenectomy) may be necessary. After splenectomy, the liver, bone marrow, and lymph nodes take over the functions of the spleen.

The **thymus gland** (Fig. 14–5, *B*) is a lymphatic organ located in the upper mediastinum between the lungs. During fetal life and childhood it is quite large, but it becomes smaller with age. The thymus gland is composed of nests of lymphoid cells resting on a platform of connective tissue. It plays an important role in the body's ability to protect itself from disease (immunity), especially in fetal life and during the early years of growth. It is known that a thymectomy (removal of the thymus gland) performed in an animal during the first weeks of life impairs the ability of the animal to make antibodies and to produce immune cells that fight against foreign antigens such as bacteria and viruses.

Early in development, in the thymus, lymphocytes learn to recognize and accept the body's own antigens as "self" or friendly. This acceptance of "self" antigens is called **tolerance.** When the tolerance process fails, immune cells react against normal cells of the body, and diseases (autoimmune) result. See page 535, under **autoimmune disease.**

IMMUNE SYSTEM

The immune system is specialized to defend the body against **antigens** or foreign organisms. This system includes the **lymphoid organs** (lymph nodes, spleen, and thymus gland) and their products (**lymphocytes** and **antibodies**) and also **macrophages** (phagocytes that are found in the blood, brain, liver, lymph nodes, and spleen).

Immunity is the body's ability to resist foreign organisms and toxins (poisons) that damage tissues and organs. **Natural immunity** is a **genetic predisposition** present in the body at birth. It is not dependent on a specific immune response or a previous contact with an infectious agent. When bacteria enter the body, natural immunity protects the body as **phagocytes** such as neutrophils (white blood cells) migrate to the site of infection and ingest the bacteria. They release proteins that attract other immune system cells and cause localized inflammation. **Macrophages** move in to clear away the dead cells and debris as the infection subsides. Other cells known as **natural killer (NK) cells** are primitive lymphocytes that destroy tumor cells and virally infected cells.

Besides possessing natural immunity, a person may **acquire immunity.** In this way, the body develops powerful, specific immunity (typically by means of antibodies and cells) against invading antigens. **Acquired active immunity** occurs in several ways. First, **having an infection** causes the production of antibodies that fight against foreign organisms and then remain in the body to protect against further infection by the same organism. Next, receiving a **vaccination** containing a modified toxin, pathogen (bacterial or viral protein), or nontoxic version of a virus stimulates lymphocytes to produce antibodies without previous exposure from an attack of the disease. An example is vaccination against smallpox, using the cowpox virus, which produces immunity but no infection. Finally, immunity also can be acquired through the **transfer of immune cells** (lymphocytes or hematopoietic stem cells) from a donor, as in a stem cell transplant, which stimulates the growth of immune cells in the bone marrow of the recipient.

When immediate protection is needed, **acquired passive immunity** can be induced. For this purpose, the patient receives immune serum (antiserum) containing antibodies produced in another animal or person. Examples are **antitoxins** given in cases of poisonous snake bites and rabies infections. Injections of **immunoglobulins** (antibodies) also provide protection against disease or lessen its severity. Newborns receive passive acquired immunity as **maternal antibodies** pass through the placenta or in breast milk after birth. Figure 14–6 reviews the various types of immunity.

The immune response involves two major disease fighters: **B lymphocytes,** or B cells, and **T lymphocytes,** or T cells. B cells are involved in **humoral immunity.** They produce antibodies in response to specific antigens. B cells originate from bone marrow stem cells. When a B cell is confronted with a specific type of antigen, it transforms into an antibody-producing cell called a **plasma cell.** Plasma cells produce antibodies called **immunoglobulins,** such as **IgA, IgD, IgE, IgG,** and **IgM.** Immunoglobulins travel to the

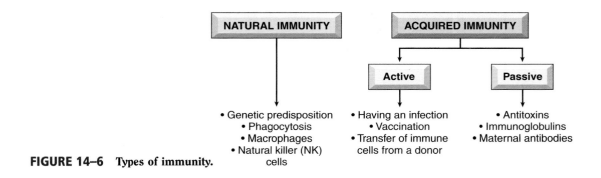

FIGURE 14–6   Types of immunity.

site of an infection to react with and neutralize antigens. IgG, the most abundant immunoglobulin, crosses the placenta to provide immunity for newborns. IgE is important in causing allergic reactions and fighting parasitic infections.

T lymphocytes are involved in **cell-mediated immunity.** They also originate from stem cells in the bone marrow but are further processed in the thymus gland, where they are acted on by thymic hormones. When a T cell encounters an antigen, the T cell multiplies rapidly to produce cells that destroy the antigen (bacteria, viruses, and cancer cells). T cells also react to transplanted tissues and skin grafts.

There are several types of T cells. One type is a **cytotoxic T cell.** Specialized cytotoxic cells are **killer T cells.** They act directly on antigens to destroy them. Cytotoxic cells also produce proteins called **cytokines (interferons and interleukins)** that aid other cells in antigen destruction. Another T cell is known as a **helper T cell.** It stimulates and promotes synthesis of antibodies by B cells and cytokines by cytotoxic T cells to enhance the immune response. **Suppressor T cells** control B and T cell activity and inhibit, or stop, the immune response when the antigen has been destroyed. Disease may occur when the normal ratio of helper to suppressor cells (2:1) is altered. For example, in AIDS (acquired immunodeficiency syndrome) the number of helper T cells is diminished. Figure 14-7 summarizes the functions of B and T lymphocytes.

Another important cell of the immune system is the **dendritic cell.** This cell, a macrophage derived from monocytes, specializes in recognizing and digesting foreign antigens. The dendritic cell then pushes the antigen to its surface (this is called antigen presentation) where T cells recognize them. This leads to proliferation of antigen-fighting T cells in **clones** (groups of identical cells from the same parent cell).

Immunotherapy is the use of immunologic techniques to treat disease. Examples are:

- Inoculation with **vaccines** to prevent infectious disease.
- **Monoclonal antibody (MoAb)** therapy for certain cancers. These antibodies are produced in a laboratory by special **cloning techniques** (making multiple copies of cells or genes). An example is the MoAb preparation rituximab (Rituxan) made to kill lymphoma cells. The antibody can be linked to various toxins or radioactive particles and delivered to tumor cells to add to the killing effect.

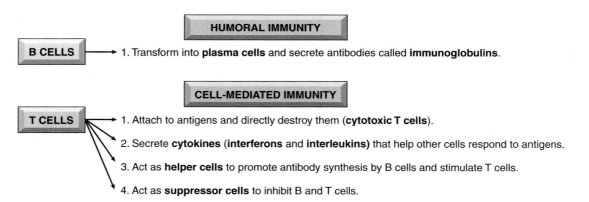

HUMORAL IMMUNITY

B CELLS ——→ 1. Transform into **plasma cells** and secrete antibodies called **immunoglobulins**.

CELL-MEDIATED IMMUNITY

T CELLS
1. Attach to antigens and directly destroy them (**cytotoxic T cells**).
2. Secrete **cytokines** (**interferons** and **interleukins**) that help other cells respond to antigens.
3. Act as **helper cells** to promote antibody synthesis by B cells and stimulate T cells.
4. Act as **suppressor cells** to inhibit B and T cells.

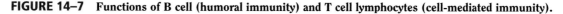

FIGURE 14–7   Functions of B cell (humoral immunity) and T cell lymphocytes (cell-mediated immunity).

VOCABULARY

This list reviews many of the new terms introduced in the text. Short definitions reinforce your understanding of the terms. Refer to the Pronunciation of Terms section for help with unfamiliar or difficult words.

acquired immunity	Formation of antibodies and lymphocytes after exposure to an antigen.
adenoids	Masses of lymphatic tissue in the nasopharynx.
antibody	Protein produced by B cell lymphocytes to destroy antigens.
antigen	Substance that the body recognizes as foreign; evokes an immune response.
axillary node	Any of the 20 to 30 lymph nodes in the armpit (underarm).
B cell	Lymphocyte that originates in the bone marrow and transforms into a plasma cell to secrete antibodies. The B refers to the bursa of Fabricius, an organ in birds in which B cell differentiation and growth were first noted to occur.
cell-mediated immunity	An immune response involving T lymphocytes; antigens are destroyed by direct action of cells, as opposed to by antibodies.
cervical node	One of many lymph nodes in the neck region.
cytokine	Protein (made by T lymphocytes) that aids antigen destruction. Examples are interferons, interleukins, and colony-stimulating factors such as granulocyte colony–stimulating factor (G-CSF) and granulocyte-macrophage colony-stimulating factor (GM-CSF).
cytotoxic T cell	T lymphocyte that directly kills foreign cells.
dendritic cell	Cell (specialized macrophage) that ingests antigens and presents them to T cells.
helper T cell	Lymphocyte that aids B cells in recognizing antigens and stimulating antibody production; also called **T4 cell** or **CD4⁺ cell.**
humoral immunity	Immune response in which B cells transform into plasma cells and secrete antibodies.
immune response	Body's capacity to resist foreign organisms and toxins that can damage tissue and organs; humoral and cell-mediated immunity.
immunoglobulins	Antibodies (gamma globulins) such as IgA, IgE, IgG, IgM, and IgD that are secreted by plasma cells in humoral immunity.
immunotherapy	Use of immunologic knowledge and techniques to treat or prevent disease. Examples are inoculation with vaccines and monoclonal antibody therapy.
inguinal node	One of several lymph nodes in the groin region (where the legs join the trunk of the body).
interferons	Antiviral proteins (cytokines) secreted by T cells; they also stimulate macrophages to ingest bacteria.
interleukins	Proteins (cytokines) that stimulate the growth of B or T lymphocytes and activate specific components of the immune response.

14

interstitial fluid	Fluid in the spaces between cells. This fluid becomes lymph when it enters lymph capillaries.
killer T cell	Cytotoxic T cell lymphocyte that recognizes and destroys foreign cells (viruses and tumor cells).
lymph	Thin, watery fluid found within lymphatic vessels and collected from tissues throughout the body. Latin *lympha* means water.
lymph capillaries	Tiniest lymphatic vessels.
lymphoid organs	Lymph nodes, spleen, and thymus gland.
lymph node	Stationary solid lymphatic tissue along lymph vessels.
lymph vessel	Carrier of lymph throughout the body; lymphatic vessels empty lymph into veins in the upper part of the chest.
macrophage	Large phagocyte found in lymph nodes and other tissues of the body.
mediastinal node	Any of many lymph nodes in the area between the lungs in the thoracic (chest) cavity.
monoclonal antibody	Antibody produced in a laboratory to attack antigens. It is useful in immunotherapy and cancer treatment.
natural immunity	An individual's own genetic ability to fight off disease.
plasma cell	Lymphoid cell that secretes an antibody and originates from B lymphocytes.
right lymphatic duct	Large lymphatic vessel in the chest that receives lymph from the upper right part of the body.
spleen	Organ near the stomach that produces, stores, and eliminates blood cells.
suppressor T cell	Lymphocyte that inhibits the activity of B and T lymphocytes.
T cell	Lymphocyte that originates in the bone marrow but matures in the thymus gland; it acts directly on antigens to destroy them or produce chemicals (cytokines) such as interferons and interleukins that are toxic to antigens.
tolerance	In the thymus, T lymphocytes learn to recognize and accept the body's own antigens as "self" or friendly.
thoracic duct	Large lymphatic vessel in the chest that receives lymph from below the diaphragm and from the left side of the body above the diaphragm; it empties the lymph into veins in the upper chest.
thymus gland	Organ in the mediastinum that produces T lymphocytes and aids in the immune response.
tonsils	Masses of lymphatic tissue in the back of the oropharynx.
toxin	Poison; a protein produced by certain bacteria, animals, or plants.
vaccination	Introduction of altered antigens (viruses or bacteria) to produce an immune response and protection against disease. The term comes from the Latin *vacca*, cow, and was used when the first inoculations were given with organisms that caused the disease cowpox to produce immunity to smallpox.
vaccine	Weakened or killed microorganisms or toxins administered to induce immunity to infection or disease.

COMBINING FORMS, PREFIXES, AND TERMINOLOGY

Write the meanings of the medical terms in the spaces provided.

COMBINING FORMS

Combining Form	Meaning	Terminology	Meaning
immun/o	protection	autoimmune disease _____	
		Examples are rheumatoid arthritis and lupus erythematosus. These are chronic, disabling diseases caused by the abnormal production of antibodies against normal body tissues. Signs and symptoms are inflammation of joints, skin rash, and fever. Glucocorticoid drugs (prednisone) and other immunosuppressants (azathioprine, methotrexate) are effective as treatment but make patients susceptible to infection.	
		immunoglobulin _____	
		immunosuppression _____	
		This may occur because of exposure to drugs (corticosteroids) or as the result of disease (AIDS and cancer). Immunosuppressed patients are susceptible to infection with fungi, Pneumocystis bacteria, and other pathogens.	
lymph/o	lymph	lymphopoiesis _____	
		lymphedema _____	
		Interstitial fluid collects within the spaces between cells as a result of obstruction of lymphatic vessels and nodes. Radiation therapy may destroy lymphatics and produce lymphedema, as in breast cancer treatment. See Figure 14–8.	
		lymphocytopenia _____	
		lymphocytosis _____	
		lymphoid _____	
		The suffix -oid means resembling or derived from. Lymphoid organs include lymph nodes, spleen, and thymus gland.	

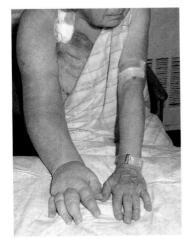

FIGURE 14–8 **Lymphedema** of right arm secondary to mastectomy, lymphadenectomy, and radiotherapy. (From Swartz MH: Textbook of Physical Diagnosis, History and Examination, 4th ed. Philadelphia, WB Saunders, 2002.)

14

Combining Form	Meaning	Terminology	Meaning
lymphaden/o	lymph node (gland)	lymphadenopathy _____	
		lymphadenitis _____	
splen/o	spleen	splenomegaly _____	
		Note that the combining form for spleen contains only one "e."	
		splenectomy _____	
		hypersplenism _____	
		A syndrome marked by splenomegaly and often associated with blood cell destruction, anemia, leukopenia, and thrombocytopenia.	
thym/o	thymus gland	thymoma _____	
		thymectomy _____	
tox/o	poison	toxic _____	

PREFIXES

Prefix	Meaning	Terminology	Meaning
ana-	again, anew	anaphylaxis _____	
		The suffix -phylaxis means protection. This is an exaggerated or unusual hypersensitivity to previously encountered foreign proteins or other antigens. Vasodilation and a decrease in blood pressure can be life threatening.	
inter-	between	interstitial fluid _____	
		The suffix -stitial means pertaining to standing or positioned.	

DISORDERS OF THE LYMPHATIC AND IMMUNE SYSTEMS

IMMUNODEFICIENCY

acquired immunodeficiency syndrome (AIDS)

Syndrome associated with suppression of the immune system and marked by opportunistic infections, secondary neoplasms, and neurologic problems.

AIDS is caused by the **human immunodeficiency virus (HIV).** HIV destroys helper T cells (also known as **CD4⁺ cells,** containing the CD4 protein antigen). This disrupts the cell-mediated immune response, allowing infections to occur. Infectious diseases associated with AIDS are **opportunistic infections** because HIV lowers resistance and allows infection by bacteria and parasites that are easily otherwise contained by normal defenses. Table 14–1 lists many of these opportunistic infections.

Table 14–1

Opportunistic Infections with AIDS

Infection	Description
Candidiasis	Yeast-like fungus *(Candida)*, normally present in the mouth, skin, intestinal tract, and vagina, overgrows, causing infection of the mouth (thrush), respiratory tract, and skin.
Cryptococcal infection (Crypto)	Yeast-like fungus *(Cryptococcus)* causes lung, brain, and blood infections. Pathogen is found in pigeon droppings, nesting places, air, water, and soil.
Cryptosporidiosis	Parasitic infection of the gastrointestinal tract and brain and spinal cord. The pathogen, *Cryptosporidium*, is a one-celled organism commonly found in farm animals.
Cytomegalovirus (CMV) infection	Virus causes enteritis and retinitis (inflammation of the retina at the back of the eye). Found in saliva, semen, cervical secretions, urine, feces, blood, and breast milk, but usually causes disease only when the immune system is compromised.
Herpes simplex	Viral infection causes small blisters on the skin of the lips or nose or on the genitals. Herpes simplex virus also can cause encephalitis.
Histoplasmosis (Histo)	Fungal infection caused by inhalation of dust contaminated with *Histoplasma capsulatum*; causes fever, chills, and lung infection. Pathogen is found in bird and bat droppings.
***Mycobacterium avium-intracellulare* (MAI) infection**	Bacterial disease manifesting with fever, malaise, night sweats, anorexia, diarrhea, weight loss, and lung and blood infections.
***Pneumocystis* pneumonia (PCP)**	One-celled organism *(P. jirovecii)* causes lung infection, with fever, cough, and chest pain. Pathogen is found in air, water, and soil and is carried by animals. Infection is treated with trimethoprim–sulfamethoxazole (Bactrim), a combination of antibiotics, or with pentamidine. Aerosolized pentamidine, which is inhaled, can prevent occurrence of PCP.
Toxoplasmosis (Toxo)	Parasitic infection involving the central nervous system (CNS) and causing fever, chills, visual disturbances, confusion, hemiparesis (slight paralysis in half of the body), and seizures. Pathogen *(Toxoplasma)* is acquired by eating uncooked lamb or pork, unpasteurized dairy products, and raw eggs or vegetables.
Tuberculosis (TB)	Bacterial disease (caused by *Mycobacterium tuberculosis*) involving the lungs. Signs and symptoms are fever, loss of weight, anorexia, and low energy.

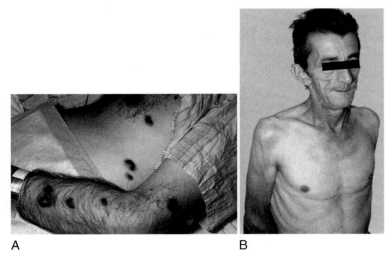

A   B

FIGURE 14–9 **A, Kaposi sarcoma. B, Wasting syndrome.** (A from Swartz MH: Textbook of Physical Diagnosis, History and Examination, 4th ed. Philadelphia, WB Saunders, 2002. **B** from Lemmi FO, Lemmi CAE: Physical Assessment Findings. CD-ROM. Philadelphia, WB Saunders, 2000.)

Malignancies associated with AIDS are **Kaposi sarcoma** (a cancer arising from the lining cells of capillaries that produces bluish-red skin nodules) and lymphoma (cancer of lymph nodes). **Wasting syndrome,** marked by weight loss and decrease in muscular strength, appetite, and mental activity also may occur with AIDS. See Figure 14–9, *A* and *B*.

Persons who were exposed to HIV and now have antibodies in their blood against this virus are **HIV-positive.** HIV is found in blood, semen, vaginal and cervical secretions, saliva, and other body fluids. Transmission of HIV may occur by three routes: sexual contact, blood inoculation (through sharing of contaminated needles, accidental needlesticks, or contact with contaminated blood or blood products), and passage of the virus from infected mothers to their newborns. Table 14–2 summarizes the common routes of transmission of HIV.

Table 14–2

Common Routes of Transmission

Route	People Affected
Receptive oral and anal intercourse	Men and women
Receptive vaginal intercourse	Women
Sharing of needles and equipment (users of intravenous drugs)	Men and women
Contaminated blood (for transfusion) or blood products (in hemophiliacs)	Men and women
From mother, in utero	Neonates

HIV-infected patients may remain asymptomatic for as long as 10 years. Signs and symptoms associated with HIV infection are lymphadenopathy, neurologic disease, oral thrush (fungal infection), night sweats, fatigue, and evidence of opportunistic infections.

Drugs that are used to treat AIDS are inhibitors of the viral enzyme called **reverse transcriptase (RT).** After invading the helper T cell (carrying the CD4$^+$ antigen), HIV releases RT to help it grow and multiply inside the cell. Examples of **RT inhibitors (RTIs)** are zidovudine and lamivudine (Epivir). A second class of anti-HIV drugs are inhibitors of the viral protease (proteolytic) enzyme. HIV needs protease to make viral proteins that are essential to its structure and reproduction. Use of combinations of **protease inhibitors** (nelfinavir, amprenavir) and RT inhibitors is called **HAART (highly active antiretroviral therapy).** This treatment approach destroys HIV in several ways and in many cases has abolished evidence of viral infection in affected people.

HYPERSENSITIVITY

Allergy

Abnormal hypersensitivity acquired by exposure to an antigen

Allergic (all/o = other) reactions occur when a sensitized person, who has previously been exposed to an agent **(allergen),** reacts violently to a subsequent exposure. This reaction varies from allergic rhinitis or hay fever (caused by pollen or animal dander) to systemic **anaphylaxis,** in which an extraordinary hypersensitivity reaction occurs throughout the body, leading to fall in blood pressure (hypotension), shock, respiratory distress, and edema of the larynx. Anaphylaxis can be life threatening, but the patient usually survives if the airways are kept open and treatment is given immediately (epinephrine and antihistamines).

Other allergies include asthma (pollens, dust, molds), hives (caused by food or drugs) and **atopic dermatitis** (rash from soaps, cosmetics, chemicals). **Atopic** means related to atopy, a hypersensitivity or allergic state arising from an inherited predisposition. A person who is atopic is prone to allergies. See Figure 14–10.

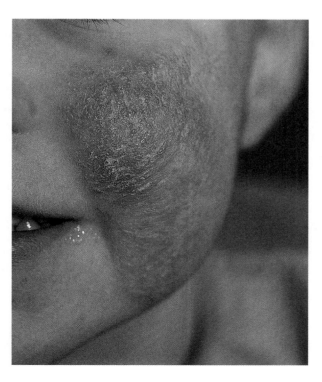

FIGURE 14–10 Atopic dermatitis. (From Zitelli BJ, Davis HW: Atlas of Pediatric Physical Diagnosis, 3rd ed., St. Louis, Mosby, 1997.)

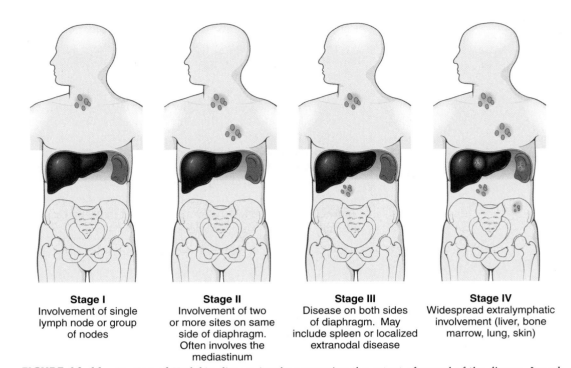

Stage I	Stage II	Stage III	Stage IV
Involvement of single lymph node or group of nodes	Involvement of two or more sites on same side of diaphragm. Often involves the mediastinum	Disease on both sides of diaphragm. May include spleen or localized extranodal disease	Widespread extralymphatic involvement (liver, bone marrow, lung, skin)

FIGURE 14–11 **Staging of Hodgkin disease** involves assessing the extent of spread of the disease. Lymph node biopsies, laparotomy with liver and lymph node biopsies, and splenectomy may be necessary for staging.

MALIGNANCIES

lymphoma

Malignant tumor of lymph nodes and lymph tissue.

There are many types of lymphoma, varying according to the particular cell type and degree of differentiation. Some examples are:

Hodgkin disease—Malignant tumor of lymphoid tissue in the spleen and lymph nodes. This disease is characterized by lymphadenopathy (lymph nodes enlarge), splenomegaly, fever, weakness, and loss of weight and appetite. The diagnosis often is made by identifying a malignant cell (Reed-Sternberg cell) in the lymph nodes. If disease is localized, the treatment may be radiotherapy or chemotherapy. If the disease is more widespread, chemotherapy is given alone. There is a very high probability of cure with available treatments. Figure 14–11 illustrates staging of Hodgkin disease.

Non-Hodgkin lymphoma—Types of this disease include **follicular lymphoma** (composed of collections of small lymphocytes in a follicle or nodule arrangement) and **large cell lymphoma** (composed of large lymphocytes that infiltrate nodes and tissues diffusely). Chemotherapy may cure or stop the progress of this disease.

multiple myeloma

Malignant tumor of bone marrow cells.

This is a tumor composed of plasma cells (antibody-producing B lymphocytes) associated with high levels of one of the specific immunoglobulins, usually IgG. **Waldenström macroglobulinemia** is another tumor of malignant B cells. This disease involves B cells that produce large quantities of IgM (a globulin of high molecular weight). Increased IgM concentration impairs the passage of blood through capillaries in the brain and eyes, causing a hyperviscosity syndrome (thickening of the blood).

thymoma	**Malignant tumor of the thymus gland.**
	Some signs and symptoms of thymoma are cough, dyspnea, dysphagia, fever, chest pain, weight loss, and anorexia. Often, the tumor is associated with disorders of the immune system that cause muscular weakness (myasthenia gravis) or anemia.
	Surgery is the principal method of treating thymoma; postoperative radiation therapy is used for patients with evidence of spread of the tumor.

STUDY SECTION

Practice spelling each term and know its meaning.

allergen	Substance capable of causing a specific hypersensitivity in the body; a type of antigen.
anaphylaxis	Exaggerated or unusual hypersensitivity to foreign protein or other substance.
atopy	Hypersensitive or allergic state involving an inherited predisposition. From the Greek word *atopia*, which means strangeness.
CD4$^+$ cells	Helper T cells that carry the CD4 protein antigen on their surface. HIV binds to CD4 and infects and kills T cells bearing this protein.
Hodgkin disease	Malignant tumor of lymph tissue in spleen and lymph nodes; Reed-Sternberg cell often is found on microscopic analysis.
human immunodeficiency virus (HIV)	Virus (retrovirus) that causes AIDS.
Kaposi sarcoma	Malignant (cancerous) condition associated with AIDS; arises from the lining of capillaries and appears as bluish-red skin nodules.
non-Hodgkin lymphoma	Group of malignant tumors involving lymphoid tissue. Examples are follicular lymphoma and large cell lymphoma.
opportunistic infections	Infectious diseases associated with AIDS; they occur because HIV infection lowers the body's resistance and allows infection by bacteria and parasites that normally are easily contained.
protease inhibitor	Drug that treats AIDS by blocking the production of protease, a proteolytic enzyme that helps to create new viral pieces for HIV.
retrovirus	RNA virus that makes copies of itself by using the host cell's DNA; this is in reverse (retro-) fashion because the regular method is for DNA to copy itself onto RNA. A retrovirus (like HIV) carries an enzyme, called **reverse transcriptase,** that enables it to reproduce within the host cell.
reverse transcriptase inhibitor	Drug that treats AIDS by blocking reverse transcriptase, an enzyme needed to make copies of HIV.

LABORATORY TESTS AND CLINICAL PROCEDURES

LABORATORY TESTS

CD4+ cell count	**Measures the number of CD4+ T cells (helper T cells) in the bloodstream of patients with AIDS.** A normal count usually is between 500 and 1500 CD4+ cells/mm³. If a CD4+ count falls below 250 to 200, it is recommended to start treatment with anti-HIV drugs.
ELISA	**Screening test to detect anti-HIV antibodies in the bloodstream.** Antibodies to HIV begin to appear within 2 weeks of infection with HIV. If the result of this test is positive, it is confirmed with a **Western blot** test, which is more specific. ELISA is an abbreviation for enzyme-linked immunosorbent assay.
immunoelectrophoresis	**Test that separates immunoglobulins (IgG, IgM, IgE, IgA, IgD).** This procedure detects the presence of abnormal levels of antibodies in patients with conditions such as multiple myeloma and Waldenström macroglobulinemia.
viral load tests	**Tests that measure the amount of AIDS virus (HIV) in the bloodstream.** Two viral load tests are a PCR (polymerase chain reaction) assay and a NASBA (nucleic acid sequence–based amplification) test.

CLINICAL PROCEDURES

computed tomography (CT) scan	**X-ray imaging in the transverse plane produces cross-sectional views of anatomic structures.** These x-ray views show abnormalities of lymphoid organs, such as lymph nodes, spleen, and thymus gland.

ABBREVIATIONS

AIDS	acquired immunodeficiency syndrome
CD4+	protein antigen on helper T cells
CMV	cytomegalovirus—causes opportunistic AIDS-related infection
Crypto	*Cryptococcus*—causes opportunistic AIDS-related infection
ELISA	enzyme-linked immunosorbent assay—test to detect anti-HIV antibodies
G-CSF	granulocyte colony-stimulating factor—a cytokine that promotes neutrophil production
GM-CSF	granulocyte-macrophage colony-stimulating factor—cytokine secreted by macrophages that promotes the growth of myeloid progenitor cells and differentiation to granulocytes
HAART	highly active antiretroviral therapy—use of combinations of drugs that are effective against AIDS
HD	Hodgkin disease
Histo	histoplasmosis—fungal infection seen in AIDS patients
HIV	human immunodeficiency virus—causes AIDS
HSV	herpes simplex virus
IgA, IgD, IgE, IgG, IgM	immunoglobulins
IL1-15	interleukins
KS	Kaposi sarcoma
MAC	*Mycobacterium avium* complex—group of pathogens that cause lung and systemic disease in immunocompromised patients

MAI	*Mycobacterium avium-intracellulare*— the bacterial species, *M. avium* and *M. intracellulare*, that have been identified in MAC
MoAb	monoclonal antibody
NHL	non-Hodgkin lymphoma
NK cell	natural killer cell—lymphocyte that recognizes and destroys foreign cells by releasing cytotoxins

PCP	*Pneumocystis* pneumonia— opportunistic AIDS-related infection
PI	protease inhibitor
RTIs	reverse transcriptase inhibitors—for example, zidovudine (Retrovir) and lamivudine (Epivir)
Toxo	toxoplasmosis—parasitic infection associated with AIDS

PRACTICAL APPLICATIONS

Answers to the questions are on page 551.

MEDICAL TERMINOLOGY IN SENTENCES

1. In addition to the opportunistic infections and malignancies that typically characterize AIDS, pathology of the central nervous system (CNS) occurs with some regularity. Specifically, CNS tumors, encephalitis, meningitis, progressive leukoencephalopathy, and myelitis have been reported in patients with HIV infection. Dementia and delirium [clouding of consciousness] also have been reported as psychiatric complications.

2. Protease inhibitors interrupt HIV replication, blocking an enzyme called protease. When protease is blocked, HIV cannot infect new cells. Protease inhibitors can reduce HIV viral load in the blood and increase CD4+ T cell counts. Examples of protease inhibitors are indinavir (Crixivan) and nelfinavir (Viracept).

3. Lymph nodes that are nontender and rock-hard are suggestive of a diagnosis of metastatic carcinoma.

4. Infectious mononucleosis and Hodgkin disease are more common in young adults, whereas non-Hodgkin lymphoma and chronic lymphocytic leukemia are more common in middle-aged and elderly people.

5. Oral candidiasis (thrush) presenting without a history of recent antibiotic therapy, chemotherapy, or immunosuppression often indicates the possibility of HIV infection.

Questions

1. What parts of the body commonly are affected by the AIDS virus?
   a. Kidney and urinary bladder
   b. Brain and spinal cord
   c. Pancreas and thyroid glands

2. Which CNS condition often is seen in AIDS patients?
   a. Inflammation of the brain and membranes around the brain
   b. Fluid collection in the brain
   c. Disk impinging on the spinal cord

3. Aside from delirium, what other psychiatric complication has been reported in AIDS patients?
   a. Loss of intellectual abilities
   b. Feelings of persecution
   c. Fears such as claustrophobia and agoraphobia

14

4. Protease is a/an
   a. Antiviral enzyme
   b. Enzyme that helps HIV infect new cells
   c. Reverse transcriptase inhibitor

5. CD4$^+$ T cell counts can be increased by:
   a. High levels of HIV in the blood
   b. Protease inhibitors
   c. Lymphocyte-inhibiting agents

6. Metastatic carcinoma means:
   a. The tumor has spread to a secondary location.
   b. Lymph nodes are not usually affected.
   c. The tumor is localized.

7. Hodgkin disease:
   a. Commonly affects elderly people
   b. Is a type of lymphoma affecting young adults
   c. Is an infectious disease

8. What condition may indicate an AIDS virus infection?
   a. High blood sugar
   b. Oral leukoplakia
   c. Fungal infection of the mouth

![EXERCISES icon] **EXERCISES**

Remember to check your answers carefully with those given in the Answers to Exercises, page 550.

A. Name the structure or fluid based on its meaning below.

1. stationary lymphatic tissue along the path of lymph vessels all over the body

    _____

2. large lymph vessel in the chest that drains lymph from the lower part and left side of the body above

    the diaphragm _____

3. organ near the stomach that produces, stores, and eliminates blood cells _____

4. mass of lymphatic tissue in the nasopharynx _____

5. organ in the mediastinum that produces T lymphocytes and helps in the immune response

    _____

6. tiniest lymph vessels _____

7. large lymph vessel in the chest that drains lymph from the upper right part of the body

    _____

8. fluid present between cells that becomes lymph as it enters lymph capillaries _____

B. Give the locations of the following lymph nodes.

1. inguinal nodes _____

2. axillary nodes _____

3. cervical nodes _____

4. mediastinal nodes _____

C. Circle the correct answer in each sentence.

1. An immune response in which B cells transform into plasma cells and secrete antibodies is **(cell-mediated immunity, humoral immunity)**.

2. Lymphocytes, formed in the thymus gland, that act on antigens are **(B cells, T cells, macrophages)**.

3. An immune response in which T cells destroy antigens is **(cell-mediated immunity, humoral immunity)**.

4. Lymphocytes that transform into plasma cells and secrete antibodies are **(B cells, T cells, macrophages)**.

14

D. Match the following cell names with their meanings as given below.

dendritic cell   macrophage   suppressor T cell
helper T cell   plasma cell

1. cell that originates from a B lymphocyte and secretes antibodies _____

2. large phagocyte found in lymph nodes and other tissues of the body _____

3. T cell that aids B cells in recognizing antigens _____

4. T cell that inhibits the activity of B lymphocytes _____

5. cell that specializes in antigen presentation and destruction of antigens by T cells

_____

E. Match the terms in Column I with their descriptions in Column II. Write your answers in the spaces provided.

Column I

1. immunoglobulins   _____

2. toxins   _____

3. helper T cells   _____

4. suppressor T cells   _____

5. cytotoxic T cells   _____

6. plasma cells   _____

7. interferons   _____

Column II

A. Antibodies—IgA, IgE, IgG, IgM, IgD
B. Lymphocyte that aids B cells; also called T4 or CD4$^+$ cell
C. Poisons (antigens)
D. T cell lymphocytes that inhibit the activity of B cell lymphocytes
E. Antiviral proteins secreted by T cells
F. Transformed B cells that secrete antibodies
G. T lymphocytes that directly kill foreign cells

F. Use the given definitions to build medical terms.

1. removal of the spleen _____

2. enlargement of the spleen _____

3. formation of lymph _____

4. tumor of the thymus gland _____

5. inflammation of lymph glands (nodes) _____

6. deficiency of lymph cells _____

7. pertaining to poison _____

8. disease of lymph glands (nodes) _____

G. Match the following terms with their meanings below.

AIDS   Hodgkin disease   lymphoid organs
allergen   hypersplenism   thymectomy
anaphylaxis   lymphedema

1. syndrome marked by enlargement of the spleen and associated with anemia, leukopenia, and

    thrombocytopenia _____

2. an extraordinary hypersensitivity to a foreign protein; marked by hypotension, shock, and

    respiratory distress _____

3. an antigen capable of causing allergy (hypersensitivity) _____

4. disorder in which the immune system is suppressed by exposure to HIV _____

5. removal of a mediastinal organ _____

6. malignant tumor of lymph nodes and spleen marked by the presence of Reed-Sternberg cells in

    lymph nodes _____

7. tissue that produces lymphocytes—spleen, thymus, tonsils, and adenoids _____

8. swelling of tissues due to interstitial fluid accumulation _____

H. Match the following terms or abbreviations related to AIDS with their meanings below.

CD4$^+$ cells   Kaposi sarcoma   RT inhibitor
ELISA   opportunistic infections   viral load test
HAART   PCP   wasting syndrome
HIV   protease inhibitor

1. a malignant condition associated with AIDS (bluish-red skin nodules appear) _____

2. human immunodeficiency virus; the retrovirus that causes AIDS _____

3. white blood cells that are destroyed by the AIDS virus _____

4. *Pneumocystis* pneumonia that occurs in AIDS patients _____

5. group of infectious diseases associated with AIDS _____

6. measures the amount of HIV in blood _____

7. weight loss with decreased muscular strength, appetite, and mental activity _____

8. drug used to treat AIDS by blocking the growth of HIV _____

9. drug used to treat AIDS by blocking the production of a proteolytic enzyme _____

10. use of combinations of drugs to treat AIDS _____

11. test to detect anti-HIV antibodies _____

14

I. Complete the following terms according to their definitions. Pay close attention to the proper spelling of each term.

1. chronic, disabling diseases caused by abnormal production of antibodies to normal tissue:

   auto_____ diseases

2. a hypersensitivity or allergic state with an inherited predisposition: a_____

3. a malignant tumor of lymph nodes; follicular and large cell are types of this disease:

   non-_____

4. fluid that lies between cells throughout the body: inter_____ fluid

5. formation of lymphocytes or lymphoid tissue: lympho_____

6. chronic swelling of a part of the body due to collection of fluid between tissues secondary to

   obstruction of lymph vessels and nodes: lymph_____

7. an unusual or exaggerated allergic reaction to a foreign protein: ana_____

8. introduction of altered antigens to produce an immune response and protection from disease:

   vac_____

9. test that separates immunoglobulins: immuno_____

J. Circle the correct term(s) to complete each sentence.

1. Mr. Blake had been HIV-positive for 5 years before he developed **(PCP, thymoma, multiple myeloma)** and was diagnosed with **(Hodgkin disease, non-Hodgkin lymphoma, AIDS)**.

2. Mary developed rhinitis, rhinorrhea, and red eyes every spring when pollen was prevalent. She consulted her doctor about her bad **(hypersplenism, allergies, lymphadenitis)**.

3. Paul felt some marble-sized lumps in his left groin. His doctor told him that he had an infection in his foot and had developed secondary **(axillary, cervical, inguinal)** lymphadenopathy.

4. Mr. Jones was referred to a dermatologist and an oncologist when his primary physician noticed purple spots on his arms and legs. Because he had AIDS, his physician was concerned about the possibility of **(Kaposi sarcoma, splenomegaly, thrombocytopenic purpura)**.

5. Fifteen-year-old Peter was allergic to peanuts. His allergy was so severe that he carried epinephrine with him at all times to prevent **(acquired immunity, anaphylaxis, immunosuppression)** in case he came in contact with peanut butter at school.

14

6. When she was in her mid-20s, Rona was diagnosed with a lymph node malignancy known as **(sarcoidosis, Kaposi sarcoma, Hodgkin disease)**. Because the disease was primarily in her chest, her **(inguinal, mediastinal, axillary)** lymph nodes were irradiated (radiation therapy), and she was cured. When she developed lung cancer in her mid-40s, her oncologist told her she had a/an **(iatrogenic, hereditary, metastatic)** radiation-induced secondary tumor.

7. Mary has suffered from hay fever, asthma, and chronic dermatitis ever since she was a young child. She has been particularly bothered by the severely pruritic (itching), erythematous (reddish) patches on her hands. Her dermatologist gave her topical steroids for her **(toxic, atopic, opportunistic)** dermatitis and told her to avoid soaps, cosmetics, and irritating chemicals.

8. Bernie noticed pain in his pelvis, spine, and ribs and was evaluated by his physician. Blood tests showed high levels of plasma cells and abnormal globulins. Increased numbers of plasma cells were revealed on **(chest x-ray, stem cell transplant, bone marrow biopsy)**. Radiologic studies showed bone loss. The physician's diagnosis was multiple **(sclerosis, thymoma, myeloma)**.

9. AIDS is caused by **(herpes simplex virus, monoclonal antibodies, human immunodeficiency virus)**. Lymphocytes called **(CD4$^+$ cells, suppressor cells, B cells)** are destroyed, which disrupts **(humoral immunity, cell-mediated immunity, natural immunity)**, leading to **(anaphylaxis, atopy, opportunistic infections)**.

10. Drugs used to treat AIDS are **(immunosuppressants, protease inhibitors, interferons)**. Other anti-AIDS drugs are **(reverse transcriptase inhibitors, monoclonal antibodies, immunoglobulins)**.

MEDICAL SCRAMBLE

Unscramble the letters to form lymphatic/immune system–related terms from the clues. Use the letters in squares to complete the bonus term. Answers are found on page 551.

14

1. *Clue:* Swelling due to fluid collection in spaces between tissue

   ☐ __ __ __ ☐ __ __ __ __ ☐   PELAMHYEMD

2. *Clue:* Enlargement of a lymphoid organ in the LUQ

   ☐☐ __ __ ☐ __ __ __ __ __ __ ☐   NASLOPYELGEM

3. *Clue:* Large phagocyte that engulfs other cells; found in lymph nodes and tissues

   __ ☐ __ __ __ __ __ ☐ __ __   GARPAMOHEC

4. *Clue:* A poison

   __ __ ☐ ☐ __   NOXIT

BONUS TERM: *Clue:* Hypersensitivity reaction

   ☐☐☐☐☐☐☐☐☐☐☐

ANSWERS TO EXERCISES

A

1. lymph nodes
2. thoracic duct
3. spleen

4. adenoids
5. thymus gland
6. lymph capillaries

7. right lymphatic duct
8. interstitial fluid

B

1. groin region
2. armpit region

3. neck (of the body) region
4. space between the lungs in the chest

C

1. humoral immunity
2. T cells

3. cell-mediated immunity
4. B cells

D

1. plasma cell
2. macrophage
3. helper T cell
4. suppressor T cell
5. dendritic cell

E

1. A
2. C
3. B
4. D
5. G
6. F
7. E

F

1. splenectomy
2. splenomegaly
3. lymphopoiesis
4. thymoma
5. lymphadenitis
6. lymphocytopenia
7. toxic
8. lymphadenopathy

G

1. hypersplenism
2. anaphylaxis
3. allergen
4. AIDS
5. thymectomy
6. Hodgkin disease
7. lymphoid organs
8. lymphedema

H

1. Kaposi sarcoma
2. HIV
3. CD4$^+$ cells
4. PCP
5. opportunistic infections
6. viral load tests
7. wasting syndrome
8. RT inhibitor
9. protease inhibitor
10. HAART
11. ELISA (enzyme-linked immunosorbent assay)

I

1. autoimmune
2. atopy
3. non-Hodgkin lymphoma
4. interstitial
5. lymphopoiesis
6. lymphedema
7. anaphylaxis
8. vaccination
9. immunoelectrophoresis

J

1. PCP; AIDS
2. allergies
3. inguinal
4. Kaposi sarcoma
5. anaphylaxis
6. Hodgkin disease; mediastinal; iatrogenic
7. atopic
8. bone marrow biopsy; myeloma
9. human immunodeficiency virus; CD4$^+$ cells; cell-mediated immunity; opportunistic infections
10. protease inhibitors; reverse transcriptase inhibitors

ANSWERS TO PRACTICAL APPLICATIONS

1. b
2. a
3. a
4. b
5. b
6. a
7. b
8. c

ANSWERS TO MEDICAL SCRAMBLE

1. LYMPHEDEMA   2. SPLENOMEGALY   3. MACROPHAGE   4. TOXIN

BONUS TERM: ANAPHYLAXIS

PRONUNCIATION OF TERMS

To test your understanding of the terminology in this chapter, write the meaning of each term in the space provided. In addition, you may wish to cover the terms and write them by looking at your definitions. Make sure your spelling is correct. The page number after each term indicates where it is defined or used in the book, so you can easily check your responses. You will find complete definitions for all of these terms and their audio pronunciations on the CD.

VOCABULARY AND TERMINOLOGY

Term	Pronunciation	Meaning
acquired immunity (533)	ă-KWĬRD ĭ-MŪ-nĭ-tē	
acquired immunodeficiency syndrome (536)	ă-KWĬRD ĭm-ū-nō-dĕ-FĬSH-ĕn-sē SĬN-drōm	
adenoids (533)	ĂD-ĕ-noydz	
allergen (541)	ĂL-ĕr-jĕn	
allergy (539)	ĂL-ĕr-jē	
anaphylaxis (536)	ăn-ă-fă-LĂK-sĭs	
antibody (533)	ĂN-tĭ-bŏ-dē	
antigen (533)	ĂN-tĭ-jĕn	
atopy (541)	ĂT-ō-pē	
autoimmune disease (535)	aw-tō-ĭ-MŪN dĭ-ZĒZ	
axillary node (533)	ĂKS-ĭ-lăr-ē nōd	
B cell (533)	B sĕl	
CD4+ cells (541)	CD4-plŭs sĕlz	
cell-mediated immunity (533)	sĕl MĒ-dē-ā-tĕd ĭ-MŪ-nĭ-tē	
cervical node (533)	SĔR-vĭ-k'l nōd	
cytokine (533)	SĪ-tō-kĭne	
cytotoxic T cell (533)	sī-tō-TŎK-sĭk T sĕl	
dendritic cell (533)	dĕn-DRĬ-tĭk sĕl	
ELISA (542)	ĕ-LĪ-ză	
helper T cell (533)	HĔL-pĕr T sĕl	
Hodgkin disease (540)	HŎJ-kĭn dĭ-ZĒZ	
human immunodeficiency virus (541)	HŪ-măn ĭm-ū-nō-dĕ-FĬSH-ĕn-sē VĪ-rŭs	

Term	Pronunciation	Meaning
humoral immunity (533)	HŪ-mŏr-ăl ĭ-MŪ-nĭ-tē	
hypersensitivity (539)	hī-pĕr-sĕn-sĭ-TĬV-ĭ-tē	
hypersplenism (536)	hī-pĕr-SPLĔN-ĭzm	
immune response (533)	ĭ-MŪN rĕ-SPŎNS	
immunoelectrophoresis (542)	ĭm-ū-nō-ē-lĕk-trō-phŏr-Ē-sĭs	
immunoglobulins (535)	ĭm-ū-nō-GLŎB-ū-lĭnz	
immunosuppression (535)	ĭm-ū-nō-sŭ-PRĔ-shŭn	
immunotherapy (533)	ĭ-mū-nō-THĔR-ă-pē	
inguinal node (533)	ĬNG-gwĭ-năl nōd	
interferons (533)	ĭn-tĕr-FĔR-ŏnz	
interleukins (533)	ĭn-tĕr-LOO-kĭnz	
interstitial fluid (534)	ĭn-tĕr-STĬSH-ăl FLOO-ĭd	
Kaposi sarcoma (538)	KĂ-pō-sē (or kă-PŌS-sē) săr-KŌ-mă	
lymph (534)	lĭmf	
lymphadenitis (536)	lĭm-FĂH-dĕ-nī-tĭs	
lymphadenopathy (536)	lĭm-făd-ĕ-NŎP-ăh-thē	
lymph capillaries (534)	lĭmf KĂP-ĭ-lă-rēz	
lymphedema (535)	lĭmf-ĕ-DĒ-mă	
lymph node (534)	lĭmf nōd	
lymphocytes (528)	LĬM-fō-sītz	
lymphocytosis (535)	lĭm-fō-sī-TŌ-sĭs	
lymphocytopenia (535)	lĭm-fō-sī-tō-PĒ-nē-ă	
lymphoid organs (535)	LĬM-foid ŎR-gănz	
lymphoma (540)	lĭm-FŌ-mă	
lymphopoiesis (535)	lĭm-fō-poy-Ē-sĭs	
lymph vessel (528)	lĭmf VĔS-ĕl	
macrophage (534)	MĂK-rō-făj	
mediastinal node (534)	mē-dē-ăs-TĪ-năl nōd	
monoclonal antibody (534)	mŏn-ō-KLŌ-năl ĂN-tĭ-bŏd-ē	
multiple myeloma (540)	MŬLT-ĭbl mī-ĕ-LŌ-mă	
natural immunity (534)	NĂ-tū-răl ĭm-MŪ-nĭ-tē	
non-Hodgkin lymphoma (540)	nŏn-HŎJ-kĭn lĭm-FŌ-ma	

Term	Pronunciation	Meaning
opportunistic infections (536)	ŏp-pŏr-tū-NĬS-tĭk ĭn-FĔK-shŭnz	_____
plasma cell (534)	PLĂZ-mă sĕl	_____
protease inhibitor (539)	PRŌ-tē-ās ĭn-HĬB-ĭ-tŏr	_____
retrovirus (541)	rĕ-trō-VĪ-rŭs	_____
reverse transcriptase inhibitor (539)	rē-VĔRS trănz-SCRĬP-tās ĭn-HĬB-ĭ-tŏr	_____
right lymphatic duct (534)	rīt lĭm-FĂ-tĭk dŭkt	_____
spleen (534)	splēn	_____
splenectomy (536)	splĕ-NĔK-tō-mē	_____
splenomegaly (536)	splĕ-nō-MĔG-ă-lē	_____
suppressor T cell (534)	sŭ-PRĔ-sŏr T sĕl	_____
T cell (534)	T sĕl	_____
thoracic duct (534)	thō-RĂ-sĭk dŭkt	_____
thymectomy (536)	thī-MĔK-tō-mē	_____
thymoma (536)	thī-MŌ-mă	_____
thymus gland (534)	THĪ-mŭs glănd	_____
tonsils (534)	TŎN-sĭlz	_____
toxic (536)	TŎK-sĭk	_____
toxin (534)	TŎK-sĭn	_____
vaccination (534)	văk-sĭ-NĀ-shŭn	_____
vaccine (534)	văk-SĒN	_____
viral load tests (542)	vī-răl lōd tĕsts	_____
wasting syndrome (538)	WĀST-ĭng SĬN-drōm	_____
Western blot (542)	WĔS-tĕrn blŏt	_____

REVIEW SHEET

Write the meaning of the word parts in the spaces provided. Check your answers with the information in the chapter or in the glossary (Medical Word Parts—English) at the end of the book.

COMBINING FORMS

Combining Form	Meaning	Combining Form	Meaning
axill/o	_____	lymphaden/o	_____
cervic/o	_____	splen/o	_____
immun/o	_____	thym/o	_____
inguin/o	_____	tox/o	_____
lymph/o	_____		

SUFFIXES

Suffix	Meaning	Suffix	Meaning
-cytosis	_____	-penia	_____
-edema	_____	-phylaxis	_____
-globulin	_____	-poiesis	_____
-megaly	_____	-stitial	_____
-oid	_____	-suppression	_____
-pathy	_____		

PREFIXES

Prefix	Meaning	Prefix	Meaning
ana-	_____	inter-	_____
auto-	_____	retro-	_____
hyper-	_____		

 Please refer to the enclosed CD for additional exercises and images related to this chapter.

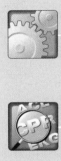

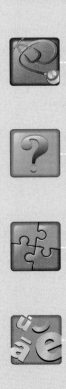

Musculoskeletal System

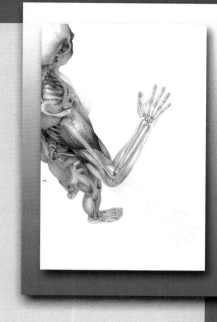

Image Description: Superior view of the human skeleton and muscles highlighting the movement of the arm.

In this chapter you will

- Define terms relating to the structure and function of bones, joints, and muscles.
- Describe the process of bone formation and growth.
- Locate and name the major bones of the body.
- Analyze the combining forms, prefixes, and suffixes used to describe bones, joints, and muscles.
- Explain various musculoskeletal disease conditions and terms related to bone fractures.
- Describe important laboratory tests and clinical procedures relating to the musculoskeletal system, and recognize relevant abbreviations.
- Apply your new knowledge to understanding medical terms in their proper contexts, such as medical reports and records.

INTRODUCTION

The musculoskeletal system includes the bones, muscles, and joints. All have important functions in the body. **Bones** provide the framework around which the body is constructed and protect and support internal organs. Bones also assist the body in movement because they are a point of attachment for muscles. The inner core of bones is composed of hematopoietic tissue (red bone marrow manufactures blood cells), whereas other parts of bone are storage areas for minerals necessary for growth, such as calcium and phosphorus.

Joints are the places at which bones come together. Several different types of joints are found within the body. The type of joint found in any specific location is determined by the need for greater or lesser flexibility of movement.

Muscles, whether attached to bones or to internal organs and blood vessels, are responsible for movement. Internal movement involves the contraction and relaxation of muscles that are a part of viscera, and external movement is accomplished by the contraction and relaxation of muscles that are attached to the bones.

Physicians (MDs) who treat bone and joint diseases are **orthopedists.** Originally, orthopedics was a branch of medicine dealing with correcting deformities in children (**orth/o** means straight, **ped/o** means child). **Rheumatologists** are physicians who primarily treat joint diseases. **Rheumat/o** means watery flow and relates to joint diseases because various forms of arthritis are marked by the collection of fluid in the joint spaces.

Osteopathic physicians, or osteopaths (DOs), practice **osteopathy**, which is a separate school of medicine using diagnostic and therapeutic measures based on the belief that the body is capable of healing itself when bones are in proper position and adequate nutrition is provided. Osteopaths are not medical doctors (MDs). **Chiropractors** (**chir/o** means hand) are neither medical doctors nor osteopaths. They use physical means to manipulate the spinal column, believing that disease is caused by pressure on nerves.

BONES

FORMATION AND STRUCTURE

Formation

Bones are complete organs composed chiefly of connective tissue called **osseous** (bony) **tissue** plus a rich supply of blood vessels and nerves. Osseous tissue consists of a combination of **osteocytes** (bone cells), dense connective tissue strands known as **collagen,** and intercellular **calcium salts.**

During fetal development, the bones of the fetus are composed of **cartilaginous tissue,** which resembles osseous tissue but is more flexible and less dense because of a lack of calcium salts in its intercellular spaces. As the embryo develops, the process of depositing calcium salts in the soft, cartilaginous tissue occurs and continues throughout the life of the individual after birth. The gradual replacement of cartilage and its intercellular substance by immature bone cells and calcium deposits is **ossification** (bone formation).

Osteoblasts are the immature osteocytes that produce the bony tissue that replaces cartilage during ossification. **Osteoclasts** (**-clast** means to break) are large cells that function to reabsorb, or digest, bony tissue. Osteoclasts (also called **bone phagocytes**) digest bone tissue from the inner sides of bones and thus enlarge the inner bone cavity so that the bone does not become overly thick and heavy. When a bone breaks, osteoblasts lay down the mineral bone matter (calcium salts) and osteoclasts remove excess bone debris (smooth out the bone).

Osteoblasts and osteoclasts work together in all bones throughout life, tearing down (osteoclasts) and rebuilding (osteoblasts) bony tissue. This allows bone to respond to mechanical stresses placed on it and thus enables it to be a living tissue, constantly rebuilding and renewing itself.

The formation of bone depends largely on a proper supply of **calcium** and **phosphorus** to the bone tissue. These minerals must be taken into the body along with a sufficient amount of vitamin D. Vitamin D helps calcium to pass through the lining of the small intestine and into the bloodstream. Once calcium and phosphorus are in the bones, osteoblastic activity produces an enzyme that forms calcium phosphate, a substance that gives bone its characteristic hard quality. It is the major calcium salt.

Not only are calcium and phosphorus part of the hard structure of bone tissue, but calcium also is stored elsewhere in bones, and small quantities are present in the blood. If the proper amount of calcium is lacking in the blood, nerve fibers are unable to transmit impulses effectively to muscles, the heart muscle becomes weak, and muscles attached to bones undergo spasms.

The necessary level of calcium in the blood is maintained by the parathyroid gland, which secretes a hormone that signals the release of calcium from bone storage. An excess of the hormone (caused by tumor or another pathologic process) will raise blood calcium at the expense of the bones, which become weakened by the loss of calcium.

Structure

There are 206 bones of various types in the body. **Long bones** are found in the thigh, lower leg, and upper and lower arm. These bones are very strong, are broad at the ends where they join with other bones, and have large surface areas for muscle attachment.

15

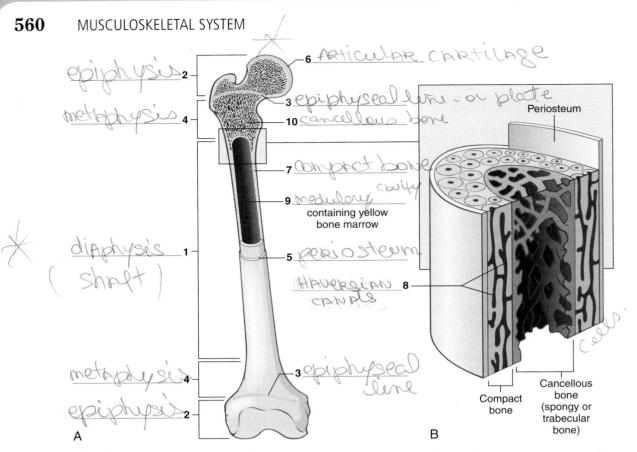

Handwritten annotations on figure:
- epiphysis 2
- metaphysis 4
- diaphysis 1 (shaft)
- metaphysis 4
- epiphysis 2
- 6 Articular cartilage
- 3 epiphyseal line or plate
- 10 cancellous bone
- 7 compact bone
- 9 medullary cavity
- 5 periosteum
- Haversian 8 canals
- 3 epiphyseal line
- cells

Printed labels on figure:
- Periosteum
- containing yellow bone marrow
- Cancellous bone (spongy or trabecular bone)
- Compact bone
- A
- B

FIGURE 15–1 **A,** Divisions of a long bone and interior bone structure. **B,** Composition of compact (cortical) bone.

Short bones are found in the wrist and ankle and are small with irregular shapes. **Flat bones** are found covering soft body parts. These are the shoulder blades, ribs, and pelvic bones. **Sesamoid bones** are small, rounded bones resembling a sesame seed in shape. They are found near joints, and they increase the efficiency of muscles near a particular joint. The kneecap is the largest example of a sesamoid bone.

Figure 15–1, *A*, shows the anatomic divisions of a long bone such as the thigh bone or upper arm bone. Label the figure as you read the following.

The shaft, or middle region, of a long bone is called the **diaphysis** [1]. Each end of a long bone is called an **epiphysis** [2]. The **epiphyseal line** or **plate** [3] represents an area of cartilage tissue that is constantly being replaced by new bone tissue as the bone grows; it also is commonly known as the growth plate. Cartilage cells at the edges of the epiphyseal plate form new bone, which is responsible for lengthening bones during childhood and adolescence. The plate calcifies and disappears when the bone has achieved its full growth. The **metaphysis** [4] is the flared portion of the bone; it lies between the epiphysis and the diaphysis. It is adjacent to the epiphysis plate.

The **periosteum** [5] is a strong, fibrous, vascular membrane that covers the surface of long bones, except at the ends of the epiphyses. It has an extensive nerve supply as well. Bones other than long bones are also covered by periosteum.

The ends of long bones and the surface of any bone that meets another bone to form a joint are covered with **articular cartilage** [6]. When two bones come together to form a joint, the bones themselves do not touch precisely. The articular cartilage that caps the end of one bone comes in contact with that of the other bone. Articular cartilage is a very smooth, strong, and slick tissue. It cushions the joint and allows it to move smoothly and efficiently. Unlike the cartilage of the epiphyseal plate, which disappears when a bone achieves its full growth, articular cartilage is present throughout life.

Compact (cortical) bone [7] is a layer of hard, dense bone that lies under the periosteum in all bones and lies chiefly around the diaphysis of long bones. Within the compact bone is a system of small canals containing blood vessels that bring oxygen and nutrients to the bone and remove waste products such as carbon dioxide. Figure 15–1, *B*, shows these channels, called **haversian canals** [8], in the compact bone. Compact bone is tunneled out in the central shaft of the long bones by a **medullary cavity** [9] that contains **yellow bone marrow.** Yellow bone marrow is composed chiefly of fat cells.

Cancellous bone [10], sometimes called **spongy** or **trabecular bone,** is much more porous and less dense than compact bone. The mineral matter in it is laid down in a series of separated bony fibers that make up a spongy latticework. These interwoven fibers, called **trabeculae,** are found largely in the epiphyses and metaphyses of long bones and in the middle portion of most other bones of the body as well. Spaces in cancellous bone contain **red bone marrow.** This marrow, as opposed to yellow marrow, which is fatty tissue, is richly supplied with blood and consists of immature and mature blood cells in various stages of development.

In an adult, the ribs, pelvic bone, sternum (breastbone), and vertebrae, as well as the epiphyses of long bones, contain red bone marrow within cancellous tissue. Red marrow in the medullary cavity of long bones is plentiful in young children but decreases through the years and is replaced by yellow marrow.

PROCESSES AND DEPRESSIONS IN BONES

Bone processes are enlarged areas that extend out from bones to serve as attachments for muscles and tendons. Label Figure 15–2, *A* and *B*, which shows the shapes of some of the common bony processes:

Bone head [1]—rounded end of a bone separated from the body of the bone by a neck; usually covered by articular cartilage. In the femur (see Fig. 15–2, *A*) the bone head is called the **femoral head**.

Greater trochanter [2]—large process on the femur for attachment of tendons and muscle. The **lesser trochanter** [3] is a smaller process.

Tubercle [4]—rounded process on many bones for attachment of tendons and muscles. A **tuberosity** is another small, rounded elevation on a bone.

Condyle [5]—rounded, knuckle-like process at the joint; usually covered by articular cartilage.

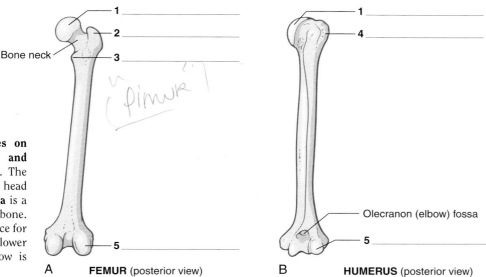

FIGURE 15–2 Bone processes on the femur (thigh bone) (**A**) and humerus (upper arm bone) (**B**). The bone neck separates the bone head from the rest of the bone. A **fossa** is a shallow depression or cavity in a bone. The fossa on the humerus is a space for the olecranon process on the lower arm bone (ulna) when the elbow is extended.

Bone neck

1 _____
2 _____
3 _____
5 _____

A **FEMUR** (posterior view)

1 _____
4 _____
Olecranon (elbow) fossa
5 _____

B **HUMERUS** (posterior view)

Many bones possess openings or hollow regions that help join one bone to another and/or that serve as passageways for blood vessels and nerves. The names of some common depressions in bone are as follows:

Fossa—shallow cavity in or on a bone
Foramen—opening for blood vessels and nerves
Fissure—narrow, deep, slit-like opening
Sinus—hollow cavity within a bone

CRANIAL BONES

The bones of the skull, or cranium, protect the brain and structures related to it, such as the sense organs. Muscles for controlling head movements and chewing motions are connected to the cranial bones. The cranial bones join each other at joints called **sutures.**

The cranial bones of a newborn child are not completely joined. There are gaps of unossified tissue in the skull at birth. These are called soft spots, or **fontanelles** (little fountains). The pulse of blood vessels can be felt (palpated) under the skin in those areas.

Figure 15–3 illustrates the bones of the cranium. Label them as you read the following descriptions:

Frontal bone [1]—forms the forehead and the roof of the bony sockets that contain the eyes.
Parietal bone [2]—the two bones (one on each side of the skull) that form the roof and upper part of the sides of the cranium.

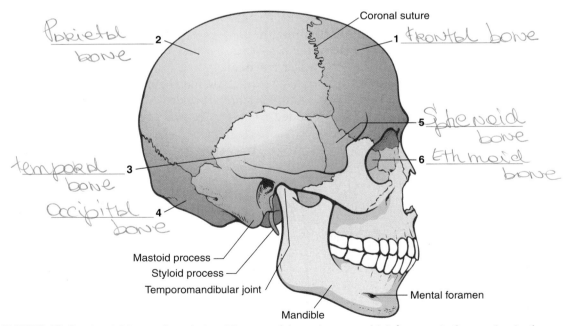

FIGURE 15–3 Cranial bones, lateral view. The **mental** (ment/o means chin) **foramen** is the opening in the mandible that allows blood vessels and nerves to enter and leave. The **coronal suture** is the connection across the skull between the two parietal bones and the frontal bone.

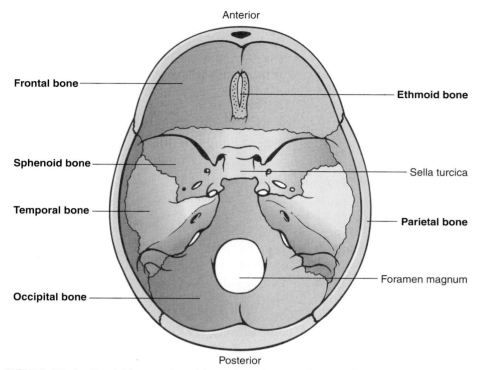

FIGURE 15–4 **Cranial bones,** viewed from above downward, to the floor of the cranial cavity.

Temporal bone [3]—the two bones that form the lower sides and base of the cranium. Each bone encloses an ear and contains a fossa for joining with the mandible (lower jaw bone). The **temporomandibular joint (TMJ)** is the area of connection between the temporal and mandibular bones. The **mastoid process** is a round (**mast/o** means breast) process of the temporal bone behind the ear. The **styloid process** (**styl/o** means pole or stake) projects downward from the temporal bone.

Occipital bone [4]—forms the back and base of the skull and joins the parietal and temporal bones, forming a suture. The inferior portion of the occipital bone has an opening called the **foramen magnum** through which the spinal cord passes (Fig. 15–4).

Sphenoid bone [5]—the bat-shaped bone that extends behind the eyes and forms part of the base of the skull. Because it joins with the frontal, occipital, and ethmoid bones, it serves as an anchor to hold those skull bones together (**sphen/o** means wedge). The **sella turcica** (meaning Turkish saddle) is a depression in the sphenoid bone in which the pituitary gland is located (see Fig. 15–4).

Ethmoid bone [6]—the thin, delicate bone that supports the nasal cavity and forms part of the orbits of the eyes. It is composed primarily of spongy, cancellous bone, which contains numerous small holes (**ethm/o** means sieve).

Study Figure 15–4, which shows these cranial bones as viewed from above downward, toward the floor of the cranial cavity.

15

FACIAL BONES

All of the facial bones except one are joined together by sutures, so they are immovable. The mandible (lower jaw bone) is the only facial bone capable of movement. This ability is necessary for activities such as mastication (chewing) and speaking.

Figure 15–5 shows the facial bones; label it as you read the following descriptions of the facial bones:

Nasal bones [1]—the two slender bones that support the bridge of the nose (**nas/o** means nose). They join with the frontal bone superiorly and form part of the nasal septum.

Lacrimal bones [2]—the two small, thin bones located at the corner of each eye. The lacrimal (**lacrim/o** means tear) bones contain fossae for the lacrimal gland (tear gland) and canals for the passage of the lacrimal duct.

Maxillary bones [3]—the two large bones that compose the massive upper jawbones **(maxillae).** They are joined by a suture in the median plane. If the two bones do not come together normally before birth, the condition known as **cleft palate** results.

Mandibular bone [4]—the lower jawbone **(mandible).** Both the maxilla and the mandible contain the sockets called **alveoli** in which the teeth are embedded. The mandible joins the skull at the region of the temporal bone, forming the temporomandibular joint (TMJ) on either side of the skull.

Zygomatic bones [5]—the two bones, one on each side of the face, that form the high portion of the cheek.

Vomer [6]—the thin, single, flat bone that forms the lower portion of the nasal septum.

Sinuses, or air cavities, are located in specific places within the cranial and facial bones to lighten the skull and warm and moisten air as it passes through. Figure 15–6 shows the sinuses of the skull.

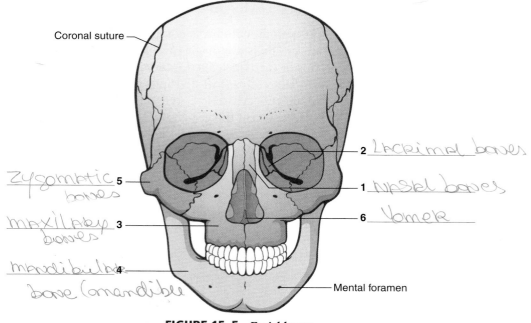

Coronal suture

2 Lacrimal bones

1 Nasal bones

6 Vomer

Zygomatic bones 5

maxillary bones 3

mandibular bone (mandible) 4

Mental foramen

FIGURE 15–5 Facial bones.

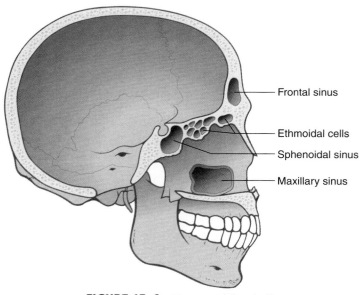

Frontal sinus

Ethmoidal cells

Sphenoidal sinus

Maxillary sinus

FIGURE 15–6 Sinuses of the skull.

VERTEBRAL COLUMN AND STRUCTURE OF VERTEBRAE

The **vertebral,** or **spinal, column** is composed of 26 bone segments, called vertebrae, that are arranged in five divisions from the base of the skull to the tailbone. The bones are separated by pads of cartilage called **intervertebral disks** (discs).

Figure 15–7 illustrates the divisions of the vertebral column: cervical, thoracic, lumbar, sacrum, and coccyx.

The first seven bones of the vertebral column, forming the bony aspect of the neck, are the **cervical (C1 to C7) vertebrae.** These vertebrae do not articulate (join) with the ribs.

The second set of 12 vertebrae are known as the **thoracic (T1 to T12) vertebrae.** These vertebrae articulate with the 12 pairs of ribs.

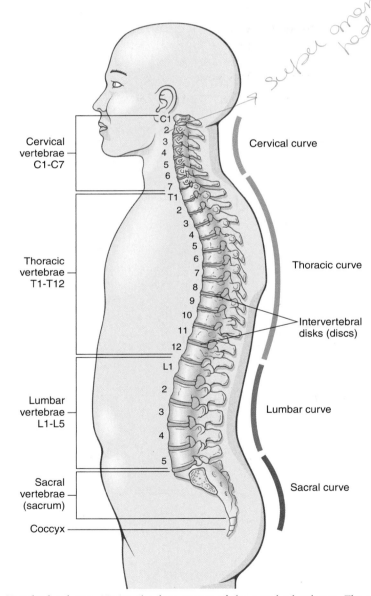

FIGURE 15–7 Vertebral column. Notice the four curves of the vertebral column. The sacral and thoracic curvatures are present at birth. The cervical curvature develops when the infant holds the head erect. The lumbar curvature develops as the infant begins to stand and walk.

The third set of five vertebral bones are the **lumbar (L1 to L5) vertebrae.** They are the strongest and largest of the backbones. Like the cervical vertebrae, these bones do not articulate with the ribs.

The **sacral vertebrae (sacrum)** are five separate bones that fuse in a young child. In an adult, the sacrum is a slightly curved, triangularly shaped bone.

The **coccyx** is the tailbone, and it, too, is a fused bone, having been formed from four small coccygeal bones.

Figure 15–8, *A*, illustrates the general structure of a vertebra. Although the individual vertebrae in the separate regions of the spinal column are all slightly different in structure, they do have several parts in common.

A vertebra is composed of an inner, thick, round anterior portion called the **vertebral body** [1]. Between the body of one vertebra and the bodies of the vertebrae lying beneath and above is an **intervertebral disk (disc).** It is a pad of cartilage that provides flexibility and shocks to the vertebral column (See Fig. 15–8, *B*).

The posterior portion of a vertebra (vertebral arch) consists of a single **spinous process** [2], a **transverse process** [3] on both sides of the spinous process, and a bar-like **lamina** [4] on either side. The **neural canal** [5] is the space between the vertebral body and the vertebral arch through which the spinal cord passes. Figure 15–8, *B*, shows a lateral view of several vertebrae. Note the location of the spinal cord running through the neural canal.

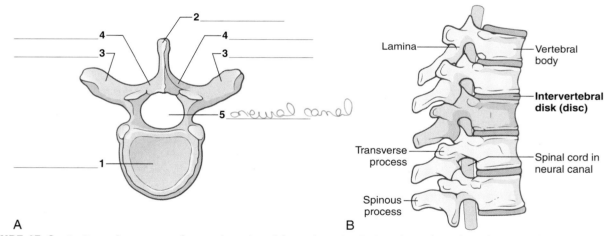

FIGURE 15–8 **A, General structure of a vertebra,** viewed from above. **B, Series of vertebrae,** lateral view, to show the position of the spinal cord behind the vertebral bodies and intervertebral discs.

BONES OF THE THORAX, PELVIS, AND EXTREMITIES

Label Figure 15–9 as you read the following descriptions of the bones of the thorax (chest cavity), pelvis (hipbone), and extremities (arms and legs):

Bones of the Thorax

Clavicle [1]—collar bone; a slender bone, ventrally, one on each side, connecting the breastbone to each shoulder blade

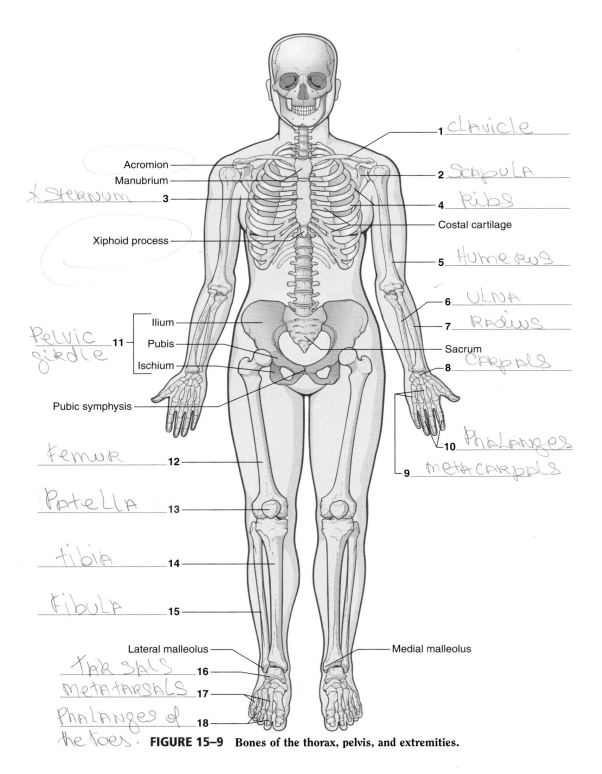

Acromion
Manubrium
Xiphoid process
Ilium
Pubis
Ischium
Pubic symphysis
Sacrum
Lateral malleolus
Medial malleolus
Costal cartilage

1 clavicle
2 scapula
4 ribs
5 humerus
6 ulna
7 radius
8 carpals
10 phalanges
9 metacarpals
11 pelvic girdle
3 sternum
12 femur
13 patella
14 tibia
15 fibula
16 tarsals
17 metatarsals
18 phalanges of the toes

(no ribs drawn)

FIGURE 15–9 Bones of the thorax, pelvis, and extremities.

Scapula [2]—shoulder blade; two flat, triangular bones, one on each dorsal side of the thorax. The extension of the scapula that joins with the clavicle to form a joint above the shoulder is called the **acromion** (**acr/o** means extremity, **om/o** means shoulder). The joint formed by these two bones is known as the acromioclavicular (AC) joint. Figure 15–10 shows a posterior view of the scapula.

Sternum [3]—breastbone; a flat bone extending down the midline of the chest. The uppermost part of the sternum articulates on the sides with the clavicle and ribs, and the lower, narrower portion is attached to the diaphragm and abdominal muscles. The lower portion of the sternum is the **xiphoid process** (**xiph/o** means sword). The upper portion is the **manubrium** (from a Latin term meaning handle).

Ribs [4]—There are 12 pairs of ribs. The first 7 pairs join the sternum anteriorly through cartilaginous attachments called **costal cartilages.** Ribs 1 to 7 are called **true ribs.** They join with the sternum anteriorly and with the vertebral column in the back. Ribs 8 to 10 are called **false ribs.** They join with the vertebral column in the back but join the 7th rib anteriorly instead of attaching to the sternum. Ribs 11 and 12 are the **floating ribs** because they are completely free at their anterior ends. Figure 15–10 shows a posterior view of the rib cage.

Bones of the Arm and Hand

These are described with the subject in the anatomic position—palms forward.

Humerus [5]—upper arm bone; the large head of the humerus is rounded and joins with the glenoid fossa of the scapula to form the shoulder joint (see Fig. 15–10).

Ulna [6]—medial lower arm bone; the proximal bony process of the ulna at the elbow is called the **olecranon** (elbow bone). The olecranon is the bony point of the elbow when the elbow is bent.

Radius [7]—lateral lower arm bone (in line with the thumb)

Carpals [8]—wrist bones; there are two rows of four bones in the wrist.

Metacarpals [9]—the five radiating bones in the fingers. These are the bones of the palm of the hand.

Phalanges [10] (singular: **phalanx**)—finger bones. Each finger (except the thumb) has three phalanges: a proximal, a middle, and a distal phalanx. The thumb has only two phalanges: a proximal and a distal phalanx.

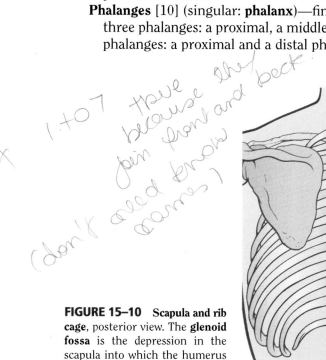

(handwritten note: X 1. to 7 true because they join front and back (don't need to know names))

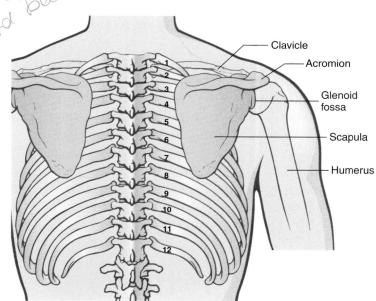

FIGURE 15–10 Scapula and rib cage, posterior view. The **glenoid fossa** is the depression in the scapula into which the humerus fits.

Clavicle
Acromion
Glenoid fossa
Scapula
Humerus

Bones of the Pelvis

Pelvic girdle [11]—pelvis. This collection of bones supports the trunk of the body and articulates with the femur to form the hip joint. The adult pelvis is composed of three pairs of fused bones: the ilium, ischium, and pubis, which articulate posteriorly with the sacrum of the vertebral column.

The **ilium** is the uppermost and largest portion. Dorsally, the two parts of the ilium do not meet. Rather, they join the sacrum on either side to form the sacroiliac joints. The connection between the iliac bones and the sacrum is very firm, and very little motion occurs at these joints. The superior part of the ilium is the **iliac crest.** It is filled with red bone marrow and serves as an attachment for abdominal wall muscles.

The **ischium** is the posterior part of the pelvis. The ischium and the muscles attached to it are what you sit on.

The **pubis** is the anterior part, and the two pubic bones join by way of a cartilaginous disk. This area is called the **pubic symphysis.** Like the sacroiliac joints, this area is quite rigid.

The region within the ring of bone formed by the pelvic girdle is the **pelvic cavity.** The rectum, sigmoid colon, bladder, and female reproductive organs lie within the pelvic cavity and are protected by the rigid architecture of the pelvic girdle.

Bones of the Leg and Foot

Femur [12]—thigh bone; this is the longest bone in the body. At its proximal end it has a rounded head that fits into a depression, or socket, in the pelvis. This socket is called the **acetabulum.** The acetabulum was named because of its resemblance to a rounded cup the Romans used for vinegar (*acetum*). The head of the femur and the acetabulum form the "ball and socket" joint otherwise known as the hip joint.

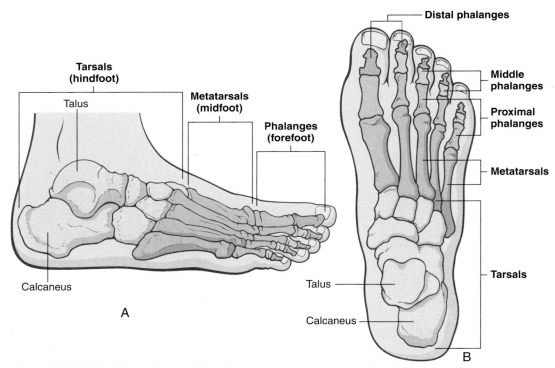

FIGURE 15–11 **A, Bones of the foot,** lateral view. **B, Bones of the foot,** viewed from above.

15

Patella [13]—kneecap; this is a small, flat bone that lies in front of the articulation between the femur and one of the lower leg bones called the tibia. It is a sesamoid bone surrounded by protective tendons and held in place by muscle attachments. Together with the femur and the tibia, it forms the knee joint.

Tibia [14]—larger of two bones of the lower leg; the tibia runs under the skin in the front part of the leg. It joins with the femur and patella proximally, and at its distal end (ankle) forms a flare that is the bony prominence (medial **malleolus**) at the inside of the ankle. The tibia commonly is called the **shin bone.**

Fibula [15]—smaller of two lower leg bones; this thin bone, well hidden under the leg muscles, runs parallel to the tibia. At its distal part, it forms a flare, which is the bony prominence (lateral **malleolus**) on the outside of the ankle. The tibia, fibula, and **talus** (the first of the tarsal bones) come together to form the **ankle joint.**

Tarsals [16]—bones of the hind part of the foot (hindfoot); these seven short bones resemble the carpal bones of the wrist but are larger. The **calcaneus** is the largest of these bones and also is called the **heel bone** (Fig. 15–11). The **talus** is one of three bones that form the ankle joint.

Metatarsals [17]—bones of the midfoot; there are five metatarsal bones, which are similar to the metacarpals of the hand. Each leads to the phalanges of the toes.

Phalanges of the toes [18]—bones of the forefoot; similar to the hand, there are two phalanges in the big toe and three in each of the other toes.

Figure 15–11 illustrates the bones of the foot. Table 15–1 reviews bones and bone processes and their common names.

Table 15–1

Bones or Processes and Their Common Names

Bone or Process	Common Name	Bone or Process	Common Name
Acetabulum	Hip socket	Metatarsals	Midfoot bones
Calcaneus	Heel	Olecranon	Elbow
Carpals	Wrist bones	Patella	Kneecap
Clavicle	Collar bone	Phalanges	Finger and toe bones
Coccyx	Tailbone	Pubis	Anterior part of the pelvic bone
Cranium	Skull		
Femur	Thigh bone	Radius	Lower arm bone (thumb side)
Fibula	Smaller lower leg bone		
Humerus	Upper arm bone	Scapula	Shoulder blade
Ilium	Upper part of pelvic bone	Sternum	Breastbone
Ischium	Posterior part of the pelvic bone	Tarsals	Hind foot bones
		Tibia	Shin bone (larger of two lower leg bones)
Malleolus	Ankle		
Mandible	Lower jaw bone	Ulna	Lower arm bone (little finger side)
Maxilla	Upper jaw bone	Vertebra	Backbone
Metacarpals	Hand bones		

VOCABULARY

This list reviews many of the new terms introduced in the text. Short definitions reinforce your understanding of the terms. Refer to the Pronunciation of Terms section for help with unfamiliar or difficult terms.

acetabulum	Rounded depression, or socket, in the pelvis, which joins the femur (thigh bone), forming the hip joint.
acromion	Outward extension of the shoulder blade forming the point of the shoulder. It overlies the shoulder joint and articulates with the clavicle.
articular cartilage	Thin layer of cartilage surrounding the bone in the joint space.
bone	Dense, hard connective tissue composing the skeleton. Examples are long bones (femur), short bones (carpals), flat bones (scapula), and sesamoid bones (patella).
calcium	One of the mineral constituents of bone. **Calcium phosphate** is the major calcium salt in bones.
cancellous bone	Spongy, porous, bone tissue in the inner part of a bone.
cartilaginous tissue	Flexible, rubbery connective tissue. It is found in the immature skeleton, at the epiphyseal growth plate, and on joint surfaces.
collagen	Dense, connective tissue protein strands found in bone and other tissues.
compact bone	Hard, dense bone tissue, usually found around the outer portion of bones.
condyle	Knuckle-like process at the end of a bone near the joint.
cranial bones	Skull bones: ethmoid, frontal, occipital, parietal, sphenoid, and temporal.
diaphysis	Shaft, or mid-portion, of a long bone.
disk (disc)	Flat, round, plate-like structure. An intervertebral disk is a fibrocartilaginous substance between two vertebrae.
epiphyseal plate	Cartilaginous area at the ends of long bones where lengthwise growth takes place in the immature skeleton.
epiphysis	Each end of a long bone; the area beyond the epiphyseal plate.
facial bones	Bones of the face: lacrimal, mandibular, maxillary, nasal, vomer, and zygomatic.
fissure	Narrow, slit-like opening in or between bones.
fontanelle	Soft spot (incomplete bone formation) between the skull bones of an infant.
foramen	Opening or passage in bones where blood vessels and nerves enter and leave. The **foramen magnum** is the opening of the occipital bone through which the spinal cord passes.
fossa	Shallow cavity in a bone.
haversian canals	Minute spaces filled with blood vessels; found in compact bone.
malleolus	Round process on both sides of the ankle joint. The lateral malleolus is part of the fibula, and the medial malleolus is part of the tibia.

manubrium	Upper portion of the sternum; articulates with the medial aspect of the clavicle.
mastoid process	Round projection on the temporal bone behind the ear.
medullary cavity	Central, hollowed-out area in the shaft of a long bone.
metaphysis	Flared portion of a long bone, between the diaphysis (shaft) and the epiphyseal plate (in this term, meta- means between).
olecranon	Large process on the proximal end of the ulna; the point of the flexed elbow.
osseous tissue	Bone tissue.
ossification	Process of bone formation.
osteoblast	Bone cell that helps form bony tissue.
osteoclast	Bone cell that absorbs and removes unwanted bony tissue.
periosteum	Membrane surrounding bones; rich in blood vessels and nerve tissue.
phosphorus	Mineral substance found in bones in combination with calcium.
pubic symphysis	Area of confluence (coming together) of the two pubic bones in the pelvis. They are joined (sym- means together, -physis means to grow) by a fibrocartilaginous disk.
red bone marrow	Found in cancellous bone; site of hematopoiesis.
ribs	Twelve pairs of curved bones that form the chest wall. True ribs are the first 7 pairs; false ribs are pairs 8 to 10; floating ribs are pairs 11 and 12.
sella turcica	Depression in the sphenoid bone where the pituitary gland is located.
sinus	Hollow air cavity within a bone.
styloid process	Pole-like process extending downward from the temporal bone on each side of the skull.
suture	Joint between bones, such as the skull (cranium).
temporomandibular joint	Connection on either side of the head between the temporal bone of the skull and mandibular bone of the jaw.
trabeculae	Supporting bundles of bony fibers in cancellous (spongy) bone.
trochanter	Large process at the neck of the femur; attachment site for muscles and tendons.
tubercle	Rounded, small process on bone; attachment site for muscles and tendons.
tuberosity	Rounded process on bone; attachment site for muscles and tendons.
vertebra	Individual backbone composed of the vertebral body, vertebral arch, spinous process, transverse process, lamina, and neural canal.
xiphoid process	Lower, narrow portion of the sternum.
yellow bone marrow	Fatty tissue found in the medullary cavity of most adult long bones.

COMBINING FORMS AND SUFFIXES

15

The following word parts pertaining to bones are divided into two groups: general terms and terms related to specific bones. Write the meanings of the medical terms in the spaces provided.

GENERAL TERMS

COMBINING FORMS

[handwritten notes:] hyper excessive / emie blood condition

Combining Forms	Meaning	Terminology	Meaning
calc/o, calci/o	calcium	hypercalcemia *[handwritten: excesso of calcium en the blood]*	
		decalcification _____ *de- means less or lack of; -fication is the process of making.*	
kyph/o	humpback, hunchback (posterior curvature in the thoracic region)	kyphosis _____ *The term (from Greek meaning hill or mountain) indicates a hump on the back. The affected person's height is reduced, and kyphosis may lead to pressure on the spinal cord or peripheral nerves. See Figure 15–12.*	
lamin/o	lamina (part of the vertebral arch)	laminectomy _____ *An operation often performed to relieve the symptoms of compression of the spinal cord or spinal nerve roots. It involves removal of the lamina and spinous process.*	
lord/o	curve, swayback (anterior curvature in the lumbar region)	lordosis _____ *The normal anterior curvature of the lumbar spine becomes exaggerated. See Figure 15–12. The word lordosis is derived from Greek, describing a person leaning backward in a lordly fashion.*	

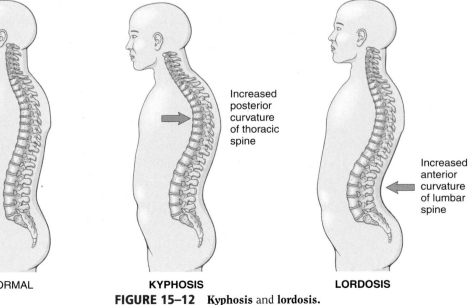

NORMAL   KYPHOSIS

Increased posterior curvature of thoracic spine

LORDOSIS

Increased anterior curvature of lumbar spine

FIGURE 15–12 **Kyphosis** and **lordosis**.

Combining Forms	Meaning	Terminology	Meaning
lumb/o	loins, lower back	lumbar _pertaining to lower back_	
		lumbosacral _____	
myel/o	bone marrow	myelopoiesis _____	
orth/o	straight	orthopedics _____	
		Ped/o means child.	
oste/o	bone	osteitis _____	
		osteodystrophy _____	
		osteogenesis _____	
		Osteogenesis imperfecta *is a genetic disorder involving defective development of bones, which are brittle and fragile; fractures occur with the slightest trauma.*	
scoli/o	crooked, bent (lateral curvature)	scoliosis _____	
		The spinal column is bent abnormally to the side. Scoliosis is the most common spinal deformity in adolescent girls (Fig. 15–13).	
spondyl/o (used to make words about conditions of the structure)	vertebra	spondylosis _____	
		Degeneration of the intervertebral disks in the cervical, thoracic, and lumbar regions. Signs and symptoms include pain and restriction of movement.	

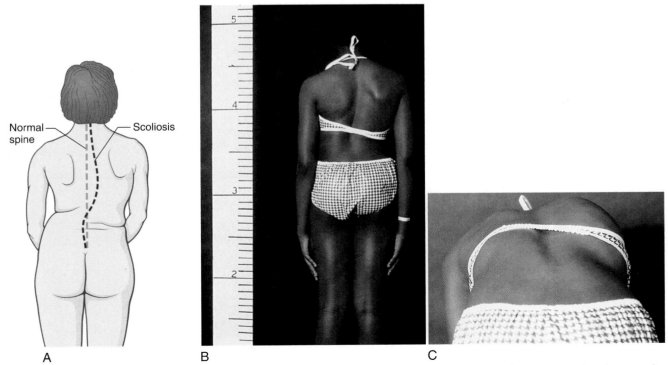

Normal spine — Scoliosis

A   B   C

FIGURE 15–13 Moderate thoracic idiopathic adolescent scoliosis. A, Normal spine and **scoliosis. B,** Notice the **scapular asymmetry** in the upright position. This results from rotation of the spine and attached rib cage. **C,** Bending forward reveals a mild rib hump deformity. (**B** and **C** from Zitelli BJ, Davis HW: Atlas of Pediatric Physical Diagnosis, 4th ed. St. Louis, Mosby, 2002, p. 756.)

15

Combining Forms	Meaning	Terminology	Meaning
vertebr/o (used to describe the structure itself)	vertebra	vertebral _____	

SUFFIXES

Suffix	Meaning	Terminology	Meaning
-blast	embryonic or immature cell	osteoblast _____ *This cell synthesizes collagen and protein to form bone tissue.*	
-clast	to break	osteoclast _____ *This cell breaks down bone to remove bone tissue.*	
-listhesis	slipping	spondylolisthesis _____ *(Pronounced spŏn-dĭ-lō-lĭs-THĒ-sĭs.) The forward slipping (subluxation) of a vertebra over a lower vertebra.*	
-malacia	softening	osteomalacia _____ *A condition in which vitamin D deficiency leads to decalcification of bones; known as rickets in children.*	
-physis	to grow	epiphysis _____ pubic symphysis _____	
-porosis	pore, passage	osteoporosis _____ *Loss of bony tissue with decreased mass of bone. See page 581.*	
-tome	instrument to cut	osteotome _____ *This surgical chisel is designed to cut bone.*	

TERMS RELATED TO SPECIFIC BONES

COMBINING FORMS

Combining Forms	Meaning	Terminology	Meaning
acetabul/o	acetabulum (hip socket)	acetabular _____	
calcane/o	calcaneus (heel)	calcaneal _____ *The calcaneus is one of the tarsal (hindfoot) bones.*	
carp/o	carpals (wrist bones)	carpal _____	
clavicul/o	clavicle (collar bone)	supraclavicular _____ *Supra- means above.*	
cost/o	ribs (true ribs, false ribs, and floating ribs)	subcostal _____ chondrocostal _____ *Cartilage that is attached to the ribs.*	

15

Combining Forms	Meaning	Terminology	Meaning
crani/o	cranium (skull)	craniotomy _____	
		craniotome _____	
femor/o	femur (thigh bone)	femoral _____	
fibul/o	fibula (smaller lower leg bone)	fibular _____ *See perone/o.*	
humer/o	humerus (upper arm bone)	humeral _____	
ili/o	ilium (upper part of pelvic bone)	iliac _____	
ischi/o	ischium (posterior part of pelvic bone)	ischial _____	
malleol/o	malleolus (process on each side of the ankle)	malleolar _____ *The medial malleolus is at the lower end of the tibia, and the lateral malleolus is at the lower end of the fibula.*	
mandibul/o	mandible (lower jaw bone)	mandibular _____	
maxill/o	maxilla (upper jaw bone)	maxillary _____	
metacarp/o	metacarpals (hand bones)	metacarpectomy _____	
metatars/o	metatarsals (foot bones)	metatarsalgia _____	
olecran/o	olecranon (elbow)	olecranal _____	
patell/o	patella (kneecap)	patellar _____	
pelv/i	pelvis (hipbone)	pelvimetry _____	
perone/o	fibula	peroneal _____	
phalang/o	phalanges (finger and/or toe bones)	phalangeal _____	
pub/o	pubis (anterior part of the pelvic bone)	pubic _____	

Peroneal/Peritoneal

Peroneal means pertaining to the fibula (smaller of two lower leg bones). Don't confuse this term with *peritoneal,* meaning pertaining to the peritoneum (membrane surrounding the abdominal organs).

Combining Forms	Meaning	Terminology	Meaning
radi/o	radius (lower arm bone—thumb side)	radial _____	
scapul/o	scapula (shoulder blade)	scapular _____	
stern/o	sternum (breastbone)	sternal _____	
tars/o	tarsals (bones of the hindfoot)	tarsectomy _____	
tibi/o	tibia (shin bone)	tibial _____	
uln/o	ulna (lower arm bone—little finger side)	ulnar _____	

PATHOLOGIC CONDITIONS INCLUDING FRACTURES

Ewing sarcoma

Malignant bone tumor.

Pain and swelling are common, especially if the tumor involves the shaft (medullary cavity) of a long bone. This tumor usually occurs at an early age (5 to 15 years old), and combined treatment with surgery, radiotherapy, and chemotherapy represents the best chance for cure (60 to 70 percent of patients are cured if metastasis has not occurred).

exostosis

Bony growth arising from the surface of bone (ex- means out, -ostosis means condition of bone).

Osteochondromas (composed of cartilage and bone) are **exostoses** and usually are found on the metaphyses of long bones near the epiphyseal plates

A **bunion** is a swelling of the metatarsophalangeal joint near the base of the big toe and is accompanied by the buildup of soft tissue and underlying bone at the distal/medial aspect of the first metatarsal.

fracture

Traumatic breaking of a bone.

A **closed fracture** means that the bone is broken but there is no open wound in the skin, whereas an **open (compound) fracture** means that the bone is broken and a fragment of bone protrudes through an open wound in the skin. A **pathologic fracture** is caused by disease of the bone such as tumor or infection, making it weak. **Crepitus** is the crackling sound produced when ends of bones rub each other or rub against roughened cartilage.

Examples of fractures (Fig. 15–14) are the following:

Colles fracture—occurs near the wrist joint at the lower end of the radius.
comminuted fracture—bone is splintered or crushed into several pieces. A simple fracture means that a bone breaks in only one place and is therefore not comminuted.
compression fracture—bone is compressed; often occurs in vertebrae.
greenstick fracture—bone is partially broken; it breaks on one surface and only bends on the other, as when a green stick breaks; occurs in children.
impacted fracture—one fragment is driven firmly into the other.

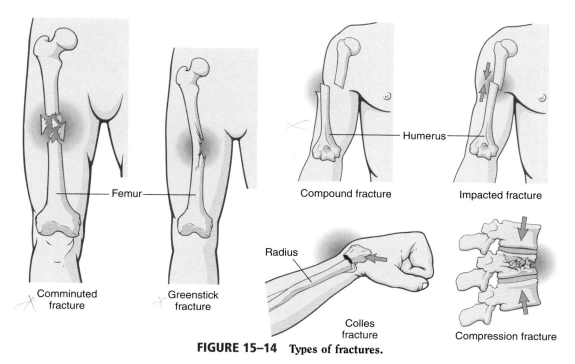

FIGURE 15–14 Types of fractures.

Treatment of fractures involves **reduction**, which is restoration of the bone to its normal position. A **closed reduction** is manipulative reduction without a surgical incision; in an **open reduction,** an incision is made into the fracture site. A **cast** (solid mold of the body part) is applied to fractures to immobilize the injured bone. The abbreviation **ORIF** means open reduction/internal fixation. Often this involves insertion of metal plates, screws, rods, or pins to stabilize the bone.

osteogenic sarcoma

Malignant tumor arising from bone (osteosarcoma).

This is the most common type of malignant bone tumor. Osteoblasts multiply, forming large, bony tumors, especially at the ends of long bones (half of the lesions are located just below or just above the knee) (Fig. 15–15). Metastasis takes place through the bloodstream, often affecting the lungs. Surgical resection followed by chemotherapy improves the survival rate.

Malignant tumors from other parts of the body (breast, prostate, lung, thyroid gland, and kidney) that metastasize to bones are **metastatic bone lesions.**

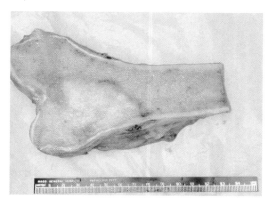

FIGURE 15–15 Osteosarcoma. The tumor has grown through the cortex of the bone and elevated the periosteum. (Courtesy of Dr. Francis Hornicek, Massachusetts General Hospital, Department of Orthopedics, Boston.)

15

osteomalacia

Softening of bone, with inadequate amounts of mineral (calcium) in the bone.

Osteomalacia occurs primarily as a disease of infancy and childhood and is then known as **rickets.** Bones fail to receive adequate amounts of calcium and phosphorus; they become soft, bend easily, and become deformed.

In affected patients, vitamin D is deficient in the diet, which prevents calcium and phosphorus from being absorbed into the bloodstream from the intestines. Vitamin D is formed by the action of sunlight on certain compounds (such as cholesterol) in the skin; thus, rickets is more common in large, smoky cities during the winter months.

Treatment most often consists of administration of large daily doses of vitamin D and an increase in dietary intake of calcium and phosphorus.

osteomyelitis

Inflammation of the bone and bone marrow secondary to infection.

Bacteria enter the body through a wound and spread to the bone. Children are affected most often, and the infection usually occurs near the ends of long bones of the legs and arms. Adults can be affected too, usually as the result of an open fracture.

The lesion begins as an inflammation with pus collection. Pus tends to spread down the medullary cavity and outward to the periosteum. Antibiotic therapy corrects the condition if the infection is treated quickly. If treatment is delayed, an **abscess** can form. An abscess is a walled-off area of infection that can be difficult or impossible to penetrate with antibiotics. Surgical drainage of an abscess usually is necessary.

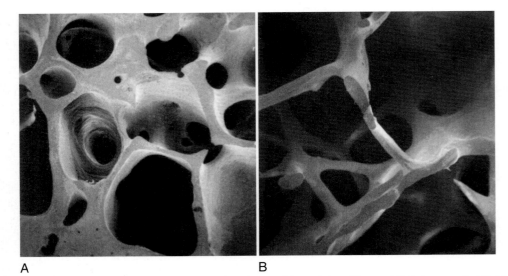

A   B

FIGURE 15–16   Scanning electron micrographs of **normal bone (A)** and **bone with osteoporosis (B)**. Notice the thinning and wide separation of the trabeculae in the osteoporotic bone. (From Dempster DW, Shane E, Horbert W, et al: A simple method for correlative light and scanning electron microscopy of human iliac crest bone biopsies: qualitative observations in normal and osteoporotic subjects. J Bone Miner Res 1:15, 1986.)

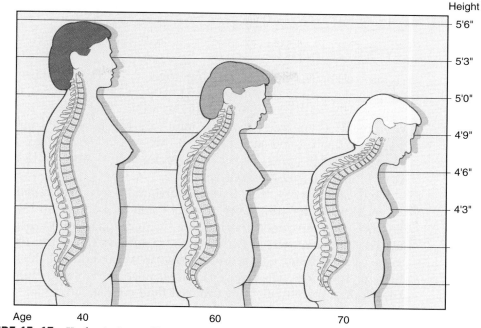

FIGURE 15–17 **Kyphosis.** Loss of bone mass due to osteoporosis produces posterior curvature of the spine in the thoracic region. A normal spine is shown at 40 years of age, and osteoporotic changes are illustrated at 60 and at 70 years of age. The changes in the spine can cause a loss of as much as 6 to 9 inches in height.

osteoporosis

Decrease in bone density (mass); thinning and weakening of bone.

This condition also is called **osteopenia** because the interior of bones is diminished in structure, as if the steel skeleton of a building had rusted and deteriorated (Fig. 15–16). Osteoporosis commonly occurs in older women as a consequence of estrogen deficiency with menopause. Lack of estrogen promotes excessive bone resorption (osteoclast activity) and less bone deposition. Weakened bones are subject to fractures (as in the hip); loss of height and kyphosis occur as vertebrae collapse (Fig. 15–17).

Estrogen replacement therapy and increased intake of calcium may be helpful for some patients. A weight-bearing daily exercise program also is important, as is the avoidance of smoking. Bisphosphonates (Fosamax) may be taken to decrease osteoclast activity and increase bone mineral content.

Osteoporosis can occur with atrophy caused by disuse, as in a limb that is in a cast, in the legs of a paraplegic, or in a bedridden patient. It also may occur in men as part of the aging process and in patients who have received corticosteroid (hormones made by the adrenal gland and used to treat inflammatory conditions) therapy.

talipes

Congenital abnormality of the hindfoot (involving the talus).

Talipes (Latin *talus* = ankle, *pes* = foot) is a congenital anomaly (abnormal positioning of the fetus in the womb). The most common form is **talipes equinovarus** (**equin/o** means horse), or **clubfoot.** The infant cannot stand with the sole of the foot flat on the ground. The defect can be corrected by orthopedic splinting in the early months of infancy or, if that fails, by surgery.

JOINTS

TYPES OF JOINTS

A joint (articulation) is a coming together of two or more bones. Some joints are immovable, such as the **suture joints** between the skull bones. Other joints, such as those between the vertebrae, are partially movable. Most joints, however, allow considerable movement. These freely movable joints are called **synovial joints.** Examples of synovial joints are the ball-and-socket type (the hip and shoulder joints) and the hinge type (elbow, knee, and ankle joints). Label the structures in Figure 15–18 as you read the following description of a synovial joint.

The bones in a synovial joint are surrounded by a **joint capsule** [1] composed of fibrous tissue. **Ligaments** (thickened fibrous bands of connective tissue) anchor one bone to another and thereby add considerable strength to the joint capsule in critical areas. Bones at the joint are covered with a smooth surface called the **articular cartilage** [2]. The **synovial membrane** [3] lies under the joint capsule and lines the **synovial cavity** [4] between the bones. The synovial cavity is filled with a special lubricating fluid produced by the synovial membrane. This **synovial fluid** contains water and nutrients that nourish as well as lubricate the joints so that friction on the articular cartilage is minimal.

BURSAE

Bursae (singular: **bursa**) are closed sacs of synovial fluid lined with a synovial membrane and are located near but not within a joint. Bursae are present wherever two types of tissue are closely opposed and need to slide past one another with as little friction as possible. Bursae serve as layers of lubrication between the tissues. Common sites of bursae are between **tendons** (connective tissue that connects a muscle to bone) and bones, between **ligaments** (connective tissue binding bone to bone) and bones, and between skin and bones in areas where bony anatomy is prominent.

Some common locations of bursae are at the elbow joint (olecranon bursa), knee joint (prepatellar bursa), and shoulder joint (subacromial bursa). Figure 15–19, *A*, shows a lateral view of the knee joint with bursae. Figure 15–19, *B*, is a frontal view of the knee showing ligaments that provide stability for the joint.

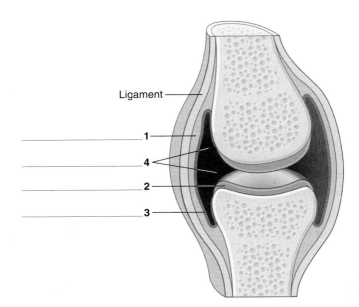

Ligament

1
4
2
3

FIGURE 15–18   Structure of a synovial joint.

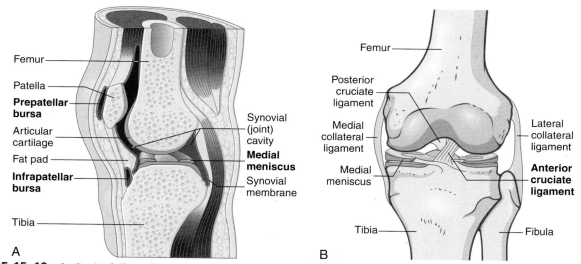

FIGURE 15–19   A, Sagittal (lateral) section of the knee showing bursae and other structures. A **meniscus** (pl., menisci) is a crescent-shaped piece of cartilage that acts as a protective cushion in a synovial joint such as the knee. A "torn cartilage" in the knee is a damaged meniscus and is frequently repaired with arthroscopic surgery. **B, Frontal view of the knee.** Notice the **anterior cruciate ligament (ACL),** which may be damaged ("torn ligament") with knee injury. Reconstruction of the ACL can require extensive surgery, and months of physical therapy may be required before return of normal function.

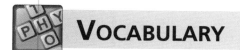 # VOCABULARY

This list reviews many new terms introduced in the text. Short definitions reinforce your understanding of the terms. Refer to the Pronunciation of Terms section for help with unfamiliar or difficult terms.

articulation	Any joint.
bursa (*plural:* **bursae**)	Sac of fluid near a joint; promotes smooth sliding of one tissue against another.
ligament	Connective tissue binding bones to other bones; supports, strengthens, and stabilizes the joint.
suture joint	Joint in which apposed surfaces are closely united; motion is minimal.
synovial cavity	Space between bones at a synovial joint; contains synovial fluid produced by the synovial membrane.
synovial fluid	Viscous (sticky) fluid within the synovial cavity. Synovial fluid is similar in viscosity to egg white; this accounts for the origin of the term (syn- means like, ov/o means egg).
synovial joint	A freely movable joint.
synovial membrane	Membrane lining the synovial cavity; it produces synovial fluid.
tendon	Connective tissue that binds muscles to bones.

COMBINING FORMS AND SUFFIXES

15

Write the meanings of the medical terms in the spaces provided.

COMBINING FORMS

Combining Form	Meaning	Terminology	Meaning
ankyl/o	stiff	ankylosis	

*A fusion of bones across a joint space by either bone tissue (**bony ankylosis**) or growth of fibrous tissue (**fibrous ankylosis**). Immobility and stiffening of the joint result; this most often occurs in rheumatoid arthritis.*

arthr/o	joint	arthroplasty	

Replacement arthroplasty is replacement of one or both bone ends by a prosthesis (artificial part) of metal or plastic. See page 596.

	arthrotomy	
	hemarthrosis	
	hydrarthrosis	

Synovial fluid collects abnormally in the joint.

	polyarthritis	

Combining Form	Meaning	Terminology	Meaning
articul/o	joint	articular cartilage	
burs/o	bursa	bursitis	

Causes of this periarticular condition may be related to stress placed on the bursa or to diseases such as gout or rheumatoid arthritis. The bursa becomes inflamed and movement is limited and painful. Intrabursal injection of corticosteroids and also rest and splinting of the limb are helpful in treatment.

Combining Form	Meaning	Terminology	Meaning
chondr/o	cartilage	achondroplasia	

This is an inherited condition in which the bones of the arms and legs fail to grow to normal size because of a defect in cartilage and bone formation. Dwarfism results, with short limbs and a normal-sized head and trunk. See page 86.

	chondroma	
	chondromalacia	

***Chondromalacia patellae** is a softening and roughening of the articular cartilaginous surface of the kneecap, resulting in pain, a grating sensation, and mechanical "catching" behind the patella.*

Ankylosis/Alkalosis
Ankylosis is a condition of joint stiffening or immobilization. Don't confuse this term with *alkalosis,* meaning increased alkalinity (pH) of blood and tissues.

Combining Form	Meaning	Terminology	Meaning
ligament/o	ligament	ligamentous _____	
rheumat/o	watery flow	rheumatologist _____	
		Various forms of arthritis are marked by collection of fluid in joint spaces.	
synov/o	synovial membrane	synovitis _____	
ten/o	tendon	tenorrhaphy _____	
		tenosynovitis _____	
		Synov/o here refers to the sheath (covering) around the tendon.	
tendin/o	tendon	tendinitis _____	
		Also spelled tendonitis.	

SUFFIXES

Suffix	Meaning	Terminology	Meaning
-desis	to bind, tie together	arthrodesis _____	
		Bones are fused across the joint space by surgery (artificial ankylosis). This operation is performed when a joint is very painful, unstable, or chronically infected.	
-stenosis	narrowing	spinal stenosis _____	
		Narrowing of the neural canal or nerve root canals in the lumbar spine. Symptoms (pain, paresthesias, urinary retention, bowel incontinence) come from compression of the cauda equina (nerves that spread out from the lower end of the spinal cord like a horse's tail).	

PATHOLOGIC CONDITIONS

arthritis

Inflammation of joints.

Some of the more common forms are:

1. ankylosing spondylitis

Chronic, progressive arthritis with stiffening of joints, primarily of the spine.

Bilateral sclerosis (hardening) of the sacroiliac joints is a diagnostic sign. Joint changes are similar to those seen in rheumatoid arthritis, and the condition can respond to corticosteroids and anti-inflammatory drugs.

2. gouty arthritis

Inflammation and painful swelling of joints caused by excessive uric acid in the body

A defect in the metabolism of uric acid causes too much of it to accumulate in blood **(hyperuricemia),** joints, and soft tissues near joints. The "pointy" uric acid crystals (salts) destroy the articular cartilage and damage the synovial membrane, often resulting in excruciating pain. The joint chiefly affected is the big toe; hence, the condition often is called **podagra** (pod/o means foot, -agra means excessive pain).

15

Treatment consists of drugs to lower uric acid production (allopurinol) and to prevent inflammation (colchicine and indomethacin) and a special diet that avoids foods that are rich in uric acid, such as red meats, red wines, and fermented cheeses.

3. osteoarthritis (OA)

Progressive, degenerative joint disease characterized by loss of articular cartilage and hypertrophy of bone (formation of osteophytes, or bone spurs) at articular surfaces.

This condition, also known as **degenerative joint disease,** occurs mainly in the hips and knees of older people and is marked by a narrowing of the joint space (due to loss of cartilage). Treatment consists of aspirin and other analgesics to reduce inflammation and pain and physical therapy to loosen impaired joints. Figure 15–20 compares a normal joint and those that have changes characteristic of osteoarthritis and rheumatoid arthritis.

End-stage osteoarthritis is the most common reason for joint replacement surgery (total joint arthroplasty).

4. rheumatoid arthritis (RA)

Chronic disease in which joints become inflamed and painful. It is believed to be caused by an immune (autoimmune) reaction against joint tissues, particularly against the synovial membrane.

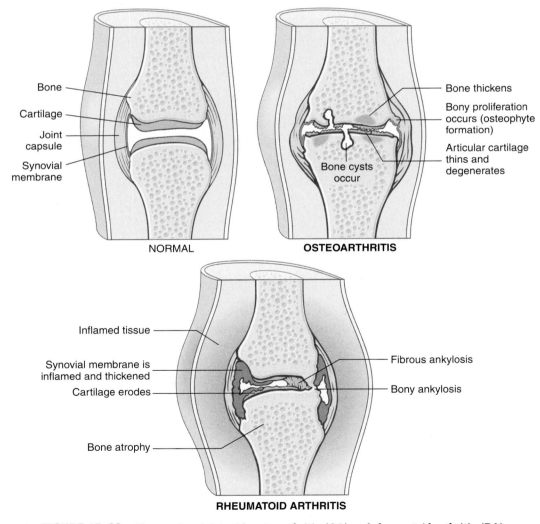

NORMAL

OSTEOARTHRITIS

- Bone
- Cartilage
- Joint capsule
- Synovial membrane

- Bone thickens
- Bony proliferation occurs (osteophyte formation)
- Articular cartilage thins and degenerates
- Bone cysts occur

RHEUMATOID ARTHRITIS

- Inflamed tissue
- Synovial membrane is inflamed and thickened
- Cartilage erodes
- Bone atrophy
- Fibrous ankylosis
- Bony ankylosis

FIGURE 15–20 Changes in a joint with **osteoarthritis (OA)** and **rheumatoid arthritis (RA).**

The small joints of the hands and feet are affected first, and larger joints later. Women are more commonly afflicted than men. Synovial membranes become inflamed and thickened, damaging the articular cartilage and preventing easy movement (see Fig. 15–20). Sometimes fibrous tissue forms and calcifies, creating a bony **ankylosis** (union) at the joint and preventing any movement at all. Swollen, painful joints accompanied by **pyrexia** (fever) are symptoms.

Diagnosis is by a blood test that shows the presence of the rheumatoid factor (an antibody) and x-ray images revealing changes around the affected joints. Treatment consists of heat applications and drugs such as aspirin or nonsteroidal anti-inflammatory drugs (NSAIDs), and corticosteroids to reduce inflammation and pain. Disease-modifying antirheumatic drugs (DMARDs) such as methotrexate and gold salts also are used.

bunion

Abnormal swelling of the medial aspect of the joint between the big toe and the first metatarsal bone.

A bursa often develops over the site, and chronic irritation from ill-fitting shoes can cause a buildup of soft tissue and underlying bone. Bunionectomy (removal of a bony exostosis and associated soft tissue) is indicated if other measures (changing shoes and use of anti-inflammatory agents) fail.

carpal tunnel syndrome (CTS)

Compression (by a wrist ligament) of the median nerve as it passes between the ligament and the bones and tendons of the wrist (the carpal tunnel) (Fig. 15–21).

This condition most often affects middle-aged women, and pain and burning sensations occur in the fingers and hand, sometimes extending to the elbow. The index (second) and long (third) fingers are affected most often, although the thumb and radial half of the ring (fourth) finger also may be symptomatic. Excessive wrist movement, arthritis, hypertrophy of bone, and swelling of the wrist can produce CTS.

Treatment consists of splinting the wrist to immobilize it, use of anti-inflammatory medications, and injection of cortisone into the carpal tunnel. If these measures fail, surgical release of the carpal ligament can be helpful.

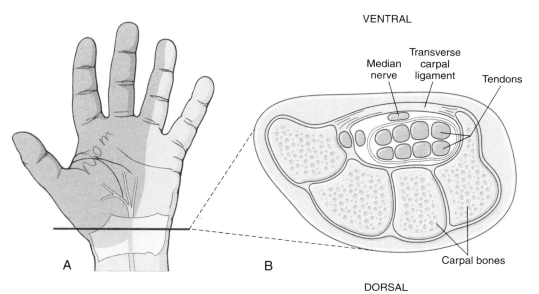

FIGURE 15–21   Carpal tunnel syndrome (CTS). A, The median nerve's sensory distribution in the thumb, first three fingers, and palm. **B,** Cross section of a right hand at the level indicated in **A.** Note the position of the median nerve between the carpal ligament and the tendons and carpal bones.

15

dislocation

Displacement of a bone from its joint.

Dislocated bones do not articulate with each other. The most common cause of dislocations is trauma. Some examples of dislocations are **acromioclavicular dislocation** (disruption of the articulation between the acromion and clavicle, also known as a shoulder separation); **shoulder dislocation** (disruption of articulation between the head of the humerus and the glenoid fossa of the scapula); and **hip dislocation** (disruption of articulation between the head of the femur and the acetabulum of the pelvis).

Treatment of dislocations involves **reduction**, which is restoration of the bones to their normal positions. A **subluxation** is a partial or incomplete dislocation.

ganglion

NO WORRY

A fluid-filled cyst arising from the joint capsule or a tendon in the wrist.

Most common in the wrist, but can occur in the shoulder, knee, hip, or ankle.

herniation of an intervertebral disk (disc)

Abnormal protrusion of a fibrocartilaginous intervertebral disk into the neural canal or spinal nerves.

This condition is commonly referred to as a **slipped disk** (disc). Pain is experienced as the protruded disk (Fig. 15–22) presses on spinal nerves or on the spinal cord. Low-back pain and **sciatica** (pain radiating down the leg) are symptoms when the disk protrudes in the lumbar spine. Neck pain and burning pain radiating down an arm are characteristic of a herniated disk in the cervical spine. Bed rest, physical therapy, and drugs for pain help in initial treatment. In patients with chronic or recurrent disk herniation, **laminectomy** (surgical removal of a portion of the vertebral arch) and open diskectomy (removal of all or part of the protruding disk) may be advised. Spinal fusion of the two vertebrae may be necessary as well. In endoscopic diskectomy the disk is removed by inserting a tube through the skin and aspirating the disk through the tube. Chemonucleolysis is injection of a disk-dissolving enzyme (such as chymopapain) into the center of a herniated disk in an effort to relieve pressure on the compressed nerve or spinal cord.

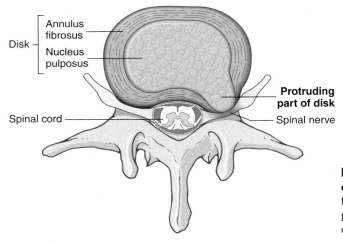

FIGURE 15–22 **Protrusion (herniation) of an intervertebral disk** (view from above the vertebra). The inner portion (nucleus pulposus) of the disk can be seen pressing on the spinal nerve.

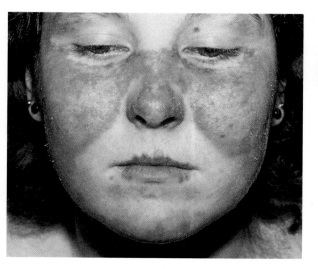

FIGURE 15–23 **Butterfly rash** that may accompany systemic lupus erythematosus. (From Lewis SM, Heitkemper MM, Dirksen SR: Medical-Surgical Nursing: Assessment and Management of Clinical Problems, 6th ed. St. Louis, Mosby, 2004, p. 1740.)

Lyme disease

A recurrent disorder marked by severe arthritis, myalgia, malaise, and neurologic and cardiac symptoms.

Also known as **Lyme arthritis.** The cause of the condition is a spirochete (bacterium) that is carried by a tick. It was first reported in Old Lyme, Connecticut, and is now found throughout the eastern coastal region of the United States. It is treated with antibiotics.

sprain

Trauma to a joint with pain, swelling, and injury to ligaments.

Sprains may also involve damage to blood vessels, muscles, tendons, and nerves. A **strain** is a less serious injury involving the overstretching of muscle. Application of ice, elevation of the joint, and application of a gentle compressive wrap are immediate measures to relieve pain and minimize swelling caused by sprains.

systemic lupus erythematosus (SLE)

Chronic inflammatory autoimmune disease involving joints, skin, kidneys, nervous system, heart, and lungs.

This condition affects connective tissue (specifically a protein component called **collagen**) in tendons, ligaments, bones, and cartilage all over the body. Typically, there is a red, scaly rash over the nose and cheeks ("butterfly" rash) (Fig. 15–23). Patients, usually women, experience joint pain in several joints (polyarthralgia), pyrexia (fever), kidney inflammation, and malaise. SLE is an autoimmune disease that is diagnosed by the presence of abnormal antibodies in the bloodstream and characteristic white blood cells called LE cells. Treatment involves giving corticosteroids, hormones made by the adrenal gland that are used to treat inflammatory conditions.

The name lupus, meaning wolf, has been used since the 13th century because affected people were thought to have the look of a wolf due to the facial changes in long-standing disease.

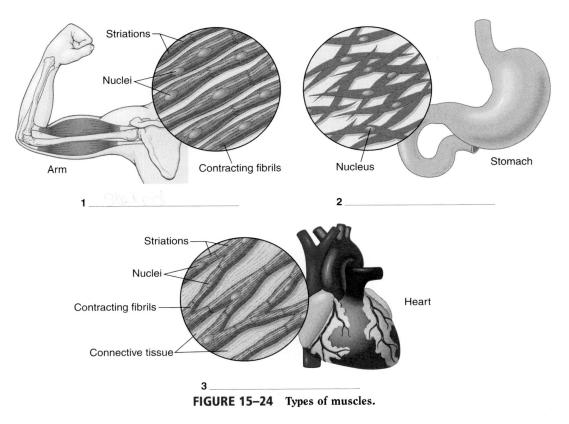

FIGURE 15–24 Types of muscles.

MUSCLES

TYPES OF MUSCLES

There are three types of muscles in the body. Label Figure 15–24 as you read the following descriptions of the various types of muscles.

Striated muscle [1] makes up the **voluntary** or **skeletal muscles** that move all bones, as well as controlling facial expression and eye movements. Through the central and peripheral nervous system, we have conscious control over these muscles. Striated muscle fibers (cells) have a pattern of dark and light bands, or fibrils, in their cytoplasm. Fibrous tissue that envelops and separates muscles is called **fascia,** which contains the muscle's blood, lymph, and nerve supply.

Smooth muscle [2] makes up the **involuntary** or **visceral muscles** that move internal organs such as the digestive tract, blood vessels, and secretory ducts leading from glands. These muscles are controlled by the autonomic nervous system. They are called smooth because they have no dark and light fibrils in their cytoplasm. Skeletal muscle fibers are arranged in bundles, whereas smooth muscle forms sheets of fibers as it wraps around tubes and vessels.

Cardiac muscle [3] is striated in appearance but is like smooth muscle in its action. Its movement cannot be consciously controlled. The fibers of cardiac muscle are branching fibers and are found in the heart.

ACTIONS OF SKELETAL MUSCLES

Skeletal (striated) muscles (more than 600 in the human body) are the muscles that move bones. Figure 15–25 shows some skeletal muscles of the head, neck, and torso and muscles of the posterior aspect of the leg. When a muscle contracts, one of the bones to which it is joined remains virtually stationary as a result of other muscles that hold it in place. The point of attachment of the muscle to the stationary bone is called the **origin (beginning)** of that muscle. When the muscle contracts, however, another bone to which it is attached does move. The point of junction of the muscle to the bone that moves is called the **insertion** of the muscle. Most often, the origin of a muscle lies proximal in the skeleton, whereas its insertion lies distal.

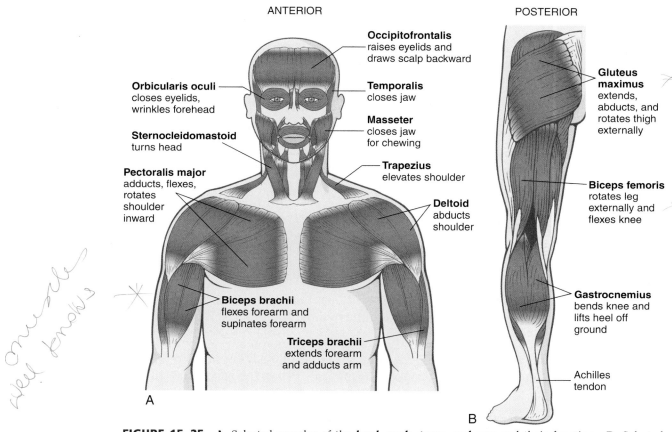

ANTERIOR

Occipitofrontalis
raises eyelids and
draws scalp backward

Orbicularis oculi
closes eyelids,
wrinkles forehead

Temporalis
closes jaw

Masseter
closes jaw
for chewing

Sternocleidomastoid
turns head

Trapezius
elevates shoulder

Pectoralis major
adducts, flexes,
rotates
shoulder
inward

Deltoid
abducts
shoulder

Biceps brachii
flexes forearm and
supinates forearm

Triceps brachii
extends forearm
and adducts arm

A

POSTERIOR

**Gluteus
maximus**
extends,
abducts, and
rotates thigh
externally

Biceps femoris
rotates leg
externally and
flexes knee

Gastrocnemius
bends knee and
lifts heel off
ground

Achilles
tendon

B

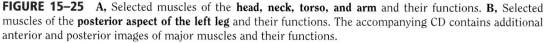

FIGURE 15–25   A, Selected muscles of the **head, neck, torso, and arm** and their functions. **B,** Selected muscles of the **posterior aspect of the left leg** and their functions. The accompanying CD contains additional anterior and posterior images of major muscles and their functions.

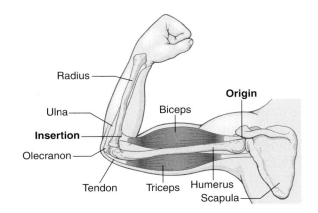

FIGURE 15–26 **Origin and insertion of the biceps in the arm.** Note also the origin of the triceps at the scapula and the insertion at the olecranon of the ulna.

Figure 15–26 shows the biceps and triceps muscles in the upper arm. One origin of the biceps is at the scapula, and its insertion is at the radius. Tendons are the connective tissue bands that connect muscles to the bones.

Muscles can perform a variety of actions. Some of the terms used to describe those actions are listed here with a short description of the specific type cf movement performed (Fig. 15–27):

Action	Meaning
flexion	Decreasing the angle between two bones; bending a limb.
extension	Increasing the angle between two bones; straightening out a limb.
abduction	Movement away from the midline of the body.
adduction	Movement toward the midline of the body.
rotation	Circular movement around an axis (central point). Internal rotation is toward the midline and external rotation is away from the midline.
dorsiflexion	Decreasing the angle of the ankle joint so that the foot bends backward (upward). This is the opposite movement of stepping on the gas pedal when driving a car.
plantar flexion	Motion that extends the foot downward toward the ground as when pointing the toes or stepping on the gas pedal. Plant/o means sole of the foot.
supination	As applied to the hand and forearm, the act of turning the palm forward, or up.
pronation	As applied to the hand and forearm, the act of turning the palm backward, or down.

know

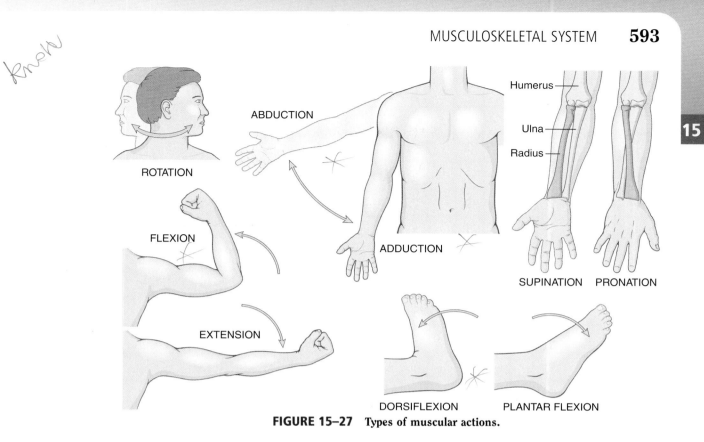

FIGURE 15–27 Types of muscular actions.

VOCABULARY

This list reviews many of the new terms introduced in the text. Short definitions reinforce your understanding of the terms. Refer to the Pronunciation of Terms section for help with unfamiliar or difficult terms.

abduction	Movement away from the midline of the body.
adduction	Movement toward the midline of the body.
dorsiflexion	Backward (upward) bending of the foot.
extension	Straightening of a flexed limb.
fascia	Fibrous membrane separating and enveloping muscles.
flexion	Bending at a joint.
insertion of a muscle	Connection of the muscle to a bone that moves.
origin of a muscle	Connection of the muscle to a stationary bone.
plantar flexion	Bending the sole of the foot downward toward the ground.
pronation	Turning the palm backward.
rotation	Circular movement around a central point.
skeletal muscle	Muscle connected to bones; voluntary or striated muscle.
smooth muscle	Muscle connected to internal organs; involuntary or visceral muscle.
striated muscle	Skeletal muscle.
supination	Turning the palm forward.
visceral muscle	Smooth muscle.

COMBINING FORMS, SUFFIXES, AND PREFIXES

15 Write the meanings of the medical terms in the spaces provided.

COMBINING FORMS

Combining Form	Meaning	Terminology	Meaning
fasci/o	fascia (forms sheaths enveloping muscles)	fasciectomy	_fascia removal_
fibr/o	fibrous connective tissue	fibromyalgia _fibrous conective tissue pain_ *Chronic pain and stiffness in muscles, joints, and fibrous tissue, especially of the back, shoulders, neck, hips, and knees. Fatigue is a common complaint.*	
leiomy/o	smooth (visceral) muscle that lines the walls of internal organs	leiomyoma leiomyosarcoma	
my/o	muscle	myalgia _muscle pain_ electromyography myopathy	
myocardi/o	heart muscle	myocardial _pertaining to the heart muscle_	
myos/o	muscle	myositis	
plant/o	sole of the foot	plantar flexion	
rhabdomy/o	skeletal (striated) muscle connected to bones	rhabdomyoma _skeletal muscle tumor_ rhabdomyosarcoma	

SUFFIXES

Suffix	Meaning	Terminology	Meaning
-asthenia	lack of strength	myasthenia gravis *Muscles lose strength because of a failure in transmission of the nervous impulse from the nerve to the muscle cell.*	
-trophy	development, nourishment	atrophy _without development_ *Decrease in size of an organ or tissue.* hypertrophy *Increase in size of an organ or tissue.*	

Suffix	Meaning	Terminology	Meaning
		amyotrophic _____	

In **amyotrophic lateral sclerosis** *(Lou Gehrig disease), muscles are affected (paralysis occurs) by degeneration of nerves in the spinal cord and lower region of the brain.*

PREFIXES

Prefix	Meaning	Terminology	Meaning
ab-	away from	abduction _movement away from the_____	

Duct/o means to lead.

ad-	toward	adduction _____	
dorsi-	back	dorsiflexion _____	
poly-	many, much	polymyalgia _____	

Polymyalgia rheumatica *is a syndrome marked by aching and morning stiffness in the shoulder, hip, or neck for more than one month.*

PATHOLOGIC CONDITIONS

muscular dystrophy	**A group of inherited diseases characterized by progressive weakness and degeneration of muscle fibers without involvement of the nervous system.** **Duchenne muscular dystrophy** is the most common form. Muscles appear to enlarge **(pseudohypertrophy)** as fat replaces functional muscle cells that have degenerated and atrophied. Onset of muscle weakness occurs soon after birth, and diagnosis can be made by muscle biopsy and electromyography.
polymyositis	**Chronic inflammatory myopathy.** This condition is marked by symmetrical muscle weakness and pain, often accompanied by a rash around the eyes and on the face and limbs. Evidence that polymyositis is an autoimmune disorder is growing stronger, and some patients recover completely with immunosuppressive therapy.

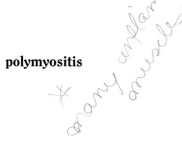

LABORATORY TESTS AND CLINICAL PROCEDURES

LABORATORY TESTS

antinuclear antibody test (ANA)	**Detects an antibody present in serum of patients with systemic lupus erythematosus (SLE).** _lupus_
erythrocyte sedimentation rate (ESR)	**Measures the rate at which erythrocytes settle to the bottom of a test tube.** Elevated ESR is associated with inflammatory disorders such as rheumatoid arthritis, tumors, and infections, and with chronic infections of bone and soft tissue.

rheumatoid factor test (RF)	**Serum is tested for the presence of an antibody found in patients with rheumatoid arthritis.**
serum calcium (Ca)	**Measurement of calcium level in serum.**
	Hypercalcemia may be caused by disorders of the parathyroid gland and malignancy that affects bone metabolism. Hypocalcemia is seen in critically ill patients with burns, sepsis, and acute renal failure.
serum creatine kinase (CK)	**Measurement of an enzyme (creatine kinase) in serum.**
	This enzyme normally is present in skeletal and cardiac muscle. Increased levels occur in muscular dystrophy, polymyositis, and traumatic injuries.
uric acid test	**Measurement of uric acid in serum.**
	High levels are associated with gouty arthritis.

CLINICAL PROCEDURES

arthrocentesis	**Surgical puncture to remove fluid from the joint space.**
	Synovial fluid is removed for analysis.
arthrography	**Process of taking x-ray images after injection of contrast material into the joint.**
arthroplasty	**Surgical repair of a joint.**
	Total hip arthroplasty or **total hip replacement (THR)** is replacement of the femoral head and acetabulum with prostheses that are fastened into the bone (Fig. 15–28).

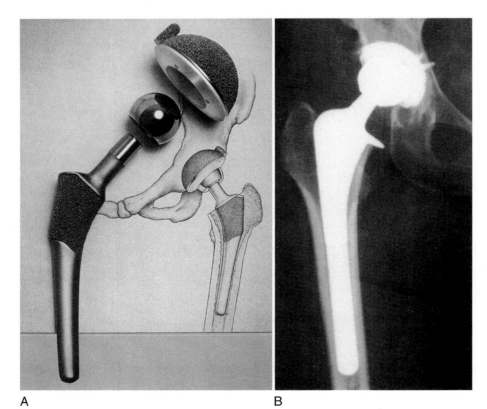

A   B

FIGURE 15–28   A, Acetabular and femoral components of a total hip arthroplasty. **B,** Radiograph showing a hip after a **Charnley total hip arthroplasty.** (**A** from Jebson LR, Coons DD: Total hip arthroplasty. Surg Technol October 1998. **B** from Mercier LR: Practical Orthopedics, 5th ed. St. Louis, Mosby, 2000, p. 237.)

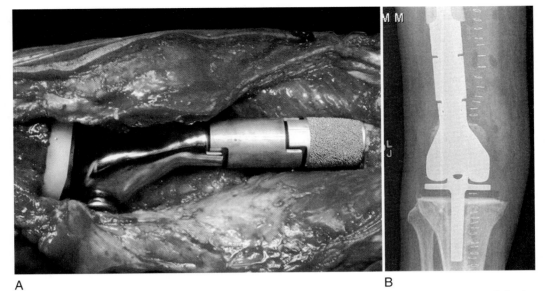

A   B

FIGURE 15–29 **A, Total knee replacement (TKR)** with prosthesis in place. **B,** X-ray image of the knee obtained during TKR surgery. (Courtesy of Dr. Francis Hornichek, Massachusetts General Hospital, Department of Orthopedics, Boston.)

In a **total knee replacement (TKR)** a metal prosthesis covers the end of the femur and a tibial component made of metal and plastic covers the tip end of the tibia. See Figure 15-29, *A* and *B.*

arthroscopy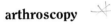

Visual examination of the inside of a joint with an endoscope and television camera.

An orthopedist passes small surgical instruments into a joint (knee, shoulder, ankle) to remove and repair damaged tissue (Fig. 15–30).

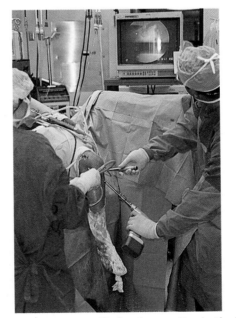

FIGURE 15–30 **Knee arthroscopy in progress.** Notice the monitor in the background. An arthroscope is used in the diagnosis of pathologic changes. (From Miller MD, Howard RF, Plancher KD: Surgical Atlas of Sports Medicine, Philadelphia, WB Saunders, 2003, p. 53.)

bone density test (bone densitometry)	**Low-energy x-ray absorption in bones of the spinal column, pelvis, and wrist to measure bone mass.** An x-ray detector measures how well x-rays penetrate through bones. See Figure 15-31. Areas of decreased density indicate osteopenia and osteoporosis. Also called **dual-energy x-ray absorptiometry (DEXA** or DXA).
bone scan	**Uptake of a radioactive substance is measured in bone.** A nuclear medicine physician uses a special scanning device to detect areas of increased uptake (tumors, infection, inflammation, stress fractures). See Figure 15–32.
computed tomography (CT)	**X-ray beam is used with a computer to provide cross-sectional images.** CT scans identify soft tissue abnormalities, bone abnormalities, and musculoskeletal trauma.
diskography	**X-ray examination of cervical or lumbar intervertebral disk after injection of contrast into nucleus pulposus (interior of the disk).**

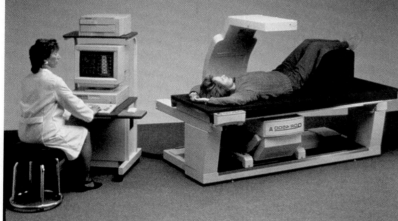

FIGURE 15–31 Patient undergoing a **bone density test** using **dual energy x-ray absorptiometry** (DEXA or DXA). (From Greer I, et al: Mosby's Color Atlas and Text of Obstetrics and Gynecology. London, Mosby, 2001.)

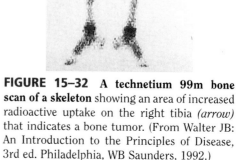

FIGURE 15–32 A technetium 99m bone scan of a skeleton showing an area of increased radioactive uptake on the right tibia *(arrow)* that indicates a bone tumor. (From Walter JB: An Introduction to the Principles of Disease, 3rd ed. Philadelphia, WB Saunders, 1992.)

electromyography (EMG)   Process of recording the strength of muscle contraction as a result of electrical stimulation.

magnetic resonance imaging (MRI)   Radio waves and a magnetic field create images of soft tissue.

muscle biopsy   Removal of muscle tissue for microscopic examination.

ABBREVIATIONS

AC joint	acromioclavicular joint	**LE cell**	lupus erythematosus cell
ACL	anterior cruciate ligament of the knee	**NSAID**	nonsteroidal anti-inflammatory drug—often prescribed to treat joint disorders
ANA	antinuclear antibody—indicator of systemic lupus erythematosus	**ORIF**	open reduction (of fracture)/internal fixation
C1–C7	cervical vertebrae	**Ortho**	orthopedics (or orthopaedics)
Ca	calcium	**OT**	occupational therapy
CK	creatine kinase—enzyme elevated in muscle disease	**P**	phosphorus
CTS	carpal tunnel syndrome	**PT**	physical therapy
DEXA or **DXA**	dual-energy x-ray absorptiometry—a test of bone density	**RA**	rheumatoid arthritis
		RF	rheumatoid factor
DMARD	disease-modifying antirheumatic drug	**ROM**	range of motion
DO	doctor of osteopathy	**sed rate**	erythrocyte sedimentation rate
DTRs	deep tendon reflexes	**SLE**	systemic lupus erythematosus
EMG	electromyography	**T1–T12**	thoracic vertebrae
ESR	erythrocyte sedimentation rate—indicates inflammation	**TKR**	total knee replacement
		THR	total hip replacement
IM	intramuscular	**TMJ**	temporomandibular joint
L1–L5	lumbar vertebrae		

PRACTICAL APPLICATIONS

15

This section contains an x-ray report and an orthopedic operating room schedule. Answers to matching questions are found on page 614.

MEDICAL REPORT: RESULTS OF CHEST X-RAY EXAMINATION

PA [posteroanterior] and lateral chest: The heart is enlarged in its transverse diameter. The lungs are fully expanded and free of active disease.

Thoracic spine shows a scoliosis of the upper thoracic spine convex to the left. There is 50 percent wedge compression fracture of T6 and slight wedge compression fracture of T5. There is also anterior wedge compression fracture of T12.

Lumbar spine shows 90 percent compression fractures of L1 and L3 with 30 percent compression fractures of L2 and L5. All bones are markedly osteoporotic. There is calcification within the aortic arch. There are gallstones in the right upper quadrant. The findings in the spine are most compatible with osteoporotic compression fractures. During the procedure, the patient had a sickable* episode and fell, striking her head. A skull series, done at no cost to the patient, shows no evidence of bony fracture. The pineal gland is calcified and has a midline location. The sella turcica is normal.

---

*This word was incorrectly transcribed. The correct term is syncopal.

OPERATING ROOM SCHEDULE

Match the operation in Column I with an accompanying diagnosis or indication for surgery from Column II.

Column I

1. Excision, osteochondroma, R calcaneus _____

2. TMJ arthroscopy with probable arthrotomy _____

3. L4–5 laminectomy and diskectomy _____

4. Arthroscopy, left knee _____

5. Open reduction, malleolar fracture _____

6. R occipital craniotomy with tumor resection _____

7. Excision, distal end right clavicle, with prob. acromioplasty _____

8. Acetabuloplasty with open reduction hip _____

Column II

A. Fracture of the ankle
B. ACL rupture
C. Neoplastic lesion in brain
D. Exostosis on heel bone
E. Pelvic fracture
F. Pain and malocclusion of jaw bones
G. Lower back pain radiating down one leg
H. Pain in shoulder joint with bone spur (exostosis) evident on x-ray

![?] **EXERCISES**

Remember to check your answers carefully with those given in the Answers to Exercises, page 611.

A. Complete the following sentences.

1. Bones are composed of bony connective tissue called _____ tissue.

2. Bone cells are called _____.

3. The bones of a fetus are composed mainly of _____.

4. During bone development, immature bone cells called _____ produce bony tissue.

5. Large bone cells called _____ digest bone tissue to shape the bone and smooth it out.

6. Two mineral substances necessary for proper development of bones are

   _____ and _____.

7. A round, small bone resembling a sesame seed in shape and covering the knee joint is called a/an

   _____ bone.

8. The shaft of a long bone is called the _____.

9. The ends of a long bone are called the _____.

10. The cartilaginous area at the end of a long bone where growth takes place is called the

    _____.

11. Red bone marrow is found in spongy or _____ bone.

12. Yellow bone marrow is composed of _____ tissue.

13. The strong membrane surrounding the surface of a bone is the _____.

14. Hard, dense bone tissue lying under the periosteum is _____.

15. A series of canals containing blood vessels lie within the outer dense tissue of bone and are called

    the _____ canals.

16. A thin layer of cartilage covering the ends of bones at the joints is _____.

17. The _____ is a central, hollowed-out area in the shaft of long bones.

18. A physician who treats bones and bone diseases is a/an _____.

19. A practitioner who uses his or her hands to manipulate the patient's spinal column (in the belief

    that diseases are caused by pressure on spinal nerves) is a/an _____.

20. A doctor who treats patients based on the belief that the body can be healed when bones are in

    proper position and adequate nutrition is provided is a/an _____.

15

B. Give a short description of each term.

1. metaphysis _____

2. sinus _____

3. tubercle _____

4. condyle _____

5. fossa _____

6. tuberosity _____

7. trochanter _____

8. foramen _____

9. fissure _____

10. bone head _____

C. Match the following cranial and facial bones with their meanings as given below.

ethmoid bone	mandible	occipital bone	temporal bone
frontal bone	maxilla	parietal bone	vomer
lacrimal bones	nasal bone	sphenoid bone	zygomatic bone

1. forms the roof and upper side parts of the skull _____

2. delicate bone, composed of spongy, cancellous tissue; supports the nasal cavity and orbits of the

   eye _____

3. forms the back and base of the skull _____

4. forms the forehead _____

5. bat-shaped bone extending behind the eyes to form the base of the skull _____

6. bone near the ear and connecting to the lower jaw _____

7. cheekbone _____

8. bone that supports the bridge of the nose _____

9. thin, flat bone forming the lower portion of the nasal septum _____

10. lower jawbone _____

11. upper jawbone _____

12. two paired bones, one located at the corner of each eye _____

D. Name the five divisions of the spinal column.

1. _____

2. _____

3. _____

4. _____

5. _____

E. Identify the following parts associated with a vertebra.

1. space through which the spinal cord passes _____

2. piece of cartilage between each vertebra _____

3. posterior part of a vertebra _____

4. anterior part of a vertebra _____

F. Give the medical names of the following bones.

1. shoulder blade _____

2. upper arm bone _____

3. breastbone _____

4. thigh bone _____

5. finger bones _____

6. hand bones _____

7. lower arm bone (little finger side) _____

8. lower arm bone (thumb side) _____

9. collar bone _____

10. wrist bones _____

11. backbone _____

12. kneecap _____

13. shin bone (larger of two lower leg bones) _____

14. smaller of two lower leg bones _____

15. three parts of the pelvis _____, _____, and

_____

16. midfoot bones _____

15

G. Give the meanings of the following terms associated with bones.

1. foramen magnum _____

2. calcaneus _____

3. acromion _____

4. xiphoid process _____

5. lamina _____

6. malleolus _____

7. acetabulum _____

8. pubic symphysis _____

9. olecranon _____

10. fontanelle _____

11. mastoid process _____

12. styloid process _____

H. Give the meanings of the following terms.

1. osteogenesis _____

2. hypercalcemia _____

3. spondylosis _____

4. epiphyseal _____

5. decalcification _____

6. ossification _____

7. osteitis _____

8. costoclavicular _____

I. Build medical terms for the following definitions.

1. pertaining to the shoulder blade _____

2. instrument to cut the skull _____

3. pertaining to the upper arm bone _____

4. pertaining to below the kneecap _____

5. softening of cartilage _____

6. pertaining to a toe bone _____

7. removal of hand bones _____

8. pertaining to the shin bone _____

9. pertaining to the heel bone _____

10. poor bone development _____

11. removal of the lamina of the vertebral arch _____

12. pertaining to the sacrum and ilium _____

J. Give medical terms for the following.

1. formation of bone marrow _____

2. clubfoot _____

3. humpback _____

4. high levels of calcium in the blood _____

5. benign tumors arising from the bone surface _____

6. brittle bone disease _____

7. lateral curvature of the spine _____

8. anterior curvature of the spine _____

9. forward slipping (subluxation) of a vertebra over a lower vertebra _____

10. instrument to cut bone _____

K. Match the term in Column I with its description in Column II. Write the letter of the description in the space provided.

Column I

1. greenstick fracture   _____

2. closed fracture   _____

3. comminuted fracture   _____

4. compound (open) fracture   _____

5. Colles fracture   _____

6. cast   _____

7. open reduction   _____

8. closed reduction   _____

9. impacted fracture   _____

10. compression fracture   _____

Column II

A. Fracture of the lower end of the radius at the wrist.

B. Break in bone with wound in the skin.

C. One side of the bone is fractured; the other side is bent.

D. Bone is put in proper place without incision of skin.

E. Mold of the bone applied to fractures to immobilize the injured bone.

F. Bone is broken by pressure from another bone; often in vertebrae, bone is partially flattened.

G. Bone is splintered or crushed.

H. Bone is put in proper place after incision through the skin.

I. Bone is broken and one side of the fracture is wedged into the other.

J. Break in the bone without an open skin wound.

L. Give the meanings of the following terms.

1. osteoporosis _____

2. osteomyelitis _____

3. osteogenic sarcoma _____

4. crepitus _____

5. osteomalacia _____

6. abscess _____

7. osteopenia _____

8. Ewing sarcoma _____

9. metastatic bone lesion _____

M. Complete the following sentences.

1. A joint in which apposed bones are closely united as in the skull bones is called a/an

   _____.

2. Connective tissue that binds muscles to bones is a/an _____.

3. Another term for a joint is a/an _____.

4. Connective tissue that binds bones to other bones is a/an _____.

5. Fluid found in a joint is called _____.

6. The membrane that lines the joint cavity is the _____.

7. A sac of fluid near a joint is a/an _____.

8. Smooth cartilage that covers the surface of bones at joints is _____.

9. Surgical repair of a joint is called _____.

10. Inflammation surrounding a joint is known as _____.

N. Complete the following terms based on the definitions provided.

1. inflammation of a tendon: _____itis

2. tumor (benign) of cartilage: _____oma

3. tumor (malignant) of cartilage: _____oma

4. incision of a joint: arthr_____

5. softening of cartilage: chondro_____

6. abnormal condition of blood in the joint: _____osis

7. inflammation of a sac of fluid near the joint: _____itis

8. a doctor who specializes in treatment of joint disorders: _____logist

9. abnormal condition of a stiffened, immobile joint: _____osis

10. suture of a tendon: ten_____

O. Select from the following terms to name the abnormal conditions below.

achondroplasia   dislocation   osteoarthritis
ankylosing spondylitis ganglion   rheumatoid arthritis
bunion   gouty arthritis   systemic lupus erythematosus
carpal tunnel syndrome Lyme disease   tenosynovitis

1. an inherited condition in which the bones of the arms and the legs fail to grow normally because

   of a defect in cartilage and bone formation; type of dwarfism _____

2. degenerative joint disease; chronic inflammation of bones and joints _____

3. inflammation of joints caused by excessive uric acid in the body (hyperuricemia)

   _____

4. chronic joint disease; inflamed and painful joints owing to autoimmune reaction against normal

   joint tissue, and synovial membranes become swollen and thickened _____

5. tick-borne bacterium causes this condition marked by arthritis, myalgia, malaise, and neurologic

   and cardiac symptoms _____

6. abnormal swelling of a metatarsophalangeal joint _____

7. cystic mass arising from a tendon in the wrist _____

8. chronic, progressive arthritis with stiffening of joints, especially of the spine (vertebrae)

   _____

9. chronic inflammatory disease affecting not only the joints but also the skin (butterfly rash on the

   face), kidneys, heart, and lungs _____

10. inflammation of a tendon sheath _____

11. compression of the median nerve in the wrist as it passes through an area between a ligament and

    tendons, bones, and connective tissue _____

12. displacement of a bone from its joint _____

P. Give the meanings of the following terms.

1. subluxation _____

2. arthrodesis _____

3. pyrexia _____

15

4. podagra _____

5. sciatica _____

6. herniation of an intervertebral disk _____

7. laminectomy _____

8. sprain _____

9. strain _____

10. hyperuricemia _____

Q. Circle the term that best fits the given definition.

1. fibrous membrane separating and enveloping muscles: **(fascia, flexion)**

2. movement away from the midline of the body: **(abduction, adduction)**

3. connection of the muscle to a stationary bone: **(insertion, origin)** of the muscle

4. connection of the muscle to a bone that moves: **(insertion, origin)** of the muscle

5. muscle that is connected to internal organs; involuntary muscle: **(skeletal, visceral)** muscle

6. muscle that is connected to bones; voluntary muscle: **(skeletal, visceral)** muscle

7. pain of many muscles: **(myositis, polymyalgia)**

8. pertaining to heart muscle: **(myocardial, myasthenia)**

9. process of recording electricity within muscles: **(muscle biopsy, electromyography)**

10. increase in development (size) of an organ or tissue: **(hypertrophy, atrophy)**

R. Match the term for muscle action in Column I with its meaning in Column II. Write the letter of your answer in the space provided.

Column I

1. extension _____

2. rotation _____

3. flexion _____

4. adduction _____

5. supination _____

6. abduction _____

7. pronation _____

8. dorsiflexion _____

9. plantar flexion _____

Column II

A. Movement away from the midline
B. Turning the palm backward
C. Turning the palm forward
D. Straightening out a limb or joint
E. Bending the sole of the foot downward
F. Circular movement around an axis
G. Bending a limb
H. Movement toward the midline
I. Backward (upward) bending of the foot

S. Give the meanings of the following abnormal conditions affecting muscles.

1. leiomyosarcoma _____

2. rhabdomyoma _____

3. polymyositis _____

4. fibromyalgia _____

5. muscular dystrophy_____

6. myasthenia gravis _____

7. amyotrophic lateral sclerosis _____

T. Match the term in Column I with its meaning in Column II. Write the letter of your answer in the space provided.

Column I

1. antinuclear antibody test _____
2. serum creatine kinase _____
3. uric acid test _____
4. rheumatoid factor test _____
5. bone scan _____
6. muscle biopsy _____
7. arthroscopy _____
8. acetylcholine _____
9. calcium _____
10. arthrography _____

Column II

A. Radioactive substance is injected and traced in dense, hard connective tissue.
B. Chemical found in myoneural space.
C. Test for presence of an antibody found in the serum of patients with rheumatoid arthritis.
D. Substance necessary for proper bone development.
E. Visual examination of a joint.
F. Test tells if patient has gouty arthritis.
G. Test tells if patient has systemic lupus erythematosus.
H. Removal of soft connective tissue for microscopic examination.
I. Process of taking x-ray pictures of a joint.
J. Elevated blood levels of this enzyme are found in muscular disorders.

U. Circle the term that best completes the meaning of the sentence.

1. Selma, a 40-year-old secretary, had been complaining of wrist pain with tingling sensations in her fingers for months. Dr. Ayres diagnosed her condition as **(osteomyelitis, rheumatoid arthritis, carpal tunnel syndrome)**.

2. Daisy tripped while playing tennis and landed on her hand. She had excruciating pain, which was due to a **(Ewing, Colles, pathologic)** fracture that required casting.

3. In her fifties, Estelle started hunching over more and more. Her doctor realized that she was developing **(gouty arthritis, osteoarthritis, osteoporosis)** and prescribed calcium pills and exercise.

4. Paul had a skiing accident and tore ligaments in his knee. Dr. Miller recommended **(electromyography, hypertrophy, arthroscopic surgery)** to repair the ligaments.

15

5. For several months after her first pregnancy Elsie noticed a red rash on her face and cheeks. Her joints were giving her pain and she had a slight fever. Her ANA was elevated and her doctor suspected that she had **(SLE, polymyositis, muscular dystrophy)**.

6. David injured his left knee while playing basketball. He was scheduled for arthroscopic repair of his **(ACL, SLE, TMJ)**. However, because his ligament was so long, his **(rheumatologist, orthopedist, chiropractor)** decided to do "open" surgery.

7. James has significant lower back pain radiating down his left leg. MRI shows an intervertebral **(disk, bunion, exostosis)** impinging on spinal nerves at the **(L5–S1, C2–C3, T3–T5)** level. Bed rest produced no improvement. His orthopedist decided to perform a **(tenorrhaphy, laminectomy, bunionectomy)** to relieve pressure on his nerves.

8. Bruce spent two weeks hiking and vacationing on Nantucket Island. A week later he developed a bull's-eye rash on his chest (from a tick bite), fever, muscle pain, and a swollen, tender right ankle. His physician ordered a blood test that revealed **(antigens, antibodies)** to a spirochete bacterium. The physician told Bruce he had contracted **(ankylosing spondylitis, polymyositis, Lyme disease)**.

9. Scott likes to eat rich food. Lately he has noticed pain and tenderness in his right toe, called **(talipes, podagra, rickets)**, and also deposits of hard lumps over his elbows. His doctor orders a serum uric acid test; the result is abnormally high, revealing **(hemarthrosis, hyperuricemia, hypercalcemia)**, consistent with a diagnosis of **(rheumatoid arthritis, gouty arthritis, osteoarthritis)**.

10. Sara, a 70-year-old widow, has persistent midback pain, and her **(CXR, ESR, EMG)** shows compression fractures of her **(scapula, femur, vertebrae)** and thinning of her bones. A bone density scan confirms the diagnosis of **(osteomyelitis, osteomalacia, osteoporosis)**, and her doctor prescribes calcium, vitamin D, and Fosamax.

V. Give meanings for the abbreviations in Column I. Then select the letter in Column II of the best association for each.

Column I

1. ROM _____ ____

2. NSAID _____ ____

3. TMJ _____ ____

4. EMG _____ ____

5. ACL _____ ____

6. SLE _____ ____

7. C1–C5 _____ ____

8. T1–T12 _____ ____

9. THR _____ ____

10. ORIF _____ ____

Column II

A. Connection between the lower jawbone and a bone of the skull.

B. Band of fibrous tissue connecting bones in the knee.

C. Bones of the spinal column in the chest region.

D. Test of strength of electrical transmission within muscle.

E. This autoimmune disease affects joints, skin, and other body tissues.

F. Measurement in degrees of a circle assesses the extent a joint can be flexed or extended.

G. Bones of the spinal column in the neck region.

H. Drug used to treat joint diseases.

I. Procedure to repair compound fracture

J. Arthroplasty

MEDICAL SCRAMBLE

Unscramble the letters to form musculoskeletal system–related terms from the clues. Use the letters in squares to complete the bonus term. Answers are found on page 614.

1. *Clue:* One of the jaw bones

□□_ _□_ _ _ BALMINED

2. *Clue:* One of the bones in the arm

_ _□□_ _ _ SUHEMUR

3. *Clue:* Group of bones at the tailbone of the spinal column

_□_ _□_ YCOCXC

4. *Clue:* Anterior bone of the skull

_ _□_ _ _□ TRAFOLN

BONUS TERM: *Clue:* Benign tumor of smooth muscle

□□□□□□□□□

ANSWERS TO EXERCISES

A

1. osseous
2. osteocytes
3. cartilage
4. osteoblasts
5. osteoclasts
6. calcium and phosphorus
7. sesamoid
8. diaphysis
9. epiphyses
10. epiphyseal plate
11. cancellous or trabecular
12. fat
13. periosteum
14. compact bone
15. haversian
16. articular cartilage
17. medullary cavity
18. orthopedist
19. chiropractor
20. osteopath

B

1. flared portion of a long bone that lies between the diaphysis and the epiphyseal plate
2. hollow cavity within the bone
3. rounded process for attachment of tendons and muscles
4. rounded, knuckle-like process at the joint
5. shallow cavity in or on a bone
6. rounded process for attachment of muscles and tendons
7. large process on the femur for attachment of tendons and muscles
8. opening in a bone for blood vessels and nerves
9. narrow, deep, slit-like opening
10. rounded end of a bone separated from the rest of the bone by a neck

C

1. parietal bone
2. ethmoid bone
3. occipital bone
4. frontal bone
5. sphenoid bone
6. temporal bone
7. zygomatic bone
8. nasal bone
9. vomer
10. mandible
11. maxilla
12. lacrimal bones

D

1. cervical
2. thoracic
3. lumbar
4. sacral
5. coccygeal

E

1. neural canal
2. intervertebral disk
3. vertebral arch
4. vertebral body

F

1. scapula
2. humerus
3. sternum
4. femur
5. phalanges
6. metacarpals
7. ulna
8. radius
9. clavicle
10. carpals
11. vertebral column
12. patella
13. tibia
14. fibula
15. ilium, ischium, pubis
16. metatarsals

G

1. opening of the occipital bone through which the spinal cord passes
2. heel bone; largest of the tarsal bones
3. lateral extension of the scapula
4. lower portion of the sternum
5. portion of the vertebral arch
6. the bulge on either side of the ankle joint; the lower end of the fibula is the lateral malleolus, and the lower end of the tibia is the medial malleolus
7. depression in the pelvis into which the femur fits
8. area of convergence of the two pubis bones, at the midline
9. bony process at the proximal end of the ulna; elbow joint
10. soft spot between the bones of the skull in an infant
11. round process on the temporal bone behind the ear
12. pole-like process projecting downward from the temporal bone

H

1. formation of bone; osteogenesis imperfecta is known as brittle bone disease
2. excessive calcium in the blood
3. abnormal condition of the vertebrae; degenerative changes in the spine
4. pertaining to the epiphysis
5. removal of calcium from bones
6. formation of bone
7. inflammation of bone; osteitis deformans (Paget disease) causes deformed bones such as an enlarged skull
8. pertaining to the ribs and clavicle

I

1. scapular
2. craniotome
3. humeral
4. subpatellar
5. chondromalacia
6. phalangeal
7. metacarpectomy
8. tibial
9. calcaneal
10. osteodystrophy
11. laminectomy
12. sacroiliac

J

1. myelopoiesis
2. talipes
3. kyphosis
4. hypercalcemia
5. exostoses
6. osteogenesis imperfecta
7. scoliosis
8. lordosis
9. spondylolisthesis
10. osteotome

K

1. C
2. J
3. G
4. B
5. A
6. E
7. H
8. D
9. I
10. F

L

1. increased porosity in bone; decrease in bone density
2. inflammation of bone and bone marrow
3. cancerous tumor of bone; osteoblasts multiply at the ends of long bones
4. crackling sensation as broken bones move against each other
5. softening of bones; rickets in children due to loss of calcium in bones
6. collection of pus
7. deficiency of bone; occurs in osteoporosis
8. malignant tumor of bone, often involving the entire shaft of a long bone
9. malignant tumor that has spread to bone from the breast, lung, kidney, or prostate gland

M

1. suture joint; a synovial joint is a freely movable joint
2. tendon
3. articulation
4. ligament
5. synovial fluid
6. synovial membrane
7. bursa
8. articular cartilage
9. arthroplasty
10. periarthritis

N

1. tendinitis or tendonitis
2. chondroma
3. chondrosarcoma
4. arthrotomy
5. chondromalacia
6. hemarthrosis
7. bursitis
8. rheumatologist
9. ankylosis
10. tenorrhaphy

O

1. achondroplasia
2. osteoarthritis
3. gouty arthritis
4. rheumatoid arthritis
5. Lyme disease
6. bunion
7. ganglion
8. ankylosing spondylitis
9. systemic lupus erythematosus
10. tenosynovitis
11. carpal tunnel syndrome
12. dislocation

P

1. partial or incomplete displacement of a bone from the joint
2. surgical fixation of a joint (binding it together by fusing the joint surfaces)
3. fever; increase in body temperature
4. pain in a big toe from gouty arthritis
5. pain radiating from the back to the leg (along the sciatic nerve); most commonly caused by a protruding intervertebral disk
6. protrusion of a disk into the neural canal or the spinal nerves
7. removal of a portion of the vertebral arch (lamina) to relieve pressure from a protruding intervertebral disk
8. trauma to a joint with pain, swelling, and injury to ligaments
9. overstretching of a muscle
10. high levels of uric acid in the bloodstream; present in gouty arthritis

Q

1. fascia
2. abduction
3. origin of the muscle
4. insertion of the muscle
5. visceral muscle
6. skeletal muscle
7. polymyalgia
8. myocardial
9. electromyography
10. hypertrophy

R

1. D
2. F
3. G
4. H
5. C
6. A
7. B
8. I
9. E

S

1. malignant tumor of smooth (involuntary, visceral) muscle
2. benign tumor of striated (voluntary, skeletal) muscle
3. inflammation of many muscles; polymyositis rheumatica is a chronic inflammatory condition causing muscle weakness and pain
4. pain of muscle and fibrous tissue (especially of the back); also called fibrositis or rheumatism
5. group of inherited muscular diseases marked by progressive weakness and degeneration of muscles without nerve involvement
6. loss of strength of muscles (often with paralysis) because of a defect at the connection between the nerve and the muscle cell
7. muscles degenerate (paralysis occurs) owing to degeneration of nerves in the spinal cord and lower region of the brain; Lou Gehrig disease

T

1. G	5. A	8. B
2. J	6. H	9. D
3. F	7. E	10. I
4. C		

U

1. carpal tunnel syndrome	5. SLE	9. podagra; hyperuricemia; gouty arthritis
2. Colles	6. ACL; orthopedist	10. CXR; vertebrae; osteoporosis
3. osteoporosis	7. disk; L5–S1; laminectomy	
4. arthroscopic surgery	8. antibodies; Lyme disease	

V

1. range of motion: F	5. anterior cruciate ligament: B	8. first thoracic vertebra to twelfth thoracic vertebra: C
2. nonsteroidal anti-inflammatory drug: H	6. systemic lupus erythematosus: E	9. total hip replacement: J
3. temporomandibular joint: A	7. first cervical vertebra to fifth cervical vertebra: G	10. open reduction, internal fixation: I
4. electromyography: D		

ANSWERS TO PRACTICAL APPLICATIONS

1. d	4. b	7. h
2. f	5. a	8. e
3. g	6. c	

ANSWERS TO MEDICAL SCRAMBLE

1. MANDIBLE   2. HUMERUS   3. COCCYX   4. FRONTAL
BONUS TERM: LEIOMYOMA

PRONUNCIATION OF TERMS

PRONUNCIATION GUIDE

ā as in āpe   ă as in ăpple
ē as in ēven   ĕ as in ĕvery
ī as in īce   ĭ as in ĭnterest
ō as in ōpen   ŏ as in pŏt
ū as in ūnit   ŭ as in ŭnder

To test your understanding of the terminology in this chapter, write the meaning of each term in the space provided. In addition, you may wish to cover the terms and write them by looking at your definitions. Make sure your spelling is correct. The page number after each term indicates where it is defined or used in the book, so you can easily check your responses. You will find complete definitions for all of these terms and their audio pronunciations on the CD.

TERMS RELATED TO BONES

Term	Pronunciation	Meaning
acetabulum (572)	ăs-ĕ-TĂB-ū-lŭm	_____
acromion (572)	ă-KRŌ-mē-ŏn	_____
articular cartilage (572)	ăr-TĬK-ū-lăr KĂR-tĭ-lăj	_____
calcaneal (576)	kăl-KĀ-nē-ăl	_____
calcaneus (576)	kăl-KĀ-nē-ŭs	_____
calcium (572)	KĂL-sē-ŭm	_____

Term	Pronunciation	Meaning
cancellous bone (572)	KĂN-sĕ-lŭs bōn	
carpals (576)	KĂR-pălz	
cartilage (572)	KĂR-tĭ-lăj	
cervical vertebrae (566)	SĔR-vĭ-kăl VĔR-tĕ-brā	
chondrocostal (576)	kŏn-drō-KŎS-tăl	
clavicle (576)	KLĂV-ĭ-k'l	
coccyx (567)	KŎK-sĭks	
collagen (572)	KŎL-ă-jĕn	
Colles fracture (578)	KŎL-ēz FRĂK-shŭr	
comminuted fracture (578)	KŎM-ĭ-nūt-ĕd FRĂK-shŭr	
compact bone (572)	KŎM-păkt bōn	
condyle (572)	KŎN-dīl	
cranial bones (572)	KRĀ-nē-ăl bōnz	
craniotome (577)	KRĀ-nē-ō-tōm	
craniotomy (577)	krā-nē-ŎT-ō-mē	
crepitus (578)	KRĔP-ĭ-tŭs	
decalcification (574)	dē-kăl-sĭ-fĭ-KĀ-shŭn	
diaphysis (572)	dī-ĂF-ĭ-sĭs	
epiphyseal plate (572)	ĕp-ĭ-FĬZ-ē-ăl plāt	
epiphysis (572)	ĕ-PĬF-ĭ-sĭs	
ethmoid bone (563)	ĔTH-moyd bōn	
Ewing sarcoma (578)	Ū-ĭng săr-KŌ-mă	
exostosis (578)	ĕk-sŏs-TŌ-sĭs	
facial bones (572)	FĀ-shăl bōnz	
femoral (577)	FĔM-ŏr-ăl	
femur (577)	FĒ-mŭr	
fibula (577)	FĬB-ū-lă	
fibular (577)	FĬB-ū-lăr	
fissure (572)	FĬSH-ŭr	
fontanelle (572)	fŏn-tă-NĔL	
foramen (572)	fōr-Ā-mĕn	
fossa (572)	FŎS-ă	
frontal bone (562)	FRŎN-tăl bōn	

15

Term	Pronunciation	Meaning
haversian canals (572)	hă-VĔR-shăn kă-NĂLZ	_____
humeral (577)	HŪ-mĕr-ăl	_____
humerus (577)	HŪ-mĕr-ŭs	_____
hypercalcemia (574)	hī-pĕr-kăl-SĒ-mē-ă	_____
iliac (577)	ĬL-ē-ăk	_____
ilium (577)	ĬL-ē-ŭm	_____
impacted fracture (579)	ĭm-PĂK-tĕd FRĂK-shŭr	_____
ischial (577)	ĬSH-ē-ăl or ĬS-kē-ăl	_____
ischium (577)	ĬSH-ē-ŭm or ĬS-kē-ŭm	_____
kyphosis (574)	kī-FŌ-sĭs	_____
lacrimal bones (564)	LĂ-krĭ-măl bōnz	_____
lamina (574)	LĂM-ĭ-nă	_____
laminectomy (574)	lăm-ĭ-NĔK-tō-mē	_____
lordosis (574)	lŏr-DŌ-sĭs	_____
lumbar vertebrae (567)	LŬM-băr VĔR-tĕ-brā	_____
lumbosacral (575)	lŭm-bō-SĀ-krăl	_____
malleolar (577)	mă-LĒ-ō-lăr	_____
malleolus (572)	măl-LĒ-ō-lŭs	_____
mandible (577)	MĂN-dĭ-b'l	_____
mandibular (577)	măn-DĬB-ū-lăr	_____
manubrium (573)	mă-NŪ-brē-ŭm	_____
mastoid process (573)	MĂS-toyd PRŎS-ĕs	_____
medullary cavity (573)	MĔD-ū-lăr-ē KĂ-vĭ-tē	_____
metacarpals (577)	mĕt-ă-KĂR-pălz	_____
metacarpectomy (577)	mĕt-ă-kăr-PĔK-tō-mē	_____
metaphysis (573)	mĕ-TĂ-fĭ-sĭs	_____
metatarsalgia (577)	mĕt-ă-tăr-SĂL-jă	_____
metatarsals (577)	mĕt-ă-TĂR-sălz	_____
myelopoiesis (575)	mī-ĕ-lō-poy-Ē-sĭs	_____
nasal bone (564)	NĀ-zăl bōn	_____
occipital bone (563)	ŏk-SĬP-ĭ-tăl bōn	_____
olecranal (577)	ō-LĔK-ră-năl	_____
olecranon (573)	ō-LĔK-ră-nŏn	_____

Term	Pronunciation	Meaning
orthopedics (575)	ŏr-thō-PĒ-dĭks	
osseous tissue (573)	ŎS-ē-ŭs TĬSH-ū	
ossification (573)	ŏs-ĭ-fĭ-KĀ-shŭn	
osteitis (575)	ŏs-tē-Ī-tĭs	
osteoblast (573)	ŎS-tē-ō-blăst	
osteoclast (573)	ŎS-tē-ō-klăst	
osteodystrophy (575)	ŏs-tē-ō-DĬS-trō-fē	
osteogenesis imperfecta (575)	ŏs-tē-ō-JĔN-ě-sĭs ĭm-pěr-FĔK-tă	
osteogenic sarcoma (579)	ŏs-tē-ō-JĔN-ĭk săr-KŌ-mă	
osteomalacia (576)	ŏs-tē-ō-mă-LĀ-shă	
osteomyelitis (580)	ŏs-tē-ō-mī-ě-LĪ-tĭs	
osteopenia (581)	ŏs-tē-ō-PĒ-nē-ă	
osteoporosis (576)	ŏs-tē-ō-pŏr-Ō-sĭs	
osteotome (576)	ŎS-tē-ō-tōm	
parietal bones (562)	pă-RĪ-ě-tăl bōnz	
patella (577)	pă-TĔL-ă	
pelvimetry (577)	pěl-VĬM-ě-trē	
periosteum (573)	pě-rē-ŎS-tē-ŭm	
peroneal (577)	pěr-ō-NĒ-ăl	
phalangeal (577)	fă-lăn-JĒ-ăl	
phalanges (577)	fă-LĂN-jēz	
phosphorus (573)	FŎS-fō-rŭs	
pubic symphysis (573)	PŪ-bĭk SĬM-fĭ-sĭs	
pubis (577)	PŪ-bĭs	
radial (578)	RĀ-dē-ăl	
radius (578)	RĀ-dē-ŭs	
red bone marrow (573)	rěd bōn MĂ-rō	
reduction (579)	rě-DŬK-shŭn	
ribs (573)	rĭbz	
sacral vertebrae (567)	SĀ-krăl VĔR-tě-brā	
scapula (578)	SKĂP-ū-lă	
scapular (578)	SKĂP-ŭ-lăr	
scoliosis (575)	skō-lē-Ō-sĭs	

15

Term	Pronunciation	Meaning
sella turcica (573)	SĔ-lă TŬR-sĭ-kă	
sinus (573)	SĪ-nŭs	
sphenoid bone (563)	SFĒ-noyd bōn	
spondylolisthesis (576)	spŏn-dĭ-lō-lĭs-THĒ-sĭs	
spondylosis (575)	spŏn-dĭ-LŌ-sĭs	
sternum (578)	STĔR-nŭm	
styloid process (573)	STĪ-loyd PRŎS-ĕs	
subcostal (576)	sŭb-KŎS-tăl	
supraclavicular (576)	sŭ-pră-klă-VĬK-ū-lăr	
suture (573)	SŪ-tŭr	
talipes (581)	TĂL-ĭ-pēz	
tarsals (578)	TĂR-sălz	
tarsectomy (578)	tăr-SĔK-tō-mē	
temporal bones (563)	TĔM-pōr-ăl bōnz	
temporomandibular joint (573)	tĕm-pŏr-ō-măn-DĬB-ŭ-lăr joynt	
thoracic vertebrae (566)	thō-RĂS-ĭk VĔR-tĕ-brā	
tibia (578)	TĬB-ē-ă	
tibial (578)	TĬB-ē-ăl	
trabeculae (573)	tră-BĔK-ū-lē	
trochanter (573)	trō-KĂN-tĕr	
tubercle (573)	TŪ-bĕr-k'l	
tuberosity (573)	tū-bĕ-RŎS-ĭ-tē	
ulna (578)	ŬL-nă	
ulnar (578)	ŬL-năr	
vertebra, pl. vertebrae (573)	VĔR-tĕ-bră; VĔR-tĕ-brā	
vomer (564)	VŌ-mĕr	
xiphoid process (573)	ZĬF-oyd PRŎS-ĕs	
yellow bone marrow (573)	YĔ-lō bōn MĂ-rō	
zygomatic bones (564)	zī-gō-MĂ-tĭk bōnz	

TERMS RELATED TO JOINTS AND MUSCLES

Term	Pronunciation	Meaning
abduction (592)	ăb-DŬK-shŭn	
achondroplasia (584)	ā-kŏn-drō-PLĀ-zē-ă	
adduction (592)	ă-DŬK-shŭn	
amyotrophic lateral sclerosis (595)	ā-mī-ō-TRŌ-fĭk LĂT-ĕr-ăl sklĕ-RŌ-sĭs	
ankylosing spondylitis (585)	ăng-kĭ-LŌ-sĭng spŏn-dĭ-LĪ-tĭs	
ankylosis (584)	ăng-kĭ-LŌ-sĭs	
arthrodesis (585)	ăr-thrō-DĒ-sĭs	
arthrotomy (584)	ăr-THRŎT-ō-mē	
articular cartilage (582)	ăr-TĬK-ū-lăr KĂR-tĭ-lĭj	
articulation (583)	ăr-tĭk-ū-LĀ-shŭn	
atrophy (594)	ĂT-rō-fē	
bunion (587)	BŬN-yŭn	
bursa; bursae (582)	BŬR-să; BŬR-sē	
bursitis (584)	bŭr-SĪ-tis	
carpal tunnel syndrome (587)	KĂR-păl TŬN-nĕl SĬN-drōm	
chondroma (584)	kŏn-DRŌ-mă	
chondromalacia (584)	kŏn-drō-mă-LĀ-shă	
dislocation (588)	dĭs-lō-KĀ-shŭn	
dorsiflexion (592)	dŏr-sē-FLĔK-shŭn	
extension (592)	ĕk-STĔN-shŭn	
fascia (590)	FĂSH-ē-ă	
fasciectomy (594)	făsh-ē-ĔK-tō-mē	
fibromyalgia (594)	fī-brō-mī-ĂL-jă	
flexion (592)	FLĔK-shŭn	
ganglion (588)	GĂNG-lē-ŏn	
gouty arthritis (585)	GŎW-tē ăr-THRĪ-tĭs	
hemarthrosis (584)	hĕm-ăr-THRŌ-sĭs	
hydrarthrosis (584)	hī-drăr-THRŌ-sĭs	
hypertrophy (594)	hī-PĔR-trō-fē	
hyperuricemia (585)	hī-pĕr-ŭr-ĭ-SĒ-mē-ă	
leiomyoma (594)	lī-ō-mī-Ō-mă	

15

Term	Pronunciation	Meaning
leiomyosarcoma (594)	lī-ō-mī-ō-săr-KŌ-mă	
ligament (582)	LĬG-ă-mĕnt	
ligamentous (585)	lĭg-ă-MĚN-tŭs	
Lyme disease (589)	līm dĭ-ZĒZ	
muscular dystrophy (595)	MŬS-kū-lăr DĬS-trŏ-fē	
myalgia (594)	mī-ĂL-jă	
myopathy (594)	mī-ŎP-ă-thē	
myositis (594)	mī-ō-SĪ-tĭs	
osteoarthritis (586)	ŏs-tē-ō-ăr-THRĪ-tĭs	
plantar flexion (592)	PLĂN-tăr FLĚK-shun	
podagra (585)	pō-DĂG-ră	
polyarthritis (584)	pŏl-ē-ărth-RĪ-tĭs	
polymyalgia (595)	pŏl-ē-mĭ-ĂL-jă	
polymyositis (595)	pŏl-ē-mī-ō-SĪ-tĭs	
pronation (592)	prō-NĀ-shŭn	
pyrexia (587)	pī-RĚK-sē-ă	
rhabdomyoma (594)	răb-dō-mī-Ō-mă	
rhabdomyosarcoma (594)	răb-dō-mī-ō-săr-KŌ-mă	
rheumatoid arthritis (586)	ROO-mă-toyd ăr-THRĪ-tĭs	
rheumatologist (585)	roo-mă-TŎL-ō-jĭst	
rotation (592)	rō-TĀ-shŭn	
spinal stenosis (585)	SPĪ-năl stĕ-NŌ-sĭs	
sprain (589)	sprān	
strain (589)	strān	
striated muscle (590)	STRĪ-ā-tĕd MŬS-l	
subluxation (588)	sŭb-lŭk-SĀ-shŭn	
supination (592)	sū-pĭ-NĀ-shŭn	
suture joint (583)	SŪ-chŭr joint	
synovial cavity (583)	sĭ-NŌ-vē-ăl KĂV-ĭ-tē	
synovial fluid (583)	sĭ-NŌ-vē-ăl FLOO-ĭd	
synovial joint (583)	sĭ-NŌ-vē-ăl joint	
synovial membrane (583)	sĭ-NŌ-vē-ăl MĚM-brān	

Term	Pronunciation	Meaning
synovitis (585)	sĭn-ō-VĪ-tĭs	_____
systemic lupus erythematosus (589)	sĭs-TĔM-ĭk LOO-pŭs ĕ-rĭ-thē-mă-TŌ-sŭs	_____
tendinitis (585)	tĕn-dĭ-NĪ-tĭs	_____
tendon (583)	TĔN-dŭn	_____
tenorrhaphy (585)	tĕn-ŎR-ă-fē	_____
tenosynovitis (585)	tĕn-ō-sī-nō-VĪ-tĭs	_____
visceral muscle (590)	VĬS-ĕr-ăl MŬS-l	_____

LABORATORY TESTS AND CLINICAL PROCEDURES

Term	Pronunciation	Meaning
antinuclear antibody test (595)	ăn-tē-NŪ-klē-ăr ĂN-tĭ-bŏd-ē tĕst	_____
arthrocentesis (596)	ăr-thrō-sĕn-TĒ-sĭs	_____
arthrography (596)	ăr-THRŎG-ră-fē	_____
arthroplasty (596)	ăr-thrō-PLĂS-tē	_____
arthroscopy (597)	ăr-THRŎS-kō-pē	_____
bone density test (598)	bōn DĔN-sĭ-tē tĕst	_____
bone scan (598)	bōn skăn	_____
computed tomography (598)	kŏm-PŪ-tĕd tō-MŎG-ră-fē	_____
diskography (598)	dĭsk-ŎG-ră-fē	_____
electromyography (599)	ē-lĕk-trō-mī-ŎG-ră-fē	_____
erythrocyte sedimentation rate (595)	ĕ-RĬTH-rō-sīt sĕd-ĭ-mĕn-TĀ-shŭn rāt	_____
magnetic resonance imaging (599)	măg-NĔT-ĭk RĔ-sō-năns ĬM-ăj-ĭng	_____
muscle biopsy (599)	MŬS-'l BĪ-ŏp-sē	_____
rheumatoid factor test (596)	ROO-mă-tŏyd FĂK-tŏr tĕst	_____
serum calcium (596)	SĔR-ŭm KĂL-sē-ŭm tĕst	_____
serum creatine kinase (596)	SĔR-ŭm KRĒ-ă-tĭn KĪ-nās	_____
uric acid test (596)	ŪR-ĭk ĂS-ĭd tĕst	_____

REVIEW SHEET

15

Write the meanings of the word parts in the spaces provided. Check your answers with the information in the chapter or in the glossary (Medical Word Parts—English) at the end of the book.

COMBINING FORMS

Combining Form	Meaning	Combining Form	Meaning
acetabul/o		mandibul/o	
ankyl/o		maxill/o	
arthr/o		metacarp/o	
articul/o		metatars/o	
burs/o		my/o	
calc/o		myel/o	
calcane/o		myocardi/o	
calci/o		myos/o	
carp/o		olecran/o	
cervic/o		orth/o	
chondr/o		oste/o	
clavicul/o		patell/o	
coccyg/o		ped/o	
cost/o		pelv/i	
crani/o		perone/o	
fasci/o		phalang/o	
femor/o		plant/o	
fibr/o		pub/o	
fibul/o		radi/o	
humer/o		rhabdomy/o	
ili/o		rheumat/o	
ischi/o		sacr/o	
kyph/o		sarc/o	
lamin/o		scapul/o	
leiomy/o		scoli/o	
ligament/o		spondyl/o	
lord/o		stern/o	
lumb/o		synov/o	
malleol/o		tars/o	

Combining Form	Meaning	Combining Form	Meaning
ten/o	_____	tibi/o	_____
tendin/o	_____	uln/o	_____
thorac/o	_____	vertebr/o	_____

SUFFIXES

Suffix	Meaning	Suffix	Meaning
-algia	_____	-penia	_____
-asthenia	_____	-physis	_____
-blast	_____	-plasty	_____
-clast	_____	-porosis	_____
-desis	_____	-stenosis	_____
-emia	_____	-tome	_____
-listhesis	_____	-trophy	_____
-malacia	_____		

PREFIXES

Prefix	Meaning	Prefix	Meaning
a-, an-	_____	hyper-	_____
ab-	_____	meta-	_____
ad-	_____	peri-	_____
dia-	_____	poly-	_____
dorsi-	_____	sub-	_____
epi-	_____	supra-	_____
exo-	_____	sym-	_____

 Please refer to the enclosed CD for additional exercises and images related to this chapter.

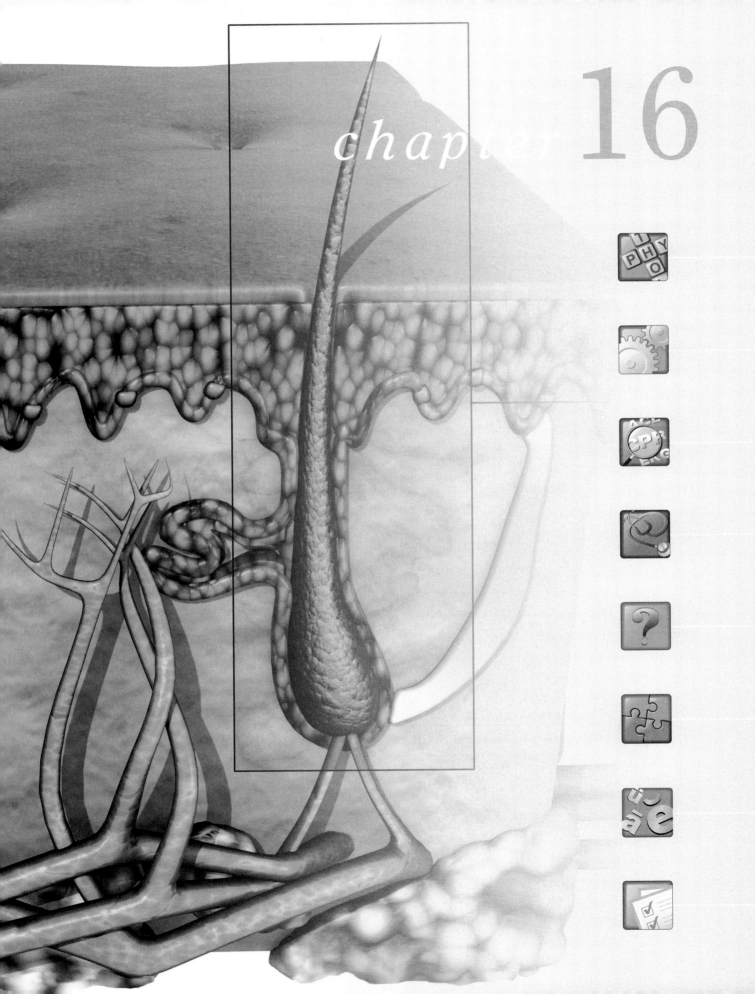

chapter 16

Skin

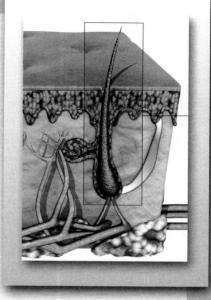

THIS CHAPTER IS DIVIDED INTO THE FOLLOWING SECTIONS

In this chapter you will

- Name the layers of the skin and the accessory structures associated with the skin.
- Build medical words using the combining forms that are related to the specialty of dermatology.
- Identify lesions, signs and symptoms, and pathologic conditions that relate to the skin.
- Describe laboratory tests and clinical procedures that pertain to the skin, and recognize relevant abbreviations.
- Apply your new knowledge to understanding medical terms in their proper contexts, such as medical reports and records.

Image Description: *Anterior illustration of a section of the skin.*

16

INTRODUCTION

The skin and its accessory organs (hair, nails, and glands) are the **integumentary system** of the body. Integument means covering, and the skin (weighing 8 to 10 pounds and extending over an area of 22 square feet in an average adult) is the outer covering for the body. It is, however, more than a simple body covering. This complex system of specialized tissues contains glands that secrete several types of fluids, nerves that carry impulses, and blood vessels that aid in the regulation of the body temperature. The following paragraphs review the many important functions of the skin.

First, as a protective membrane over the entire body, the skin guards the deeper tissues of the body against excessive loss of water, salts, and heat and against invasion of pathogens and their toxins. Secretions from the skin are slightly acidic in nature, which contributes to the skin's ability to prevent bacterial invasion. Specialized cells (Langerhans cells) react to the presence of antigens and have an immune function.

Second, the skin contains two types of glands that produce important secretions. These glands under the skin are the **sebaceous** and the **sweat glands.** Sebaceous glands produce **sebum,** an oily secretion, and sweat glands produce **sweat,** a watery secretion. Sebum and sweat pass to the outer edges of the skin through ducts and leave the skin through openings, or pores. Sebum lubricates the surface of the skin, and sweat cools the body as it evaporates from the skin surface.

Third, nerve fibers under the skin are receptors for sensations such as pain, temperature, pressure, and touch. Thus, the body's adjustment to the environment depends on sensory messages relayed to the brain and spinal cord by sensitive nerve endings in the skin.

Fourth, different tissues in the skin maintain body temperature (thermoregulation). Nerve fibers coordinate thermoregulation by carrying messages to the skin from heat centers in the brain that are sensitive to increases and decreases in body temperature. Impulses from these fibers cause blood vessels to dilate to bring blood to the surface and cause sweat glands to produce the watery secretion that carries heat away.

STRUCTURE OF THE SKIN

Figure 16–1, *A*, shows three layers of the skin. Label them from the outer surface inward:

Epidermis [1]—a thin, cellular membrane layer; containing keratin
Dermis [2]—dense, fibrous, connective tissue layer; containing collagen
Subcutaneous layer [3]—thick, fat-containing tissue

EPIDERMIS

The epidermis is the outermost, totally cellular layer of the skin. It is composed of **squamous epithelium.** Epithelium is the covering of both the internal and the external surfaces of the body. Squamous epithelial cells are flat and scale-like. In the outer layer of the skin, these cells are arranged in several layers **(strata)** to form **stratified squamous epithelium.**

The epidermis lacks blood vessels, lymphatic vessels, and connective tissue (elastic fibers, cartilage, fat) and is therefore dependent on the deeper dermis (also called corium) layer and its rich network of capillaries for nourishment. In fact, oxygen and nutrients seep out of the capillaries in the dermis, pass through tissue fluid, and supply nourishment to the deeper layers of the epidermis.

16

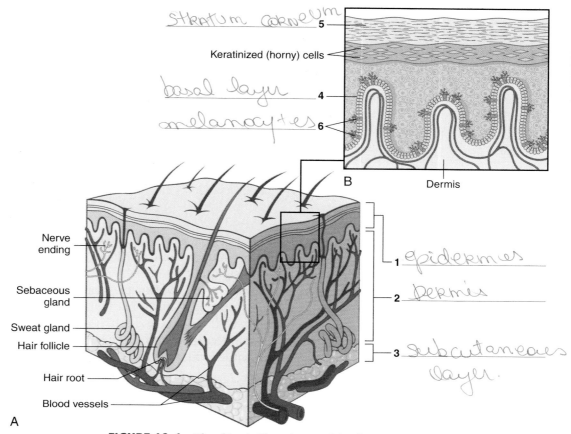

[Handwritten annotations: Stratum corneum (5), basal layer (4), melanocytes (6), epidermis (1), dermis (2), subcutaneous layer (3)]

Keratinized (horny) cells

B

Dermis

Nerve ending

Sebaceous gland

Sweat gland

Hair follicle

Hair root

Blood vessels

A

FIGURE 16–1 **The skin. A,** Three layers of the skin. **B,** Epidermis.

Figure 16–1, *B,* illustrates the multilayered cells of the epidermis. The deepest layer is called the **basal layer** [4]. The cells in the basal layer are constantly growing and multiplying and give rise to all the other cells in the epidermis. As the basal layer cells divide, they are pushed upward and away from the blood supply of the dermal layer by a steady stream of younger cells. In their movement toward the most superficial layer of the epidermis, called the **stratum corneum** [5], the cells flatten, shrink, lose their nuclei, and die, becoming filled with a hard protein material called **keratin.** The cells are then called horny cells, reflecting their composition of keratin. Finally, within 3 to 4 weeks after beginning as a basal cell in the deepest part of the epidermis, the keratinized cell is sloughed off from the surface of the skin. The epidermis is thus constantly renewing itself, cells dying at the same rate at which they are replaced.

The basal layer of the epidermis contains special cells called **melanocytes** [6]. Melanocytes form and contain a brown-black pigment called **melanin** that is transferred to other epidermal cells and gives color to the skin. The number of melanocytes in all human races is the same, but the amount of melanin within each cell accounts for the color differences among the races. Individuals with darker skin possess more melanin within the melanocytes, not a greater number of melanocytes. The presence of melanin in the epidermis is vital for protection against the harmful effects of ultraviolet radiation, which can manifest themselves as skin cancer. Individuals who are incapable of forming melanin are called **albino.** Skin and hair are white. Their pupils (circular opening in the eye) are red because in the absence of pigment in the retina, the tiny blood vessels are visible in the iris (normally pigmented portion) of the eye.

16

Melanin production increases with exposure to strong ultraviolet light, and this creates a suntan, which is a protective response. When the melanin cannot absorb all of the ultraviolet rays, the skin becomes sunburned and inflamed (redness, swelling, and pain). Over a period of years, excessive exposure to sun can tend to cause wrinkles, permanent pigmenting changes, and even cancer of the skin. Because dark-skinned people have more melanin, they acquire fewer wrinkles and they are less likely to develop skin cancer.

DERMIS

The dermis, directly below the epidermis, is composed of blood and lymph vessels and nerve fibers, as well as the accessory organs of the skin, which are the hair follicles, sweat glands, and sebaceous glands. To support the elaborate system of nerves, vessels, and glands, the dermis contains connective tissue cells and fibers that account for the extensibility and elasticity of the skin.

The dermis is composed of interwoven elastic and **collagen** fibers. Collagen (**colla** means glue) is a fibrous protein material found in bone, cartilage, tendons, and ligaments, as well as in the skin. It is tough and resistant but also flexible. In the infant, collagen is loose and delicate; it becomes harder as the body ages. During pregnancy, overstretching of a woman's skin may break the elastic fibers, resulting in linear markings called striae ("stretch marks"). Collagen fibers support and protect the blood and nerve networks that pass through the dermis. Collagen diseases affect connective tissues of the body. Examples of these connective tissue collagen disorders are systemic lupus erythematosus and scleroderma.

SUBCUTANEOUS LAYER

The subcutaneous layer (epidermis and dermis are the cutaneous layers) specializes in the formation of fat. **Lipocytes** (fat cells) are predominant in the subcutaneous layer, and they manufacture and store large quantities of fat. Obviously, areas of the body and individuals vary so far as fat deposition is concerned. Functionally, this layer of the skin is important in protection of the deeper tissues of the body, as a heat insulator, and for energy storage.

ACCESSORY ORGANS OF THE SKIN

HAIR

A hair fiber is composed of a tightly fused meshwork of cells filled with the hard protein called **keratin.** Hair growth is similar to the growth of the epidermal layer of the skin. Deep-lying cells in the hair root (see Fig. 16-2) produce keratinized cells that move upward through **hair follicles** (sacs within which each hair fiber grows). Melanocytes (see Fig. 16-2) are located at the root of the hair follicle, and they donate the melanin pigment to the cells of the hair fiber. A type of melanin containing iron is responsible for red hair. Hair turns gray when with advancing age the melanocytes stop producing melanin.

Of the 5 million hairs on the body, about 100,000 are on the head. They grow about ½ inch (1.3 cm) per month. Cutting the hair has no effect on its rate of growth.

NAILS

Nails are hard keratin plates covering the dorsal surface of the last bone of each toe and finger. They are composed of horny cells that are cemented together tightly and can extend indefinitely unless cut or broken. A nail grows in thickness and length as a result of division of cells in the region of the nail root, which is at the base (proximal portion) of the nail plate.

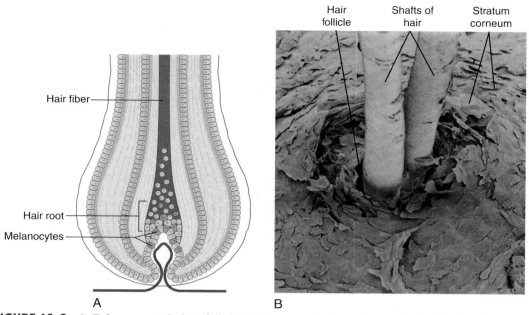

FIGURE 16–2   **A,** Enlargement of a **hair follicle. B,** Scanning electron micrograph of **shafts** (visible parts of hair) extending from their hair follicles. (**B** from Thibodeau GA, Patton KT: Anatomy & Physiology, 6th ed. St. Louis, Mosby, 2007, p. 212.)

Fingernails grow about 1 mm per week, which means that they can regrow in 3 to 5 months. Toenails grow more slowly than fingernails; it takes 12 to 18 months for toenails to be replaced completely.

The **lunula** is a semilunar (half-moon–shaped) whitish region at the base of the nail plate. It generally can be seen in the thumbnail of most people and is evident to varying degrees in other fingers. Air mixed in with keratin and cells rich in nuclei give the lunula its whitish color. The **cuticle,** a narrow band of epidermis (layer of keratin), is at the base and sides of the nail plate. The **paronychium** is the soft tissue surrounding the nail border. Figure 16–3, *A*, illustrates the anatomic structure of a nail.

Nail growth and appearance commonly alter during systemic disease. For example, grooves in nails may occur with high fevers and serious illness, and spoon nails (flattening of the nail plate) occur in iron deficiency anemia. **Onycholysis (onych/o** means nail) is the loosening of the nail plate with separation from the nail bed. It may occur with infection of the nail (see Fig. 16–3, *B*).

FIGURE 16–3   **A, Anatomic structure of a nail. B, Onycholysis.** Infection or trauma to the nail may be the cause of the detachment of the nail from its plate. (**B** from Seidel HM: Mosby's Guide to Physical Examination, 5th ed. St. Louis, Mosby, 2003, p. 214.)

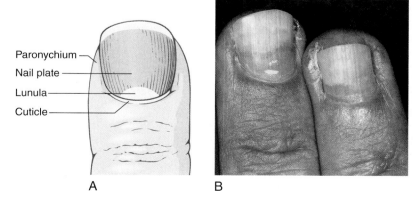

GLANDS

Sebaceous Glands

Sebaceous glands are located in the dermal layer of the skin over the entire body, with the exception of the palms (hands) and soles (feet). They secrete an oily substance called **sebum.** Sebum, containing lipids, lubricates the skin and minimizes water loss. Sebaceous glands are closely associated with hair follicles, and their ducts open into the hair follicle through which the sebum is released. Figure 16–4 shows the relationship of the sebaceous gland to the hair follicle. The sebaceous glands are influenced by sex hormones, which cause them to hypertrophy at puberty and atrophy in old age. Overproduction of sebum during puberty contributes to blackhead (comedo) formation and acne in some people.

Sweat Glands

Sweat glands (the most common type are **eccrine sweat glands**) are tiny, coiled glands found on almost all body surfaces (about 2 million in the body). They are most numerous in the palm of the hand (3000 glands per square inch) and in the sole of the foot. As illustrated in Figure 16–4, the coiled eccrine sweat gland originates deep in the dermis and straightens out to extend up through the epidermis. The tiny opening on the surface is a **pore.**

Sweat, or perspiration, is almost pure water, with dissolved materials such as salt making up less than 1 percent of the total composition. It is colorless and odorless. The odor produced when sweat accumulates on the skin is caused by the action of bacteria on the sweat.

Sweat cools the body as it evaporates into the air. Perspiration is controlled by the sympathetic nervous system, whose nerve fibers are activated by the heart regulatory center in the hypothalamic region of the brain, which stimulates sweating.

A special variety of sweat gland, active only from puberty onward and larger than the ordinary kind, is concentrated in a few areas of the body near the reproductive organs and in the armpits. These glands (**apocrine sweat glands**) secrete an odorless sweat, containing substances easily broken down by bacteria on the skin. The bacterial waste products produce a characteristic human body odor. The milk-producing mammary gland is another type of apocrine sweat gland; it secretes milk after the birth of a child.

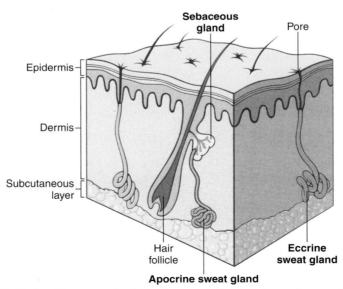

FIGURE 16–4 Sebaceous gland, eccrine sweat gland, and apocrine sweat gland.

VOCABULARY

This list reviews many of the new terms introduced in the text. Short definitions reinforce your understanding of the terms. Refer to the Pronunciation of Terms section for help with unfamiliar or difficult words.

albino	Person with skin deficient in pigment (melanin).
apocrine sweat gland	One of the large dermal exocrine glands located in the axilla and genital areas. It secretes sweat that, in action with bacteria, is responsible for human body odor.
basal layer	Deepest region of the epidermis; it gives rise to all the epidermal cells.
collagen	Structural protein found in the skin and connective tissue.
cuticle	Band of epidermis at the base and sides of the nail plate.
dermis	Middle layer of the skin.
eccrine sweat gland	Most numerous sweat-producing exocrine gland in the skin.
epidermis	Outermost layer of the skin.
epithelium	Layer of skin cells forming the outer and inner surfaces of the body.
hair follicle	Sac within which each hair grows.
integumentary system	The skin and its accessory structures such as hair and nails.
keratin	Hard protein material found in the epidermis, hair, and nails. Keratin means horn and commonly is found in the horns of animals.
lipocyte	A fat cell.
lunula	The half-moon–shaped, whitish area at the base of a nail.
melanin	Major skin pigment. It is formed by melanocytes in the epidermis.
paronychium	Soft tissue surrounding the nail border.
pore	Tiny opening on the surface of the skin.
sebaceous gland	Oil-secreting gland in the dermis that is associated with hair follicles.
sebum	Oily substance secreted by sebaceous glands.
squamous epithelium	Flat, scale-like cells composing the epidermis.
stratified	Arranged in layers.
stratum (*plural:* **strata**)	A layer (of cells).
stratum corneum	Outermost layer of the epidermis, which consists of flattened, keratinized (horny) cells.
subcutaneous layer	Innermost layer of the skin, containing fat tissue.

COMBINING FORMS AND SUFFIXES

16

Write the meanings of the medical terms in the spaces provided.

COMBINING FORMS

Combining Form	Meaning	Terminology	Meaning
adip/o	fat (see **lip/o** and **steat/o**)	adipose _____	
albin/o	white	albinism _____ *Table 16–1 lists combining forms for colors and examples of terms using those combining forms.*	
caus/o	burn, burning	causalgia _____ *Intensely unpleasant burning sensation in skin and muscles when there is damage to nerves.*	
cauter/o	heat, burn	electrocautery _____ *An instrument containing a needle or blade used during surgery to burn through tissue by means of an electrical current. Electrocauterization is very effective in minimizing blood loss.*	

Table 16–1

Colors

Combining Form	Meaning	Terminology
albin/o	white	*albinism*
anthrac/o	black (as coal)	*anthracosis*
chlor/o	green	*chlorophyll*
cirrh/o	tawny yellow	*cirrhosis*
cyan/o	blue	*cyanosis*
eosin/o	rosy	*eosinophil*
erythr/o	red	*erythrocyte*
jaund/o	yellow	*jaundice*
leuk/o	white	*leukoderma*
lute/o	yellow	corpus *luteum*
melan/o	black	*melanocyte*
poli/o	gray	*poliomyelitis*
xanth/o	yellow	*xanthoma*

16

Combining Form	Meaning	Terminology	Meaning
cutane/o	skin (see **derm/o**)	subcutaneous _____ *Epidermis and dermis are the cutaneous layers of the skin.*	
derm/o, dermat/o	skin	epidermis _____	
		dermatitis _____ **Atopic dermatitis** *is marked by intense itching and excoriation (scratching). Atopic means pertaining to a genetic tendency to experience an allergic reaction. See Figure 16–5, A.*	
		dermatoplasty _____ *Skin is transplanted to a body surface damaged by disease or injury.*	
		dermatologist _____	
		dermabrasion _____ *Abrasion means a scraping away. Dermabrasion using a sandpaper-like material removes acne scars and fine wrinkles.*	
		epidermolysis _____ *Loosening of the epidermis with the development of large blisters; occurs after injury, or with blister-producing diseases.*	
diaphor/o	profuse sweating (see **hidr/o**)	diaphoresis _____ *Commonly called sweating.*	
erythem/o, erythemat/o	redness	erythema _____ *Flushing; widespread redness of the skin.* **Erythema infectiosum** *(fifth disease) is a benign infectious disease, mainly of children. It is marked by fever and an* **erythematous** *rash that begins on the cheeks and later appears on the arms, buttocks, and trunk. It is caused by a parvovirus. See Figure 16–5, B.*	

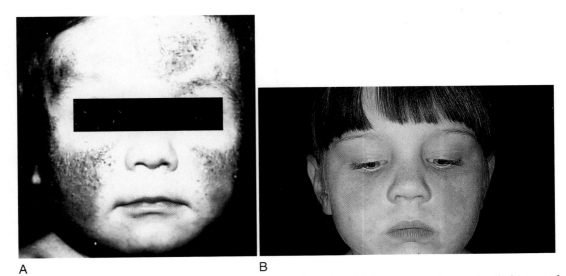

A   B

FIGURE 16–5 **A, Atopic dermatitis (eczema)** in an infant. Over 70% of patients have a family history of other atopic conditions such as allergic rhinitis, hay fever, and asthma. **B, Erythema infectiosum.** (**A** from Zitelli BJ, Davis HW: Atlas of Pediatric Physical Diagnosis, 4th ed. St. Louis, Mosby, 2002. **B** from Callen JP, et al: Color Atlas of Dermatology, 2nd ed. Philadelphia, WB Saunders, 2000.)

16

Combining Form	Meaning	Terminology	Meaning
hidr/o	sweat	anhidrosis _____ *Do not confuse hidr/o with hydr/o (water)!*	
ichthy/o	scaly, dry (fish-like)	ichthyosis _____ *A hereditary condition in which the skin is dry, rough, and scaly (resembling fish scales) because of a defect in keratinization. Ichthyosis also can be acquired, appearing with malignancies such as lymphomas and multiple myeloma. Greek* ichthys *means fish. See Figure 16–6, A.*	
kerat/o	hard, horny tissue	keratosis _____ *See page 646.*	
leuk/o	white	leukoplakia _____ *The suffix -plakia means plaques. See Figure 16–6, B.*	
lip/o	fat	lipoma _____ liposuction _____ *Removal of subcutaneous fat tissue through a tube that is introduced into the fatty area via a small incision. The fat is aspirated (suctioned) out.*	
melan/o	black	melanocyte _____ melanoma _____ *This is a malignant skin tumor. See page 647.*	

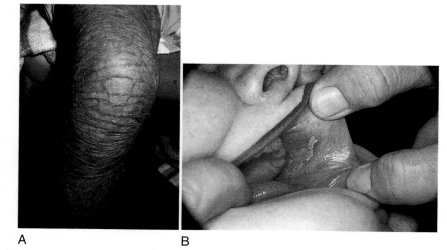

A   B

FIGURE 16–6   A, Ichthyosis. B, Leukoplakia. (A from Kanski JJ: Systemic Diseases and the Eye. St. Louis, Mosby, 2001. **B** from Callen JP, et al: Color Atlas of Dermatology, 2nd ed. Philadelphia, WB Saunders, 2000.)

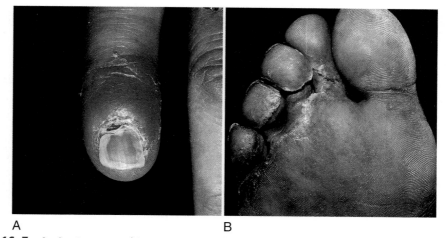

A   B

FIGURE 16–7 **A, Acute paronychia** most commonly occurs from nail biting, finger sucking, aggressive manicuring, or penetrating trauma. The most common infecting organism is *Staphylococcus aureus*. **B, Dermatophytosis** (tinea pedis, or "athlete's foot"). (**A** from Callen JP, et al: Color Atlas of Dermatology, 2nd ed. Philadelphia, WB Saunders, 2000. **B** from Zitelli BJ, Davis HW: Atlas of Pediatric Physical Diagnosis, 4th ed. St. Louis, Mosby, 2002.)

Combining Form	Meaning	Terminology	Meaning
myc/o	fungus (fungi include yeasts, molds, and mushrooms)	mycosis _____ *Examples of mycoses (fungal infections) are tinea pedis, commonly called "athlete's foot." See Figure 16–7, B. Another fungal infection is tinea corporis (ringworm). See page 644.*	
onych/o	nail (see **ungu/o**)	onycholysis _____ *Separation of the nail plate from the nail bed in fungal infections or after trauma. See Figure 16–3, B.*	
		onychomycosis _____ *Fungal infection of the nails, which become white, opaque, thick, and brittle.*	
		paronychia _____ *Par- means near or beside. Paronychia is the inflammation and swelling of the soft tissue around the nail and is associated with torn cuticles or ingrown nails. See Figure 16–7, A.*	
phyt/o	plant	dermatophytosis _____ *Examples are fungal infections (mycoses). See Figure 16–7, B.*	
pil/o	hair (see **trich/o**), hair follicle	pilosebaceous _____ *Sebace/o means a gland that secretes sebum.*	

16

Combining Form	Meaning	Terminology	Meaning
py/o	pus	pyoderma _____	
		Pus is within the skin (-derma). Impetigo is a purulent (pus containing) skin disease caused by bacterial infection. See Figure 16–8, A. Also see page 642.	
rhytid/o	wrinkle	rhytidectomy _____	
		Reconstructive plastic surgery to remove wrinkles and signs of aging skin; also called rhytidoplasty or face lift. Laser treatments and **Botox** *(purified botulinum toxin) injections are used to soften facial lines and wrinkles.*	
seb/o	sebum (oily secretion from sebaceous glands)	seborrhea _____	
		Excessive secretion from sebaceous glands. **Seborrheic dermatitis** *commonly is known as* **dandruff.**	
squam/o	scale-like	squamous epithelium _____	
		Cells are flat and scale-like; pavement epithelium.	
steat/o	fat	steatoma _____	
		A cystic collection of sebum (fatty material) that forms in a sebaceous gland and can become infected; **sebaceous cyst.**	
trich/o	hair	trichomycosis _____	
ungu/o	nail	subungual _____	
xanth/o	yellow	xanthoma _____	
		Nodules develop under the skin owing to excess lipid deposits. Usually associated with a high cholesterol level. Plaques that appear on the eyelids are **xanthelasmas** *(-elasma means a flat plate). See Figure16–8, B.*	
xer/o	dry	xeroderma _____	
		The suffix -derma means skin. This is a mild form of ichthyosis.	

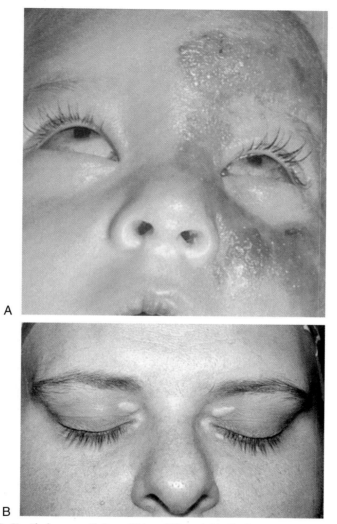

FIGURE 16–8   A, Impetigo. B, Xanthelasmas. (A from Phipps WJ et al: Medical-Surgical Nursing, 7th ed., St. Louis, Mosby, 2003, p. 1951; **B** from Seidel HM et al: Mosby's Guide to Physical Examination, 5th ed., St. Louis, Mosby, 2003.)

16

LESIONS, SIGNS AND SYMPTOMS, ABNORMAL CONDITIONS, AND SKIN NEOPLASMS

CUTANEOUS LESIONS

A **lesion** is an area of damaged tissue anywhere on or in the body. It may be caused by disease or trauma (external forces). The following terms describe common skin lesions, which are illustrated in Figure 16–9, *A–L*.

A. crust
Collection of dried serum and cellular debris.
A scab is a crust. It forms from the drying of a body exudate, as in eczema, impetigo, and seborrhea.

B. cyst
Thick-walled, closed sac or pouch containing fluid or semisolid material.
Examples of cysts are the **pilonidal cyst,** which is found over the sacral area of the back in the midline and contains hairs (**pil/o** means hair, **nid/o** means nest); and a **sebaceous cyst,** a collection of yellowish, cheesy sebum commonly found on the scalp, vulva, and scrotum.

C. erosion
Wearing away or loss of epidermis.
Erosions do not penetrate below the dermoepidermal junction. They occur as a result of inflammation or injury and heal without scarring.

D. fissure
Groove or crack-like sore.
An anal fissure is a break in the skin lining of the anal canal.

E. macule
Discolored (often reddened) flat lesion.
Freckles, tattoo marks, and flat moles are examples.

F. nodule
Solid, round or oval elevated lesion more than 1 cm in diameter.
An enlarged lymph node and solid growths are examples.

G. papule
Small (less than 1 cm in diameter), solid elevation of the skin.
Pimples are examples of papules. Papules may become confluent (run together) and form **plaques.**

H. polyp
Benign growth extending from the surface of mucous membrane.
Polyps commonly are found in the nose and sinuses, urinary bladder, and uterus.

I. pustule
Small elevation of the skin containing pus.
A pustule is a small **abscess** (collection of pus) on the skin.

J. ulcer
Open sore on the skin or mucous membranes within the body.
Decubitus ulcers (bedsores) are caused by pressure that results from lying in one position (Latin *decubitus* means lying down). Pressure ulcers usually involve loss of tissue substance and pus or exudate formation.

K. vesicle
Small collection of clear fluid (serum); blister.
Vesicles form in burns, allergies, and dermatitis. A **bulla** (*plural*: bullae) is a large vesicle.

L. wheal
Smooth, slightly elevated, edematous (swollen) area that is redder or paler than the surrounding skin.
Wheals may be circumscribed, as in a mosquito bite, or may involve a wide area, as in allergic reactions. Wheals often are accompanied by itching and are seen in hives, anaphylaxis, and insect bites.

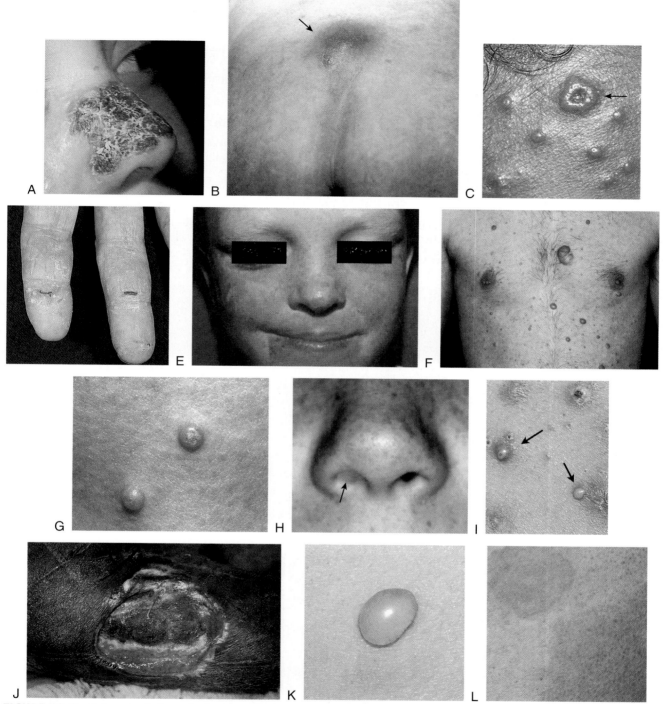

FIGURE 16–9 Cutaneous lesions. **A, Crust**—scab. **B, Cyst**—pilonidal cyst. **C, Erosion**—in varicella (chickenpox after rupture of blister). **D, Fissures. E, Macule**—freckles. **F, Nodules. G, Papules. H, Polyp**—nasal polyp. **I, Pustules**—acne. **J, Ulcer**—decubitus ulcer. **K, Vesicle**—bulla. **L, Wheals**—urticaria.

(**A** from Seidel HM, et al: Mosby's Guide to Physical Examination, 5th ed. St. Louis, Mosby, 2003. **B** from Zitelli BJ, Davis HW: Atlas of Pediatric Physical Diagnosis, 4th ed. St. Louis, Mosby, 2002. **C** from Cohen BA: Atlas of Pediatric Dermatology. London, Wolfe, 1993. **D** from Callen JP, et al: Color Atlas of Dermatology, 2nd ed. Philadelphia, WB Saunders, 2000. **E** and **I** from Weston WL, et al: Color Textbook of Pediatric Dermatology, 3rd ed. St. Louis, Mosby, 2002. **F** from Habif TP: Clinical Dermatology, 4th ed., St. Louis, Mosby, 2004, p. 906. **G** courtesy Dr. Bruce A. Chabner; **H** from Frazier MS, et al: Essentials of Human Diseases and Conditions, 3rd ed. Philadelphia, WB Saunders, 2004; **J** from Gould BE: Pathophysiology for the Health Professions, 3rd ed. Philadelphia, WB Saunders, 2006. **K** from White GM: Color Atlas of Regional Dermatology. London, Times-Mirror, 1994. **L** from Farrar WE: Atlas of Infections of the Nervous System. London, Mosby-Wolfe, 1993.)

SIGNS AND SYMPTOMS

alopecia

Absence of hair from areas where it normally grows.

Alopecia, or baldness, may be hereditary (usual progressive loss of scalp hair in men) or it may be caused by disease, injury, or treatment (chemotherapy) or may occur in old age. **Alopecia areata** is an idiopathic condition in which hair falls out in patches. See Figure 16–10, *A*.

ecchymosis (*plural:* **ecchymoses**)

Bluish-black mark (bruise) on the skin.

Ecchymoses (**ec-** means out, **chym/o** means to pour) are caused by hemorrhages into the skin from injury or spontaneous leaking of blood from vessels. See Figure 16–10, *B*.

petechia (*plural:* **petechiae**)

Small, pinpoint hemorrhage.

Petechiae are smaller versions of ecchymoses. See Figure 16–10, *C*. Both ecchymoses and petechiae are forms of **purpura** (bleeding into the skin).

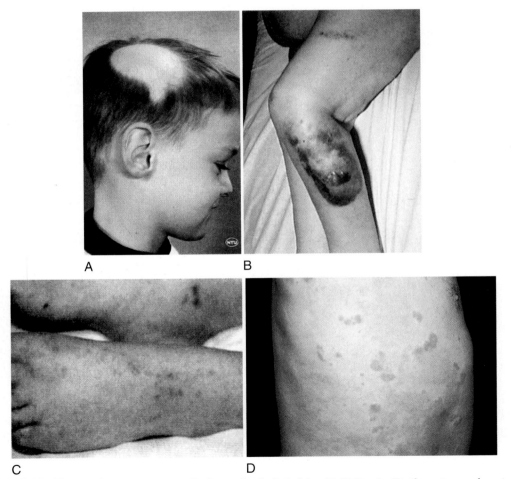

A B
C D

FIGURE 16–10   A, Alopecia areata. B, Ecchymosis. C, Petechiae. D, Urticaria. Erythematous, edematous, often circular plaques. (**A** from Barkauskas VH, et al: Health and Physical Assessment, 2nd ed. St. Louis, Mosby, 1998. **B** from Moll JMH: Rheumatology, 2nd ed. London, Churchill Livingstone, 1997. **C** from Mosby's Medical, Nursing and Allied Health Dictionary, 5th ed. St. Louis, Mosby, 1998. **D** from Habif TP: Clinical Dermatology, 4th ed., St. Louis, Mosby, 2004, p. 130.)

pruritus	**Itching.**

Pruritus is a symptom associated with most forms of dermatitis and with other conditions as well. It arises as a result of stimulation of nerves in the skin by substances released in allergic reactions or by irritation caused by substances in the blood or by foreign bodies. Be careful to spell pruri*tus* correctly. It is a condition, not an inflammation (-itis).

urticaria (hives)

Acute allergic reaction in which red, round wheals develop on the skin. See Figure 16–10, *D.*

Pruritus may be intense, and the cause is commonly allergy to foods (such as shellfish or strawberries). Localized edema (swelling) occurs as well.

ABNORMAL CONDITIONS

acne

Chronic papular and pustular eruption of the skin with increased production of sebum.

Acne vulgaris (Latin *vulgaris* means ordinary) is caused by the buildup of sebum and keratin in the pores of the skin. A **blackhead** or **comedo** (*plural*: **comedones**) is a sebum plug partially blocking the pore (Fig. 16–11). If the pore becomes completely blocked, a **whitehead** forms. Bacteria in the skin break down the sebum, producing inflammation in the surrounding tissue. Papules, pustules, and cysts can thus form. Treatment consists of long-term antibiotic use and medications to dry the skin. Benzoyl peroxide and tretinoin (Retin-A) are medications used to prevent comedo formation; isotretinoin (Accutane) is used in severe cystic acne.

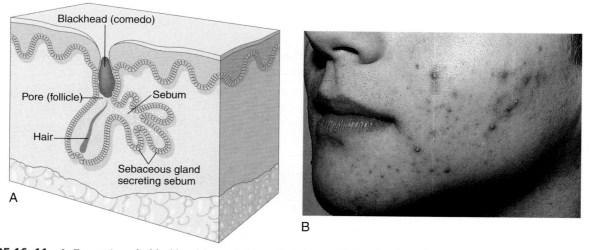

FIGURE 16–11 **A,** Formation of a **blackhead (comedo)** in a dilated pore filled with sebum, bacteria, and pigment. **B, Acne vulgaris** on the face. (**B** from Callen JP, Paller AS, Greer KE, Swinyer LJ: Color Atlas of Dermatology, 2nd ed. Philadelphia, WB Saunders, 2000, p. 151.)

Pruritus/Pleuritis
Pruritus means itching. Don't confuse it with *pleuritis,* which is inflammation of the pleura.

burns

Injury to tissues caused by heat contact.

Burns may be caused by dry heat (fire), moist heat (steam or liquid), chemicals, lightning, electricity, or radiation. Burns usually are classified as follows:

> **first-degree burns**—superficial epidermal lesions, erythema, hyperesthesia, and no blisters. Sunburn is an example.
>
> **second-degree burns (partial-thickness burn injury)**—epidermal and dermal lesions, erythema, blisters, and hyperesthesia (Fig. 16–12, *A*).
>
> **third-degree burns (full-thickness burn injury)**—epidermis and dermis are destroyed (necrosis of skin), and subcutaneous layer is damaged, leaving charred, white tissue (see Fig. 16–12, *B*).

cellulitis

Diffuse, acute infection of the skin marked by local heat, redness, pain, and swelling.

Abscess and tissue destruction can occur if antibiotics are not taken. Areas of poor lymphatic drainage are susceptible to this skin infection.

eczema

Inflammatory skin disease with erythematous, papulovesicular lesions.

This chronic or acute atopic dermatitis (rash occurs on face, neck, elbows, and knees) is accompanied by pruritus and tends to occur in patients with a family history of allergic conditions. Treatment depends on the cause but usually includes the use of corticosteroids.

exanthematous viral diseases

Rash (exanthema) of the skin due to a viral infection.

Examples are **rubella** (German measles), **rubeola** (measles), and **varicella** (chickenpox).

gangrene

Death of tissue associated with loss of blood supply.

In this condition, ischemia resulting from injury, inflammation, frostbite, diseases such as diabetes, or arteriosclerosis can lead to necrosis of tissue followed by bacterial invasion and putrefaction (proteins are decomposed by bacteria).

impetigo

Bacterial inflammatory skin disease characterized by vesicles, pustules, and crusted-over lesions.

This is a contagious **pyoderma** (**py/o** means pus) and usually is caused by staphylococci or streptococci. Systemic use of antibiotics and proper cleansing of lesions are effective treatments. See Figure 16–8, *A*.

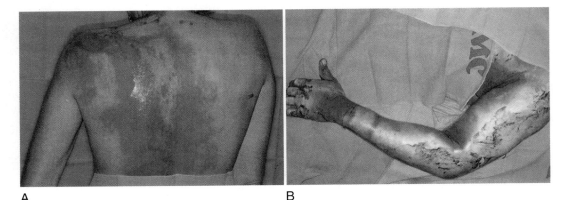

A   B

FIGURE 16–12   Burns. A, Second-degree burn. Wound is painful and very sensitive to touch and air currents. **B, Third-degree burn** showing variable color (deep-red, white, black, and brown). The wound itself is insensate (patient does not respond to pinprick). (From Black JM, Hawks JH, Keene AM: Medical-Surgical Nursing: Clinical Management for Positive Outcomes, 6th ed. Philadelphia, WB Saunders, 2001, pp. 1335–1336.)

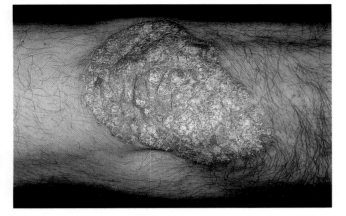

FIGURE 16–13 **Psoriasis.** Thick red plaques have a sharply defined border and an adherent silvery scale. (From Habif TP, et al: Skin Disease: Diagnosis and Treatment. St. Louis, Mosby, 2001.)

psoriasis	**Chronic, recurrent dermatosis marked by itchy, scaly, red plaques covered by silvery gray scales** (Fig. 16–13).

Psoriasis commonly involves the forearms, knees, legs, and scalp. It is neither infectious nor contagious but is caused by an increased rate of growth of the basal layer of the epidermis. The cause is unknown, but the condition runs in families and may be worsened by anxiety. Treatment is palliative (relieving but not curing) and includes topical lubricants, keratolytics, and steroids. Psoralen–ultraviolet A (PUVA) light therapy is also used.

scabies

A contagious, parasitic infection of the skin with intense pruritus.

Scabies (from Latin *scabere*, to scratch) commonly affects areas such as the groin, nipples, and skin between the fingers. Treatment is topical medicated cream to destroy the scabies mites (tiny parasites).

scleroderma

A chronic progressive disease of the skin with hardening and shrinking of connective tissue.

Fibrous scar tissue infiltrates the skin, and the heart, lungs, kidneys, and esophagus may be affected as well. Skin is thick, hard, and rigid, and pigmented patches may occur. The cause is not known. Palliative treatment consists of drugs, such as immunosuppressives and anti-inflammatory agents, and physical therapy.

systemic lupus erythematosus (SLE)

Chronic autoimmune inflammatory disease of collagen in the skin, of joints, and of internal organs.

Lupus, meaning wolf-like (the shape and color of the skin lesions resembles the bite of a wolf), produces a characteristic "butterfly" pattern of redness over the cheeks and nose. In more severe cases, the extent of erythema increases, and all exposed areas of the skin may be involved. Primarily a disease of females, lupus is an autoimmune condition. High levels of certain antibodies are found in the patient's blood. Corticosteroids and immunosuppressive drugs are used to control symptoms.

SLE should be differentiated from chronic **discoid lupus erythematosus (DLE),** which is a milder, scaling, plaque-like, superficial eruption of the skin confined to the face, scalp, ears, chest, arms, and back. The reddish patches heal and leave scars.

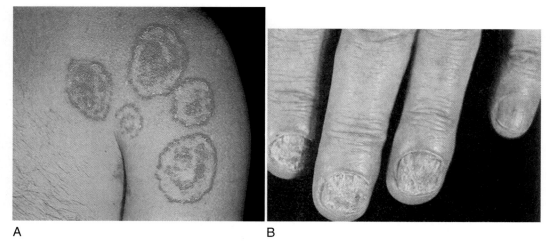

A   B

FIGURE 16–14 **A, Tinea corporis (ringworm). B, Tinea unguium.** Fungal infection of the nail causes the distal nail plate to turn yellow or white. Hyperkeratotic debris accumulates, causing the nail to separate from the nail bed (onycholysis). (**A** from Lewis SM, Heitkemper MM, Dirksen SR: Medical–Surgical Nursing: Assessment and Management of Clinical Problems, 6th ed. St. Louis, Mosby, 2004, p. 497. **B** courtesy of the American Academy of Dermatology and Institute for Dermatologic Communication and Education, Evanston, IL. From Seidel HM: Mosby's Guide to Physical Examination, 5th ed. St. Louis, Mosby, 2003, p. 213.)

tinea

Infection of the skin caused by a fungus.

Tinea corporis, or ringworm, so called because the infection is in a ring-like pattern (see Fig. 16–14, *A*), is highly contagious and causes severe pruritus. Other examples are **tinea pedis** (athlete's foot), which affects the skin between the toes, tinea capitis (on the scalp), **tinea barbae,** affecting the skin under a beard), and **tinea unguium** (affecting the nails) (see Fig. 16–14, *B*). Treatment is with antifungal agents. (Latin *tinea* means worm or moth—apparently the Romans thought that skin affected with tinea looked "moth-eaten.")

vitiligo (vĭt-ĭl-Ĭ-gō)

Loss of pigment (depigmentation) in areas of the skin (milk-white patches).

Also known as **leukoderma** (Fig. 16–15). There is an increased association of vitiligo with certain autoimmune conditions such as thyroiditis, hyperthyroidism, and diabetes mellitus.

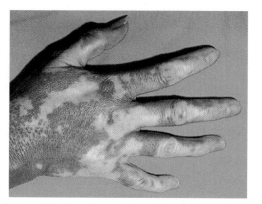

FIGURE 16–15 **Vitiligo** on the hand (Latin *vitium*, a blemish). Epidermal melanocytes are completely lost in depigmented areas through an autoimmune process. (From Jarvis C: Physical Examination and Health Assessment, 3rd ed. Philadelphia, WB Saunders, 2000, p. 223.)

SKIN NEOPLASMS

Benign Neoplasms

callus

Increased growth of cells in the keratin layer of the epidermis caused by pressure or friction.

The feet (Fig. 16–16, *A*) and the hands are common sites for callus formation. A **corn** is a type of callus that develops a hard core (a whitish, corn-like central kernel).

keloid

Hypertrophied, thickened scar that occurs after trauma or surgical incision.

Keloids (see Fig. 16–16, *B*) result from excessive collagen formation in the skin during connective tissue repair. The term comes from the Greek *kelis*, meaning blemish. Surgical excision often is combined with intralesional steroid injections or low-dose radiotherapy.

A normal scar left by a healed wound is called a **cicatrix** (SĬK-ă-trĭks).

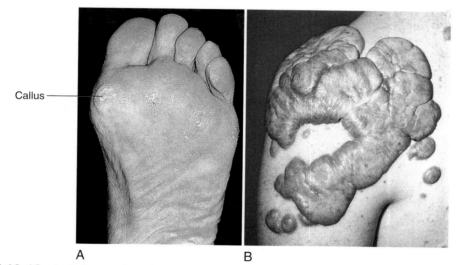

Callus

A   B

FIGURE 16–16   A, Callus on the sole of the foot. **B, Keloid. (A** from Mosby's Medical, Nursing, and Allied Health Dictionary, 6th ed. St. Louis, Mosby, 2002, p. 265. **B** from Ignatavicius DD, Workman ML: Medical-Surgical Nursing: Critical Thinking for Collaborative Care, 4th ed. Philadelphia, WB Saunders, 2002, p. 1544.)

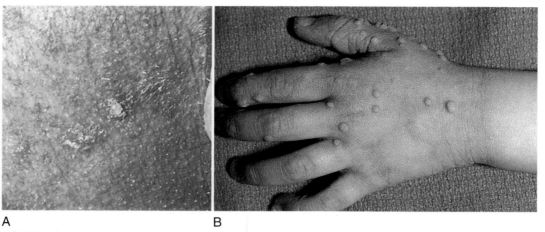

FIGURE 16–17   **A, Actinic (solar) keratosis. B, Verruca vulgaris. Warts** are multiple papules with rough, pebble-like surfaces. (**A** from Ignatavicius DD, Workman ML: Medical-Surgical Nursing: Critical Thinking for Collaborative Care, 4th ed. Philadelphia, WB Saunders, 2002, p. 1502. **B** from Cotran RS, Kumar V, Collins T [eds]: Robbins Pathologic Basis of Disease, 6th ed. Philadelphia, WB Saunders, 1999, p. 1208.)

keratosis	**Thickened and reddened area of the epidermis, usually associated with aging or skin damage.**
	Actinic keratoses are caused by excessive exposure to light and are precancerous lesions. See Figure 16–17, *A*. **Seborrheic keratoses** result from overgrowth of basal cells and are dark in color.
leukoplakia	**White, thickened patches on mucous membrane tissue of the tongue or cheek.**
	This precancerous lesion is common in smokers and may be caused by chronic inflammation.
nevus (*plural:* **nevi**)	**Pigmented lesion of the skin.**
	Nevi include dilated blood vessels radiating out from a point (vascular spiders), hemangiomas, and moles. Many are present at birth, but some are acquired.
	Dysplastic nevi are moles that do not form properly and may progress to form a type of skin cancer called melanoma (see **malignant melanoma**).
verruca	**Epidermal growth (wart) caused by a virus.**
	Verruca vulgaris (common wart) is the most frequent type of wart (see Fig. 16–17, *B*). Plantar warts (verrucae) occur on the soles of the feet, juvenile warts occur on the hands and face of children, and venereal warts occur on the genitals and around the anus. Warts are removed with acids, electrocautery, or freezing with liquid nitrogen (cryosurgery). If the virus remains in the skin, the wart frequently regrows.

Cancerous Lesions

basal cell carcinoma	**Malignant tumor of the basal cell layer of the epidermis.**
	This is the most frequent type of skin cancer. It is a slow-growing tumor that usually occurs on the face, especially near or on the nose. See Figure 16–18, *A*. It almost never metastasizes.

SKIN **647**

16

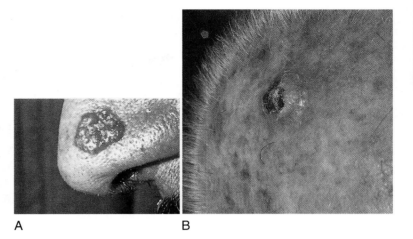

FIGURE 16–18 **A, Basal cell carcinoma. B, Squamous cell carcinoma.** Lesions are often nodular and ulcerated. (**A** from Mosby's Medical, Nursing, and Allied Health Dictionary, 6th ed. St. Louis, Mosby, 2002, p. 184. **B** from Cotran RS, Kumar V, Collins T [eds]: Robbins Pathologic Basis of Disease, 6th ed. Philadelphia, WB Saunders, 1999, p. 1186.)   A   B

squamous cell carcinoma	**Malignant tumor of the squamous epithelial cells of the epidermis.**

This tumor may grow in places other than the skin, wherever squamous epithelium is found (mouth, larynx, bladder, esophagus, lungs). **Actinic** (sun-related) **keratoses** are premalignant lesions in people with sun-damaged skin. Progression to squamous cell carcinoma (see Fig. 16–18, *B*) may occur if lesions are not removed. Treatment is surgical excision, cryotherapy, curettage and electrodesiccation, or radiotherapy.

malignant melanoma   **Cancerous growth composed of melanocytes.**

This malignancy is attributed to the intense exposure to sunlight that many people experience. Melanoma usually begins as a mottled, light brown to black, flat macule with irregular borders (Fig. 16–19). The lesion may turn shades of red, blue, and white and may crust on the surface and bleed. Melanomas often arise in preexisting moles (dysplastic nevi) and frequently appear on the upper back, lower legs, arms, head, and neck.

Biopsy is required to confirm the diagnosis of melanoma, and prognosis is commonly determined by measuring tumor thickness in millimeters.

Melanomas often metastasize to the lung, liver, bone, and brain. Treatment includes excision of the tumor, regional lymphadenectomy, chemotherapy/immunotherapy, or radiotherapy.

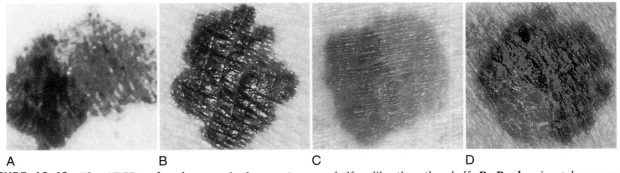

A   B   C   D

FIGURE 16–19 **The ABCDs of melanoma. A, Asymmetry:** one half unlike the other half. **B, Border:** irregular or poorly circumscribed border. **C, Color:** varies from one area to another; shades of tan and brown; black; sometimes white, red, or blue. **D, Diameter:** usually larger than 6 mm (diameter of a pencil eraser). (From Lewis SM, Heitkemper MM, Dirksen SR: Medical-Surgical Nursing: Assessment and Management of Clinical Problems, 6th ed. St. Louis, Mosby, 2004, p. 493.)

16

Kaposi sarcoma	**Malignant, vascular, neoplastic growth characterized by cutaneous nodules.**
	Frequently arising on the lower extremities, nodules range in color from deep pink to dark blue and purple. The condition is associated with acquired immunodeficiency syndrome (AIDS).

LABORATORY TESTS AND CLINICAL PROCEDURES

LABORATORY TESTS

bacterial analyses	**Samples of skin are sent to a laboratory to detect presence of microorganisms.**
	Purulent (pus-filled) material or **exudate** (fluid that accumulates) often are taken for examination.
fungal tests	**Scrapings from skin lesions, hair specimens, or nail clippings are sent to a laboratory for culture and microscopic examination.**
	The specimen also may be treated with a potassium hydroxide (KOH) preparation and examined microscopically. A positive result on a KOH test often eliminates the need for a culture.

CLINICAL PROCEDURES

cryosurgery	**Use of subfreezing temperature via liquid nitrogen application to destroy tissue.**
curettage	**Use of a sharp dermal curette to scrape away a skin lesion.**
	A curette is shaped like a spoon or scoop.
electrodesiccation	**Tissue is destroyed by burning with an electric spark.**
	This procedure is used along with curettage to remove and destroy small cancerous lesions with well-defined borders.
Mohs surgery	**Thin layers of a malignant growth are removed, and each is examined under a microscope.**
	Mohs surgery is a specialized form of excision to treat basal squamous cell carcinomas and other tumors. It is also known as **microscopically controlled surgery.**
skin biopsy	**Suspected malignant skin lesions are removed and sent to the pathology laboratory for microscopic examination.**
	In a **punch biopsy,** a surgical instrument removes a core of tissue by rotation of its sharp, circular edge. In a **shave biopsy,** tissue is excised using a cut parallel to the surface of the surrounding skin.
skin test	**Reaction of the body to a substance by observing the results of injecting the substance intradermally or applying it topically to the skin.**
	Skin tests are used to diagnose allergies and disease. In the **patch test,** an allergen-treated piece of gauze or filter paper is applied to the skin. If the skin becomes red or swollen, the result is positive. In the **scratch test,** several scratches are made in the skin, and a very minute amount of test material is inserted into the scratches. The Schick test (for diphtheria) and the Mantoux and purified protein derivative (PPD) tests (for tuberculosis) are other skin tests.

ABBREVIATIONS

ABCD	asymmetry (of shape), border (irregularity), color (variation with one lesion), diameter (greater than 6 mm)—characteristics associated with skin cancer	**PPD**	purified protein derivative— skin test for tuberculosis
		PUVA	psoralen–ultraviolet A light therapy; treatment for psoriasis and other skin conditions
bx	biopsy		
Derm.	dermatology	**SLE**	systemic lupus erythematosus
DLE	discoid lupus erythematosus	**SC**	subcutaneous

PRACTICAL APPLICATIONS

This section contains disease descriptions and a medical report using terms that you have studied in this and previous chapters. Explanations of more difficult terms are added in brackets. Answers to the questions are on page 661.

DISEASE DESCRIPTIONS

1. **Candidiasis** (*Candida* is a yeast-like fungus): This fungus is normally found on mucous membranes, skin, and vaginal mucosa. Under certain circumstances (excessive warmth; administration of birth control pills, antibiotics, and corticosteroids; debilitated states; infancy), it can change to a pathogen and cause localized or generalized mucocutaneous disease. Examples are paronychial lesions, lesions in areas of the body where the rubbing of opposed surfaces is common (groin, perianal, axillary, inframammary, and interdigital), thrush (white plaques attached to oral or vaginal mucous membranes), and vulvovaginitis.

2. **Cellulitis:** This is a common nonsuppurative infection of connective tissue with severe inflammation of the dermal and subcutaneous layers of the skin. Cellulitis appears on an extremity as a reddish-brown area of edematous skin. A surgical wound, puncture, insect bite, skin ulcer, or patch of dermatitis is the usual means of entry for bacteria (most cases are caused by streptococci). Therapy includes rest, elevation, hot wet packs, and antibiotics. Any cellulitis on the face should be given special attention because the infection may extend directly to the brain.

3. **Mycosis fungoides (cutaneous T cell lymphoma):** This rare, chronic skin condition is caused by the infiltration of the skin by malignant lymphocytes. Contrary to its name (myc/o = fungus), it is not caused by a fungus but was formerly thought to be of fungal origin. It is characterized by generalized erythroderma and large, reddish, raised tumors that spread and ulcerate. In some cases, the malignant cells may involve lymph nodes and other organs. Treatment with cortisone ointments, topical nitrogen mustard, and ultraviolet light (PUVA) can be effective in controlling the disease.

16

MEDICAL REPORT: FINDINGS ON DERMATOLOGIC EXAMINATION

A wide variety of lesions are seen on the face, shoulders, and back. The predominant lesions are pustules on an inflammatory base. Many pustules are confluent [running together] over the chin and forehead. Comedones are present on the face, especially along the nasolabial folds. Inflammatory papules are present on the lower cheeks and chin. Large abscesses and ulcerated cysts are present over the upper shoulder area. Numerous scars are present over the face and upper back.

Questions about the Medical Report

1. In this skin condition, the dominant damage to tissue involves:
   a. Discolored flat lesions
   b. Grooves or crack-like sores
   c. Small elevations containing pus

2. Comedones are:
   a. Sebum plugs partially blocking skin pores
   b. Contagious, infectious plugs of sebum
   c. Small, pinpoint hemorrhages

3. Papules also are known as:
   a. Purpura
   b. Pimples
   c. Freckles

4. In the scapular region, lesions are:
   a. Large pigmented areas
   b. Numerous collections of blisters
   c. Large collections of sacs containing pus with erosion of skin

5. A hypertrophied scar (cicatrix) also is known as a:
   a. Wheal
   b. Keloid
   c. Polyp

6. What is your diagnosis of this skin condition, based on the physical examination?
   a. Acne vulgaris
   b. Leukoplakia
   c. Scabies

EXERCISES

Remember to check your answers carefully with those given in the Answers to Exercises, page 660.

A. Select from the following terms to complete the sentences below.

basal layer	dermis	lunula	sebum
collagen	keratin	melanin	stratum corneum
cuticle	lipocyte		

1. A fat cell is a/an _____.

2. The half-moon–shaped white area at the base of a nail is the _____.

3. A structural protein found in skin and connective tissue is _____.

4. A black pigment found in the epidermis is_____.

5. The deepest region of the epidermis is the _____.

6. The outermost layer of the epidermis, which consists of flattened, keratinized cells, is the

   _____.

7. An oily substance secreted by sebaceous glands is_____.

8. The middle layer of the skin is the _____.

9. A hard, protein material found in epidermis, hair, and nails is_____.

10. A band of epidermis at the base and sides of the nail plate is the _____.

B. Complete the following terms based on their meanings as given below.

1. the outermost layer of skin: epi_____

2. profuse sweating: dia_____

3. excessive secretion from sebaceous glands: sebo_____

4. inflammation and swelling of soft tissue around a nail: par_____

5. fungal infections of hands and feet: dermato_____

6. burning sensation (pain) in skin: caus_____

C. Match the terms in Column I with the descriptive meanings in Column II. Write the letter of the answer in the space provided.

16

Column I

1. squamous epithelium   _____

2. sebaceous gland   _____

3. albinism   _____

4. electrocautery   _____

5. subcutaneous tissue   _____

6. collagen   _____

7. dermis   _____

8. melanocyte   _____

9. erythema   _____

10. dermabrasion   _____

Column II

A. Connective tissue layer of skin
B. Surgical procedure to scrape away tissue
C. Flat, scale-like cells
D. Connective tissue protein
E. Pigment deficiency of the skin
F. Contains a dark pigment
G. Redness of skin
H. Contains lipocytes
I. Oil-producing organ
J. Knife used to burn through tissue

D. Build medical terms based on the definitions and word parts given.

1. surgical repair of the skin: dermato_____

2. pertaining to under the skin: sub_____

3. abnormal condition of lack of sweat: an_____

4. abnormal condition of proliferation of horny, keratinized cells: kerat_____

5. abnormal condition of dry, scaly skin: _____osis

6. loosening of the epidermis: epidermo_____

7. yellow tumor (nodule under the skin): _____oma

8. pertaining to under the nail: sub_____

9. abnormal condition of fungus in the hair: _____mycosis

10. abnormal condition of nail fungus: onycho_____

11. removal of wrinkles: _____ectomy

E. Give the meanings for the following combining forms.

1. melan/o _____

2. adip/o _____

3. squam/o _____

4. xanth/o _____

5. myc/o _____

6. onych/o _____

7. pil/o _____

8. xer/o _____

9. trich/o _____

10. erythem/o _____

11. albin/o _____

12. ichthy/o _____

13. hidr/o _____

14. ungu/o _____

15. cauter/o _____

16. steat/o _____

17. rhytid/o _____

F. Match each of the following lesions with their illustrations below (see Fig. 16–20).

cyst   macule   pustule
crust (scab)   nodule   ulcer
erosion   papule   vesicle
fissure   polyp   wheal

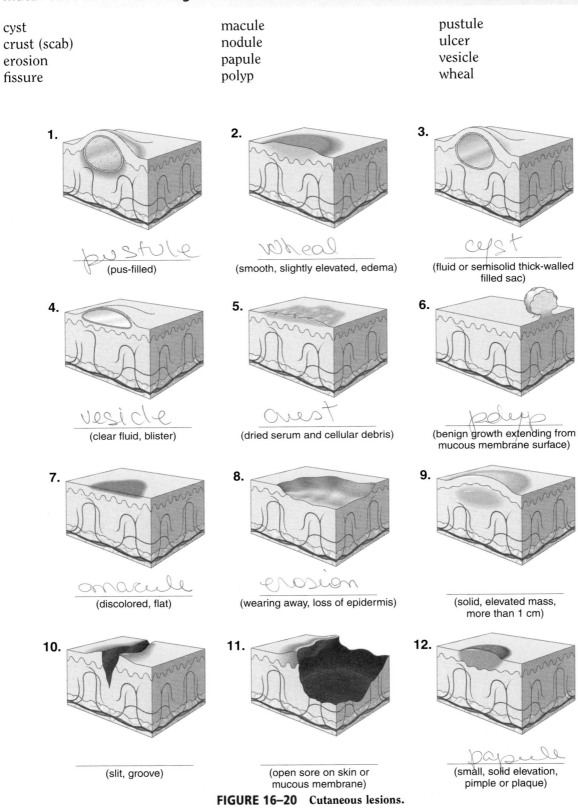

1. *pustule*
   (pus-filled)

2. *wheal*
   (smooth, slightly elevated, edema)

3. *cyst*
   (fluid or semisolid thick-walled filled sac)

4. *vesicle*
   (clear fluid, blister)

5. *crust*
   (dried serum and cellular debris)

6. *polyp*
   (benign growth extending from mucous membrane surface)

7. *macule*
   (discolored, flat)

8. *erosion*
   (wearing away, loss of epidermis)

9. (solid, elevated mass, more than 1 cm)

10. (slit, groove)

11. (open sore on skin or mucous membrane)

12. *papule*
    (small, solid elevation, pimple or plaque)

FIGURE 16–20 Cutaneous lesions.

G. Give the medical terms for the following.

1. baldness _____

2. bluish-black mark (macule) caused by hemorrhages into the skin _____

3. itching _____

4. acute allergic reaction in which red, round wheals develop on the skin _____

5. blackhead _____

6. small, pinpoint hemorrhages _____

H. Match the pathologic skin condition with its description below.

acne vulgaris   gangrene   scleroderma
basal cell carcinoma   impetigo   squamous cell carcinoma
decubitus ulcer   malignant melanoma   systemic lupus erythematosus
eczema   psoriasis   tinea

1. malignant neoplasm originating in scale-like cells of the epidermis _____

2. buildup of sebum and keratin in pores of the skin leading to papular and pustular eruptions

   _____

3. fungal skin infection _____

4. chronic disease marked by hardening and shrinking of connective tissue in the skin

   _____

5. bedsore _____

6. necrosis of skin tissue resulting from ischemia _____

7. chronic or acute inflammatory skin disease with erythematous, pustular, or papular lesions

   _____

8. widespread inflammatory disease of the joints and collagen of the skin with "butterfly" rash on the

   _____ face

9. cancerous tumor composed of melanocytes _____

10. chronic, recurrent dermatosis marked by silvery-gray scales covering red patches on the skin

    _____

11. malignant neoplasm originating in the basal layer of the epidermis _____

12. contagious, infectious pyoderma _____

16

I. Circle the term that best fits the definition given.

1. contagious parasitic infection with intense pruritus: **(scleroderma, scabies)**

2. measles: **(rubella, rubeola)**

3. chickenpox: **(varicella, eczema)**

4. thickened cicatrix (scar): **(tinea, keloid)**

5. white patches on mucous membrane of tongue or inner cheek: **(leukoplakia, albinism)**

6. characterized by a rash: **(gangrene, exanthematous)**

7. thickening of epidermis related to sunlight exposure: **(actinic keratosis, callus)**

8. small, pinpoint hemorrhages: **(psoriasis, petechiae)**

9. large blisters: **(bullae, pustules)**

10. colored pigmentation of skin (mole): **(nevus, verruca)**

11. sac of fluid and hair over sacral region: **(ecchymosis, pilonidal cyst)**

12. acute allergic reaction in which hives develop: **(vitiligo, urticaria)**

J. Describe the following types of burns.

1. second-degree burn _____

2. first-degree burn _____

3. third-degree burn _____

K. Match the following medical terms with their more common meanings below.

alopecia   exanthem   tinea pedis
comedones   nevi   urticaria
decubitus ulcer   pruritus   verrucae
ecchymosis   seborrheic dermatitis   vesicles

1. blackheads _____

2. moles _____

3. baldness _____

4. itching _____

5. hives _____

6. bedsore _____

7. warts _____

8. athlete's foot _____

9. "black-and-blue" mark _____

10. dandruff _____

11. blisters _____

12. rash _____

L.   Describe how the following conditions affect the skin.

1. pyoderma _____

2. xeroderma _____

3. leukoderma _____

4. erythema _____

5. callus _____

6. keloid _____

7. gangrene _____

M.   Give short answers for the following.

1. Two skin tests for allergy are _____ and _____.

2. The _____ test is an intradermal test for diphtheria.

3. The _____ test and the _____ test are skin tests for tuberculosis.

4. Purulent means _____.

5. A surgical procedure to core out a disk of skin for microscopic analysis is a/an _____.

6. The procedure in which thin layers of a malignant growth are removed and each is examined under the microscope is _____.

7. A type of skin cancer associated with AIDS and marked by dark blue-purple lesions over the skin is _____.

8. Abnormal, premalignant moles are _____.

9. Removal of skin tissue using a cut parallel to the surface of the surrounding skin is called a/an

   _____.

10. Destruction of tissue by use of intensely cold temperatures is _____.

11. Scraping away skin to remove acne scars and fine wrinkles on the skin is _____.

12. Removal of subcutaneous fat tissue by aspiration is _____.

13. Destruction of tissue using an electric spark is _____.

14. Use of a sharp spoon-like instrument to scrape away tissue is _____.

N. Circle the term that best completes the meaning of the sentence.

1. Since he had been a teenager, Jim had had red, scaly patches on his elbows and behind his knees. Dr. Horn diagnosed Jim's dermatologic condition as **(vitiligo, impetigo, psoriasis)** and prescribed a special cream.

2. Clarissa noticed a rash across the bridge of her nose and aching in her joints. She saw a rheumatologist, who did some blood work and diagnosed her condition as **(rheumatoid arthritis, systemic lupus erythematosus, scleroderma)**.

3. Bea had large, red patches all over her trunk and neck after eating shrimp. The doctor prescribed hydrocortisone cream to relieve her itching **(seborrhea, acne, urticaria)**.

4. The poison ivy she touched caused very uncomfortable **(pruritus, calluses, keratosis)**, and Maggie was scratching her arms raw.

5. Kelly was fair-skinned with red hair. She had many benign nevi on her arms and legs, but Dr. Keefe was especially worried about one pigmented lesion with an irregular, raised border, which he biopsied and found to be malignant **(melanoma, Kaposi sarcoma, pyoderma)**.

6. After five days of high fever, 3-year-old Sadie developed a red rash all over her body. The pediatrician described it as a viral **(eczema, purpura, exanthem)** and told her mother it was a case of **(rubeola, impetigo, scabies)**.

7. Several months after her surgery, Mabel's scar became raised and thickened. It had **(atrophied, stratified, hypertrophied)**, and her physician described it as a **(nevus, verruca, keloid)**.

8. Perry had a bad habit of biting his nails and picking at the **(follicle, cuticle, subcutaneous tissue)** surrounding his nails. Often, he developed inflammation and swelling of the soft tissue around the nail, a condition known as **(onychomycosis, onycholysis, paronychia)**.

9. Brenda noticed a small papillomatous wart on her hand. Her **(oncologist, dermatologist, psychologist)** explained that it was a **(pustule, polyp, verruca)** and was caused by a **(bacterium, virus, toxin)**. The doctor suggested removing it by **(Mohs surgery, cryosurgery, dilation and curettage)**.

10. Sarah, a teenager, was self-conscious about the inflammatory lesions of papules and pustules on her face. She noticed blackheads or **(wheals, bullae, comedones)** and whiteheads (collections of pus). She was advised to begin taking antibiotics and medications to dry her **(acne vulgaris, scleroderma, gangrene)**.

MEDICAL SCRAMBLE

Unscramble the letters to form dermatologic terms from the clues. Use the letters in squares to complete the bonus term. Answers are found on page 661.

1. *Clue:* Small skin elevation containing pus

___ ___ ___ [ ] ___ ___ [ ] UPESLUT

2. *Clue:* Contagious, parasitic infection with intense pruritus

___ ___ [ ] ___ ___ [ ] ___ IBSACES

3. *Clue:* Epidermal growth caused by a virus

___ ___ [ ] ___ [ ] [ ] ___ CRERAVU

4. *Clue:* Loss of pigmentation

___ ___ [ ] ___ ___ ___ [ ] ___ IGILOVTI

BONUS TERM: *Clue:* Procedure using a sharp instrument to scrape away skin lesions

[ ] [ ] [ ] [ ] [ ] [ ] [ ] [ ] [ ]

16

ANSWERS TO EXERCISES

A

1. lipocyte
2. lunula
3. collagen
4. melanin

5. basal layer
6. stratum corneum
7. sebum

8. dermis
9. keratin
10. cuticle

B

1. epidermis
2. diaphoresis
3. seborrhea
4. paronychia

5. dermatophytosis or dermatomycosis (tinea)
6. causalgia

C

1. C
2. I
3. E
4. J

5. H
6. D
7. A

8. F
9. G
10. B

D

1. dermatoplasty
2. subcutaneous
3. anhidrosis
4. keratosis

5. ichthyosis
6. epidermolysis
7. xanthoma
8. subungual

9. trichomycosis
10. onychomycosis
11. rhytidectomy

E

1. black
2. fat
3. scale-like
4. yellow
5. fungus
6. nail

7. hair
8. dry
9. hair
10. redness
11. white
12. scaly, dry

13. sweat
14. nail
15. heat, burn
16. fat
17. wrinkle

F

1. pustule
2. wheal
3. cyst
4. vesicle

5. crust (scab)
6. polyp
7. macule
8. erosion

9. nodule
10. fissure
11. ulcer
12. papule

G

1. alopecia
2. ecchymosis
3. pruritus

4. urticaria
5. comedo
6. petechiae

H

1. squamous cell carcinoma
2. acne vulgaris
3. tinea
4. scleroderma

5. decubitus ulcer
6. gangrene
7. eczema
8. systemic lupus erythematosus

9. malignant melanoma
10. psoriasis
11. basal cell carcinoma
12. impetigo

I

1. scabies
2. rubeola
3. varicella
4. keloid

5. leukoplakia
6. exanthematous
7. actinic keratosis
8. petechiae

9. bullae
10. nevus
11. pilonidal cyst
12. urticaria

16

J

1. damage to the epidermis and dermis with blisters, erythema, and hyperesthesia
2. damage to the epidermis with erythema and hyperesthesia; no blisters
3. destruction of both epidermis and dermis and damage to subcutaneous layer

K

1. comedones
2. nevi
3. alopecia
4. pruritus
5. urticaria
6. decubitus ulcer
7. verrucae
8. tinea pedis
9. ecchymosis
10. seborrheic dermatitis
11. vesicles
12. exanthem

L

1. collections of pus in the skin
2. dry skin
3. white patches of skin (vitiligo)
4. redness of skin
5. increased growth of epidermal horny-layer cells due to excess pressure or friction
6. thickened, hypertrophied scar tissue
7. necrosis (death) of skin tissue

M

1. scratch test; patch test
2. Schick
3. Mantoux; PPD
4. pus-filled
5. punch biopsy
6. Mohs surgery
7. Kaposi sarcoma
8. dysplastic nevi
9. shave biopsy
10. cryosurgery
11. dermabrasion
12. liposuction
13. electrodesiccation
14. curettage

N

1. psoriasis
2. systemic lupus erythematosus
3. urticaria
4. pruritus
5. melanoma
6. exanthem; rubeola
7. hypertrophied; keloid
8. cuticle; paronychia
9. dermatologist; verruca virus; cryosurgery
10. comedones; acne vulgaris

ANSWERS TO PRACTICAL APPLICATIONS

1. c
2. a
3. b
4. c
5. b
6. a

ANSWERS TO MEDICAL SCRAMBLE

1. PUSTULE 2. SCABIES 3. VERRUCA 4. VITILIGO
BONUS TERM: CURETTAGE

PRONUNCIATION OF TERMS

PRONUNCIATION GUIDE

ā as in āpe   ă as in ăpple
ē as in ēven   ĕ as in ĕvery
ī as in īce   ĭ as in ĭnterest
ō as in ōpen   ŏ as in pŏt
ū as in ūnit   ŭ as in ŭnder

To test your understanding of the terminology in this chapter, write the meaning of each term in the space provided. In addition, you may wish to cover the terms and write them by looking at your definitions. Make sure your spelling is correct. The page number after each term indicates where it is defined or used in the book, so you can easily check your responses. You will find complete definitions for all of these terms and their audio pronunciations on the CD.

VOCABULARY, COMBINING FORMS, AND SUFFIXES

Term	Pronunciation	Meaning
adipose (632)	ĂD-ĭ-pōs	_____
albinism (632)	ĂL-bĭ-nĭzm	_____
albino (631)	ăl-BĪ-nō	_____
alopecia (640)	ăl-ō-PĒ-shē-ă	_____
anhidrosis (634)	ăn-hī-DRŌ-sĭs	_____
apocrine sweat gland (631)	ĂP-ō-krĭn swĕt glănd	_____
atopic dermatitis (633)	ā-TŎP-ĭk dĕr-mă-TĪ-tĭs	_____
basal layer (631)	BĀ-săl LĀ-ĕr	_____
causalgia (632)	kăw-ZĂL-jă	_____
collagen (631)	KŎL-ă-jĕn	_____
cuticle (631)	KŪ-tĭ-k'l	_____
dermabrasion (633)	dĕrm-ă-BRĀ-zhŭn	_____
dermatologist (633)	dĕr-mă-TŎL-ō-jĭst	_____
dermatophytosis (635)	dĕr-mă-tō-fī-TŌ-sĭs	_____
dermatoplasty (633)	DĔR-mă-tō-plăs-tē	_____
dermis (631)	DĔR-mĭs	_____
diaphoresis (633)	dī-ă-fŏr-RĒ-sĭs	_____
eccrine sweat gland (631)	Ĕ-krĭn swĕt glănd	_____
electrocautery (632)	ĕ-lĕk-trō-KĂW-tĕr-ē	_____
epidermis (631)	ĕp-ĭ-DĔR-mĭs	_____
epidermolysis (633)	ĕp-ĭ-dĕr-MŎL-ĭ-sĭs	_____
epithelium (631)	ĕp-ĭ-THĒL-ē-ŭm	_____
erythema (633)	ĕr-ĭ-THĒ-mă	_____

16

Term	Pronunciation	Meaning
erythematous (633)	ĕr-ĭ-THĒ-mă-tŭs	_____
hair follicle (631)	hār FŎL-ĭ-k'l	_____
ichthyosis (634)	ĭk-thē-Ō-sĭs	_____
integumentary system (631)	ĭn-tĕg-ū-MĔN-tăr-ē SĬS-tĕm	_____
keratin (631)	KĔR-ă-tĭn	_____
keratosis (634)	kĕr-ă-TŌ-sĭs	_____
leukoderma (644)	lū-kō-DĔR-mă	_____
leukoplakia (634)	lū-kō-PLĀ-kē-ă	_____
lipocyte (631)	LĬP-ō-sīt	_____
lipoma (634)	lī-PŌ-mă _or_ lĭ-PŌ-mă	_____
liposuction (634)	lī-pō-SŬK-shun	_____
lunula (631)	LŪ-nū-lă	_____
melanin (631)	MĔL-ă-nĭn	_____
melanocyte (632)	mĕ-LĂN-ō-sīt	_____
mycosis (635)	mī-KŌ-sĭs	_____
onycholysis (635)	ŏn-ĭ-KŎL-ĭ-sĭs	_____
onychomycosis (635)	ŏn-ĭ-kō-mī-KŌ-sĭs	_____
paronychia (635)	păr-ō-NĬK-ē-ă	_____
paronychium (631)	păr-ŏn-NĬK-ē-um	_____
pilosebaceous (635)	pī-lō-sĕ-BĀ-shŭs	_____
pyoderma (636)	pī-ō-DĔR-mă	_____
rhytidectomy (636)	rĭt-ĭ-DĔK-tō-mē	_____
sebaceous gland (631)	sĕ-BĀ-shŭs glănd	_____
seborrhea (636)	sĕb-ō-RĒ-ă	_____
seborrheic dermatitis (636)	sĕb-ō-RĒ-ĭk dĕr-mă-TĪ-tĭs	_____
sebum (631)	SĒ-bŭm	_____
squamous epithelium (631)	SKWĀ-mŭs ĕp-ĭ-THĒ-lē-ŭm	_____
steatoma (636)	stē-ă-TŌ-mă	_____
stratified (631)	STRĂT-ĭ-fīd	_____
stratum; strata (631)	STRĂ-tŭm; STRĂ-tă	_____
stratum corneum (631)	STRĂ-tŭm KŎR-nē-ŭm	_____
subcutaneous layer (631)	sŭb-kū-TĀ-nē-ŭs LĀ-ĕr	_____
subungual (636)	sŭb-ŬNG-wăl	_____

16

Term	Pronunciation	Meaning
trichomycosis (636)	trĭk-ō-mī-KŌ-sĭs	_____
xanthoma (632)	zăn-THŌ-mă	_____
xeroderma (636)	zē-rō-DĔR-mă	_____

LESIONS, SYMPTOMS, ABNORMAL CONDITIONS, AND NEOPLASMS; LABORATORY TESTS AND CLINICAL PROCEDURES

Term	Pronunciation	Meaning
abscess (638)	ĂB-sĕs	_____
acne (641)	ĂK-nē	_____
actinic keratosis (646)	ăk-TĬN-ĭk kĕr-ă-TŌ-sis	_____
alopecia areata (640)	ăl-ō-PĒ-shē-ă ăr-ē-ĂT-ă	_____
basal cell carcinoma (646)	BĀ-săl sĕl kăr-sĭ-NŌ-mă	_____
bulla; bullae (638)	BŬL-ă; BŬL-ē	_____
burns (642)	bŭrnz	_____
callus (645)	KĂL-ŭs	_____
cellulitis (642)	sĕl-ū-LĪ-tĭs	_____
cicatrix (645)	SĬK-ă-trĭks	_____
comedo; comedones (641)	KŎM-ĕ-dō; kŏm-ĕ-DŌNZ	_____
crust (638)	krŭst	_____
curettage (648)	kū-rĕ-TOZH	_____
cyst (638)	sĭst	_____
decubitus ulcer (638)	dē-KŪ-bĭ-tŭs ŬL-sĕr	_____
dysplastic nevi (646)	dĭs-PLĂS-tik NĒ-vī	_____
ecchymosis; ecchymoses (640)	ĕk-ĭ-MŌ-sĭs; ĕk-ĭ-MŌ-sēz	_____
eczema (642)	ĔK-zĕ-mă	_____
electrodesiccation (648)	ĕ-lĕk-trō-dĕ-sĭ-KĀ-shun	_____
erosion (638)	ĕ-RŌ-zhŭn	_____
exanthematous viral disease (642)	ĕg-zăn-THĔM-ă-tŭs VĪ-răl dĭ-ZĒZ	_____
fissure (638)	FĬSH-ŭr	_____
fungal tests (648)	FŬNG-ăl tĕsts	_____
gangrene (642)	găng-GRĒN	_____
impetigo (642)	ĭm-pĕ-TĪ-gō	_____
Kaposi sarcoma (648)	KĂH-pō-sē săr-KŌ-mă	_____

Term	Pronunciation	Meaning
keloid (645)	KĒ-lŏyd	
macule (638)	MĂK-ūl	
malignant melanoma (647)	mă-LĬG-nănt mĕ-lă-NŌ-mă	
Mohs surgery (648)	mōz SŬR-jĕ-rē	
nevus; nevi (646)	NĒ-vŭs; NĒ-vī	
nodule (638)	NŎD-ūl	
papule (638)	PĂP-ūl	
petechia; petechiae (640)	pĕ-TĒ-kē-ă; pĕ-TĒ-kē-ī	
pilonidal cyst (638)	pī-lō-NĪ-dăl sĭst	
polyp (638)	PŎL-ĭp	
pruritus (641)	proo-RĪ-tŭs	
psoriasis (643)	sō-RĪ-ă-sĭs	
purpura (640)	PŬR-pŭr-ă	
purulent (648)	PŪ-roo-lĕnt	
pustule (638)	PŬS-tūl	
rubella (642)	roo-BĔL-ă	
rubeola (642)	roo-bē-Ō-lă	
scabies (643)	SKĀ-bēz	
scleroderma (643)	sklĕr-ō-DĔR-mă	
sebaceous cyst (638)	sĕ-BĀ-shŭs sĭst	
skin biopsy (648)	skĭn BĪ-ŏp-sē	
skin test (648)	skĭn tĕst	
squamous cell carcinoma (647)	SKWĀ-mŭs sĕl kăr-sĭ-NŌ-mă	
systemic lupus erythematosus (643)	sĭs-TĔM-ĭk LOO-pŭs ĕr-ĭ-thē-mă-TŌ-sŭs	
tinea (644)	TĬN-ē-ă	
ulcer (638)	ŬL-sĕr	
urticaria (641)	ŭr-tĭ-KĀ-rē-ă	
varicella (642)	văr-ĭ-SĔL-ă	
verruca; verrucae (646)	vĕ-ROO-kă; vĕ-ROO-kē	
vesicle (638)	VĔS-ĭ-k'l	
vitiligo (644)	vĭt-ĭl-Ī-gō	
wheal (638)	wēl	

REVIEW SHEET

16

Write the meanings of the word parts in the spaces provided and test yourself. Check your answers with the information in the chapter or in the glossary (Medical Word Parts—English) at the end of the book.

COMBINING FORMS

Combining Form	Meaning	Combining Form	Meaning
adip/o	_____	melan/o	_____
albin/o	_____	myc/o	_____
caus/o	_____	onych/o	_____
cauter/o	_____	phyt/o	_____
cutane/o	_____	pil/o	_____
derm/o	_____	py/o	_____
dermat/o	_____	rhytid/o	_____
diaphor/o	_____	seb/o	_____
erythem/o	_____	sebace/o	_____
erythemat/o	_____	squam/o	_____
hidr/o	_____	steat/o	_____
hydr/o	_____	trich/o	_____
ichthy/o	_____	ungu/o	_____
kerat/o	_____	xanth/o	_____
leuk/o	_____	xer/o	_____
lip/o	_____		

SUFFIXES

Suffix	Meaning	Suffix	Meaning
-algia	_____	-osis	_____
-derma	_____	-ous	_____
-esis	_____	-plakia	_____
-lysis	_____	-plasty	_____
-ose	_____	-rrhea	_____

GIVE COMBINING FORMS FOR THE FOLLOWING (FIRST LETTERS ARE GIVEN).

fat	a_____		sweat	d_____	
	l_____			h_____	
	s_____		yellow	x_____	
white	a_____		dry	x_____	
	l_____		scaly, dry	i_____	
skin	c_____		redness	e_____	
	d_____			e_____	
nail	o_____		hard, horny	k_____	
	u_____		burn, burning	c_____	
hair	p_____		black	m_____	
	t_____		fungus	m_____	
plant	p_____				

Please refer to the enclosed CD for additional exercises and images related to this chapter.

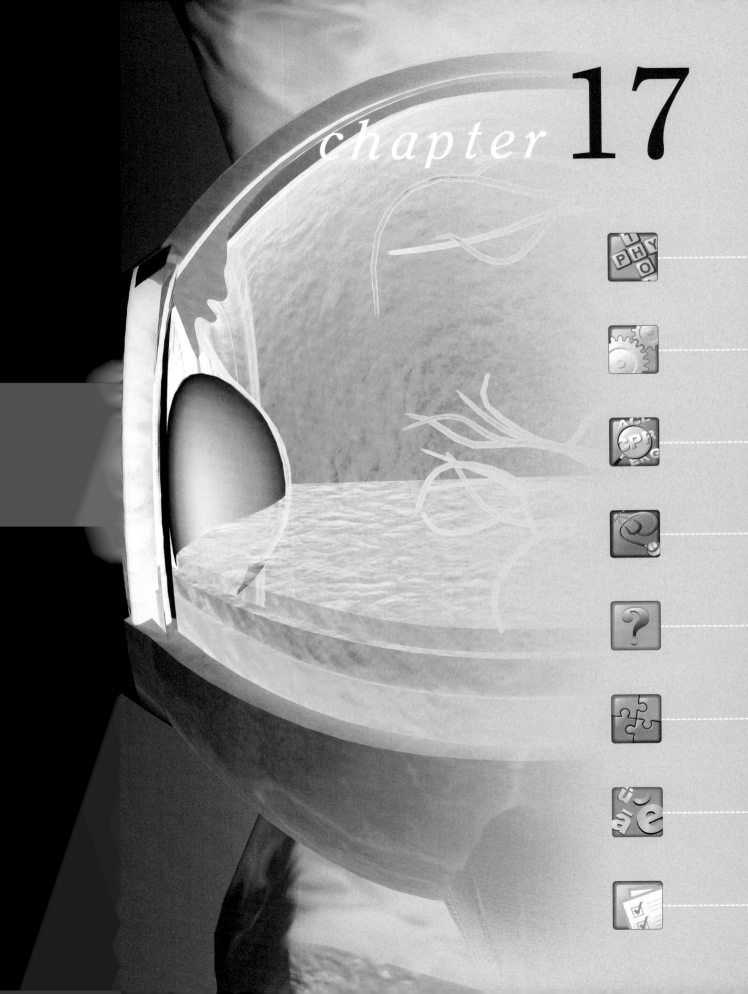

chapter 17

Sense Organs: The Eye and the Ear

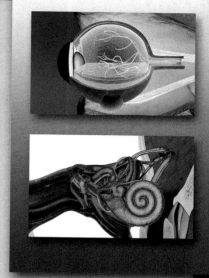

THIS CHAPTER IS DIVIDED INTO THE FOLLOWING SECTIONS

In this chapter you will

- Identify locations and functions of the major parts of the eye and the ear.
- Name the combining forms, prefixes, and suffixes most commonly used to describe these organs and their parts.
- Describe the abnormal conditions that may affect the eye and ear.
- Identify clinical procedures that pertain to ophthalmology and otology.
- Apply your new knowledge to understanding medical terms in their proper contexts, such as medical reports and records.

Image Description: EYE: Lateral view of the eyeball.
EAR: Stylized view showing inner anatomy.

17

INTRODUCTION

The **eye** and the **ear** are sense organs, like the skin, taste buds, and **olfactory** (centers of smell in the nose) regions. As such, they are receptors whose sensitive cells may be activated by a particular form of energy or stimulus in the external or internal environment. The sensitive cells in the eye and ear respond to the stimulus by initiating a series of nerve impulses along sensory nerve fibers that lead to the brain.

No matter what stimulus affects a particular receptor, the sensation felt is determined by regions in the brain connected to that receptor. Thus, mechanical injury that stimulates receptor cells in the eye and ear produces sensations of vision (flashes of light) and sound (ringing in the ears). If one could make a nerve connection between the sensitive receptor cells of the ear and the area in the brain associated with sight, it would be possible to perceive, or "see," sounds.

Figure 17–1 reviews the general pattern of events when such stimuli as light and sound are applied to sense organs such as the eye and the ear.

THE EYE

ANATOMY AND PHYSIOLOGY

Label Figure 17–2 as you read the following:

Light rays enter the dark opening of the eye, the **pupil** [1], which is surrounded by the colored portion of the eye, or **iris** (see the photo inset). The **conjunctiva** [2] is a membrane lining the inner surfaces of the eyelids and anterior portion of the eyeball over the white of the eye. The conjunctiva is clear and colorless except when blood vessels are dilated. Dust and smoke may cause the blood vessels to dilate, giving the conjunctiva a reddish appearance—commonly known as bloodshot eyes.

Before entering the eye through the pupil, light passes through the **cornea** [3]. The cornea is a fibrous, transparent tissue that extends like a dome over the pupil and colored portion of the eye. The function of the cornea is to bend, or **refract,** the rays of light, so they are focused properly on the sensitive receptor cells in the posterior region of the eye. The normal, healthy cornea is avascular (has no blood vessels) but receives nourishment from blood vessels near its junction with the opaque white of the eye, the **sclera** [4]. Corneal transplants for people with scarred or opaque corneas are often successful because antibodies responsible for rejection of foreign tissue usually do not reach the avascular, transplanted corneal tissue. The sclera is a tough, fibrous, supportive, connective tissue that extends from the cornea on the anterior surface of the eyeball to the optic nerve in the back of the eye.

The **choroid** [5] is a dark brown membrane inside the sclera. It contains many blood vessels that supply nutrients to the eye. The choroid is continuous with the pigment-containing **iris** [6] and the **ciliary body** [7] on the anterior surface of the eye.

The iris is the colored (it can appear blue, green, hazel, gray, or brown) portion of the eye, which has a circular opening in the center that forms the pupil. Muscles of the iris

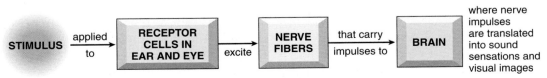

FIGURE 17–1 Pattern of events in the stimulation of a sense organ.

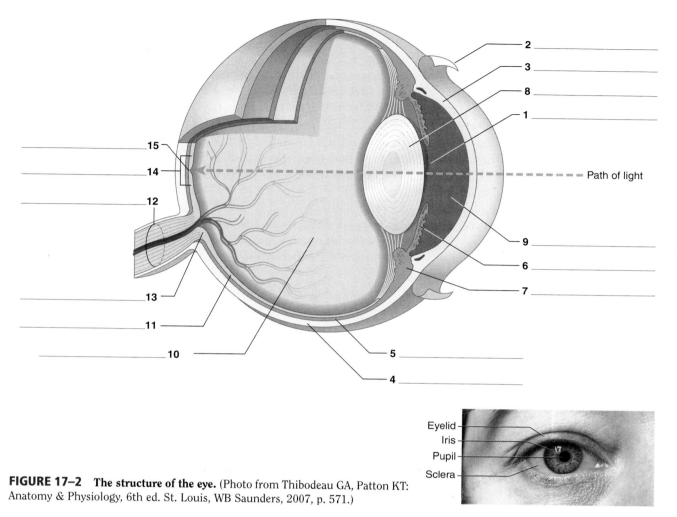

FIGURE 17–2   The structure of the eye. (Photo from Thibodeau GA, Patton KT: Anatomy & Physiology, 6th ed. St. Louis, WB Saunders, 2007, p. 571.)

constrict the pupil in bright light and dilate the pupil in dim light, thereby regulating the amount of light entering the eye.

The ciliary body surrounds the outside of the **lens** [8] in a circular fashion for 360 degrees. There are fine thread-like attachments (zonules), which connect the ciliary body and the lens and allow the muscles in the ciliary body to adjust the shape and thickness of the lens. These changes in the shape of the lens cause **refraction** of light rays. Refraction is the bending of rays as they pass through the cornea, lens, and other tissues. Muscles of the ciliary body produce flattening of the lens (for distant vision) and thickening and rounding (for close vision). This refractory adjustment for close vision is **accommodation.**

Besides regulating the shape of the lens, the ciliary body also secretes a fluid called **aqueous humor,** which is found in the **anterior chamber** [9] of the eye. Aqueous humor maintains the shape of the anterior portion of the eye and nourishes the structures in that region. The fluid is constantly produced and leaves the eye through a canal that carries it into the bloodstream. Another cavity of the eye is the **vitreous chamber,** which is a large region behind the lens filled with a soft, jelly-like material, the **vitreous humor** [10]. Vitreous humor maintains the shape of the eyeball and is not constantly re-formed. Its escape (due to trauma or surgical damage) may result in significant damage to the eye, leading to possible retinal damage and blindness. Both the aqueous and the vitreous humors further refract light rays.

The **retina** [11] is the thin, delicate, and sensitive nerve layer of the eye. As light energy, in the form of waves, travels through the eye, it is refracted (by the cornea, lens, and fluids),

17

so that it focuses on sensitive receptor cells of the retina called the **rods** and **cones.** There are approximately 6.5 million cones and 120 million rods in the retina. The cones function in bright levels of light and are responsible for color and central vision. There are three types of cones, each stimulated by one of the primary colors in light (red, green, or blue). Most cases of color blindness affect either the green or the red receptors, so that the two colors cannot be distinguished from each other. Rods function at reduced levels of light and are responsible for peripheral vision.

When light rays are focused on the retina, a chemical change occurs in the rods and cones, initiating nerve impulses that then travel from the eye to the brain via the **optic nerve** [12]. The region in the eye where the optic nerve meets the retina is called the **optic disc** [13]. Because there are no light receptor cells in the optic disc, it is known as the blind spot of the eye. The **macula** [14] is a small, oval, yellowish area to the side of the optic disc. It contains a central depression called the **fovea centralis** [15], which is composed largely of cones and is the location of the sharpest vision in the eye. If a portion of the fovea or macula is damaged, vision is reduced and central-vision blindness occurs. Figure 17–3 shows the retina of a normal eye as seen through an ophthalmoscope. The **fundus** of the eye is this posterior, inner part that is visualized through the ophthalmoscope.

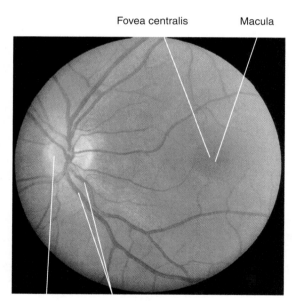

Fovea centralis   Macula

Optic disc   Retinal vessels

FIGURE 17–3   **The posterior, inner part (fundus) of the eye,** showing the retina as seen through an ophthalmoscope. (From Thibodeau GA, Patton KT: Anatomy & Physiology, 6th ed. St. Louis, Mosby, 2007, p. 571.)

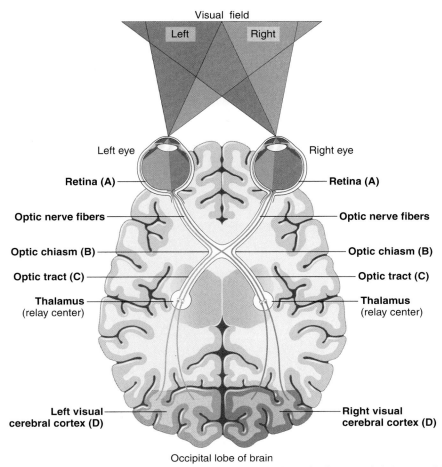

Visual field

Left   Right

Left eye — Retina (A)

Optic nerve fibers

Optic chiasm (B)

Optic tract (C)

Thalamus
(relay center)

Left visual
cerebral cortex (D)

Right eye — Retina (A)

Optic nerve fibers

Optic chiasm (B)

Optic tract (C)

Thalamus
(relay center)

Right visual
cerebral cortex (D)

Occipital lobe of brain

FIGURE 17–4   Visual pathway from the retina (A) to the visual cerebral cortex (D) (occipital lobe of the brain). Objects in the left visual field are "seen" by the right side of the brain, whereas objects in the right visual field are projected into the left visual cerebral cortex.

Figure 17–4 illustrates what happens when you look at an object and "see" it. If an object is in your left visual field (purple area), sensitive cells, rods and cones, in the right half of each **retina** (A) are stimulated. Similarly, if an object is in your right visual field (orange color), rods and cones are stimulated in the left half of each retina. Nervous impulses then travel via optic nerve fibers from each retina to an area of the brain, the **optic chiasm** (B). Here, medial optic nerve fibers cross so that fibers from the right half of each retina (purple color) form an **optic tract** (C) leading, via the **thalamus** (relay center), to the **right visual cerebral cortex** (D). Similarly, fibers from the left half of each retina (orange color) form an optic tract leading to the **left visual cerebral cortex** (D). Images (one from each eye) are then fused in the occipital lobe of the brain producing a single visual sensation with the three-dimensional effect. This is **binocular vision**.

Brain damage to nerve cells in the right visual cerebral cortex (such as in a stroke) causes loss of vision in the left visual field, whereas damage in the left cerebral cortex causes loss of vision in the right visual field. This loss of vision in the contralateral (opposite side) visual field is **hemianopsia** (**hemi-** means half, **an-** means without, **-opsia** means vision).

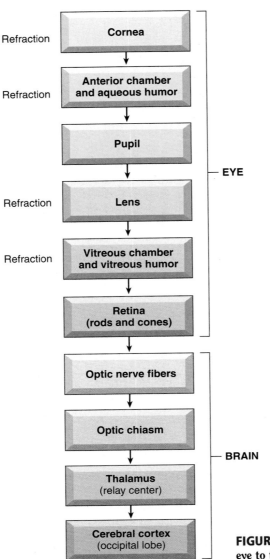

FIGURE 17–5 Pathway of light rays from the cornea of the eye to the cerebral cortex of the brain.

Figure 17–5 reviews the pathway of light rays from the cornea to the cerebral cortex of the brain.

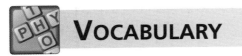 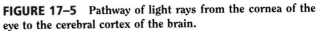

VOCABULARY

This list reviews many new terms introduced in the text. Short definitions reinforce your understanding of the terms. Refer to the Pronunciation of Terms section for help with unfamiliar or difficult words.

accommodation	Normal adjustment of the eye to focus on objects from far to near. The ciliary body adjusts the lens (rounding it) and the pupil constricts. When the eye disaccommodates, it focuses from near to far. The ciliary body flattens the lens and the pupil dilates.
anterior chamber	Area behind the cornea and in front of the lens and iris. It contains aqueous humor.

aqueous humor	Fluid produced by the ciliary body and found in the anterior chamber. A humor (Latin *humidus* means moist) is any body fluid, including blood and lymph.
biconvex	Having two sides that are rounded, elevated, and curved evenly, like part of a sphere. The lens of the eye is a biconvex body.
choroid	Middle, vascular layer of the eye, between the retina and the sclera.
ciliary body	Structure on each side of the lens that connects the choroid and iris. It contains ciliary muscles, which control the shape of the lens, and it secretes aqueous humor.
cone	Photoreceptor cell in the retina that transforms light energy into a nerve impulse. Cones are responsible for color and central vision.
conjunctiva	Delicate membrane lining the eyelids and covering the anterior eyeball.
cornea	Fibrous transparent layer of clear tissue that extends over the anterior portion of the eyeball. Derived from the Latin *corneus*, meaning horny, perhaps because as it protrudes outward, it was thought to resemble a horn.
fovea centralis	Tiny pit or depression in the retina that is the region of clearest vision.
fundus of the eye	Posterior, inner part of the eye.
iris	Colored pigmented membrane surrounding the pupil of the eye.
lens	Transparent, biconvex body behind the pupil of the eye. It bends (refracts) light rays to bring them into focus on the retina.
macula	Yellowish region on the retina lateral to and slightly below the optic disc; contains the fovea centralis, which is the area of clearest vision.
optic chiasm	Point at which optic nerve fibers cross in the brain (**chiasm** means crossing).
optic disc	Region at the back of the eye where the optic nerve meets the retina. It is the blind spot of the eye because it contains only nerve fibers, no rods or cones, and is thus insensitive to light.
optic nerve	Cranial nerve carrying impulses from the retina to the brain (cerebral cortex).
pupil	Dark opening of the eye, surrounded by the iris, through which light rays pass.
refraction	Bending of light rays by the cornea, lens, and fluids of the eye to bring the rays into focus on the retina. **Refract** means to break (-fract) back (re-).
retina	Light-sensitive nerve cell layer of the eye containing photoreceptor cells (rods and cones).
rod	Photoreceptor cell of the retina essential for vision in dim light and for peripheral vision.
sclera	Tough, white outer coat of the eyeball.
thalamus	Relay center of the brain. Optic nerve fibers pass through the thalamus on their way to the cerebral cortex.
vitreous humor	Soft, jelly-like material behind the lens in the vitreous chamber; helps maintain the shape of the eyeball.

COMBINING FORMS, SUFFIXES, AND TERMINOLOGY: STRUCTURES AND FLUIDS; CONDITIONS

Write the meanings of the medical terms in the spaces provided.

STRUCTURES AND FLUIDS

COMBINING FORMS

Combining Form	Meaning	Terminology	Meaning
aque/o	water	aqueous humor _____	
blephar/o	eyelid (see also **palpebr/o**)	blepharitis _____ *See Figure 17–6, A.*	
		blepharoptosis _____ *Pronounced blĕf-ă-rŏp-TŌ-sĭs. Also called ptosis. This condition may be caused by abnormalities of the eyelid muscle or by nerve damage.*	
conjunctiv/o	conjunctiva	conjunctivitis _____ *Commonly called pinkeye. See Figure 17–6, B.*	
cor/o	pupil (see also **pupill/o**)	anisocoria _____ *Anis/o means unequal. Anisocoria may be an indication of neurologic injury or disease. See Figure 17–7, A.*	
corne/o	cornea (see also **kerat/o**)	corneal abrasion _____	
cycl/o	ciliary body or muscle of the eye	cycloplegic _____	

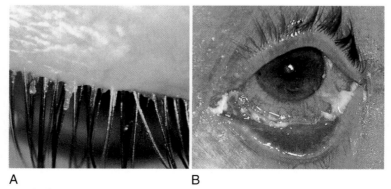

A   B

FIGURE 17–6 **A, Blepharitis.** Notice the crusting on the eyelid. **B, Acute bacterial conjunctivitis.** Notice the discharge of pus characteristic of this highly contagious infection of the conjunctiva. (**A** from Frazier MS, Drzymkowski J: Essentials of Human Disease and Conditions, 3rd ed., Philadelphia, WB Saunders, 2004, p. 189; **B** from Newell FW: Ophthalmology: Principles and Concepts, 8th ed., St. Louis, Mosby, 1996.)

Combining Form	Meaning	Terminology	Meaning
dacry/o	tears, tear duct (see also **lacrim/o**)	dacryoadenitis _____ *Figure 17–7, B, shows the lacrimal gland and lacrimal ducts.*	
ir/o, irid/o	iris (colored portion of the eye around the pupil)	iritis _____ *Characterized by pain, sensitivity to light, and lacrimation. A corticosteroid is prescribed to reduce inflammation.*	
		iridic _____	
		iridectomy _____ *A portion of the iris is removed to improve drainage of aqueous humor or to extract a foreign body.*	
kerat/o	cornea	keratitis _____ *Note that kerat/o here does not refer to keratin (protein in skin tissue).*	
lacrim/o	tears	lacrimal _____	
		lacrimation _____	
ocul/o	eye	intraocular _____	
ophthalm/o	eye	ophthalmologist _____ *A medical doctor who specializes in treating disorders of the eye.*	
		ophthalmic _____	
		ophthalmoplegia _____	

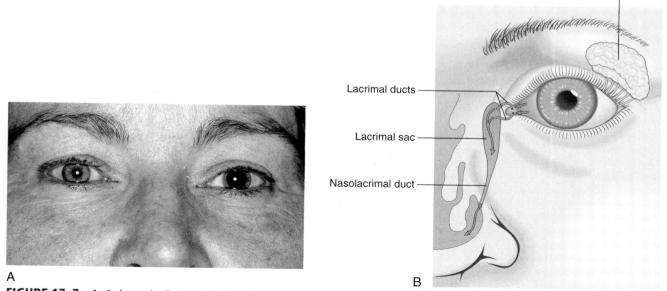

FIGURE 17–7 **A, Anisocoria. B, Lacrimal (tear) gland and ducts.** (**A** from Thibodeau GA, Patton KT: Anatomy and Physiology, 6th ed., St. Louis, Mosby, 2007, p. 575.)

17

Combining Form	Meaning	Terminology	Meaning
opt/o, optic/o	eye, vision	optic _____	
		optometrist _____ *Nonmedical professional who can examine eyes to determine vision problems and prescribe lenses (doctor of optometry; OD).*	
		optician _____ *Nonmedical professional who grinds lenses and fits glasses but cannot prescribe lenses.*	
palpebr/o	eyelid	palpebral _____	
papill/o	optic disc; nipple-like	papilledema _____ *The suffix -edema means swelling. This condition is associated with increased intracranial pressure and hyperemia (increased blood flow) in the region of the optic disc.*	
phac/o, phak/o	lens of the eye	phacoemulsification _____ *Technique of cataract extraction using ultrasonic vibrations to fragment (emulsify) the lens and aspirate it from the eye.*	
		aphakia _____ *This may be congenital, but most often it is the result of extraction of a cataract (clouded lens) without placement of an artificial lens (pseudophakia).*	
pupill/o	pupil	pupillary _____	
retin/o	retina	retinitis _____ **Retinitis pigmentosa** *is a genetic disorder (pigmented scar forms on the retina) that destroys retinal rods. Decreased vision and night blindness (nyctalopia) occur.*	
		hypertensive retinopathy _____ *Lesions such as narrowing of arterioles, microaneurysms, hemorrhages, and exudates (fluid leakage) are found on examination of the fundus.*	
scler/o	sclera (white of the eye)	corneoscleral _____	
		scleritis _____	
uve/o	uvea; vascular layer of the eye (iris, ciliary body, and choroid)	uveitis _____	
vitre/o	glassy	vitreous humor _____	

Palpebral/Palpable
Don't confuse *palpebral* with *palpable*, which means the ability to distinguish by touch.

CONDITIONS

COMBINING FORMS

Combining Form	Meaning	Terminology	Meaning
ambly/o	dull, dim	amblyopia _____	
		The suffix -opia means vision. Amblyopia is partial loss of sight and is also known as lazy eye because it is associated with failure of the eyes to work together to focus on the same point.	
dipl/o	double	diplopia _____	
glauc/o	gray	glaucoma _____	
		Here, -oma means mass or collection of fluid (aqueous humor). The term comes from the dull gray-green color of the affected eye in advanced cases. See page 682.	
mi/o	smaller, less	miosis _____	
		*Contraction of the pupil. A **miotic** is a drug (such as pilocarpine) that causes the pupil to contract.*	
mydr/o	widen, enlarge	mydriasis _____	
		Enlargement of pupils. Atropine and cocaine cause dilation, or enlargement, of pupils.	
nyct/o	night	nyctalopia _____	
		-opia means vision; -al comes from ala, meaning blindness. Night blindness is poor vision at night, but good vision on bright days. Deficiency of vitamin A leads to nyctalopia.	
phot/o	light	photophobia _____	
		Sensitivity to light.	
presby/o	old age	presbyopia _____	
		See page 681.	
scot/o	darkness	scotoma _____	
		An area of depressed vision surrounded by an area of normal vision; a blind spot. This can result from damage to the retina or the optic nerve.	
xer/o	dry	xerophthalmia _____	

SUFFIXES

Suffix	Meaning	Terminology	Meaning
-opia	vision	hyperopia _____	
		Hypermetropia (farsightedness).	
-opsia	vision	hemianopsia _____	
		Absence of vision in half of the visual field (space of vision of each eye). Stroke victims frequently have damage to the brain on one side of the visual cortex and experience hemianopsia (the visual loss is in the right or left visual field of both eyes).	

17

Suffix	Meaning	Terminology	Meaning
-tropia	to turn	esotropia _____	*Inward (eso-) turning of an eye.* **Exotropia** *is an outward turning of an eye. These conditions are examples of* **strabismus** *(defect in eye muscles so that both eyes cannot be focused on the same point at the same time).*

ERRORS OF REFRACTION

astigmatism

Defective curvature of the cornea or lens of the eye.

This problem results from one or more abnormal curvatures of the cornea or lens. This causes light rays to be unevenly and not sharply focused on the retina, so that the image is distorted. A cylindrical lens placed in the proper position in front of the eye can correct this problem (Fig. 17–8, *A*).

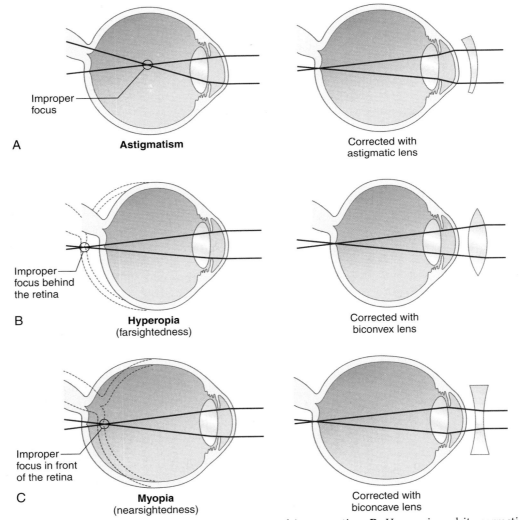

A **Astigmatism** | Corrected with astigmatic lens

Improper focus

B **Hyperopia** (farsightedness) | Corrected with biconvex lens

Improper focus behind the retina

C **Myopia** (nearsightedness) | Corrected with biconcave lens

Improper focus in front of the retina

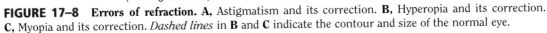

FIGURE 17–8 **Errors of refraction. A,** Astigmatism and its correction. **B,** Hyperopia and its correction. **C,** Myopia and its correction. *Dashed lines* in **B** and **C** indicate the contour and size of the normal eye.

hyperopia (hypermetropia)	**Farsightedness.**

As Figure 17–8, *B*, illustrates, the eyeball in this condition is too short or the refractive power of the lens is too weak. Parallel rays of light tend to focus behind the retina, which results in a blurred image. A convex lens (thicker in the middle than at the sides) bends the rays inward before they reach the cornea, and thus the rays can be focused properly on the retina.

myopia	**Nearsightedness.**

In myopia ◩, the eyeball is too long or the refractive power of the lens so strong that light rays do not properly focus on the retina. The image perceived is blurred because the light rays are focused in front of the retina. Concave glasses (thicker at the periphery than in the middle) correct this condition because the lenses spread the rays out before they reach the cornea, so that they can be properly focused directly on the retina (Fig. 17–8, *C*).

presbyopia	**Impairment of vision as a result of old age.**

With increasing age, loss of elasticity of the ciliary body impairs its ability to adjust the lens for accommodation to near vision. The lens of the eye cannot become fat to bend the rays coming from near objects (less than 20 feet). The light rays focus behind the retina, as in hyperopia. Therefore, a convex lens is needed to refract the rays coming from objects closer than 20 feet.

ABNORMAL CONDITIONS

cataract	**Clouding of the lens, causing decreased vision** (Fig. 17–9).

A cataract is a type of degenerative eye disease (protein in the lens aggregates and clouds vision) and is linked to the process of aging (senile cataracts). Some cataracts, however, are present at birth, and others occur with diabetes mellitus, ocular trauma, and prolonged high-dose corticosteroid administration. Vision appears blurred as the lens clouds over and becomes opaque. Lens cloudiness can be seen with an ophthalmoscope or the naked eye. Surgical removal of the lens with implantation of an artificial lens behind the iris (the preferred position) is the method of treatment. If an intraocular lens cannot be inserted, the patient may wear eyeglasses or contact lenses to help refraction.

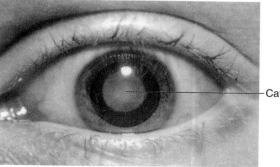

FIGURE 17–9 **Cataract.** The lens appears cloudy. (Courtesy of Ophthalmic Photography at the University of Michigan, WK Kellogg Eye Center, Ann Arbor, MI. From Black JM, Hawks JH: Medical-Surgical Nursing: Clinical Management for Positive Outcomes, 7th ed. Philadelphia, WB Saunders, 2005, p. 1950.)

Myopia/Miotic

In this term, my- comes from Greek *myein*, meaning to shut, referring to the observation that myopic persons frequently peer through half-closed eyelids. Don't confuse myopia with miotic, which is a drug that contracts the pupil of the eye.

17

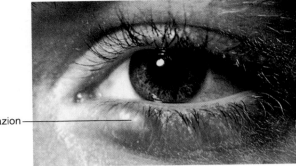

Chalazion

FIGURE 17–10 **Chalazion.** (Courtesy of Ophthalmic Photography at the University of Michigan, WK Kellogg Eye Center, Ann Arbor, MI. From Black JM, Hawks JH, Keene AM: Medical-Surgical Nursing, 5th ed. Philadelphia, WB Saunders, 1997.)

chalazion

Small, hard, cystic mass (granuloma) on the eyelid; formed as a result of chronic inflammation of a sebaceous gland (meibomian gland) along the margin of the eyelid (Fig. 17–10).

Chalazions (kă-LĀ-zē-ŏnz) often require incision and drainage.

diabetic retinopathy

Retinal effects of diabetes mellitus include microaneurysms, hemorrhages, dilation of retinal veins, and neovascularization (new blood vessels form in the retina).

Edema (macular edema) occurs as fluid leaks from blood vessels into the retina and vision is blurred. **Exudates** (fluid leaking from the blood) appear in the retina as yellow-white spots. Laser photocoagulation and vitrectomy (see pages 687 and 689) are helpful to patients in whom hemorrhaging has been severe.

glaucoma

Increased intraocular pressure results in damage to the retina and optic nerve with loss of vision.

Intraocular pressure is elevated because of the inability of aqueous humor to drain from the eye and enter the bloodstream. Normally, aqueous humor is formed by the ciliary body, flows into the anterior chamber, and leaves the eye at the angle where the cornea and the iris meet. If fluid cannot leave or too much fluid is produced, pressure builds up in the anterior chamber (Fig. 17–11).

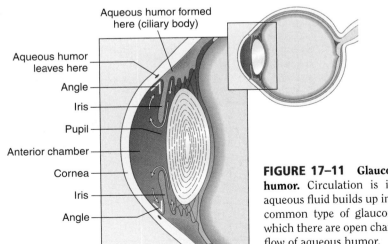

Aqueous humor formed here (ciliary body)

Aqueous humor leaves here

Angle

Iris

Pupil

Anterior chamber

Cornea

Iris

Angle

FIGURE 17–11 **Glaucoma and circulation of aqueous humor.** Circulation is impaired in glaucoma, so that aqueous fluid builds up in the anterior chamber. The most common type of glaucoma is **open-angle glaucoma**, in which there are open chamber angles but resistance to the flow of aqueous humor.

17

Glaucoma is diagnosed by means of **tonometry** (see page 686), with an instrument applied externally to the eye after administration of local anesthetic. Acute glaucoma is marked by extreme ocular pain, blurred vision, redness of the eye, and dilation of the pupil. If untreated, it causes blindness. Chronic glaucoma may produce no symptoms initially. A patient with glaucoma may experience a gradual loss of peripheral vision, with headaches, blurred vision, and halos around bright lights.

Administration of drugs to lower intraocular pressure can control the condition. Sometimes, laser therapy is used to treat glaucoma by creating a hole in the periphery of the iris (iridotomy), which allows aqueous humor to flow more easily to the anterior chamber and reduces intraocular pressure. Laser therapy for chronic glaucoma causes scarring in the drainage angle, which improves aqueous humor outflow and reduces intraocular pressure.

hordeolum (stye or sty)   **Localized, purulent, inflammatory staphylococcal infection of a sebaceous gland in the eyelid.**

Hot compresses may help localize the infection and promote drainage. In some cases, surgical incision may be necessary. Latin *hordeolum* (hŏr-DĒ-ō-lŭm) means barley corn. See Table 17–1 for a list of common eyelid abnormalities.

Table 17–1

Eyelid Abnormalities

Abnormality	Description
Blepharitis	Inflammation of eyelid, causing redness, crusting, and swelling along lid margins
Chalazion	Granuloma formed around an inflamed sebaceous gland
Dacryocystitis	Blockage, inflammation, and infection of a nasolacrimal duct and lacrimal sac, causing redness and swelling of lower lid
Ectropion	Outward sagging and eversion of the eyelid, leading to improper lacrimation and corneal drying and ulceration
Entropion	Inversion of the eyelid, causing the lashes to rub against the eye; corneal abrasion may result
Hordeolum (stye)	Infection of a sebaceous gland producing a small, superficial white nodule along lid margin
Ptosis	Drooping of upper lid margin as a result of neuromuscular problems
Xanthelasma	Raised yellowish plaque on eyelid caused by lipid disorder (**xanth/o** = yellow, **-elasma** = plate)

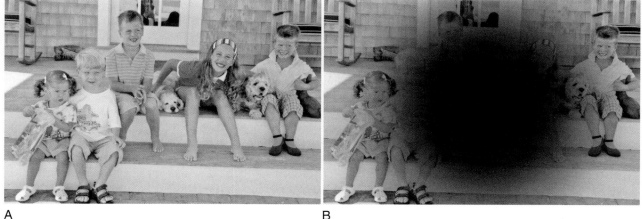

A   B

FIGURE 17–12 **A,** Picture as seen with **normal vision. B,** The same picture as it would appear to someone with **macular degeneration.** (Photograph shows the author's grandchildren: Louisa, Ben, Solomon, Bebe, and Gus, as well as Lilly and Owen. August 2005.)

macular degeneration	**Progressive damage to the macula of the retina.**

Macular degeneration is one of the leading causes of blindness in the elderly. It causes severe loss of central vision (Fig. 17–12). Peripheral vision (using the part of the retina that is outside the macular region) is retained.

Macular degeneration occurs in both a "dry" and "wet" form. The dry form (affecting about 85 percent of patients) is marked by atrophy and degeneration of retinal cells and deposits of clumps of extracellular debris, or **drusen**. The wet form results from development of new (neovascular) and leaky (exudative) blood vessels close to the macula.

There is no treatment for dry macular degeneration. Wet macular degeneration may be treated with laser photocoagulation of the leaking vessels. Unfortunately, in many cases, patients with wet macular degeneration have more severe vision loss and success of treatment is limited.

nystagmus — **Repetitive rhythmic movements of one or both eyes.**

Brain tumors or diseases of the inner ear may cause nystagmus. Nystagmus is normal in newborns.

retinal detachment — **Two layers of the retina separate from each other.**

Trauma to the eye, head injuries, bleeding, scarring from infection, or shrinkage of the vitreous humor can produce holes or tears in the retina and result in the separation of layers. Patients often see bright flashes of light **(photopsia)** and then later notice a shadow or "curtain" falling across the field of vision. **Floaters** are black spots, usually composed of vitreous clumps that detach from the retina. In some cases, floaters may be a sign of a retinal hole, tear, or detachment caused by pigmented cells from the damaged retina or bleeding that has occurred as a result of a detachment.

Photocoagulation (making pinpoint burns to form scar tissue and seal holes) and cryotherapy (creating a "freezer burn" that forms a scar and knits a tear together) are used to repair smaller retinal tears. For larger retinal detachments, a **scleral buckle** (see page 689) made of silicone is sutured to the sclera directly over the detached portion of the retina to push the two retinal layers together. In selected retinal detachments, a procedure called **pneumatic retinopexy** is performed. A gas bubble is injected into the vitreous cavity to put pressure on the area of retinal tear until the retina is reattached.

strabismus

Abnormal deviation of the eye.

A failure of the eyes to look in the same direction because of weakness of a muscle controlling the position of one eye. Different forms of strabismus include **esotropia** (one eye turns inward; cross-eyed), **exotropia** (one eye turns outward; wall-eyed), **hypertropia** (upward deviation of one eye), and **hypotropia** (downward deviation of one eye). Treatment includes medications in the form of eye drops, corrective lenses, eye exercises and patching of the normal eye, or surgery to restore muscle balance.

In children, strabismus may lead to **amblyopia** (partial loss of vision or lazy eye). Amblyopia is reversible until the retina is fully developed at about 7 years of age. When strabismus develops in an adult, **diplopia** (double vision) is a common problem.

CLINICAL PROCEDURES

DIAGNOSTIC

fluorescein angiography

Intravenous injection of fluorescein (a dye) followed by serial photographs of the retina through dilated pupils.

This test provides diagnostic information about blood flow in the retina, detects vascular changes in diabetic and hypertensive retinopathy, and identifies lesions in the macular area of the retina (Fig. 17–13).

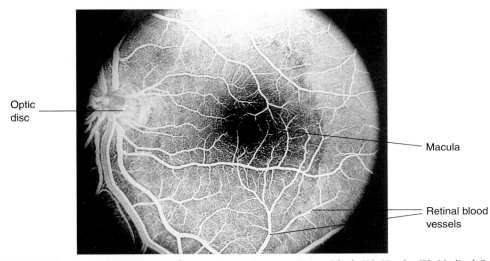

FIGURE 17–13   Normal eye seen on fluorescein angiogram. (From Black JM, Hawks JH: Medical-Surgical Nursing: Clinical Management for Positive Outcomes, 7th ed. Philadelphia, WB Saunders, 2005, p. 1930.)

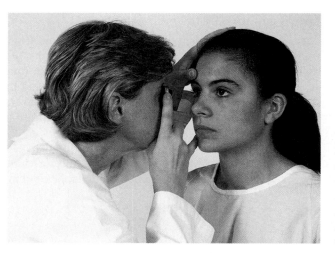

FIGURE 17–14 Ophthalmoscopy. In addition to examining the cornea, lens, and vitreous humor for opacities (cloudiness), the examiner can see the blood vessels at the back of the eye (fundus) and note degenerative changes in the retina. (From Jarvis C: Physical Examination and Health Assessment, 3rd ed. Philadelphia, WB Saunders, 2000, p. 318.)

ophthalmoscopy	**Visual examination of the interior of the eye.**

Ideally, the pupil is dilated and the physician holds the ophthalmoscope close to the patient's eye, shining the light into the back of the eye (Fig. 17–14).

slit lamp microscopy	**Examination of anterior ocular structures under microscopic magnification.**

This procedure provides a magnified view of the conjunctiva, sclera, cornea, anterior chamber, iris, lens, and vitreous. Devices attached to a slit lamp expand the scope of the examination. **Tonometry** (ton/o = tension) measures intraocular pressure to detect glaucoma (Fig. 17–15). Special magnifying lenses also permit examination of the fundus, as with a direct ophthalmoscope.

visual acuity test	**Clarity of vision is assessed** (Fig. 17–16, *A*).

A patient reads from a **Snellen chart** at 20 feet (distance vision test). Visual acuity is expressed as a ratio, such as 20/20. The first number is the distance the patient is standing from the chart. The second number is the distance at which a person with normal vision could read the same line of the chart. If the best a patient can see is the 20/200 line, then at 20 feet the patient can see what a "healthy eye" sees at 200 feet.

Mirrors are used so that measurements can be taken at less than 20 feet and still are equivalent to vision measured at 20 feet.

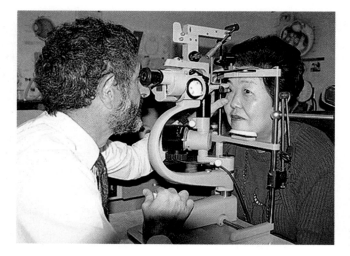

FIGURE 17–15 Slit-lamp examination measuring intraocular pressure by tonometry. (From Lewis SM, Heitkemper MM, Dirksen SR: Medical-Surgical Nursing: Assessment and Management of Clinical Problems, 5th ed. St. Louis, Mosby, 2000.)

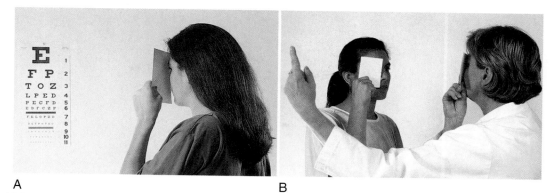

A   B

FIGURE 17–16 **A,** The **Snellen chart** assesses visual acuity. **B, Visual fields** are examined by comparing the patient's field of vision with that of the examiner's (assuming that the examiner's is normal). (From Jarvis C: Physical Examination and Health Assessment, 3rd ed. Philadelphia, WB Saunders, 2000, pp. 307 and 309.)

visual field test	**Measures the area within which objects are seen when the eyes are fixed, looking straight ahead without movement of the head** (Fig. 17–16, *B*).

TREATMENT

enucleation	**Removal of the entire eyeball.**
	This surgical procedure is necessary to treat tumors such as ocular melanoma (malignant tumor of pigmented cells in the choroid layer) or if an eye has become blind and painful from trauma or disease, such as glaucoma.
keratoplasty	**Surgical repair of the cornea.**
	Also known as a **corneal transplant** procedure (penetrating keratoplasty). The ophthalmic surgeon removes the patient's scarred or opaque cornea and replaces it with a donor cornea ("button" or graft), which is sutured into place (Fig. 17–17).
laser photocoagulation	**Intense, precisely focused light beam (argon laser) creates an inflammatory reaction that seals retinal tears and leaky retinal blood vessels.**
	This procedure is useful to treat retinal tears, diabetic retinopathy, and macular degeneration. Laser is an acronym for <u>l</u>ight <u>a</u>mplification by <u>s</u>timulated <u>e</u>mission of <u>r</u>adiation.

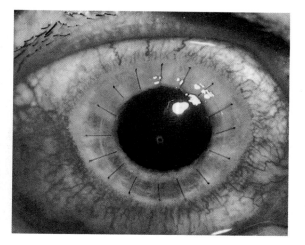

FIGURE 17–17 **Clinical appearance of the eye after keratoplasty.** (Courtesy of Ophthalmic Photography at the University of Michigan, WK Kellogg Eye Center, Ann Arbor, MI. From Black JM, Hawks JH: Medical-Surgical Nursing: Clinical Management for Positive Outcomes, 7th ed. Philadelphia, WB Saunders, 2005, p. 1958.)

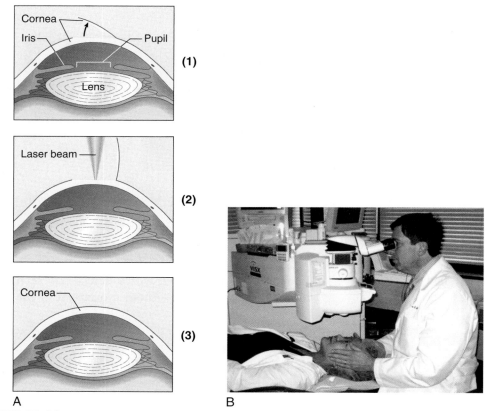

FIGURE 17–18 A, LASIK refractive eye surgery. 1. An instrument to cut the cornea (microkeratome) creates a hinged cap of tissue, which then is lifted off the corneal surface. 2. An excimer laser vaporizes and reshapes the cornea to correct the refraction. 3. Corneal flap is replaced. **B,** Ophthalmologists typically perform LASIK surgery as an office procedure. The patient with corrected vision returns home that day and is visually functioning normally the next day. (**B** courtesy Eric R. Mandel, MD, PC.)

LASIK

Use of an excimer laser to correct errors of refraction (myopia, hyperopia, and astigmatism).

Performed as an outpatient procedure with use of local anesthesia. The surgeon lifts the top layer of the cornea (a flap is made) and uses a laser to sculpt the cornea. The corneal flap is then repositioned. LASIK is an acronym for l̲aser i̲n situ k̲eratomileusis (shaping the cornea). See Figure 17–18.

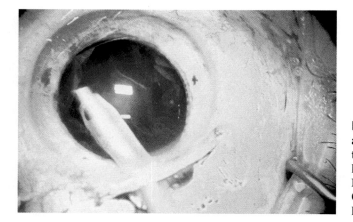

FIGURE 17–19 Phacoemulsification of a cataractous lens through a small scleral tunnel incision. (From Lewis SM, Heitkemper MM, Dirksen SR: Medical-Surgical Nursing: Assessment and Management of Clinical Problems, 6th ed. Mosby, St. Louis, 2004, p. 451.)

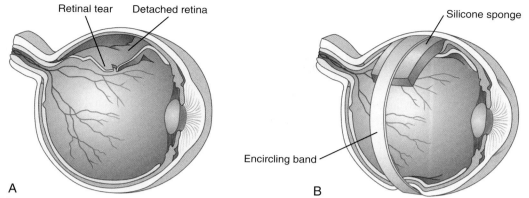

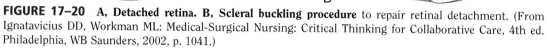

FIGURE 17–20   A, Detached retina. B, Scleral buckling procedure to repair retinal detachment. (From Ignatavicius DD, Workman ML: Medical-Surgical Nursing: Critical Thinking for Collaborative Care, 4th ed. Philadelphia, WB Saunders, 2002, p. 1041.)

phacoemulsification	**Ultrasonic vibrations break up the lens, which then is aspirated through the ultrasonic probe** (Fig. 17–19).
	This is the typical surgery for cataract removal. The ophthalmic surgeon uses a small, scleral tunnel or self-sealing corneal incision. In most patients, a foldable intraocular lens (IOL) is implanted at the time of surgery.
scleral buckle	**Suture of a silicone band to the sclera over a detached portion of the retina.**
	The band pushes the two parts of the retina against each other to bring together the two layers of the detached retina (Fig. 17–20).
vitrectomy	**Removal of the vitreous humor.**
	The vitreous is replaced with a clear solution. This is necessary when blood and scar tissue accumulate in the vitreous humor (a complication of diabetic retinopathy).

ABBREVIATIONS

AMD	age-related macular degeneration	**PERRLA**	pupils equal, round, reactive to light and accommodation
HEENT	head, eyes, ears, nose, and throat		
IOL	intraocular lens		
IOP	intraocular pressure	**POAG**	primary open-angle glaucoma
LASIK	laser in situ keratomileusis	**PRK**	photorefractive keratectomy—a laser beam flattens the cornea to correct myopia
OD	right eye (Latin, *oculus dexter*); doctor of optometry (optometrist)		
OS	left eye (Latin, *oculus sinister*)	**VA**	visual acuity
OU	both eyes (Latin, *oculus uterque*)	**VF**	visual field

THE EAR

ANATOMY AND PHYSIOLOGY

Sound waves are received by the outer ear, conducted to special receptor cells within the ear, and transmitted by those cells to nerve fibers that lead to the auditory region of the brain in the cerebral cortex. Sensations of sound are perceived within the nerve fibers of the cerebral cortex.

Label Figure 17–21 as you read the following paragraphs describing the anatomy and physiology of the ear.

The ear can be divided into three separate regions: outer ear, middle ear, and inner ear. The outer and middle ears function in the conduction of sound waves through the ear, and the inner ear contains structures that receive the auditory waves and relay them to the brain.

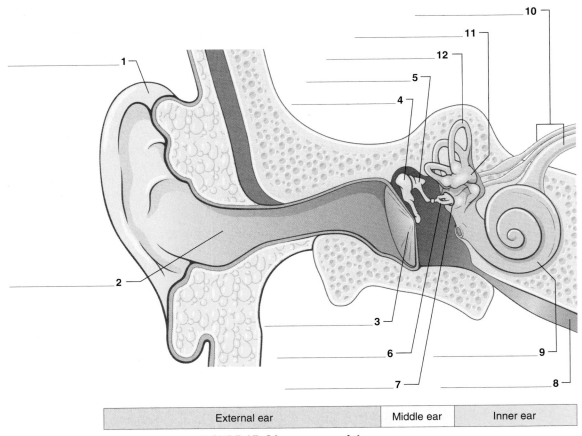

| External ear | Middle ear | Inner ear |

FIGURE 17–21 **Anatomy of the ear.**

Outer Ear

Sound waves enter the ear through the **pinna,** or **auricle** [1], which is the projecting part, or flap, of the ear. The **external auditory meatus (auditory canal)** [2] leads from the pinna and is lined with numerous glands that secrete a yellowish-brown, waxy substance called **cerumen.** Cerumen lubricates and protects the ear.

Middle Ear

Sound waves travel through the auditory canal and strike a membrane between the outer and the middle ear. This is the **tympanic membrane, or eardrum** [3]. As the eardrum vibrates, it moves three small bones, or **ossicles,** that conduct the sound waves through the middle ear. These bones, in the order of their vibration, are the **malleus** [4], the **incus** [5], and the **stapes** [6]. As the stapes moves, it touches a membrane called the **oval window** [7], which separates the middle from the inner ear.

Before proceeding with the pathway of sound conduction and reception into the inner ear, an additional structure that affects the middle ear should be mentioned. The **auditory** or **eustachian tube** [8] is a canal leading from the middle ear to the pharynx. It normally is closed but opens on swallowing. In an efficient way, this tube can prevent damage to the eardrum and shock to the middle and inner ears. Normally the pressure of air in the middle ear is equal to the pressure of air in the external environment; however, if you ascend in the atmosphere, as in flying in an airplane, climbing a high mountain, or riding a fast elevator, the atmospheric pressure, and that in the outer ear, drops, while the pressure in the middle ear remains the same—greater than that in the outer ear. This inequality of air pressure on the inside and outside of the eardrum forces the eardrum to bulge outward and potentially burst if the difference in pressures increases. Swallowing opens the eustachian tube so that air can leave the middle ear and enter the throat until the atmospheric and middle ear pressures are balanced. The eardrum then relaxes, and the danger of its bursting is averted.

Inner Ear

Sound vibrations, having been transmitted by the movement of the eardrum to the bones of the middle ear, reach the inner ear via the fluctuations of the oval window that separates the middle and inner ears. The inner ear is also called the **labyrinth** because of its circular, maze-like structure. The part of the labyrinth that leads from the oval window is a bony, snail-shaped structure called the **cochlea** [9]. The cochlea contains special auditory liquids called **perilymph** and **endolymph** through which the vibrations travel. Also present in the cochlea is a sensitive auditory receptor area called the **organ of Corti.** In the organ of Corti, tiny hair cells receive vibrations from the auditory liquids and relay the sound waves to **auditory nerve fibers** [10], which end in the auditory center of the cerebral cortex, where these impulses are interpreted and "heard."

17

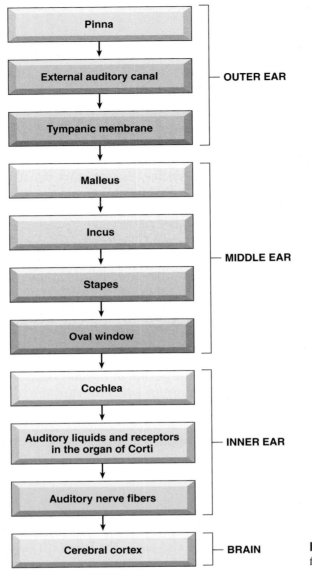

OUTER EAR

MIDDLE EAR

INNER EAR

BRAIN

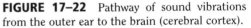

FIGURE 17–22 Pathway of sound vibrations from the outer ear to the brain (cerebral cortex).

Study Figure 17–22, which is a schematic representation of the pathway of sound vibrations from the outer ear to the brain.

The ear is an important organ of equilibrium (balance), as well as an organ for hearing. Refer back to Figure 17–21. The **vestibule** [11] connects the cochlea (for hearing) to three **semicircular canals** [12] for balance. The semicircular canals (containing two membranous sacs called the saccule and utricle) contain a fluid, endolymph, as well as sensitive hair cells. In an intricate manner, the fluid and hair cells fluctuate in response to the movement of the head. This sets up impulses in nerve fibers that lead to the brain. Messages are then sent to muscles in all parts of the body to ensure that equilibrium is maintained.

VOCABULARY

This list reviews many new terms introduced in the text. Short definitions reinforce your understanding of the terms. Refer to the Pronunciation of Terms section for help with unfamiliar or difficult words.

auditory canal	Channel that leads from the pinna to the eardrum.
auditory meatus	Auditory canal.
auditory nerve fibers	Carry impulses from the inner ear to the brain (cerebral cortex). These fibers compose the vestibulocochlear nerve (cranial nerve VIII).
auditory tube	Channel between the middle ear and the nasopharynx; **eustachian tube.**
auricle	Flap of the ear; the protruding part of the external ear, or **pinna.**
cerumen	Waxy substance secreted by the external ear; also called **ear wax.**
cochlea	Snail-shaped, spirally wound tube in the inner ear; contains hearing-sensitive receptor cells.
endolymph	Fluid within the labyrinth of the inner ear.
eustachian tube	Auditory tube.
incus	Second ossicle (bone) of the middle ear; incus means **anvil.**
labyrinth	Maze-like series of canals of the inner ear. This includes the cochlea, vestibule, and semicircular canals.
malleus	First ossicle of the middle ear; malleus means **hammer.**
organ of Corti	Sensitive auditory receptor area found in the cochlea of the inner ear.
ossicle	Small bone of the ear; includes the malleus, incus, and stapes.
oval window	Membrane between the middle ear and the inner ear.
perilymph	Fluid contained in the labyrinth of the inner ear.
pinna	Auricle; flap of the ear.
semicircular canals	Passages in the inner ear associated with maintaining equilibrium.
stapes	Third ossicle of the middle ear. Stapes means stirrup.
tympanic membrane	Membrane between the outer and the middle ear; also called the **eardrum.**
vestibule	Central cavity of the labyrinth, connecting the semicircular canals and the cochlea. The vestibule contains two structures, the saccule and utricle, that help to maintain equilibrium.

COMBINING FORMS, SUFFIXES, AND TERMINOLOGY

17

Write the meaning of the medical term in the space provided.

COMBINING FORMS

Combining Form	Meaning	Terminology	Meaning
acous/o	hearing	acoustic	
audi/o	hearing; the sense of hearing	audiogram	
audit/o	hearing	auditory	
aur/o, auricul/o	ear (see also **ot/o**)	aural	
		postauricular	
cochle/o	cochlea	cochlear	
mastoid/o	mastoid process	mastoiditis	
		The mastoid process is the posterior portion of the temporal bone extending downward behind the external auditory meatus. Mastoiditis, caused by bacterial infection, spreads from the middle ear.	
myring/o	eardrum, tympanic membrane (see also **tympan/o**)	myringotomy	
		See Figure 17–24, D.	
		myringitis	
ossicul/o	ossicle	ossiculoplasty	
ot/o	ear	otic	
		otomycosis	
		otopyorrhea	
		otolaryngologist	
salping/o	eustachian tube, auditory tube	salpingopharyngeal	
		In the context of female reproductive anatomy, salping/o means the fallopian tubes.	
staped/o	stapes (third bone of the middle ear)	stapedectomy	
		After stapedectomy a prosthetic device is used to connect the incus and the oval window (Fig. 17–23). See otosclerosis, page 697.	
tympan/o	eardrum, tympanic membrane	tympanoplasty	
		Surgical reconstruction of the bones of the middle ear with reconnection of the eardrum to the oval window. Figure 17–24, A, shows a normal tympanic membrane (eardrum).	
vestibul/o	vestibule	vestibulocochlear	

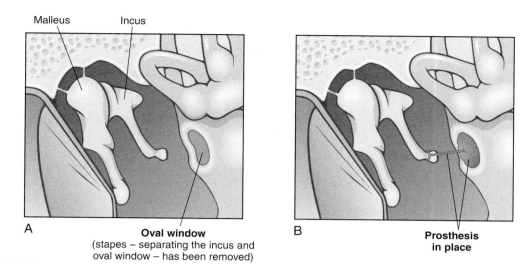

Malleus   Incus

A

B

Oval window
(stapes – separating the incus and
oval window – has been removed)

**Prosthesis
in place**

FIGURE 17–23 **A, Stapedectomy.** Using microsurgical technique and a laser, the stapes bone is removed from the middle ear. **B,** A **prosthetic device** (wire, Teflon, or metal) is placed into the incus and attached to a hole in the oval window.

SUFFIXES

Suffix	Meaning	Terminology	Meaning	
-acusis *or* **-cusis**	hearing	hyperacusis _____ *Abnormally acute sensitivity to sounds.*		
		presbycusis _____ *This type of nerve deafness occurs with the process of aging.*		
-meter	instrument to measure	audiometer _____		

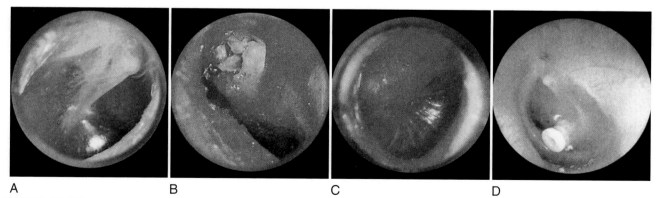

A   B   C   D

FIGURE 17–24 **A,** Healthy tympanic membrane. **B,** Tympanic membrane with **cholesteatoma. C,** Tympanic membrane with **acute otitis media. D, Myringotomy** with tympanostomy tube. (**A–C** courtesy of Richard A. Buckingham, Clinical Professor, Otolaryngology, Abraham Lincoln School of Medicine, University of Illinois, Chicago. From Barkauskas VH, et al: Health and Physical Assessment, 3rd ed. St. Louis, Mosby, 2002, pp. 278 and 290. **D** from Fireman P, Slavin RG: Atlas of Allergies, 2nd ed. London, Glower Medical Publishing, 1996.)

17

Suffix	Meaning	Terminology	Meaning
-otia	ear condition	macrotia _____	
		Abnormally large ears; congenital anomaly.	
		microtia _____	
		Abnormally small ears; congenital anomaly.	

SYMPTOMS AND PATHOLOGIC CONDITIONS

acoustic neuroma

Benign tumor arising from the acoustic vestibulocochlear nerve (eighth cranial nerve) in the brain.

Initially, this tumor causes tinnitus (ringing in the ears), vertigo (dizziness), and decreased hearing. Small tumors are resected by microsurgical techniques or ablated (removed) by radiosurgery (using powerful and precise x-ray beams rather than a surgical incision).

cholesteatoma

Collection of skin cells and cholesterol in a sac within the middle ear.

These cyst-like masses produce a foul-smelling discharge and are most often the result of chronic otitis media. They are associated with perforations of the tympanic membrane (see Fig. 17–24, *B*).

deafness

Loss of the ability to hear.

Nerve deafness (sensorineural hearing loss) results from impairment of the cochlea or auditory (acoustic) nerve. **Conductive deafness** results from impairment of the middle ear ossicles and membranes transmitting sound waves into the cochlea. Hearing aids help people with conductive or sensorineural hearing loss. These devices have a microphone to pick up sounds, an amplifier to increase their volume, and a speaker to transmit amplified sounds.

Meniere disease

Disorder of the labyrinth of the inner ear; elevated endolymph pressure within the cochlea (cochlear hydrops) and semicircular canals (vestibular hydrops).

Signs and symptoms are tinnitus, heightening sensitivity to loud sounds, progressive loss of hearing, headache, nausea, and vertigo. Attacks last minutes or continue for hours. The cause is unknown, and treatment is bed rest, sedation, and drugs to combat nausea and vertigo. Surgery may be necessary to relieve accumulation of fluid from the inner ear.

otitis media

Inflammation of the middle ear.

Acute otitis media is infection of the middle ear, often following an upper respiratory infection (URI). Pain and fever with redness and loss of mobility of the tympanic membrane occur (see Fig. 17–24, *C*). As bacteria invade the middle ear, pus formation occurs **(suppurative otitis media).** It is treated with antibiotics, but if the condition becomes chronic, myringotomy may be required to ventilate the middle ear.

Serous **otitis media** is a noninfectious inflammation with accumulation of serous fluid. It often results from a dysfunctional or obstructed auditory tube. Treatment includes myringotomy to aspirate fluid and tympanostomy tubes placed in the eardrum to allow ventilation of the middle ear. See Figure 17–24, *D*.

17

otosclerosis

Hardening of the bony tissue of the middle ear.

The result of this hereditary condition is that bone forms around the oval window and causes fixation or **ankylosis** (stiffening) of the stapes bone (ossicle). Conduction deafness occurs, as the ossicles cannot pass on vibrations when sound enters the ear. Stapedectomy with replacement by a **prosthesis** (artificial part) is effective in restoring hearing (see Fig. 17–23). In order to perform this operation, the oval window must be **fenestrated** (opened) using a laser.

tinnitus

Sensation of noises (ringing, buzzing, whistling, booming) in the ears.

Caused by irritation of delicate hair cells in the inner ear, this disease symptom may be associated with presbycusis, Meniere disease, otosclerosis, chronic otitis, labyrinthitis, and other disorders. Tinnitus can be persistent and severe and can interfere with a patient's daily life. Treatment includes biofeedback to help the patient relax and exert control over stress and anxiety if these are contributing factors.

Tinnitus, a Latin-derived term, means tinkling.

vertigo

Sensation of irregular or whirling motion either of oneself or of external objects.

Vertigo can result from disease in the labyrinth of the inner ear or in the nerve that carries messages from the semicircular canals to the brain. Equilibrium and balance are affected, and nausea may occur as well.

CLINICAL PROCEDURES

audiometry

Testing the sense of hearing.

An **audiometer** is an electrical device that delivers acoustic stimuli of specific frequencies to determine a patient's hearing loss for each frequency. See Figure 17–25, *A*. Results are shown on a chart or **audiogram**. (See Fig. 17–25, *B*).

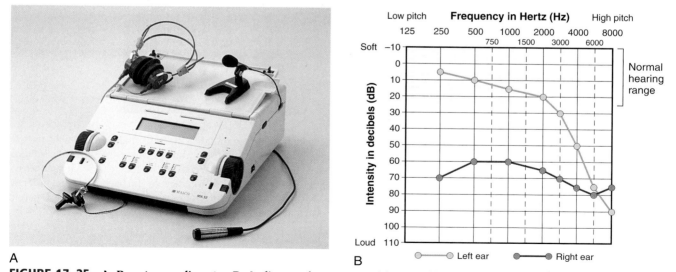

FIGURE 17–25 **A, Pure-tone audiometer. B, Audiogram** for a person with normal hearing in low frequencies (pitch). Notice the blue line sloping downward, showing severe high-frequency hearing loss in the left ear. There is moderate to severe hearing loss in the right ear. The decibel (dB) level of the softest sound you are able to hear is called your threshold. Thresholds of 0 to 25 dB *(yellow area)* are considered normal (for adults). (**A** courtesy of Maico, Inc., Minneapolis, MN. In Ignatavicius DD, Workman ML: Medical-Surgical Nursing: Critical Thinking for Collaborative Care, 5th ed. Philadelphia, WB Saunders, 2005, p. 1120.)

17

cochlear implant	**Surgically implanted device allowing sensorineural hearing–impaired persons to understand speech.**

Electrical signals are sent directly into the auditory nerve by means of multiple electrodes inserted into the cochlea. An external microphone and speech processor pick up sound signals and convert them to electrical impulses. See Figure 17–26, A.

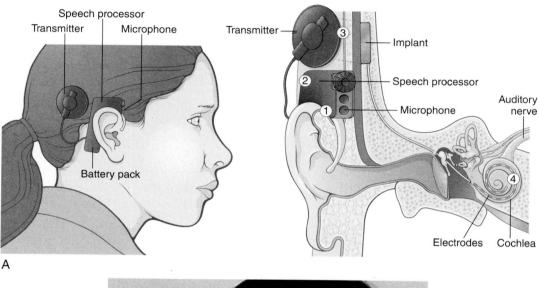

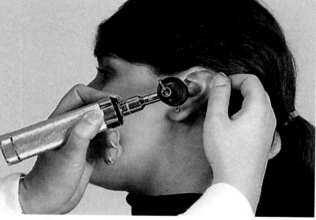

FIGURE 17–26   A, Cochlear implant. 1. Microphone receives sound. 2. Speech processor corrects sounds into digital signals. 3. Signals sent to transmitter that relays them to an implant where they are converted to electrical impulses. 4. Impulses sent to electrodes that stimulate nerve cells in the cochlea, which send them to the auditory nerve and brain. **B, Otoscopic examination.** The auricle is pulled up and back. The hand holding the otoscope is braced against the patient's face for stabilization. (**B** from Lewis SM, Heitkemper MM, Dirksen SR: Medical-Surgical Nursing: Assessment and Management of Clinical Problems, 6th ed. Mosby, St. Louis, 2004, p. 434.)

ear thermometry	**Measurement of the temperature of the tympanic membrane by detection of infrared radiation from the eardrum.** A device is inserted into the auditory canal, and results, which reflect the body's temperature, are obtained within 2 seconds.
otoscopy	**Visual examination of the ear with an otoscope.** (See Fig. 17–26, *B*.)
tuning fork test	**Test of ear conduction using a vibration source (tuning fork).** To perform the **Rinne test,** the examiner places the base of the vibrating fork against the patient's mastoid bone (bone conduction) and in front of the auditory meatus (air conduction). In the **Weber test,** the tuning fork is placed on the center of the forehead. The loudness of sound is equal in both ears if hearing is normal.

ABBREVIATIONS

AD	right ear (Latin, *auris dextra*)	**ENT**	ears, nose, and throat
AOM	acute otitis media	**HEENT**	head, eyes, ears, nose, and throat
AS	left ear (Latin, *auris sinistra*)	**PE tube**	pressure-equalizing tube—a polyethylene ventilating tube placed in the eardrum
EENT	eyes, ears, nose, and throat		
ENG	electronystagmography—a test of the balance mechanism of the inner ear by assessing eye movements (**nystagmus** is rapidly twitching eye movement)	**SOM**	serous otitis media

PRACTICAL APPLICATIONS

17

This section contains an operating room schedule and an operative report. Explanations of more difficult terms are added in brackets. Answers to the questions are on page 713.

OPERATING ROOM SCHEDULE: EYE AND EAR PROCEDURES

Match the operation in Column I with a diagnosis/surgical indication in Column II.

Column I		Column II
1. phacoemulsification with IOL; OS	_____	A. Scarred and torn cornea
2. blepharoplasty	_____	B. Ptosis of eyelid skin
3. scleral buckle	_____	C. Retinal detachment
4. vitrectomy	_____	D. Diabetic retinopathy
5. radical mastoidectomy	_____	E. Macular degeneration
6. keratoplasty	_____	F. Chronic stye
7. cochlear implant	_____	G. Chronic infection of a bone behind the ear
8. laser photocoagulation of the macula	_____	H. Severe deafness
9. incision and drainage of hordeolum	_____	I. Senile cataract; left eye

OPERATIVE REPORT

Preoperative Diagnosis. Bilateral chronic serous otitis media; tonsilloadenoiditis.

Operation. Bilateral myringotomies and ventilation tube insertion; T and A.

Procedure. With the patient in the supine position and under general endotracheal anesthesia, inspection of AD was made under the operating microscope. The external canal was clear, tympanic membrane was divided. A purulent discharge appeared to be present. This drainage was suctioned out and the ear thoroughly lavaged [washed out]. A ventilating tube was put in place and otic drops were administered. Same procedure for AS.

The patient was placed in the Rose position [supine with the head over the table edge in full extension] and the adenoids removed with adenoid curettes and adenoid biopsy forceps. A nasopharyngeal sponge was put in place. The right tonsil was then grasped with tonsil forceps, dissected free, and removed with snare. Bleeding was controlled with suction cautery. The nasopharyngeal sponge was removed and no further bleeding noted. The patient tolerated the procedure well and left the OR in good condition.

Remember to check your answers carefully with those given in the Answers to Exercises, page 711.

A. Match the structure of the eye with its description below. Write the letter of the description in the space provided.

Column I

1. pupil _____
2. conjunctiva _____
3. cornea _____
4. sclera _____
5. choroid _____
6. iris _____
7. ciliary body _____
8. lens _____
9. retina _____
10. vitreous humor _____

Column II

A. Contains sensitive cells called rods and cones that transform light energy into nerve impulses.
B. Contains muscles that control the shape of the lens and secretes aqueous humor.
C. Transparent structure behind the iris and in front of the vitreous humor; it refracts light rays onto the retina.
D. Jelly-like material behind the lens that helps to maintain the shape of the eyeball.
E. Dark center of the eye through which light rays enter.
F. Vascular layer of the eyeball that is continuous with the iris.
G. Delicate membrane lining the eyelids and covering the anterior eyeball.
H. Fibrous layer of clear tissue that extends over the anterior portion of the eyeball.
I. Colored portion of the eye; surrounds the pupil.
J. Tough, white, outer coat of the eye.

B. Supply the terms that complete the following sentences.

1. The region at the back of the eye where the optic nerve meets the retina is the _____.

2. The normal adjustment of the lens (becoming fatter) to bring an object into focus for near vision on the retina is _____.

3. A yellowish region on the retina lateral to the optic disc is the _____.

4. The tiny pit or depression in the retina that is the region of clearest vision is the

   _____.

5. The bending of light rays by the cornea, lens, and fluids of the eye is _____.

6. The point at which the fibers of the optic nerve cross in the brain is the _____.

7. The photoreceptor cells in the retina that make the perception of color possible are the

   _____.

8. The photoreceptor cells in the retina that make vision in dim light possible are the

   _____.

9. The _____ is the area behind the cornea and in front of the lens and iris. It contains aqueous humor.

10. The posterior, inner part of the eye is the _____.

17

C. Arrange the following terms in proper sequence to show the pathway of light rays to the visual region of the brain.

anterior chamber and aqueous humor
cerebral cortex (occipital lobe)
cornea
lens
optic chiasm

optic nerve fibers
pupil
retina
thalamus
vitreous chamber and vitreous humor

1. _____ fibrous transparent layer of clear tissue over the eyeball

2. _____ space and fluid in the front of the eye

3. _____ dark opening of the eye

4. _____ transparent, biconvex body that refracts light rays

5. _____ space and soft, jelly-like material in the middle of eye

6. _____ light-sensitive inner nerve cell layer; rods and cones

7. _____ cranial nerve

8. _____ area of brain where optic nerve fibers cross

9. _____ relay center of the brain

10. _____ visual region of the brain

D. Give the meanings of the following terms.

1. optic nerve _____

2. biconvex _____

3. anisocoria _____

4. cycloplegic _____

5. palpebral _____

6. mydriasis _____

7. miosis _____

8. papilledema _____

9. photophobia _____

10. scotoma _____

E. Complete the medical terms based on their meanings and the word parts given.

1. inflammation of an eyelid: _____itis

2. inflammation of the conjunctiva: _____itis

3. inflammation of a tear gland: _____itis

4. inflammation of the iris: _____itis

5. inflammation of the cornea: _____itis

6. inflammation of the white of the eye: _____itis

7. inflammation of the retina: _____itis

8. prolapse of the eyelid: blephar_____

9. pertaining to tears: _____al

10. pertaining to within the eye: intra_____

F. Select from the following terms to match the meanings below.

aphakia	hemianopsia	optometrist
corneal ulcer	hypertropia	retinitis
esotropia	ophthalmologist	uveitis
exotropia	optician	xerophthalmia

1. fibrous layer of clear tissue over the front of the eyeball has a defect resulting from infection

   _____

2. inflammation of the vascular layer of the eye (iris, ciliary body, and choroid) _____

3. condition of dry eyes _____

4. absence of vision in half of the visual field _____

5. eye abnormally turns outward _____

6. medical doctor who treats diseases of the eyes _____

7. nonmedical professional who can examine eyes and prescribe glasses _____

8. nonmedical professional who grinds lenses and fits glasses _____

9. absence of the lens of the eye _____

10. eye abnormally turns inward _____

G. Describe the following visual conditions.

1. amblyopia _____

2. hyperopia _____

3. presbyopia _____

4. myopia _____

5. nyctalopia_____

6. diplopia _____

7. astigmatism_____

17

H. Complete the following sentences.

1. In the myopic eye, light rays do not focus properly on the _____. Either the eyeball is too _____ or the refractive power of the lens is too _____, so that the image is blurred and comes to a focus in _____ of the retina. The type of lens used to correct this refractive error is called a/an _____ lens.

2. In the hyperopic eye, the eyeball is too _____ or the refractive power of the lens too _____, so that the image is blurred and focused in _____ of the retina. The type of lens used to correct this refractive error is called a/an _____ lens.

3. A miotic is a drug that _____ the pupil of the eye.

4. A mydriatic is a drug that _____ the pupil of the eye.

I. Match the following abnormal conditions of the eye with their meanings as given below.

cataract	hordeolum (stye)	retinitis pigmentosa
chalazion	macular degeneration	strabismus
diabetic retinopathy	nystagmus	
glaucoma	retinal detachment	

1. retinal microaneurysms, hemorrhages, dilation of retinal veins, and neovascularization occur secondary to an abnormal endocrine condition _____

2. two layers of the retina separate from each other _____

3. abnormal deviations of the eye occur (esotropia and exotropia) _____

4. clouding of the lens causes decreased vision _____

5. loss of central vision caused by deterioration of the macula of the retina _____

6. localized, purulent infection of a sebaceous gland in the eyelid _____

7. small, hard, cystic mass on the eyelid; formed as a result of chronic inflammation of a sebaceous gland _____

8. increased intraocular pressure results in optic nerve damage _____

9. pigmented scarring forms throughout the retina and leads to nyctalopia; an inherited condition _____

10. repetitive rhythmic movements of one or both eyes _____

J. **The picture shows how a patient with one of the following conditions would view the scene. Circle the correct term for this condition.**

A. glaucoma

B. cataract

C. stroke (hemianopsia)

D. macular degeneration

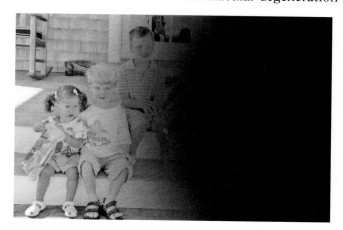

K. **Give the meaning of the following combining forms.**

1. lacrim/o _____

2. dacry/o _____

3. kerat/o _____

4. corne/o _____

5. blephar/o _____

6. palpebr/o _____

7. cor/o _____

8. pupill/o _____

9. phac/o _____

10. phak/o _____

11. ocul/o _____

12. ophthalm/o _____

13. opt/o _____

14. scot/o _____

L. Match the following clinical procedures with their meanings as given below.

17

fluorescein angiography	ophthalmoscopy	tonometry
keratoplasty	phacoemulsification	visual acuity test
laser photocoagulation	scleral buckle	visual field test
LASIK	slit lamp microscopy	vitrectomy

1. ultrasonic vibrations break up the lens, and it is aspirated from the eye _____

2. test of clearness of vision _____

3. measurement of tension or pressure within the eye; glaucoma test _____

4. high-energy light radiation beams are used to stop retinal hemorrhaging _____

5. a laser removes corneal tissue (sculpts it) to correct myopia _____

6. intravenous injection of dye followed by photographs of the eye through dilated pupils

   _____

7. suture of a silicone band to the sclera to correct retinal detachment _____

8. test to measure central and peripheral vision (area within which objects are seen) when the eyes

   are looking straight ahead _____

9. removal (and replacement) of diseased fluid in the chamber behind the lens of the eye

   _____

10. visual examination of the interior of the eye after dilation of the pupil _____

11. use of an instrument for microscopic examination of parts of the eye _____

12. corneal transplant surgery _____

M. Give the meanings of the following abbreviations.

1. OU _____

2. VA _____

3. OD _____

4. OS _____

5. VF _____

6. IOL _____

7. IOP _____

8. PERRLA _____

N. Arrange the following terms in the correct order to indicate their sequence in the transmission of sound waves to the brain from the outer ear.

auditory liquids and receptors   external auditory canal   pinna (auricle)
auditory nerve fibers   incus   stapes
cerebral cortex   malleus   tympanic membrane
cochlea   oval window

1. _____

2. _____

3. _____

4. _____

5. _____

6. _____

7. _____

8. _____

9. _____

10. _____

11. _____

O. Give the meanings of the following medical terms.

1. labyrinth _____

2. semicircular canals _____

3. auditory (eustachian) tube _____

4. stapes _____

5. organ of Corti _____

6. perilymph and endolymph _____

7. cerumen _____

8. vestibule _____

9. oval window _____

10. tympanic membrane _____

17

P. Complete the following terms based on their definitions.

1. instrument to examine the ear: _____scope

2. removal of the third bone of the middle ear: _____ectomy

3. pertaining to the auditory tube and throat: _____pharyngeal

4. flow of pus from the ear: oto_____

5. instrument to measure hearing: _____meter

6. incision of the eardrum: _____tomy

7. surgical repair of the eardrum: _____plasty

8. deafness due to old age: _____cusis

9. small ear: micr_____

10. inflammation of the middle ear: ot_____

Q. Give the meanings of the following medical terms.

1. vertigo _____

2. Meniere disease _____

3. otosclerosis _____

4. tinnitus _____

5. labyrinthitis _____

6. cholesteatoma _____

7. suppurative otitis media _____

8. acoustic neuroma _____

9. mastoiditis _____

10. myringitis _____

R. Give the meanings of the following abbreviations relating to otology.

1. ENG _____

2. AS _____

3. AD _____

4. EENT _____

5. ENT _____

6. PE tube _____

S. Circle the correct term(s) to complete each sentence.

1. Dr. Jones specializes in pediatric ophthalmology. His examination of children with poor vision often leads to the diagnosis of **(cataract, amblyopia, glaucoma),** or lazy eye.

2. Stella's near vision became progressively worse as she aged. Her physician told her that she had a common condition called **(presbyopia, detached retina, anisocoria),** which many middle-aged patients develop.

3. Matthew rubbed his itchy eyes constantly and thus spread his "pinkeye" or **(conjunctivitis, blepharitis, myringitis)** from one eye to the other. Dr. Chang prescribed antibiotics for this common condition, since he had a purulent discharge suggestive of an infection.

4. As Paul's **(mastoiditis, otitis media, tinnitus)** became progressively worse, his doctor worried that this ringing in his ears might be caused by a benign brain tumor, a/an **(cholesteatoma, acoustic neuroma, glaucoma).**

5. Before her second birthday, Sally had so many episodes of **(vertigo, otosclerosis, suppurative otitis media)** that Dr. Sills recommended the placement of PE tubes.

6. Sixty-eight-year-old Bob experienced blurred vision in the central portion of his visual field. After careful examination of his **(cornea, sclera, retina),** his **(ophthalmologist, optician, optometrist)** diagnosed his condition as **(glaucoma, iritis, macular degeneration).** The doctor explained that the form of this condition was atrophic or **(dry, wet),** causing photoreceptor rods and cones to die.

7. If Bob's condition had been diagnosed as the **(dry, wet)** form, it might have been treated with **(cryotherapy, intraocular lenses, laser photocoagulation)** to seal leaky blood vessels.

8. Sarah suddenly experienced bright flashes of light in her right eye. She also told her physician that she had a sensation of a curtain being pulled over part of the visual field in that eye. Her doctor examined her eye with **(keratoplasty, ophthalmoscopy, tonometry)** and determined that she had **(retinal refraction, retinal detachment, diabetic retinopathy).** Surgery, known as **(enucleation, vitrectomy, scleral buckling),** was recommended.

9. Carol awakened with a sensation of dizziness or **(vertigo, tinnitus, presbycusis)** as she tried to get out of bed. She was totally incapacitated for several days and noticed hearing loss in her left ear. Her physician explained that fluid called **(pus, endolymph, mucus)** had accumulated in her **(auditory tube, middle ear, cochlea)** and her condition was **(otosclerosis, cholesteatoma, Meniere disease).** He prescribed drugs to control her dizziness and nausea.

10. Patients with conductive hearing loss are helped by reconstruction of the **(labyrinth, tympanic membrane, auditory tube),** a procedure known as **(myringoplasty, audiometry, otoscopy).** Patients with sensorineural hearing loss may be helped by a **(hearing aid, cochlear implant, stapedectomy).**

MEDICAL SCRAMBLE

Unscramble the letters to form terms relating to eye or ear abnormalities from the clues. Use the letters in squares to complete the bonus term. Answers are found on page 713.

1. *Clue:* The lens appears cloudy

   □ __ __ __ □ __ __   ATCRTACA

2. *Clue:* Increased intraocular pressure

   __ □ __ □ __ __ __ □   AUGMOLAC

3. *Clue:* The eardrum is inflamed

   □ __ __ __ __ __ __ __ __ __   YSIMIGRTNI

4. *Clue:* You feel as if objects are whirling around you

   __ __ □ __ __ __ __   OVTEGIR

BONUS TERM: *Clue:* Age-related, gradual loss of central vision is _____ degeneration.

□ □ □ □ □ □ □

ANSWERS TO EXERCISES

A

1. E
2. G
3. H
4. J

5. F
6. I
7. B

8. C
9. A
10. D

B

1. optic disc
2. accommodation
3. macula
4. fovea centralis

5. refraction
6. optic chiasm
7. cones

8. rods
9. anterior chamber
10. fundus

C

1. cornea
2. aqueous chamber and aqueous humor
3. pupil
4. lens

5. vitreous chamber and vitreous humor
6. retina
7. optic nerve fibers

8. optic chiasm
9. thalamus
10. cerebral cortex (occipital lobe)

D

1. cranial nerve that carries impulses from the retina to the brain
2. having two sides that are rounded, elevated, and curved evenly
3. condition of pupils of unequal (anis/o) size

4. pertaining to paralysis of the ciliary muscles
5. pertaining to the eyelid
6. condition of enlargement of the pupil
7. condition of constriction of the pupil
8. swelling in the region of the optic disc

9. condition of sensitivity to ("fear of") light
10. blind spot; area of darkened (diminished) vision surrounded by clear vision

E

1. blepharitis
2. conjunctivitis
3. dacryoadenitis
4. iritis

5. keratitis
6. scleritis
7. retinitis

8. blepharoptosis
9. lacrimal
10. intraocular

F

1. corneal ulcer
2. uveitis
3. xerophthalmia
4. hemianopsia

5. exotropia
6. ophthalmologist
7. optometrist

8. optician
9. aphakia
10. esotropia

G

1. decreased (dim) vision; lazy eye (resulting from strabismus and diplopia)
2. farsightedness

3. decreased vision at near resulting from old age
4. nearsightedness
5. night blindness; decreased vision at night

6. double vision
7. defective curvature of the lens and cornea leading to blurred vision

H

1. retina; long; strong; front; concave
2. short; weak; back; convex

3. constricts
4. dilates

I

1. diabetic retinopathy
2. retinal detachment
3. strabismus
4. cataract

5. macular degeneration
6. hordeolum (stye)
7. chalazion

8. glaucoma
9. retinitis pigmentosa
10. nystagmus

17

J

C. Stroke (hemianopsia)—loss of half of the visual field caused by a stroke affecting the left visual cortex.

Glaucoma would cause loss of peripheral vision first (darkness around the edges of the picture).

A cataract would cause blurred vision. Macular degeneration would produce loss of central vision.

K

1. tears
2. tears
3. cornea
4. cornea
5. eyelid
6. eyelid
7. pupil
8. pupil
9. lens
10. lens
11. eye
12. eye
13. eye
14. darkness

L

1. phacoemulsification
2. visual acuity test
3. tonometry
4. laser photocoagulation
5. LASIK
6. fluorescein angiography
7. scleral buckle
8. visual field examination
9. vitrectomy
10. ophthalmoscopy
11. slit lamp ocular examination
12. keratoplasty

M

1. both eyes
2. visual acuity
3. right eye
4. left eye
5. visual field
6. intraocular lens
7. intraocular pressure
8. pupils equal, round, reactive to light and accommodation

N

1. pinna (auricle)
2. external auditory canal
3. tympanic membrane
4. malleus
5. incus
6. stapes
7. oval window
8. cochlea
9. auditory liquids and receptors
10. auditory nerve fibers
11. cerebral cortex

O

1. cochlea and organs of equilibrium (semicircular canals and vestibule)
2. organ of equilibrium in the inner ear
3. passageway between the middle ear and the throat
4. third ossicle (little bone) of the middle ear
5. region in the cochlea that contains auditory receptors
6. auditory fluids circulating within the inner ear
7. wax in the external auditory meatus
8. central cavity of the inner ear that connects the semicircular canals and the cochlea
9. delicate membrane between the middle and the inner ears
10. eardrum

P

1. otoscope
2. stapedectomy
3. salpingopharyngeal
4. otopyorrhea
5. audiometer
6. myringotomy (tympanotomy)
7. tympanoplasty (myringoplasty)
8. presbycusis
9. microtia
10. otitis media

Q

1. sensation of irregular or whirling motion either of oneself or of external objects
2. disorder of the labyrinth marked by elevation of ear fluids and pressure within the cochlea (tinnitus, vertigo, and nausea result)
3. hardening in the bony tissue of the ossicles of the middle ear
4. noise (ringing, buzzing) in the ears
5. inflammation of the labyrinth of the inner ear
6. collection of skin cells and cholesterol in a sac within the middle ear
7. inflammation of the middle ear with bacterial infection and pus collection
8. benign tumor arising from the acoustic nerve in the brain
9. inflammation of the mastoid process (behind the ear)
10. inflammation of the eardrum

R

1. electronystagmography; a test of balance
2. left ear
3. right ear
4. eyes, ears, nose, and throat
5. ears, nose, and throat
6. pressure-equalizing tube; ventilating tube placed in the eardrum

S

1. amblyopia
2. presbyopia
3. conjunctivitis
4. tinnitus; acoustic neuroma
5. suppurative otitis media

6. retina; ophthalmologist; macular degeneration; dry
7. wet; laser photocoagulation
8. ophthalmoscopy; retinal detachment; scleral buckling

9. vertigo; endolymph; cochlea; Meniere disease
10. tympanic membrane; myringoplasty; cochlear implant

17

ANSWERS TO PRACTICAL APPLICATIONS

1. I	4. D	7. H
2. B	5. G	8. E
3. C	6. A	9. F

ANSWERS TO MEDICAL SCRAMBLE

1. CATARACT   2. GLAUCOMA   3. MYRINGITIS   4. VERTIGO

BONUS TERM: MACULAR

PRONUNCIATION OF TERMS

PRONUNCIATION GUIDE

ā as in āpe   ă as in ăpple
ē as in ēven   ě as in ěvery
ī as in īce   ĭ as in ĭnterest
ō as in ōpen   ŏ as in pŏt
ū as in ūnit   ŭ as in ŭnder

To test your understanding of the terminology in this chapter, write the meaning of each term in the space provided. In addition, you may wish to cover the terms and write them by looking at your definitions. Make sure your spelling is correct. The page number after each term indicates where it is defined or used in the book, so you can easily check your responses. You will find complete definitions for all of these terms and their audio pronunciations on the CD.

VOCABULARY AND TERMINOLOGY: EYE

Term	Pronunciation	Meaning
accommodation (674)	ă-kŏm-ō-DĀ-shŭn	
amblyopia (679)	ăm-blē-Ō-pē-ă	
anisocoria (676)	ăn-ī-sō-KŌ-rē-ă	
anterior chamber (674)	ăn-TĒ-rē-ŏr CHĀM-běr	
aphakia (678)	ă-FĀ-kē-ă	
aqueous humor (675)	ĂK-wē-ŭs or Ā-kwē-ŭs HŪ-měr	
astigmatism (680)	ă-STĬG-mă-tĭzm	
biconvex (675)	bī-KŎN-věks	
blepharitis (676)	blěf-ă-RĪ-tĭs	
blepharoptosis (676)	blěf-ă-rŏp-TŌ-sĭs	
cataract (681)	KĂT-ă-răkt	
chalazion (682)	kă-LĀ-zē-ŏn	
choroid (675)	KŎR-oyd	
ciliary body (675)	SĬL-ē-ăr-ē BŎD-ē	

17

Term	Pronunciation	Meaning
cone (675)	kōn	
conjunctiva (675)	kŏn-jŭnk-TĪ-vă	
conjunctivitis (676)	kŏn-jŭnk-tĭ-VĪ-tĭs	
cornea (675)	KŎR-nē-ă	
corneal abrasion (676)	KŎR-nē-ăl ă-BRĀ-zhŭn	
corneoscleral (678)	kŏr-nē-ō-SKLĔ-răl	
cycloplegic (676)	sī-klō-PLĒ-jĭk	
dacryoadenitis (677)	dăk-rē-ō-ăd-ĕ-NĪ-tĭs	
diabetic retinopathy (682)	dī-ă-BĔT-ĭk rĕ-tĭn-NŎP-ă-thē	
diplopia (679)	dĭp-LŌ-pē-ă	
enucleation (687)	ē-nū-klē-Ā-shun	
esotropia (680)	ĕs-ō-TRŌ-pē-ă	
exotropia (685)	ĕk-sō-TRŌ-pē-ă	
fluorescein angiography (685)	floo-ō-RĔS-ē-ĭn ăn-jē-ŎG-ră-fē	
fovea centralis (675)	FŌ-vē-ă sĕn-TRĂ-lĭs	
fundus (675)	FŬN-dŭs	
glaucoma (679)	glaw-KŌ-mă	
hemianopsia (679)	hĕ-mē-ă-NŎP-sē-ă	
hordeolum (683)	hŏr-DĒ-ō-lŭm	
hyperopia (679)	hī-pĕr-Ō-pē-ă	
hypertensive retinopathy (678)	hī-pĕr-TĔN-sĭv rĕ-tĭ-NŎP-ă-thē	
intraocular (677)	ĭn-tră-ŎK-ū-lăr	
iridectomy (677)	ĭr-ĭ-DĔK-tō-mē	
iridic (677)	ĭ-RĪD-ĭk	
iris (675)	Ī-rĭs	
iritis (677)	ī-RĪ-tĭs	
keratitis (677)	kĕr-ă-TĪ-tĭs	
keratoplasty (687)	kĕr-ă-tō-PLĂS-tē	
lacrimal (677)	LĂK-rĭ-măl	
lacrimation (677)	lă-krĭ-MĀ-shŭn	
laser photocoagulation (687)	LĀ-zĕr fō-tō-kō-ăg-ū-LĀ-shŭn	
lens (675)	lĕnz	
macula (675)	MĂK-ū-lă	

Term	Pronunciation	Meaning
macular degeneration (684)	MĂK-ū-lăr dē-jĕn-ĕ-RĀ-shŭn	
miosis (679)	mī-Ō-sĭs	
miotic (679)	mī-ŎT-ĭk	
mydriasis (679)	mĭ-DRĪ-ă-sĭs	
myopia (681)	mī-Ō-pē-ă	
nyctalopia (679)	nĭk-tă-LŌ-pē-ă	
nystagmus (684)	nĭ-STĂG-mŭs	
ophthalmic (677)	ŏf-THĂL-mĭk	
ophthalmologist (677)	ŏf-thăl-MŎL-ō-jĭst	
ophthalmoplegia (677)	ŏf-thăl-mō-PLĒ-jă	
ophthalmoscopy (686)	ŏf-thăl-MŎS-kō-pē	
optic chiasm (675)	ŎP-tĭk KĪ-ăzm	
optic disc (675)	ŎP-tĭk dĭsk	
optician (678)	ŏp-TĬSH-ăn	
optic nerve (675)	ŎP-tĭk nĕrv	
optometrist (678)	ŏp-TŎM-ĕ-trĭst	
palpebral (678)	PĂL-pĕ-brăl	
papilledema (678)	păp-ĕ-lĕ-DĒ-mă	
phacoemulsification (678)	făk-ō-ĕ-mŭl-sĭ-fĭ-KĀ-shŭn	
photophobia (679)	fō-tō-FŌ-bē-ă	
presbyopia (679)	prĕz-bē-Ō-pē-ă	
pupil (675)	PŪ-pĭl	
pupillary (678)	PŪ-pĭ-lăr-ē	
refraction (675)	rē-FRĂK-shŭn	
retina (675)	RĔT-ĭ-nă	
retinal detachment (684)	RĔ-tĭ-năl dē-TĂCH-mĕnt	
retinitis pigmentosa (678)	rĕt-ĭ-NĪ-tĭs pĭg-mĕn-TŌ-să	
rod (675)	rŏd	
sclera (675)	SKLĔ-ră	
scleral buckle (689)	SKLĔ-răl BŬ-k'l	
scleritis (678)	sklĕ-RĪ-tĭs	
scotoma (679)	skō-TŌ-mă	
slit lamp microscopy (686)	slĭt lămp mī-KRŎS-kō-pē	

17

Term	Pronunciation	Meaning
strabismus (685)	stră-BĬZ-mŭs	_____
thalamus (675)	THĂL-ă-mŭs	_____
tonometry (683)	tō-NŎM-ĕ-trē	_____
uveitis (678)	ū-vē-Ī-tĭs	_____
visual acuity test (686)	VĬZ-ū-ăl ă-KŪ-ĭ-tē tĕst	_____
visual field test (687)	VĬZ-ū-ăl fēld tĕst	_____
vitrectomy (689)	vĭ-TRĔK-tō-mē	_____
vitreous humor (675)	VĬT-rē-ŭs HŪ-mŏr	_____
xerophthalmia (679)	zĕr-ŏf-THĂL-mē-ă	_____

VOCABULARY AND TERMINOLOGY: EAR

Term	Pronunciation	Meaning
acoustic (694)	ă-KOOS-tĭk	_____
acoustic neuroma (696)	ă-KOOS-tĭk nū-RŌ-mă	_____
audiogram (694)	ĂW-dē-ō-grăm	_____
audiometer (695)	ăw-dē-ŎM-ĕ-tĕr	_____
audiometry (697)	ăw-dē-ŎM-ĕ-trē	_____
auditory canal (693)	ĂW-dĭ-tō-rē kă-NĂL	_____
auditory meatus (693)	ĂW-dĭ-tō-rē mē-Ā-tŭs	_____
auditory nerve fibers (693)	ĂW-dĭ-tō-re nĕrv FĬ-bĕrz	_____
auditory tube (693)	ĂW-dĭ-tō-rē toob	_____
aural (694)	ĂW-răl	_____
auricle (693)	ĂW-rĭ-k'l	_____
cerumen (693)	sĕ-ROO-mĕn	_____
cholesteatoma (696)	kō-lē-stē-ă-TŌ-mă	_____
cochlea (693)	KŎK-lē-ă	_____
cochlear (694)	KŎK-lē-ăr	_____
deafness (696)	DĔF-nĕs	_____
ear thermometry (699)	ēr thĕr-MŎM-ĕ-trē	_____
endolymph (693)	ĔN-dō-lĭmf	_____
eustachian tube (693)	ū-STĀ-shŭn toob	_____
hyperacusis (695)	hī-pĕr-ă-KŪ-sis	_____
incus (693)	ĬNG-kŭs	_____
labyrinth (693)	LĂB-ĭ-rĭnth	_____

Term	Pronunciation	Meaning
macrotia (696)	măk-RŌ-shē-ă	_____
malleus (693)	MĂL-ē-ŭs	_____
mastoiditis (694)	măs-toy-DĪ-tĭs	_____
Meniere disease (696)	měn-ē-ĀR dĭ-ZĒZ	_____
microtia (696)	mī-KRŌ-shē-ă	_____
myringitis (694)	mĭr-ĭn-JĪ-tĭs	_____
myringotomy (694)	mĭr-ĭn-GŎT-ō-mē	_____
ossicle (693)	ŎS-ĭ-k'l	_____
ossiculoplasty (694)	ŏs-ĭ-kū-lō-PLĂS-tē	_____
otic (694)	Ō-tĭk	_____
otolaryngologist (694)	ō-tō-lă-rĭn-GŎL-ō-jĭst	_____
otomycosis (694)	ō-tō-mī-KŌ-sĭs	_____
otopyorrhea (694)	ō-tō-pī-ō-RĒ-ă	_____
otosclerosis (697)	ō-tō-sklĕ-RŌ-sĭs	_____
otoscopy (699)	ō-TŎS-kō-pē	_____
oval window (693)	Ō-văl WĬN-dō	_____
perilymph (693)	PĔR-ĭ-lĭmf	_____
pinna (693)	PĬN-ă	_____
postauricular (694)	pōst-aw-RĬK-ū-lăr	_____
presbycusis (695)	prĕz-bē-KŪ-sĭs	_____
salpingopharyngeal (694)	săl-pĭng-gō-fă-RĬN-gē-ăl	_____
semicircular canals (693)	sĕ-mē-SĔR-kū-lăr kă-NĂLZ	_____
serous otitis media (696)	SĔR-ŭs ō-TĪ-tĭs MĒ-dē-ă	_____
stapedectomy (694)	stā-pĕ-DĔK-tō-mē	_____
stapes (693)	STĀ-pēz	_____
suppurative otitis media (696)	SŬ-pŭr-ă-tĭv ō-TĪ-tĭs MĒ-dē-ă	_____
tinnitus (697)	tĭ-NĪ-tŭs	_____
tuning fork tests (699)	TOO-nĭng fŏrk tĕsts	_____
tympanic membrane (693)	tĭm-PĂN-ĭk MĔM-brān	_____
tympanoplasty (694)	tĭm-pă-nō-PLĂS-tē	_____
vertigo (697)	VĔR-tĭ-gō	_____
vestibule (693)	VĔS-tĭ-būl	_____
vestibulocochlear (694)	vĕs-tĭb-ū-lō-KŌK-lē-ăr	_____

REVIEW SHEET

17

Write the meaning of the word parts in the spaces provided and test yourself. Check your answers with the information in the chapter or in the glossary (Medical Word Parts—English) at the end of the book.

COMBINING FORMS

Combining Form	Meaning	Combining Form	Meaning
acous/o	_____	myring/o	_____
ambly/o	_____	nyct/o	_____
anis/o	_____	ocul/o	_____
aque/o	_____	ophthalm/o	_____
audi/o	_____	opt/o	_____
audit/o	_____	optic/o	_____
aur/o	_____	ossicul/o	_____
auricul/o	_____	ot/o	_____
blephar/o	_____	palpebr/o	_____
cochle/o	_____	papill/o	_____
conjunctiv/o	_____	phac/o	_____
cor/o	_____	phak/o	_____
corne/o	_____	phot/o	_____
cycl/o	_____	presby/o	_____
dacry/o	_____	pupill/o	_____
dipl/o	_____	retin/o	_____
glauc/o	_____	salping/o	_____
ir/o	_____	scler/o	_____
irid/o	_____	scot/o	_____
kerat/o	_____	staped/o	_____
lacrim/o	_____	tympan/o	_____
mastoid/o	_____	uve/o	_____
mi/o	_____	vestibul/o	_____
myc/o	_____	vitre/o	_____
mydr/o	_____	xer/o	_____

SUFFIXES

Suffix	Meaning	Suffix	Meaning
-acusis	_____	-opsia	_____
-cusis	_____	-otia	_____
-meter	_____	-phobia	_____
-metry	_____	-plegic	_____
-opia	_____	-tropia	_____

17

 Please refer to the enclosed CD for additional exercises and images related to this chapter.

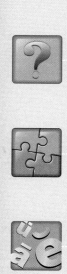

chapter 18

Endocrine System

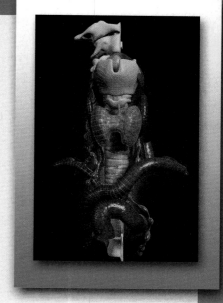

In this chapter you will

- Identify the endocrine glands and their hormones.
- Gain an understanding of the functions of these hormones in the body.
- Analyze medical terms related to the endocrine glands and their hormones.
- Identify the abnormal conditions resulting from excessive and deficient secretions of the endocrine glands.
- Describe laboratory tests and clinical procedures related to endocrinology, and recognize relevant abbreviations.
- Apply your new knowledge to understanding medical terms in their proper contexts, such as medical reports and records.

Image Description: Anterior semi-wireframe view
highlighting the thyroid gland.

721

INTRODUCTION

The endocrine system is an information signaling system much like the nervous system. However, the nervous system uses nerves to conduct information, whereas the endocrine system uses blood vessels as information channels. **Glands** located in many regions of the body release into the bloodstream specific chemical messengers called **hormones** (from the Greek word *hormōn*, meaning urging on), which regulate the many and varied functions of an organism. For example, one hormone stimulates the growth of bones, another causes the maturation of sex organs and reproductive cells, and another controls the metabolic rate (metabolism) within all the individual cells of the body. In addition, one powerful endocrine gland below the brain secretes a wide variety of different hormones that travel through the bloodstream and regulate the activities of other endocrine glands.

Hormones produce their effects by binding to **receptors,** which are recognition sites in the various **target tissues** on which the hormones act. The receptors initiate specific biologic effects when the hormones bind to them. Each hormone has its own receptor, and binding of a receptor by a hormone is much like the interaction of a key and a lock.

Endocrine glands, no matter which hormones they produce, secrete their hormones directly into the bloodstream. **Exocrine glands** send chemical substances (tears, sweat, milk, saliva) via ducts to the outside of the body. Examples of exocrine glands are sweat, mammary, mucous, salivary, and lacrimal (tear) glands.

The ductless, internally secreting **endocrine glands** are listed as follows. Locate these glands on Figure 18–1.

[1] thyroid gland	[6] ovaries in female (one pair)
[2] parathyroid glands (four glands)	[7] testes in male (one pair)
[3] adrenal glands (one pair)	[8] pineal gland
[4] pancreas (islets of Langerhans)	[9] thymus gland
[5] pituitary gland	

The last two glands on this list, the pineal and the thymus glands, are included as endocrine glands because they are ductless, although little is known about their endocrine function in the human body. The **pineal gland,** located in the central portion of the brain, secretes melatonin. **Melatonin** functions to support the body's "biological clock" and is thought to induce sleep. The pineal gland has been linked to a mental condition, seasonal affective disorder (SAD), in which a person suffers depression in winter months. Melatonin secretion increases with deprivation of light and is inhibited by sunlight. Calcification of the pineal gland can occur and can be an important radiological landmark when x-rays of the brain are examined.

The **thymus gland,** located behind the sternum in the mediastinum, resembles a lymph gland in structure. It contains lymphatic tissue and T-cell lymphocytes. The gland produces a hormone, **thymosin,** and is important in the development of immune responses in newborns (it is large in childhood but shrinks in adulthood). Removal of the thymus gland is helpful in treating a muscular-neurological disorder called myasthenia gravis.

Hormones are also secreted by endocrine tissue apart from the major glands. Examples are **erythropoietin** (kidney), **human chorionic gonadotropin** (placenta), and **cholecystokinin** (gallbladder). **Prostaglandins** are hormone-like substances that affect the body in many ways. First found in semen (produced by the prostate gland) but now recognized in cells throughout the body, prostaglandins (1) stimulate the contraction of the uterus; (2) regulate body temperature, platelet aggregation, and acid secretion in the stomach; and (3) have the ability to lower blood pressure.

Endocrine tissue (apart from the major glands) is reviewed in Table 18–1. Use it as a reference.

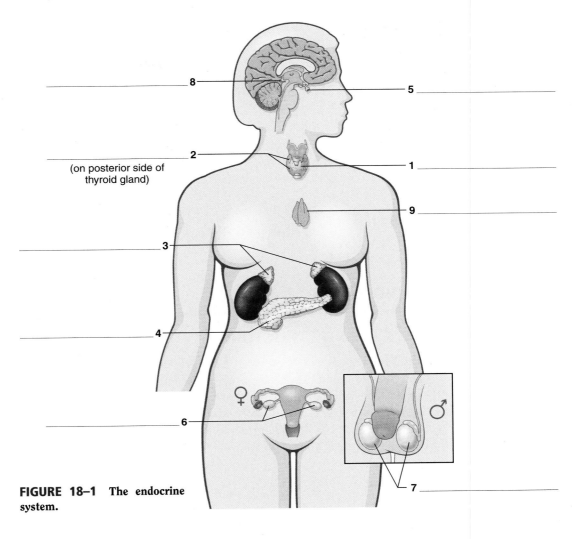

FIGURE 18–1 The endocrine system.

(on posterior side of thyroid gland)

Table 18–1

Endocrine Tissue (Apart from Major Glands): Location, Secretion, and Action

Location	Secretion	Action
Body cells	Prostaglandins	Aggregation of platelets Contract uterus Lower acid secretion in stomach Lower blood pressure
Gastrointestinal tract	Cholecystokinin Gastrin Secretin	Contracts gallbladder Stimulates gastric secretion Stimulates pancreatic enzymes
Kidney	Erythropoietin	Stimulates erythrocyte production
Pineal gland	Melatonin	Induces sleep and affects mood
Placenta	human chorionic gonadotropin	Sustains pregnancy
Skin	Vitamin D	Affects absorption of calcium
Thymus gland	Thymosin	Affects immune response

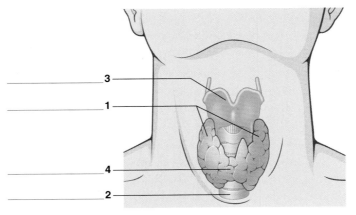

FIGURE 18–2 **The thyroid gland,** anterior view.

THYROID GLAND

LOCATION AND STRUCTURE

Label Figure 18–2.

The **thyroid gland** [1] is composed of a right and a left lobe on either side of the **trachea** [2], just below a large piece of cartilage called the **thyroid cartilage** [3]. The thyroid cartilage covers the larynx and produces the prominence on the neck known as the "Adam's apple." The **isthmus** [4] of the thyroid gland is a narrow strip of glandular tissue that connects the two lobes on the ventral (anterior) surface of the trachea.

FUNCTION

Two of the hormones secreted by the thyroid gland are **thyroxine** or **tetraiodothyronine (T_4)** and **triiodothyronine (T_3).** These hormones are synthesized in the thyroid gland from **iodine,** which is picked up from the blood circulating through the gland, and from an amino acid called tyrosine. T_4 (containing four atoms of iodine) is much more concentrated in the blood, whereas T_3 (containing three atoms of iodine) is far more potent in affecting the metabolism of cells. Most thyroid hormone is bound to protein molecules as it travels in the bloodstream.

T_4 and T_3 are necessary in the body to maintain a normal level of metabolism in all body cells. Cells need oxygen to carry on metabolic processes, one aspect of which is burning food to release the energy stored within it. Thyroid hormone aids cells in their uptake of oxygen and thus supports the metabolic rate in the body. Injections of thyroid hormone raise the metabolic rate, whereas removal of the thyroid gland, diminishing thyroid hormone content in the body, results in a lower metabolic rate, heat loss, and poor physical and mental development.

A more recently discovered hormone produced by the thyroid gland is **calcitonin.** Calcitonin is secreted when calcium levels in the blood are high. It stimulates calcium to leave the blood and enter the bones, thus lowering blood calcium back to normal. Calcitonin contained in a nasal spray may be used for treatment of osteoporosis (loss of bone density). By increasing calcium storage in bone, calcitonin strengthens weakened bone tissue and prevents spontaneous bone fractures. Figure 18–3 summarizes the hormones secreted by the thyroid gland.

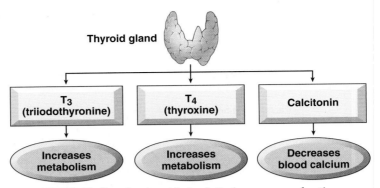

FIGURE 18–3   The thyroid gland: its hormones and actions.

PARATHYROID GLANDS

LOCATION AND STRUCTURE

Label Figure 18–4.

The **parathyroid glands** [1] are four small, oval bodies located on the dorsal aspect of the **thyroid gland** [2].

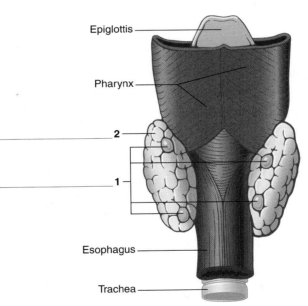

FIGURE 18–4   **The parathyroid glands,** posterior view.

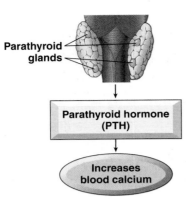

Parathyroid glands

Parathyroid hormone (PTH)

Increases blood calcium

FIGURE 18–5 The parathyroid glands: their hormone and action.

FUNCTION

Parathyroid hormone (PTH) is secreted by the parathyroid glands. This hormone (also known as **parathormone**) mobilizes **calcium** (a mineral substance) from bones into the bloodstream, where calcium is necessary for proper functioning of body tissues, especially muscles. Normally, calcium in the food we eat is absorbed from the intestine and carried by the blood to the bones, where it is stored. The adjustment of the level of calcium in the blood is a good example of the way hormones in general control the **homeostasis** (equilibrium or constancy in the internal environment) of the body. If blood calcium decreases (as in pregnancy or in vitamin D deficiency), parathyroid hormone secretion increases, causing calcium to leave bones and enter the bloodstream. Thus blood calcium levels are brought back to normal (Fig. 18–5).

ADRENAL GLANDS

LOCATION AND STRUCTURE

Label Figure 18–6.

The **adrenal glands** are two small glands, one on top of each **kidney** [1]. Each gland consists of two parts: an outer portion, the **adrenal cortex** [2], and an inner portion, the **adrenal medulla** [3]. The adrenal cortex and adrenal medulla are two glands in one, secreting different hormones. The adrenal cortex secretes **steroids** or **corticosteroids** (complex chemicals derived from cholesterol), while the adrenal medulla secretes **catecholamines** (chemicals derived from amino acids).

FUNCTION

The adrenal cortex secretes three types of corticosteroids.

1. **Glucocorticoids**—These steroid hormones have an important influence on the metabolism of sugars, fats, and proteins within all body cells and have a powerful anti-inflammatory effect.

    Cortisol helps regulate glucose, fat, and protein metabolism. It raises blood glucose as part of a response to stress. **Cortisone** is a hormone very similar to cortisol and can be prepared synthetically. Cortisone is useful in treating inflammatory conditions such as rheumatoid arthritis.

2. **Mineralocorticoids**—The major mineralocorticoid is **aldosterone**. It regulates the concentration of mineral **salts (electrolytes)** in the body. Aldosterone acts on the kidney to reabsorb **sodium** (an important **electrolyte**) and water and to excrete

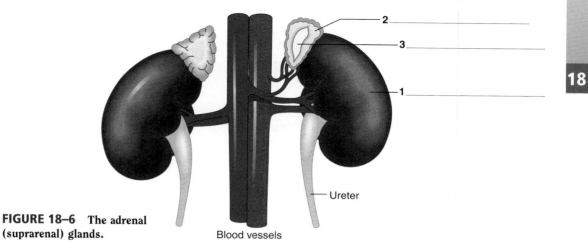

FIGURE 18–6 The adrenal (suprarenal) glands.

potassium (another major **electrolyte**). Thus, it regulates blood volume and pressure and electrolyte concentration.

3. **Sex hormones—Androgens** (testosterone) and **estrogens** are secreted in small amounts and influence sex characteristics, such as pubic and axillary hair in boys and girls. In females, the masculinizing effects of adrenal androgens (increased body hair), may appear when levels of ovarian estrogen decrease after menopause.

Remember the three S's: hormones from the adrenal cortex influence sugar (cortisol), salt (aldosterone), and sex (androgens and estrogens)!

The **adrenal medulla** secretes two types of **catecholamine** hormones:

1. **Epinephrine (adrenaline)**—Increases heart rate and blood pressure, dilates bronchial tubes, and releases glucose (sugars) from glycogen (storage substance) when the body needs it for more energy.
2. **Norepinephrine (noradrenaline)**—Constricts blood vessels to raise blood pressure.

Both epinephrine and norepinephrine are **sympathomimetic** agents because they mimic, or copy, the actions of the sympathetic nervous system. They are released to help the body meet the challenges of stress in response to stimulation by the sympathetic nervous system.

Figure 18–7 summarizes the hormones that are secreted by the adrenal glands and their actions.

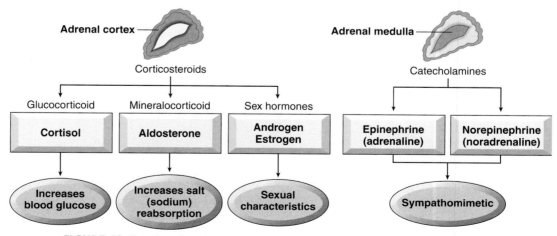

FIGURE 18–7 The adrenal cortex and adrenal medulla: their hormones and actions.

18

PANCREAS

LOCATION AND STRUCTURE

Label Figure 18–8.

The **pancreas** [1] is located near and partly behind the **stomach** [2] in the region of the first and second lumbar vertebrae. The endocrine tissue of the pancreas consists of specialized hormone-producing cells called the **islets of Langerhans** [3]. More than 98 percent of the pancreas consists of exocrine cells (glands and ducts). These cells secrete digestive enzymes into the gastrointestinal tract.

FUNCTION

The islets of Langerhans produce **insulin** (produced by beta cells) and **glucagon** (produced by alpha cells). Both play a role regulating blood **glucose** (sugar) levels. When blood glucose rises, insulin, released from beta cells, lowers blood glucose by promoting its entrance into body cells and use as fuel for energy. Also, insulin lowers blood sugar by causing conversion of **glucose** to **glycogen** (a starch-storage form of sugar) in the liver. When blood glucose levels fall, glucagon acts on liver cells to promote conversion of glycogen back to glucose, so that blood sugar rises.

Figure 18–9 reviews the secretions of the islet cells and their actions.

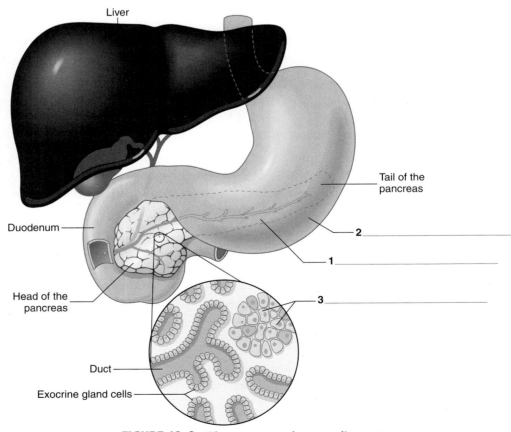

FIGURE 18–8 The pancreas and surrounding organs.

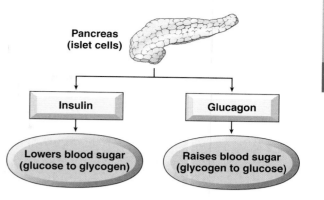

FIGURE 18–9 The pancreas (islets of Langerhans): its hormones and actions. Insulin is the only hormone that lowers blood sugar levels.

PITUITARY GLAND

LOCATION AND STRUCTURE

Label Figure 18–10.

The **pituitary gland,** also called the **hypophysis,** is a small, pea-sized gland located at the base of the brain in a small, pocket-like depression of the skull called the **sella turcica.** It is a well-protected gland, with the entire mass of the brain above it and the nasal cavity below. The ancient Greeks incorrectly imagined that its function was to produce *pituita* or nasal secretion.

The pituitary consists of two distinct parts: an **anterior lobe** or **adenohypophysis** [1], composed of glandular epithelial tissue, and a **posterior lobe** or **neurohypophysis** [2], composed of nervous tissue. The **hypothalamus** [3] is a region of the brain under the thalamus and above the pituitary gland. Signals transmitted from the hypothalamus control secretions by the pituitary gland. Special secretory neurons in the hypothalamus send releasing and inhibiting factors (hormones) via capillaries to the anterior pituitary gland.

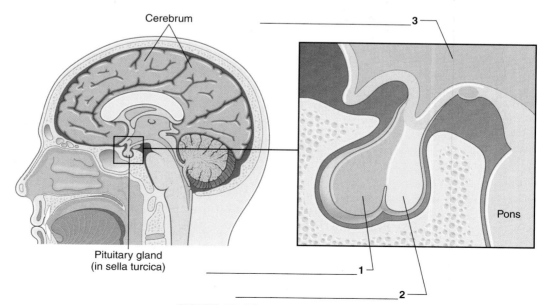

FIGURE 18–10 The pituitary gland.

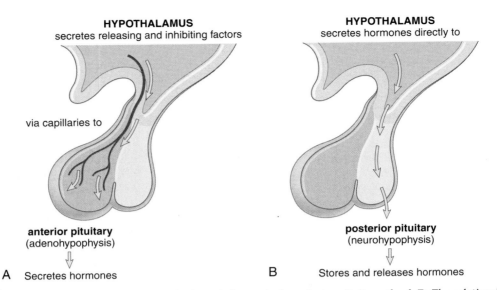

HYPOTHALAMUS
secretes releasing and inhibiting factors

HYPOTHALAMUS
secretes hormones directly to

via capillaries to

anterior pituitary
(adenohypophysis)

posterior pituitary
(neurohypophysis)

A   Secretes hormones

B   Stores and releases hormones

FIGURE 18–11   A, The relationship of the hypothalamus to the anterior pituitary gland. **B,** The relationship of the hypothalamus to the posterior pituitary gland.

These factors stimulate or inhibit secretion of hormones from the anterior pituitary (Fig. 18–11, *A*). The hypothalamus also produces and secretes hormones directly to the posterior pituitary gland, where the hormones are stored and then released (see Fig. 18–11, *B*).

FUNCTION

The major hormones of the **anterior pituitary gland** are:

1. **Growth hormone (GH)** or **somatotropin (STH)**—Promotes protein synthesis that results in the growth of bones, muscles, and other tissues. GH also stimulates the liver to make insulin-like growth factor, which stimulates the growth of bones. It increases blood glucose levels and is secreted during exercise, sleep, and hypoglycemia.
2. **Thyroid-stimulating hormone (TSH; thyrotropin)**—Stimulates the growth of the thyroid gland and secretion of thyroxine (T_4) and triiodothyronine (T_3).
3. **Adrenocorticotropic hormone (ACTH; adrenocorticotropin)**—Stimulates the growth of the adrenal cortex and increases its secretion of steroid hormones (primarily cortisol).
4. **Gonadotropic hormones**—Several gonadotropic hormones influence the growth and hormone secretion of the ovaries in females and the testes in males. In the female, **follicle-stimulating hormone (FSH)** and **luteinizing hormone (LH)** stimulate the growth of eggs in the ovaries, the production of hormones, and ovulation.

    In the male, FSH influences the production of sperm, and LH (as interstitial cell–stimulating hormone) stimulates the testes to produce testosterone.
5. **Prolactin (PRL)**—Stimulates breast development during pregnancy and sustains milk production after birth.

The **posterior pituitary gland** stores and releases two important hormones that are synthesized in the hypothalamus:

1. **Antidiuretic hormone (ADH),** also called **vasopressin**—Stimulates the reabsorption of water by the kidney tubules. In addition, ADH also increases blood pressure by constricting arterioles.

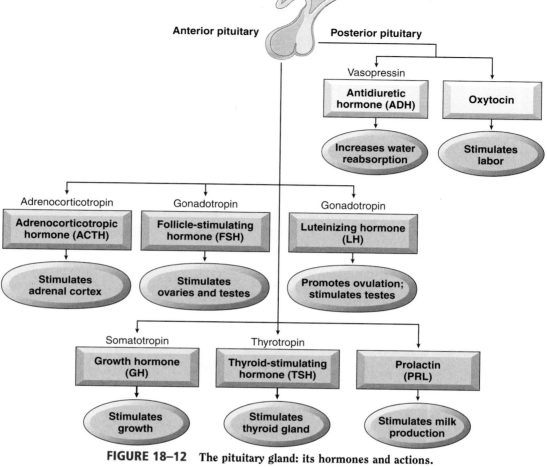

FIGURE 18–12   **The pituitary gland: its hormones and actions.**

2. **Oxytocin (OT)**—Stimulates the uterus to contract during childbirth and maintains labor during childbirth. Oxytocin is also secreted during suckling and causes the production of milk from the mammary glands.

Figure 18–12 reviews hormones secreted by the pituitary gland and their functions.

OVARIES

LOCATION AND STRUCTURE

The **ovaries** are two small glands located in the lower abdominal region of the female. The ovaries produce the female gamete, the ovum, as well as hormones that are responsible for female sex characteristics and regulation of the menstrual cycle.

FUNCTION

The ovarian hormones are **estrogens** (**estradiol** and estrone) and **progesterone.** Estrogens stimulate development of ova (eggs) and development of female secondary sex characteristics. Progesterone is responsible for the preparation and maintenance of the uterus in pregnancy.

TESTES

LOCATION AND STRUCTURE

The **testes** are two small, ovoid glands suspended from the inguinal region of the male by the spermatic cord and surrounded by the scrotal sac. The testes produce the male gametes, spermatozoa, as well as the male hormone called **testosterone.**

Table 18–2

Major Endocrine Glands, the Hormones They Produce, and Their Actions

Endocrine Gland	Hormone	Action
Thyroid	• Thyroxine (T_4); triiodothyronine (T_3)	Increases metabolism in body cells
	• Calcitonin	Lowers blood calcium
Parathyroids	• Parathyroid hormone	Increases blood calcium
Adrenals		
Cortex	• Cortisol (glucocorticoid)	Increases blood sugar
	• Aldosterone (mineralocorticoid)	Increases reabsorption of sodium
	• Androgens, estrogens (sex hormones)	Secondary sex characteristics
Medulla	• Epinephrine (adrenaline)	Sympathomimetic
	• Norepinephrine (noradrenaline)	Sympathomimetic
Pancreas		
Islet cells	• Insulin	Decreases blood sugar (glucose to glycogen)
	• Glucagon	Increases blood sugar (glycogen to glucose)
Pituitary		
Anterior lobe	• Growth hormone (GH; somatotropin)	Increases bone and tissue growth
	• Thyroid-stimulating hormone (TSH)	Stimulates thyroid gland and thyroxine secretion
	• Adrenocorticotropic hormone (ACTH)	Stimulates adrenal cortex, especially cortisol secretion
	• Gonadotropins	
	Follicle-stimulating hormone (FSH)	Oogenesis and spermatogenesis
	Luteinizing hormone (LH)	Promotes ovulation; testosterone secretion
	• Prolactin (PRL)	Promotes growth of breast tissue and milk secretion
Posterior lobe	• Antidiuretic hormone (ADH; vasopressin)	Stimulates reabsorption of water by kidney tubules
	• Oxytocin	Stimulates contraction of the uterus during labor and childbirth
Ovaries	• Estrogens	Promote development of ova and female secondary sex characteristics
	• Progesterone	Prepares and maintains the uterus in pregnancy
Testes	• Testosterone	Promotes development of sperm and male secondary sex characteristics

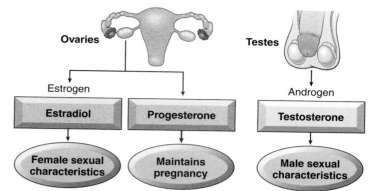

FIGURE 18–13 The ovaries and testes: their hormones and actions.

FUNCTION

Testosterone is an **androgen** (male steroid hormone) that stimulates development of sperm and secondary sex characteristics in the male (development of beard and pubic hair, deepening of voice, and distribution of fat).

Figure 18–13 reviews the hormones secreted by the ovaries and testes.

Table 18–2 lists the major endocrine glands, their hormones, and the actions they produce.

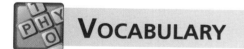 ## VOCABULARY

This list reviews many new terms introduced in the text. Short definitions reinforce your understanding of the terms. Refer to the Pronunciation of Terms section for help with unfamiliar or difficult words.

MAJOR ENDOCRINE GLANDS	
adrenal cortex	Outer section (cortex) of each adrenal gland; secretes cortisol, aldosterone, and sex hormones.
adrenal medulla	Inner section (medulla) of each adrenal gland; secretes epinephrine and norepinephrine
ovaries	Located in the lower abdomen of a female; responsible for egg production and estrogen and progesterone secretion.
pancreas	Located behind the stomach. Islet (alpha and beta) cells (islets of Langerhans) secrete hormones from the pancreas. The pancreas also contains cells that are exocrine in function. They secrete enzymes, via a duct into the small intestine to aid digestion.
parathyroid glands	Four small glands on the posterior of the thyroid gland. Some patients may have 3 or 5 parathyroid glands.
pituitary gland (hypophysis)	Located at the base of the brain in the sella turcica; composed of an anterior lobe **(adenohypophysis)** and a posterior lobe **(neurohypophysis).** It weighs only 1/16th of an ounce and is a half inch across.
testes	Two glands enclosed in the scrotal sac of a male; responsible for sperm production and testosterone secretion.
thyroid gland	Located in the neck on either side of the trachea; secretes thyroxine.

18

HORMONES

adrenaline (epinephrine)	Secreted by the adrenal medulla; increases heart rate and blood pressure.
adrenocorticotropic hormone (ACTH)	Secreted by the anterior lobe of the pituitary gland (adenohypophysis); also called **adrenocorticotropin**. ACTH stimulates the adrenal cortex.
aldosterone	Secreted by the adrenal cortex; increases salt (sodium) reabsorption.
androgen	Male hormone secreted by the testes and to a lesser extent by the adrenal cortex; testosterone is an example.
antidiuretic hormone (ADH)	Secreted by the posterior lobe of the pituitary gland (neurohypophysis). ADH **(vasopressin)** increases reabsorption of water by the kidney.
calcitonin	Secreted by the thyroid gland; decreases blood calcium levels.
cortisol	Secreted by the adrenal cortex; increases blood sugar. It is secreted in times of stress and has an anti-inflammatory effect.
epinephrine (adrenaline)	Secreted by the adrenal medulla; increases heart rate and blood pressure and dilates airways (sympathomimetic). It is part of the body's "fight or flight" reaction.
estradiol	Estrogen (female hormone) secreted by the ovaries.
estrogen	Female hormone secreted by the ovaries and to a lesser extent by the adrenal cortex. Examples are estradiol and estrone.
follicle-stimulating hormone (FSH)	Secreted by the anterior lobe of the pituitary gland (adenohypophysis). FSH stimulates hormone secretion and egg production by the ovaries and sperm production by the testes.
glucagon	Secreted by alpha islet cells of the pancreas; increases blood sugar by conversion of glycogen (starch) to glucose.
growth hormone (GH); somatotropin	Secreted by the anterior lobe of the pituitary gland (adenohypophysis); stimulates growth of bones and soft tissues.
insulin	Secreted by beta islet cells (Latin *insula* means island) of the pancreas. Insulin lowers blood sugar by transport and conversion of glucose to glycogen (starch).
luteinizing hormone (LH)	Secreted by the anterior lobe of the pituitary gland (adenohypophysis); stimulates ovulation in females and testosterone secretion in males.
norepinephrine	Secreted by the adrenal medulla; increases heart rate and blood pressure (sympathomimetic). Nor- in chemistry means a parent compound from which another is derived.
oxytocin (OT)	Secreted by the posterior lobe of the pituitary gland (neurohypophysis); stimulates contraction of the uterus during labor and childbirth.
parathormone (PTH)	Secreted by the parathyroid glands; increases blood calcium.
progesterone	Secreted by the ovaries; prepares the uterus for pregnancy.
prolactin (PRL)	Secreted by the anterior lobe of the pituitary gland (adenohypophysis); promotes milk secretion.
somatotropin (STH)	Secreted by the anterior lobe of the pituitary gland (adenohypophysis); **growth hormone.**
testosterone	Male hormone secreted by the testes.

thyroid-stimulating hormone (TSH); thyrotropin	Secreted by the anterior lobe of the pituitary gland (adenohypophysis). TSH acts on the thyroid gland to promote its functioning. Note: TSH is not secreted by the thyroid gland.
thyroxine (T_4)	Secreted by the thyroid gland; also called **tetraiodothyronine.** T_4 increases metabolism in cells.
triiodothyronine (T_3)	Secreted by the thyroid gland; T_3 increases metabolism in cells.
vasopressin	Secreted by the posterior lobe of the pituitary gland (neurohypophysis); **antidiuretic hormone** (ADH).

RELATED TERMS

catecholamines	Hormones derived from an amino acid and secreted by the adrenal medulla. Epinephrine is a catecholamine.
corticosteroids	Hormones (steroids) produced by the adrenal cortex. Examples are cortisol (raises sugar levels), aldosterone (raises salt reabsorption by kidneys), and androgens and estrogens (sex hormones).
electrolyte	Mineral salt found in the blood and tissues and necessary for proper functioning of cells; potassium, sodium, and calcium are electrolytes.
glucocorticoid	Steroid hormone secreted by the adrenal cortex; regulates glucose, fat, and protein metabolism. Cortisol raises blood sugar and is part of the stress response.
homeostasis	Tendency of an organism to maintain a constant internal environment.
hormone	Substance, secreted by an endocrine gland, that travels through the blood to a distant organ or gland where it influences the structure or function of that organ or gland.
hypothalamus	Region of the brain lying below the thalamus and above the pituitary gland. It secretes releasing factors and hormones that affect the pituitary gland.
mineralocorticoid	Steroid hormone secreted by the adrenal cortex to regulate mineral salts (electrolytes) and water balance in the body. Aldosterone is an example.
receptor	Cellular or nuclear protein that binds to a hormone so that a response can be elicited.
sella turcica	Cavity in the skull that contains the pituitary gland.
sex hormones	Steroids (androgens and estrogens) produced by the adrenal cortex to influence male and female sexual characteristics.
steroid	Complex substance related to fats (derived from a sterol, such as cholesterol), and of which many hormones are made. Examples of steroids are estrogens, androgens, glucocorticoids, and mineralocorticoids. **Ster/o** means solid; **-ol** means oil.
sympathomimetic	Pertaining to mimicking or copying the effect of the sympathetic nervous system. Adrenaline is a sympathomimetic hormone (it raises blood pressure and heart rate and dilates airways).
target tissue	Cells of an organ that are affected or stimulated by specific hormones.

COMBINING FORMS, SUFFIXES, PREFIXES, AND TERMINOLOGY: GLANDS AND RELATED TERMS

Write the meanings of the medical terms in the spaces provided.

GLANDS

COMBINING FORMS

Combining Form	Meaning	Terminology	Meaning
aden/o	gland	adenectomy _____	
adren/o	adrenal glands	adrenopathy _____	
adrenal/o	adrenal glands	adrenalectomy _____	
gonad/o	sex glands (ovaries and testes)	gonadotropin _____ *Here, -tropin means to act on. Gonadotropins act on (stimulate) gonads. Examples are FSH and LH, secreted by the pituitary gland.*	
		hypogonadism _____ *Deficiency of gonadotropins can produce hypogonadism.*	
pancreat/o	pancreas	pancreatectomy _____	
parathyroid/o	parathyroid gland	parathyroidectomy _____	
pituitar/o	pituitary gland, hypophysis	hypopituitarism _____ *Pituitary dwarfism (see page 747) is caused by hypopituitarism*	
thyr/o	thyroid gland	thyrotropin hormone _____ *Thyroid-stimulating hormone (TSH) is secreted by the pituitary gland.*	
thyroid/o	thyroid gland	thyroiditis _____ *May result from bacterial or viral infection, or an autoimmune reaction. Symptoms are throat pain, swelling, tenderness, and signs of hyperthyroidism. The condition may progress to destruction of the thyroid gland and hypothyroidism. In **Hashimoto disease** or autoimmune thyroiditis, antibodies trigger lymphocytes to destroy follicular cells in the thyroid gland, producing hypothyroidism.*	

RELATED TERMS

COMBINING FORMS

Combining Form	Meaning	Terminology	Meaning	
andr/o	male	androgen _____		
		Androgens are produced by the testes in males and by the adrenal cortex in males and females.		
calc/o, calci/o	calcium	hypercalcemia _____		
		hypocalcemia _____		
		hypercalciuria _____		
cortic/o	cortex, outer region	corticosteroid _____		
crin/o	secrete	endocrinologist _____		
dips/o	third	polydipsia _____		
		Symptom associated with both diabetes mellitus and diabetes insipidus (see page 744).		
estr/o	female	estrogenic _____		
gluc/o	sugar	glucagon _____		
		In this term, -agon means to assemble or gather together. Glucagon raises blood sugar by stimulating its release from glycogen into the bloodstream.		
glyc/o	sugar	hyperglycemia _____		
		glycemic _____		
		A patient with diabetes mellitus requires glycemic control.		
		glycogen _____		
		Glycogen is animal starch that can be converted to glucose by the liver. Glucagon promotes glycogenolysis.		
home/o	sameness	homeostasis _____		
		The suffix -stasis means to control.		
hormon/o	hormone	hormonal _____		
kal/i	potassium (an electrolyte)	hypokalemia _____		
		This condition can occur in dehydration and with excessive vomiting and diarrhea. The heart is particularly sensitive to potassium loss.		
lact/o	milk	prolactin _____		
		The suffix -in means a substance.		

18

18

Combining Form	Meaning	Terminology	Meaning
myx/o	mucus	myxedema *Mucus-like material accumulates under the skin. See page 741.*	
natr/o	sodium (an electrolyte)	hyponatremia *Occurs with hyposecretion of the adrenal cortex as salts and water leave the body.*	
phys/o	growing	hypophysectomy *The hypophysis is the pituitary gland, which is so named because it grows from the undersurface (hypo-) of the brain. See Figure 18–14.*	
somat/o	body	somatotropin *Growth hormone.*	
ster/o	solid structure	steroid *This complex, solid, ring-shaped molecule resembles a sterol (such as cholesterol); many hormones (androgens, estrogens, glucocorticoids, and mineralocorticoids) are steroids.*	
toc/o	childbirth	oxytocin *Oxy- means swift, rapid.*	
toxic/o	position	thyrotoxicosis *Condition caused by excessive thyroid gland activity and oversecretion of thyroid hormone. Symptoms are sweating, weight loss, tachycardia, and nervousness.*	
ur/o	urine	antidiuretic hormone *Posterior pituitary hormone that affects the kidneys and reduces water loss.*	

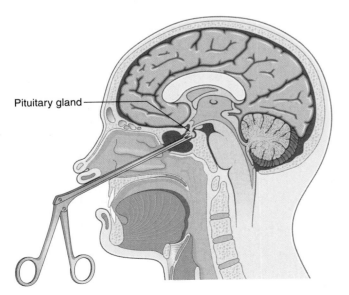

Pituitary gland

FIGURE 18–14 Hypophysectomy. Abnormal pituitary gland tissue is removed through the nasal passages and sphenoid bone (transsphenoidal hypophysectomy). The gland is removed to slow the growth of endocrine-dependent malignant tumors or to excise a pituitary tumor. Other treatments to destroy pituitary tissue include radiation therapy, radioactive implants, and cryosurgery.

18

SUFFIXES

Suffix	Meaning	Terminology	Meaning
-agon	assemble, gather together	glucagon _____	
-emia	blood condition	hypoglycemia _____	
-in, -ine	a substance	epinephrine _____	
-tropin	stimulating the function of (to turn or act on)	adrenocorticotropin _____ _The ending -tropic is the adjective form (adrenocorticotropic hormone)._	
-uria	urine condition	glycosuria _____ _Sign of diabetes mellitus._	

PREFIXES

Prefix	Meaning	Terminology	Meaning
eu-	good, normal	euthyroid _____	
hyper-	excessive; above	hyperkalemia _____ _Seen in acute renal failure, massive trauma, and major burns._	
hypo-	deficient; below; under; less than normal	hypoinsulinism _____	
oxy-	rapid, sharp, acid	oxytocin _____	
pan-	all	panhypopituitarism _____	
tetra-	four	tetraiodothyronine _____ _Iod/o means iodine._	
tri-	three	triiodothyronine _____	

ABNORMAL CONDITIONS

THYROID GLAND

Enlargement of the thyroid gland is **goiter** (Fig. 18–15, *A*). **Endemic** (**en-** means in; **dem/o** means people) **goiter** occurs in certain regions and peoples where there is a lack of **iodine** in the diet. Goiter occurs when low iodine levels lead to low T_3 and T_4 levels. This causes feedback to the hypothalamus and adenohypophysis, stimulating them to secrete releasing factors and TSH. TSH then promotes the thyroid gland to secrete T_3 and T_4, but because there is no iodine available, the only effect is to increase the size of the gland (goiter). Prevention includes increasing the supply of iodine (as iodized salt) in the diet.

Another type of goiter is **nodular** or **adenomatous goiter,** in which hyperplasia occurs as well as nodules and adenomas. Some patients with nodular goiter develop hyperthyroidism and symptoms such as rapid pulse, tremors, nervousness, and excessive sweating. Treatment is thyroid-blocking drugs or radioactive iodine to suppress thyroid functioning.

Hypersecretion

hyperthyroidism

Overactivity of the thyroid gland; thyrotoxicosis.

The most common form of this condition is **Graves disease** (resulting from autoimmune processes). Because metabolism is faster; the condition is marked by an increase in heart rate (with irregular beats), higher body temperature, hyperactivity, weight loss, and increased peristalsis (diarrhea occurs). In addition, **exophthalmos** (protrusion of the eyeballs or **proptosis**) occurs as a result of swelling of tissue behind the eyeball, pushing it forward. Treatment of Graves disease includes management with antithyroid drugs to reduce the amount of thyroid hormone produced by the gland and administration of radioactive iodine, which destroys the overactive glandular tissue. Figure 18–15, *B*, shows a patient with Graves disease.

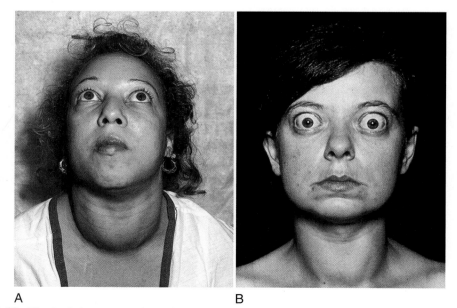

A   B

FIGURE 18–15 **A, Goiter.** Notice the wide neck, indicating enlargement of the thyroid gland. Goiter comes from the Latin *guttur*, meaning throat. **B, Exophthalmos** in Graves disease. Note the staring or startled expression as a result of periorbital edema (swelling of tissue around the eyeball or orbit of the eye). (**A** from Jarvis C: Physical Examination and Health Assessment, 3rd ed. Philadelphia, WB Saunders, 2000, p. 294. **B** from Seidel H, et al: Mosby's Guide to Physical Examination, 4th ed. St. Louis, Mosby, 1998, p. 264.)

Hyposecretion

hypothyroidism

Underactivity of the thyroid gland.

Any one of several conditions can produce hypothyroidism (thyroidectomy, thyroiditis, endemic goiter, destruction of the gland by irradiation), but all have similar physiological effects. These include fatigue, muscular and mental sluggishness, weight gain, fluid retention, slow heart rate, low body temperature, and constipation. Two examples of hypothyroidism are:

Myxedema—This is advanced hypothyroidism in adulthood. Atrophy of the thyroid gland occurs, and practically no hormone is produced. The skin becomes dry and puffy (edema) because of the collection of mucus-like (myx/o means mucus) material under the skin. Many patients also develop atherosclerosis because lack of thyroid hormone increases the quantity of blood lipids (fats). Recovery may be complete if thyroid hormone is given soon after symptoms appear. Figure 18–16, *A*, shows a patient with myxedema.

Cretinism—Extreme hypothyroidism during infancy and childhood leads to a lack of normal physical and mental growth. Skeletal growth is more inhibited than soft tissue growth, so the affected person has the appearance of an obese, short, and stocky child. Treatment consists of administration of thyroid hormone, which may be able to reverse some of the hypothyroid effects.

Neoplasms

thyroid carcinoma

Cancer of the thyroid gland.

More than half of thyroid malignancies are slow-growing papillary carcinomas and about one third are slow-growing follicular carcinomas. Others include rapidly growing anaplastic (widely metastatic) tumors. Radioactive iodine scans distinguish hyperfunctioning areas from hypofunctioning areas. "Hot" tumor areas (those collecting more radioactivity than surrounding tissues) usually indicate hyperthyroidism and benign growth; "cold," nonfunctional nodules can be either benign or malignant. Ultimately, fine-needle aspiration, surgical biopsy, or excision is required to make the diagnosis. Total or subtotal thyroidectomy with lymph node removal is required for most thyroid carcinomas. Postsurgical treatment with radioactive iodine destroys remaining tissue, and high doses of exogenous thyroid hormone are given to suppress TSH, in an effort to cause regression of residual tumor dependent on TSH.

PARATHYROID GLANDS

Hypersecretion

hyperparathyroidism

Excessive production of parathormone.

Hypercalcemia occurs as calcium leaves the bones and enters the bloodstream, where it can produce damage to the kidneys and heart. Bones become decalcified with generalized loss of bone density (osteoporosis) and susceptibility to fractures and cysts. Kidney stones can occur as a result of hypercalcemia and hypercalciuria. The cause is parathyroid hyperplasia or a parathyroid tumor. Treatment is resection of the overactive tissue. Medical therapy is another option for a patient who is not a surgical candidate. Drugs (bisphosphonates such as Fosamax) decrease bone turnover and decrease hypercalcemia.

Hyposecretion

hypoparathyroidism

Deficient production of parathyroid hormone.

Hypocalcemia results as calcium remains in bones and is unable to enter the bloodstream. This leads to muscle and nerve weakness with spasms of muscles, a condition called **tetany** (constant muscle contraction). Administration of calcium plus large quantities of vitamin D (to promote absorption of calcium) can control the calcium level in the bloodstream.

ADRENAL CORTEX

Hypersecretion

adrenal virilism

Excessive secretion of adrenal androgens.

Adrenal hyperplasia or more commonly adrenal adenomas or carcinomas can cause **virilization** in adult women. Signs and symptoms include amenorrhea, **hirsutism** (excessive hair on the face and body), acne, and deepening of the voice. Drug therapy to suppress androgen production and adrenalectomy are possible treatments.

Cushing syndrome

Group of symptoms produced by excess cortisol from the adrenal cortex.

A number of signs and symptoms occur as a result of increased cortisol secretion, including obesity, moon-like fullness of the face, excess deposition of fat in the thoracic region of the back (so-called buffalo hump), hyperglycemia, hypernatremia, hypokalemia, osteoporosis, virilization, and hypertension. The cause may be excess ACTH secretion or tumor of the adrenal cortex. Tumors and disseminated cancers can be associated with ectopic secretion of hormone, such as ectopic ACTH produced by nonendocrine neoplasms (lung and thyroid tumors). Figure 18–16, *B*, shows a woman with Cushing syndrome.

In clinical practice, most cases of Cushing syndrome result from prolonged administration of steroids (young athletes seeking to improve their performance or patients treated for autoimmune disorders, asthma, kidney, and skin conditions). Steroids are never discontinued abruptly because the adrenal cortex and pituitary gland (the ACTH producers) need time to "restart" after long periods of prescribed cortisol use (adrenal gland stops producing cortisol when cortisol is given as therapy).

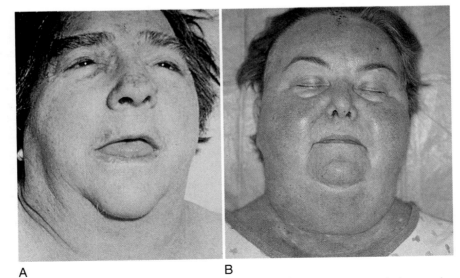

A   B

FIGURE 18–16   A, Myxedema. Note the dull, puffy, yellowed skin; course, sparse hair; prominent tongue. **B, Cushing syndrome.** Elevated plasma levels of cortisol (steroids) produce obesity, rounded facial appearance (moon-face), thin skin that bruises easily, and muscle weakness. (**A** courtesy of Paul W Ladenson, MD, The Johns Hopkins University and Hospital, Baltimore, MD. **A** and **B** from Seidel HM, et al: Mosby's Guide to Physical Examination, 5th ed. St. Louis, Mosby, 2003, p. 270.)

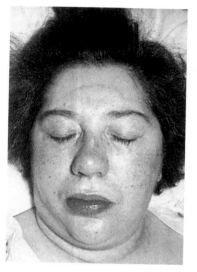

FIGURE 18–17   **Addison disease.** Notice the bronze colorization of the facial features. (From Moll JMH: Rheumatology, 2nd ed. London, Churchill Livingstone, 1997.)

Hyposecretion

Addison disease

Hypofunctioning of the adrenal cortex.

The adrenal cortex is essential to life. When aldosterone and cortisol blood levels are low a patient experiences generalized malaise, weakness, muscle atrophy, severe loss of fluids and electrolytes (with hypoglycemia, low blood pressure, and hypoglycemia). An insufficient supply of cortisol signals the pituitary to secrete more ACTH, which increases coloration of scars, skin folds, and breast nipples (hyperpigmentation). See Figure 18–17.

Primary insufficiency is believed to be due to autoimmune adrenalitis. Treatment consists of daily cortisone administration and intake of salts or administration of a synthetic form of aldosterone.

ADRENAL MEDULLA

Hypersecretion

pheochromocytoma

Benign tumor of the adrenal medulla (tumor cells stain a dark or dusky [phe/o] color [chrom/o]).

The tumor cells produce excess secretion of epinephrine and norepinephrine. Symptoms are hypertension, palpitations, severe headaches, sweating, flushing of the face, and muscle spasms. Surgery to remove the tumor and administration of antihypertensive drugs are possible treatments.

PANCREAS

Hypersecretion

hyperinsulinism

Excess secretion of insulin causing hypoglycemia.

The cause may be a tumor of the pancreas (benign adenoma or carcinoma) or an overdose of insulin. Hypoglycemia occurs as insulin draws sugar out of the bloodstream. Fainting spells, convulsions, and loss of consciousness are common because a minimal level of blood sugar is necessary for proper mental functioning.

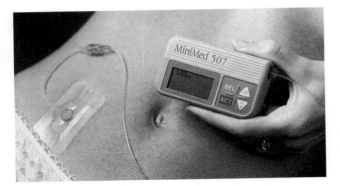

FIGURE 18–18 Insulin pump. It can be programmed to deliver doses of insulin according to varying body needs. (From Mosby's Medical, Nursing, and Allied Health Dictionary, 7th ed. St. Louis, Mosby, 2006, p. 988.)

Hyposecretion

diabetes mellitus (DM)

Lack of insulin secretion or resistance of insulin in promoting sugar, starch, and fat metabolism in cells.

In diabetes mellitus (mellitus means sweet or sugary), insulin insufficiency or ineffectiveness prevents sugar from leaving the blood and entering the body cells, where it is used to produce energy. There are two types of diabetes mellitus.

Type 1 diabetes, with onset usually in childhood, involves destruction of the beta islet cells of the pancreas and complete deficiency of insulin in the body. Patients usually are thin and require frequent injections of insulin to maintain a normal level of glucose in the blood. It is also possible to administer insulin through a portable pump, which infuses the drug continuously through a needle indwelling under the skin (Fig. 18–18).

Type 2 diabetes is a separate disease from type 1 and has a different inheritance pattern. Patients usually are older, and obesity is very common. The islet cells are not initially destroyed, and there is a relative deficiency of insulin secretion with a resistance by target tissues to the action of insulin. **Insulin resistance is the primary defect in type 2 diabetes.** A condition called **metabolic syndrome** is closely associated with insulin resistance and may be present for 5 to 10 years before type 2 is diagnosed. The following are symptoms associated with metabolic syndrome: central abdominal obesity, hypertriglyceridemia, insulin resistance, and high blood pressure. Treatment of type 2 diabetes is diet, weight reduction, exercise, and, if necessary, insulin or oral hypoglycemic agents. Oral hypoglycemic agents stimulate the release of insulin from the pancreas and improve the body's sensitivity to insulin.

Table 18–3

Comparison of Type 1 and Type 2 Diabetes Mellitus

Category	Type 1	Type 2
Clinical features	Usually occurs **before age 30** **Abrupt, rapid onset** **Little or no insulin** production **Thin** or normal body weight at onset **Ketoacidosis often occurs**	Usually occurs **after age 30** **Gradual onset;** asymptomatic **Insulin usually present** 85% are **obese** **Ketoacidosis seldom occurs**
Symptoms	**Polyuria** (glycosuria promotes loss of water) **Polydipsia** (dehydration causes thirst) **Polyphagia** (tissue breakdown causes hunger)	**Polyuria** sometimes seen **Polydipsia** sometimes seen **Polyphagia** sometimes seen
Treatment	**Insulin**	**Diet; oral hypoglycemics or insulin**

Table 18–3 compares the features, signs and symptoms, and treatments of type 1 and type 2 diabetes.

Both type 1 and type 2 diabetes are associated with primary and secondary complications. **Primary complications** of type 1 include **ketoacidosis** (fats are improperly burned, leading to an accumulation of ketones and acids in the body) and coma when blood sugar concentration gets too high or the patient receives an insufficient amount of insulin. **Hypoglycemia** occurs when too much insulin is taken by the patient. **Insulin shock** is severe hypoglycemia caused by an overdose of insulin, decreased intake of food, or excessive exercise. Symptoms are sweating, trembling, nervousness, irritability, and numbness. Treatment requires an immediate dose of glucose orally or parenterally (other than through the gastrointestinal tract). Convulsions, coma, and death can result if the diabetic person is not treated.

Secondary (long-term) **complications** appear many years after the patient develops diabetes. These include eye disorders such as glaucoma and cataract and destruction of the blood vessels of the retina **(diabetic retinopathy),** causing visual loss and blindness; destruction of the kidneys **(diabetic nephropathy),** causing renal insufficiency and often requiring hemodialysis or renal transplantation; destruction of blood vessels, with **atherosclerosis** leading to stroke, heart disease, and peripherovascular ischemia (gangrene, infection, and loss of limbs); and destruction of nerves **(diabetic neuropathy)** involving pain or loss of sensation, most commonly in the extremities. Loss of gastric motility **(gastroparesis)** also occurs. Figure 18–19 reviews the secondary complications of diabetes mellitus.

As a result of hormonal changes during pregnancy, **gestational diabetes** can occur in women with a predisposition to diabetes during the second or third trimester of pregnancy. After delivery, blood glucose usually returns to normal. Type 2 diabetes may develop in these women later in life.

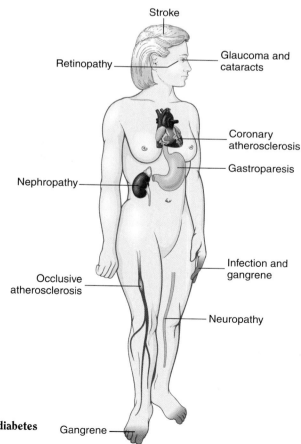

FIGURE 18–19 **Secondary complications of diabetes mellitus.**

PITUITARY GLAND: ANTERIOR LOBE

Hypersecretion

18

acromegaly

Enlargement of the extremities (acr/o means extremities) **caused by hypersecretion of the anterior pituitary after puberty.**

An excess of growth hormone (GH) is produced by adenomas of the pituitary gland that occur during adulthood. This excess GH stimulates the liver to secrete a hormone (somatomedin C, or insulin-like growth factor [IGF]) that causes the

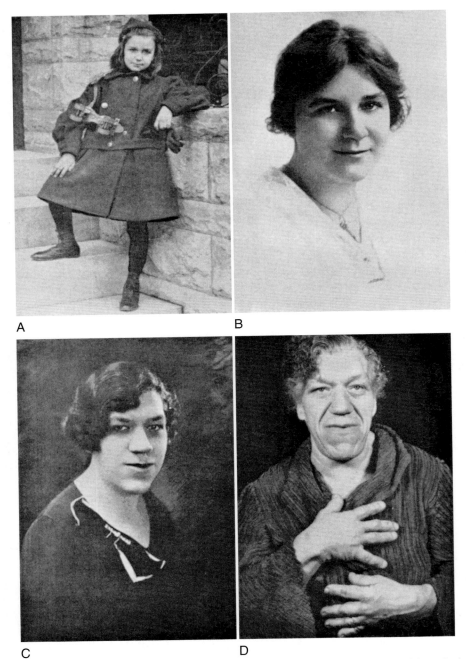

FIGURE 18–20 **Progression of acromegaly: A,** patient at age 9; **B,** age 16, with possible early features of acromegaly; **C,** age 33, well-established acromegaly; **D,** age 52, end-stage acromegaly. (From Clinical Pathological Conference. Am J Med 1956; 20:133.)

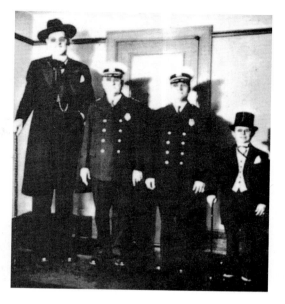

FIGURE 18–21 Gigantism *(far left),* normal individuals *(middle),* and **dwarfism** *(far right).* (From Thibodeau GA, Patton KT: Anatomy & Physiology, 6th ed. St. Louis, Mosby, 2007, p. 607.)

clinical manifestations of acromegaly. Bones in the hands, feet, face, and jaw grow abnormally large, producing a characteristic "Frankenstein"-type facial appearance. The pituitary adenoma can be irradiated or surgically removed. Figure 18–20 shows a woman with acromegaly. Measurement of blood levels of somatomedin C as GH fluctuates is a test for acromegaly.

gigantism

Hypersecretion of growth hormone from anterior lobe of the pituitary gland before puberty, leading to abnormal overgrowth of body tissues.

Benign adenomas of the pituitary gland that occur before a child reaches puberty produce an excess of growth hormone. Gigantism can be corrected by early diagnosis in childhood, followed by resection of the tumor or irradiation of the pituitary. See Figure 18–21.

Hyposecretion

dwarfism

Congenital hyposecretion of growth hormone; hypopituitary dwarfism. (See Figure 18–21).

Children who are affected are normal mentally, but their bones remain small. Treatment consists of administration of growth hormone. Achondroplastic dwarfs differ from hypopituitary dwarfs in that they have a genetic defect in cartilage formation that limits the growth of long bones.

panhypopituitarism

All pituitary hormones are deficient.

Tumors of the sella turcica as well as arterial aneurysms may be etiologic factors, causing a failure of the pituitary to secrete hormones that stimulate major glands in the body.

PITUITARY GLAND: POSTERIOR LOBE

Hypersecretion

syndrome of inappropriate ADH (SIADH)

Excessive secretion of antidiuretic hormone.

Hypersecretion of ADH produces excess water retention in the body. Treatment consists of dietary water restriction. Tumor, drug reactions, and head injury are some of the possible causes.

Abnormal Conditions of Endocrine Glands

Endocrine Gland	Hypersecretion	Hyposecretion
Adrenal cortex	Adrenal virilism Cushing syndrome	Addison disease
Adrenal medulla	Pheochromocytoma	
Pancreas	Hyperinsulinism	Diabetes mellitus
Parathyroid glands	Hyperparathyroidism (osteoporosis, kidney stones)	Hypoparathyroidism (tetany, hypocalcemia)
Pituitary—anterior lobe	Acromegaly Gigantism	Dwarfism Panhypopituitarism
Pituitary—posterior lobe	Syndrome of inappropriate antidiuretic hormone	Diabetes insipidus
Thyroid gland	Exophthalmic goiter (Graves disease, thyrotoxicosis) Nodular (adenomatous) goiter	Cretinism (children) Endemic goiter Myxedema (adults)

Hyposecretion

diabetes insipidus (DI) **Insufficient secretion of antidiuretic hormone (vasopressin).**

Deficient antidiuretic hormone causes the kidney tubules to fail to hold back (reabsorb) needed water and salts. Clinical symptoms include polyuria and polydipsia. Synthetic preparations of ADH are administered with nasal sprays or intramuscularly as treatment. **Insipidus** means tasteless, reflecting the condition of dilute urine as opposed to **mellitus** meaning sweet or honey, reflecting the sugar content of urine in diabetes mellitus. The term diabetes comes from the Greek *diabainein*, meaning to pass through. Both DI and DM are characterized by polyuria.

Table 18–4 reviews the abnormal conditions associated with hypersecretions and hyposecretions of the endocrine glands.

LABORATORY TESTS

fasting blood sugar (FBS) **Measures circulating glucose level in a patient who has fasted at least 4 hours.**

This test can diagnose diabetes mellitus. A nonfasting test is the **oral glucose tolerance test,** in which the patient drinks 75 grams of glucose and samples for glucose are drawn immediately and at 30, 60, 90, and 120 minutes. This test also is used to diagnose gestational diabetes.

The **glycosylated hemoglobin test** (**HbA1c,** or **A1c**) measures long-term glucose control. A high level indicates poor glucose control in diabetic patients.

serum and urine tests	**Measurement of hormones, electrolytes, glucose, and other substances in serum (blood) and urine as indicators of endocrine function.** Serum studies include growth hormone, somatomedin C (insulin-like growth factor), prolactin level, gonadotropin levels, parathyroid hormone, calcium, and cortisol. Urine studies include glucose (Clinistix, Labstix), ketone (Acetest, Ketostix), and 17-ketosteroids (adrenal and gonadal function). A **urinary microalbumin test** measures small quantities of albumin in urine as a marker or harbinger of diabetic nephropathy.
thyroid function tests	**Measurement of T_3, T_4, and TSH in the bloodstream.**

CLINICAL PROCEDURES

exophthalmometry	**Measurement of eyeball protrusion (as in Graves disease) with an exophthalmometer.**
computed tomography (CT) scan	**X-ray imaging of endocrine glands in cross section, to assess size and infiltration by tumor.**
magnetic resonance imaging	**Magnetic and radiofrequency pulses produce images of the hypothalamus and pituitary gland to locate abnormalities.**
radioactive iodine uptake scan	**Radioactive iodine is administered orally, and its uptake by the thyroid gland is imaged to assess thyroid function.**
thyroid scan	**A scanner detects radioactivity and visualizes the thyroid gland after intravenous administration of a radioactive (technetium) compound.** Nodules and tumors can be evaluated.
ultrasound examination	**Sound waves show images of endocrine organs.** Thyroid ultrasound is the best method to evaluate thyroid structures and abnormalities (nodules).

ABBREVIATIONS

18

A1C	blood test that measures glycosylated hemoglobin (HbA1c) to assess glucose control
ACTH	adrenocorticotropic hormone
ADH	antidiuretic hormone—vasopressin
BGM	blood glucose monitoring
BMR	basal metabolic rate—an indicator of thyroid function, but not in current use
DI	diabetes insipidus
DM	diabetes mellitus
FBG	fasting blood glucose
FBS	fasting blood sugar
FSH	follicle-stimulating hormone
GH	growth hormone
GTT	glucose tolerance test—measures ability to respond to a glucose load; a test for diabetes
HbA1C	test for the presence of glucose attached to hemoglobin (glycosylated hemoglobin test); a high level indicates poor glucose control in diabetic patients
hCG	human chorionic gonadotropin
ICSH	interstitial cell–stimulating hormone
IDDM	insulin-dependent diabetes mellitus—type 1 diabetes
IGF	insulin-like growth factor—also called somatomedin (produced in the liver, it stimulates the growth of bones)

K^+	potassium—an important electrolyte
LH	luteinizing hormone
MEN	multiple endocrine neoplasia—hereditary hormonal disorder marked by adenomas and carcinomas
Na^+	sodium—an important electrolyte
NIDDM	non–insulin-dependent diabetes mellitus—type 2 diabetes
17-OH	17-hydroxycorticosteroids
OT	oxytocin
PRL	prolactin
PTH	parathyroid hormone (parathormone)
RAI	radioactive iodine—treatment for Graves disease
RIA	radioimmunoassay—measures hormone levels in plasma
SIADH	syndrome of inappropriate ADH
STH	somatotropin—growth hormone
T_3	triiodothyronine
T_4	thyroxine—tetraiodothyronine
TFT	thyroid function test
TSH	thyroid-stimulating hormone—secreted by the anterior pituitary gland

PRACTICAL APPLICATIONS

Answers to all questions are on page 761.

CASE REPORT 1

A 24-year-old college student, known diabetic, was admitted for treatment of ketoacidosis. He had a several-year history of diabetes and had been taking insulin in the morning and in the evening. After the history was pieced together from the patient and his friends, it appeared that he had been getting progressively ill over several days following a flu-like episode and may well not have taken his insulin on the day of admission. He was found, slightly drowsy and confused, by classmates. His respirations were rapid, his pulse was 126, and he offered no sensible answers to questions. Blood sugar level was elevated at 728 mg/dL [100 mg/dL is normal], and blood ketones were positive. The patient was treated with insulin intravenously, and over the course of the next 24 hours the ketoacidosis cleared.

Questions

1. Ketoacidosis is a serious complication of
   a. Diabetes insipidus
   b. Diabetes mellitus, type 1
   c. Diabetes mellitus, type 2

2. A clinical sign of ketoacidosis is
   a. Tachypnea
   b. Bradycardia
   c. Hypoglycemia

3. Ketoacidosis occurs when
   a. Insulin blood levels are high
   b. Sugar is not transported to cells and fats are burned improperly
   c. Insulin is given intravenously

CASE REPORT 2

A 42-year-old woman presented with a 6-month history of progressive weakness. She had facial and central obesity with muscle wasting in the extremities. As an initial screening test, a 24-hour urine collection for cortisol determination revealed high levels. Her ACTH level was low. On CT scan a 3-cm mass was found in the left adrenal. When the mass was resected, it proved to be a smooth, yellow adrenocortical adenoma that secreted cortisol. The patient's condition [Cushing syndrome] normalized after surgery.

Questions

1. Signs and symptoms of Cushing syndrome are
   a. Hypoglycemia and hypergonadism
   b. Palpitations
   c. Moon-like fullness of the face and deposition of fat

2. What factors pointed to a diagnosis of Cushing syndrome?
   a. Pituitary gland tumor on CT scan
   b. Hypersecretion of ACTH
   c. Hypersecretion of cortisol and adrenal mass on CT scan

3. Surgery performed to correct this condition was
   a. Adrenocortical adenoma resection
   b. Hypophysectomy
   c. Both a and b

CASE REPORT 3

Graves disease, as characterized by exophthalmos and stare, was diagnosed in a 51-year-old man. Examination revealed a history of nervousness, palpitation, weight loss, diarrhea, dyspnea on exertion, insomnia, heat intolerance, and fatigue. An ECG showed atrial fibrillation with a ventricular rate of about 180 beats per minute, which was treated with digoxin and propranolol. A chest x-ray film disclosed cardiomegaly. Thyroid function tests showed T_4 and T_3 levels to be elevated, and a thyroid scan showed diffuse enlargement of the gland. The patient was treated with radioactive iodine and is now euthyroid. The exophthalmos has not resolved, however.

Questions

1. Symptoms of Graves disease are
   a. Bulging eyeballs
   b. Difficult breathing on exertion
   c. Both a and b

2. Atrial fibrillation means that
   a. The heart is enlarged
   b. The heart rate is less than 180 beats per minute
   c. The heart rate is rapid and irregular

3. Blood tests revealed that
   a. The thyroid gland was hypersecreting
   b. The thyroid gland was hyposecreting
   c. Goiter was present

4. The patient was treated and
   a. Exophthalmos has regressed
   b. Is still having palpitations
   c. His thyroid gland is functioning normally

EXERCISES

Remember to check your answers carefully with those given in the Answers to Exercises, page 760.

A. Match the endocrine gland with its location.

adrenal cortex   pancreas   testis
adrenal medulla   parathyroid   thyroid
ovary   pituitary (hypophysis)

1. Behind the stomach _____

2. Posterior side of the thyroid gland _____

3. Inner section of glands above each kidney _____

4. In the scrotal sac _____

5. On either side of the trachea _____

6. Outer section of gland above each kidney _____

7. Lower abdomen of a female _____

8. Below the brain in the sella turcica _____

B. Name the endocrine organs (including the appropriate lobe or region) that produce the following hormones.

1. follicle-stimulating hormone _____

2. vasopressin _____

3. aldosterone _____

4. insulin _____

5. thyroxine _____

6. cortisol _____

7. gonadotropic hormones _____

8. epinephrine _____

9. oxytocin _____

10. prolactin _____

11. growth hormone _____

12. glucagon _____

13. adrenocorticotropic hormone _____

14. estradiol _____

18

15. progesterone _____

16. testosterone _____

17. thyroid-stimulating hormone _____

C. Give the meanings of the following abbreviations for hormones.

1. ADH _____

2. ACTH _____

3. LH _____

4. FSH _____

5. TSH _____

6. PTH _____

7. GH _____

8. PRL _____

9. T_4 _____

10. T_3 _____

11. OT _____

12. STH _____

D. Match the following hormones with their actions.

ACTH   epinephrine   parathyroid hormone
ADH   estradiol   testosterone
aldosterone   insulin   thyroxine
cortisol

1. sympathomimetic; raises heart rate and blood pressure _____

2. promotes growth and maintenance of male sex characteristics _____

3. stimulates water reabsorption by kidney tubules; decreases urine output _____

4. increases metabolism in body cells _____

5. raises blood calcium _____

6. increases reabsorption of sodium by kidney tubules _____

7. stimulates secretion of hormones from the adrenal cortex _____

8. increases blood sugar _____

9. helps transport glucose to cells; decreases blood sugar _____

10. develops and maintains female sex characteristics _____

E. Indicate whether the following conditions are related to hypersecretion or hyposecretion. Also, select from the following the endocrine gland and hormone involved in each disease.

Glands

adenohypophysis	pancreas
adrenal cortex	parathyroid gland
adrenal medulla	testes
neurohypophysis	thyroid
ovaries	

Hormones

ADH	GH
aldosterone	insulin
cortisol	parathyroid hormone
epinephrine	thyroxine

Condition	Hypo or Hyper	Gland and Hormone
1. Cushing syndrome	_____	_____
2. tetany	_____	_____
3. Graves disease	_____	_____
4. diabetes insipidus	_____	_____
5. acromegaly	_____	_____
6. myxedema	_____	_____
7. diabetes mellitus	_____	_____
8. Addison disease	_____	_____
9. gigantism	_____	_____
10. endemic goiter	_____	_____
11. cretinism	_____	_____
12. pheochromocytoma	_____	_____

F. Build medical terms based on the definitions and word parts given.

1. abnormal condition (poison) of the thyroid gland: thyro_____
2. removal of the pancreas: _____ectomy
3. condition of deficiency or underdevelopment of the sex organs: hypo_____
4. pertaining to producing female (characteristics): _____genic
5. removal of the pituitary gland: _____ectomy
6. deficiency of calcium in the blood: hypo_____
7. excessive sugar in the blood: _____emia
8. inflammation of the thyroid gland: _____itis
9. specialist in the study of hormone disorders: _____ist
10. disease condition of the adrenal glands: adren_____

G. Give the meanings of the following conditions.

1. hyponatremia _____

2. polydipsia _____

3. hyperkalemia _____

4. hypercalcemia _____

5. hypoglycemia _____

6. glycosuria _____

7. euthyroid _____

8. hyperthyroidism _____

9. tetany _____

10. ketoacidosis _____

H. The following hormones are all produced by the anterior lobe of the pituitary gland (note that they all have the same suffix, -tropin). Name the target tissue they act on or stimulate in the body.

1. gonadotropins _____

2. somatotropin _____

3. thyrotropin _____

4. adrenocorticotropin _____

I. Give the meanings of the following medical terms.

1. steroids _____

2. catecholamines _____

3. adenohypophysis _____

4. tetany _____

5. exophthalmos _____

6. mineralocorticoids _____

7. homeostasis _____

8. sympathomimetic _____

9. glucocorticoids _____

10. epinephrine _____

11. glycogen _____

18

18

12. androgen _____

13. corticosteroid_____

14. oxytocin _____

15. tetraiodothyronine _____

16. adrenal virilism _____

17. thyroid carcinoma _____

18. hirsutism _____

19. acromegaly_____

20. estradiol _____

J. Give the meanings of the following terms related to diabetes mellitus.

1. type 1 _____

2. diabetic neuropathy_____

3. ketoacidosis _____

4. hypoglycemia _____

5. type 2 _____

6. diabetic retinopathy_____

7. diabetic coma _____

8. diabetic nephropathy_____

9. atherosclerosis_____

10. hyperglycemia _____

11. gastroparesis _____

12. insulin shock _____

K. Explain the following laboratory tests or clinical procedures related to the endocrine system.

1. thyroid scan_____

2. fasting blood sugar _____

3. radioactive iodine uptake _____

4. exophthalmometry _____

L. Circle the term that best fits the meaning of the sentence.

1. Phyllis was diagnosed with Graves disease when her husband noticed her **(panhypopituitarism, hirsutism, exophthalmos)**. Her eyes seemed to be bulging out of their sockets.

2. Helen had a primary brain tumor called a **(pituitary, thyroid, adrenal)** adenoma. Her entire endocrine system was disrupted, and her physician recommended surgery and radiation to help relieve her symptoms.

3. Bessie's facial features gradually became "rough" in her late thirties and forties. By the time she was 50, her children noticed her very large hands and recommended that she see an endocrinologist, who diagnosed her chronically progressive condition as **(hyperinsulism, gigantism, acromegaly)**.

4. Bobby was brought into the emergency room because he was found passed out in the kitchen. He had forgotten his insulin and had developed **(Cushing disease, hyperparathyroidism, diabetic ketoacidosis)**.

5. Because her 1-hour test of blood sugar was slightly abnormal, Selma's obstetrician ordered a **(glucose tolerance test, thyroid function test, Pap smear)** to rule out gestational **(hyperthyroidism, chlamydial infection, diabetes)**.

6. Bill noticed that he was passing his urine more frequently **(polyphagia, polyuria, hyperglycemia)** and experiencing increased thirst **(polydipsia, hypernatremia, polyphagia)**. His wife urged him to see a physician, who performed a **(serum calcium test, urinalysis, serum sodium test)** that revealed inappropriately dilute **(blood, sweat, urine)**. Measurement of a hormone **(PTH, ADH, STH)** in his blood showed low levels. His diagnosis was **(DI, DM, SIADH)**. Treatment with **(oxytocin, cortisol, vasopressin)** was prescribed via nasal spray, and his condition improved.

7. Mary noticed that she had gained weight recently and that her face had a moon-like fullness with new heavy hair growth. Blood and urine tests showed excessive secretion of adrenal **(mineralocorticoids, catecholamines, glucocorticoids)**. Her diagnostic work-up included a/an **(CT scan of the abdomen, MRI study of the head, chest x-ray)**, which revealed enlargement of both **(kidneys, adrenal glands, lobes of the brain)**. Her doctor made the diagnosis of **(Graves disease, Cushing syndrome, Addison disease)**.

8. Jack had several fractures of ribs and vertebrae in a skiing accident. X-ray images of his bones revealed a generalized decrease in bone density **(osteoporosis, tetany, acromegaly)**. A blood test showed high serum **(sodium, calcium, growth hormone)** and high levels of **(mineralocorticoids, somatotropin, parathyroid hormone)**. A CT scan of the neck revealed a **(thymus, parathyroid, thyroid)** adenoma, which was removed surgically, and he recovered fully. His bone disease and other abnormalities were all related to **(hypoparathyroidism, hyperparathyroidism, hypothyroidism)**

MEDICAL SCRAMBLE

Unscramble the letters to form endocrine system–related terms from the clues. Use the letters in squares to complete the bonus term. Answers are found on page 761.

1. *Clue:* Condition caused by increased growth hormone after puberty

   ☐ __ __ __ ☐ __ __ __ __ __   ECGYARLAOM

2. *Clue:* Hormone stimulating childbirth

   __ ☐ ☐ __ __ __ __ __   ITCXONYO

3. *Clue:* The "flight or fight" hormone

   __ ☐ __ ☐ __ __ __ __ __ ☐   ELEANDIRNA

4. *Clue:* Inner portion of the gland above the kidney

   ☐ __ __ __ __ __ __   UAMLELD

BONUS TERM: *Clue:* A condition caused by deficiency of thyroid hormone in an adult

☐ ☐ ☐ ☐ ☐ ☐ ☐ ☐

ANSWERS TO EXERCISES

18

A

1. pancreas
2. parathyroid
3. adrenal medulla
4. testis
5. thyroid gland
6. adrenal cortex
7. ovary
8. pituitary (hypophysis)

B

1. anterior pituitary gland (adenohypophysis)
2. posterior pituitary gland (neurohypophysis)
3. adrenal cortex
4. beta islet cells of the pancreas
5. thyroid gland
6. adrenal cortex
7. anterior pituitary gland; these hormones are FSH and LH
8. adrenal medulla
9. posterior pituitary gland
10. anterior pituitary gland
11. anterior pituitary gland
12. alpha islet cells of the pancreas
13. anterior pituitary gland
14. ovaries
15. ovaries
16. testes
17. anterior pituitary gland

C

1. antidiuretic hormone
2. adrenocorticotropic hormone
3. luteinizing hormone
4. follicle-stimulating hormone
5. thyroid-stimulating hormone
6. parathyroid hormone
7. growth hormone
8. prolactin
9. thyroxine; tetraiodothyronine
10. triiodothyronine
11. oxytocin
12. somatotropin (growth hormone)

D

1. epinephrine
2. testosterone
3. ADH
4. thyroxine
5. parathyroid hormone
6. aldosterone
7. ACTH
8. cortisol
9. insulin
10. estradiol

E

1. hypersecretion; adrenal cortex; cortisol
2. hyposecretion; parathyroid gland; parathyroid hormone
3. hypersecretion; thyroid gland; thyroxine
4. hyposecretion; neurohypophysis; ADH
5. hypersecretion; adenohypophysis; GH
6. hyposecretion; thyroid gland; thyroxine
7. hyposecretion; pancreas; insulin
8. hyposecretion; adrenal cortex; aldosterone and cortisol
9. hypersecretion; adenohypophysis; GH
10. hyposecretion; thyroid gland; thyroxine
11. hyposecretion; thyroid gland; thyroxine
12. hypersecretion; adrenal medulla; epinephrine

F

1. thyrotoxicosis
2. pancreatectomy
3. hypogonadism
4. estrogenic
5. hypophysectomy
6. hypocalcemia
7. hyperglycemia
8. thyroiditis
9. endocrinologist
10. adrenopathy

G

1. deficient sodium in the blood
2. condition of excessive thirst
3. excessive potassium in the blood
4. excessive calcium in the blood
5. deficient sugar in the blood
6. condition of sugar in the urine
7. normal thyroid function
8. condition of increased secretion from the thyroid gland
9. constant muscle contraction (result of hypoparathyroidism)
10. condition of excessive ketones (acids) in the blood as a result of diabetes mellitus

H

1. the male and female sex organs (ovaries and testes); examples of gonadotropins are FSH and LH
2. bones; another name for somatotropin is growth hormone
3. thyroid gland; another name for thyrotropin is thyroid-stimulating hormone
4. adrenal cortex; another name for adrenocorticotropin is adrenocorticotropic hormone (ACTH)

I

1. complex substances derived from cholesterol; hormones from the adrenal cortex and sex hormones are steroids
2. complex substances derived from an amino acid; epinephrine (adrenaline) and norepinephrine (noradrenaline) are examples
3. anterior lobe of the pituitary gland
4. continuous contractions of muscles associated with low levels of parathyroid hormone
5. eyeballs that bulge outward; associated with hyperthyroidism
6. steroid hormones from the adrenal cortex (outer region of the adrenal gland) that influence salt (minerals such as sodium and potassium) metabolism
7. tendency of an organism to maintain a constant internal environment
8. a substance that mimics the action of the sympathetic nerves; epinephrine (adrenaline) is an example
9. steroid hormones from the adrenal cortex that influence sugar metabolism in the body
10. catecholamine hormone from the adrenal medulla; adrenaline
11. animal starch; storage form of glucose
12. male hormone; testosterone is an example
13. hormone secreted by the adrenal cortex; cortisol is an example
14. hormone from the posterior lobe of the pituitary that stimulates
contraction of the uterus during labor
15. major hormone from the thyroid gland; thyroxine (contains four iodine atoms)
16. abnormal secretion of androgens from the adrenal cortex produces masculine characteristics in a female
17. cancerous tumor of the thyroid gland
18. excessive hair on the body (result of excessive secretion of androgens)
19. enlargement of extremities (excessive secretion of growth hormone after puberty)
20. female hormone; an estrogen

J

1. destruction of the beta islets of Langerhans; insulin is not produced (insulin-dependent diabetes mellitus, IDDM)
2. Destruction of nerves as a secondary complication of diabetes mellitus
3. abnormal condition of high levels of ketones (acids) in the blood as a result of improper burning of fats; fats are burned because the cells do not have sugar available as a result of lack of insulin or inability of insulin to act
4. too little sugar in the blood; this can occur if too much insulin is taken by a diabetic patient
5. insulin deficiency and resistance by target tissue to the action of insulin; (non–insulin-dependent diabetes mellitus, NIDDM)
6. destruction of blood vessels in the retina as a secondary complication of diabetes mellitus
7. unconsciousness caused by high levels of sugar in the blood; water leaves cells to balance the large amounts of sugar in the blood, leading to cellular dehydration
8. destruction of the kidneys as a secondary complication of diabetes mellitus
9. collection of fatty plaque in arteries
10. high level of sugar in the blood; insulin is unavailable or unable to transport sugar from the blood into cells
11. decreased gastric motility (-paresis means slight paralysis); secondary complication of diabetes
12. Hypoglycemic shock caused by an overdose of insulin, decreased intake of food, or excessive exercise.

K

1. A radioactive compound is given, and the thyroid gland is imaged using a scanning device.
2. Measurement of blood sugar levels in a fasting patient (at least 4 hours)
and after intervals of 30 minutes and 1, 2, and 3 hours after ingestion of glucose.
3. Radioactive iodine is given orally, and uptake by the thyroid gland assesses thyroid function.
4. Measurement of eyeball protrusion (symptom of Graves disease).

L

1. exophthalmos
2. pituitary
3. acromegaly
4. diabetic ketoacidosis
5. glucose tolerance test; diabetes
6. polyuria; polydipsia; urinalysis; urine; ADH; DI; vasopressin
7. glucocorticoids; CT scan of the abdomen; adrenal glands; Cushing syndrome
8. osteoporosis; calcium; parathyroid hormone; parathyroid; hyperparathyroidism

ANSWERS TO PRACTICAL APPLICATIONS

Case Report 1
1. b   2. a   3. b

Case Report 2
1. c   2. c   3. a

Case Report 3
1. c   2. c   3. a   4. c

ANSWERS TO MEDICAL SCRAMBLE

1. ACROMEGALY   2. OXYTOCIN   3. ADRENALINE   4. MEDULLA
BONUS TERM: MYXEDEMA

PRONUNCIATION OF TERMS

18

To test your understanding of the terminology in this chapter, write the meaning of each term in the space provided. In addition, you may wish to cover the terms and write them by looking at your definitions. Make sure your spelling is correct. The page number after each term indicates where it is defined or used in the book, so you can easily check your responses. You will find complete definitions for all of these terms and their audio pronunciations on the CD.

VOCABULARY AND TERMINOLOGY

Term	Pronunciation	Meaning
adenectomy (736)	ăd-ĕ-NĔK-tō-mē	
adenohypophysis (733)	ăd-ĕ-nō-hī-PŎF-ĭ-sĭs	
adrenal cortex (733)	ă-DRĒ-năl KŎR-tĕks	
adrenalectomy (736)	ă-drē-năl-ĔK-tō-mē	
adrenaline (734)	ă-DRĔN-ă-lĭn	
adrenal medulla (733)	ă-DRĒ-năl mĕ-DŪ-lă	
adrenocorticotropic hormone (734)	ă-drē-nō-kŏr-tĭ-kō-TRŌP-ĭk HŎR-mōn	
adrenocorticotropin (734)	ă-drē-nō-kŏr-tĭ-kō-TRŌ-pĭn	
adrenopathy (736)	ă-drē-NŎP-ă-thē	
aldosterone (734)	ăl-DŎS-tĕ-rōn	
androgen (734)	ĂN-drō-jĕn	
antidiuretic hormone (734)	ăn-tĭ-dī-ū-RĔT-ĭk HŎR-mōn	
calcitonin (734)	kăl-sĭ-TŌ-nĭn	
catecholamines (735)	kăt-ĕ-KŌL-ă-mēnz	
corticosteroid (735)	kŏr-tĭ-kō-STĔ-royd	
cortisol (734)	KŎR-tĭ-sōl	
electrolyte (735)	ĕ-LĔK-trō-līt	
endocrinologist (737)	ĕn-dō-krĭ-NŎL-ō-jĭst	
epinephrine (734)	ĕp-ĭ-NĔF-rĭn	
estradiol (734)	ĕs-tră-DĪ-ŏl	
estrogen (734)	ĔS-trō-jĕn	
estrogenic (737)	ĕs-trō-JĔN-ĭk	
euthyroid (739)	ū-THĪ-royd	

18

Term	Pronunciation	Meaning
follicle-stimulating hormone (734)	FŎL-ĭ-k'l STĬM-ū-lā-tĭng HŎR-mōn	
glucagon (734)	GLOO-kă-gŏn	
glucocorticoid (735)	gloo-kō-KŎR-tĭ-koyd	
glycemic (737)	glī-SĒ-mĭk	
glycogen (737)	GLĬ-kō-jĕn	
glycosuria (739)	glī-kōs-Ū-rē-ă	
gonadotropin (736)	gō-năd-ō-TRŌ-pĭn	
growth hormone (734)	grōth HŎR-mōn	
homeostasis (735)	hō-mē-ō-STĀ-sĭs	
hormonal (737)	hŏr-MŌ-năl	
hormone (735)	HŎR-mōn	
hypercalcemia (737)	hī-pĕr-kăl-SĒ-mē-ă	
hypercalciuria (737)	hī-pĕr-kăl-sē-ŪR-ē-ă	
hyperglycemia (737)	hī-pĕr-glī-SĒ-mē-ă	
hypocalcemia (737)	hī-pō-kăl-SĒ-mē-ă	
hypoglycemia (739)	hī-pō-glī-SĒ-mē-ă	
hypogonadism (736)	hī-pō-GŌ-năd-ĭzm	
hypoinsulinism (739)	hī-pō-ĬN-sū-lĭn-ĭzm	
hypokalemia (737)	hī-pō-kā-LĒ-mē-ă	
hyponatremia (738)	hī-pō-nā-TRĒ-mē-ă	
hypophysectomy (738)	hī-pō-fĭ-ZĔK-tō-mē	
hypophysis (733)	hī-PŎF-ĭ-sĭs	
hypopituitarism (736)	hī-pō-pĭ-TOO-ĭ-tă-rĭzm	
hypothalamus (735)	hī-pō-THĂL-ă-mŭs	
insulin (734)	ĬN-sū-lĭn	
luteinizing hormone (734)	LOO-tē-ĭn-īz-ĭng HŎR-mōn	
mineralocorticoid (735)	mĭn-ĕr-ăl-ō-KŎR-tĭ-koyd	
neurohypophysis (733)	noo-rō-hī-PŎF-ĭ-sĭs	
norepinephrine (734)	nŏr-ĕp-ĭ-NĔF-rĭn	
oxytocin (734)	ŏk-sĕ-TŌ-sĭn	
pancreas (733)	PĂN-krē-ăs	
pancreatectomy (736)	păn-krē-ă-TĔK-tō-mē	

Term	Pronunciation	Meaning
parathormone (734)	păr-ă-THŎR-mōn	_____
parathyroidectomy (736)	păr-ă-thī-roy-DĔK-tō-mē	_____
parathyroid glands (733)	păr-ă-THĬ-royd glănz	_____
pineal gland (722)	pī-NĒ-ăl glănd	_____
pituitary gland (733)	pĭ-TOO-ĭ-tĕr-ē glănd	_____
polydipsia (737)	pŏl-ē-DĬP-sē-ă	_____
progesterone (734)	prō-JĔS-tĕ-rōn	_____
prolactin (734)	prō-LĂK-tĭn	_____
receptor (735)	rē-SĔP-tor	_____
sella turcica (735)	SĔL-ă TŬR-sĭ-kă	_____
somatotropin (734)	sō-mă-tō-TRŌ-pĭn	_____
steroid (735)	STĔR-oyd	_____
sympathomimetic (735)	sĭm-pă-thō-mĭ-MĔT-ĭk	_____
target tissue (735)	TĂR-gĕt TĬS-ū	_____
testosterone (734)	tĕs-TŎS-tĕ-rōn	_____
tetraiodothyronine (735)	tĕ-tră-ī-ō-dō-THĬ-rō-nēn	_____
thyroid gland (733)	THĬ-royd glănd	_____
thyroiditis (736)	thī-royd-Ī-tĭs	_____
thyrotropin (736)	thī-rō-TRŌ-pĭn	_____
thyroxine (735)	thī-RŎK-sĭn	_____
triiodothyronine (735)	trī-ī-ō-dō-THĬ-rō-nēn	_____
vasopressin (735)	văz-ō-PRĔS-ĭn	_____

ABNORMAL CONDITIONS, LABORATORY TESTS, AND CLINICAL PROCEDURES

Term	Pronunciation	Meaning
acromegaly (746)	ăk-rō-MĔG-ă-lē	_____
Addison disease (743)	ĂD-ĭ-sŏn dĭ-ZĒZ	_____
adrenal virilism (742)	ă-DRĒ-năl VĬR-ĭ-lĭzm	_____
cretinism (741)	KRĒ-tĭn-ĭzm	_____
Cushing syndrome (742)	KŬSH-ĭng SĬN-drōm	_____
diabetes insipidus (748)	dī-ă-BĒ-tēz ĭn-SĬP-ĭ-dŭs	_____
diabetes mellitus (744)	dī-ă-BĒ-tēz MĔL-ĭ-tŭs _or_ mĕ-LĪ-tŭs	_____
dwarfism (747)	DWĂRF-ĭzm	_____

18

Term	Pronunciation	Meaning
endemic goiter (740)	ĕn-DĔM-ĭk GOY-tĕr	
exophthalmometry (749)	ĕk-sŏf-thăl-MŎM-ĕ-trē	
exophthalmos (740)	ĕk-sŏf-THĂL-mōs	
fasting blood sugar (748)	FĂS-tĭng blŭd SHŬG-ăr	
gastroparesis (745)	găs-trō-păr-Ē-sĭs	
gigantism (747)	JĪ-găn-tĭzm	
glucose tolerance test (748)	GLOO-kōs TŎL-ĕr-ăns tĕst	
goiter (740)	GOY-tĕr	
Graves disease (740)	GRĀVZ dĭ-ZĒZ	
hirsutism (742)	HĔR-soot-ĭzm	
hyperinsulinism (741)	hī-pĕr-ĬN-sū-lĭn-ĭzm	
hyperparathyroidism (741)	hī-pĕr-pă-ră-THĪ-royd-ĭzm	
hyperthyroidism (740)	hī-pĕr-THĪ-royd-ĭsm	
hypoparathyroidism (741)	hī-pō-pă-ră-THĪ-royd-ĭzm	
hypothyroidism (741)	hī-pō-THĪ-royd-ĭzm	
ketoacidosis (745)	kē-tō-ă-sĭ-DŌ-sĭs	
myxedema (741)	mĭk-sĕ-DĒ-mă	
nodular goiter (740)	NŎD-ū-lăr GOY-tĕr	
panhypopituitarism (747)	păn-hī-pō-pĭ-TŪ-ĭ-tăr-ĭzm	
pheochromocytoma (743)	fē-ō-krō-mō-sī-TŌ-mă	
radioactive iodine uptake (749)	rā-dē-ō-ĂK-tĭv Ī-ō-dīn ŬP-tāk	
syndrome of inappropriate ADH (747)	SĬN-drōm ŏf ĭn-ă-PRŌ-prē-ĭt A-D-H	
tetany (741)	TĔT-ă-nē	
thyroid carcinoma (741)	THĪ-royd kăr-sĭ-NŌ-mă	
thyroid function tests (749)	THĪ-royd FŬNK-shŭn tĕsts	
thyroid scan (749)	THĪ-royd skăn	
thyrotoxicosis (738)	thī-rō-tŏk-sĭ-KŌ-sĭs	

REVIEW SHEET

18

Write the meanings of the word parts in the spaces provided and test yourself. Check your answers with the information in the chapter or in the glossary (Medical Word Parts—English) at the end of the book.

COMBINING FORMS

Combining Form	Meaning	Combining Form	Meaning
aden/o	_____	insulin/o	_____
adren/o	_____	lact/o	_____
adrenal/o	_____	myx/o	_____
andr/o	_____	natr/o	_____
calc/o, calci/o	_____	pancreat/o	_____
cortic/o	_____	parathyroid/o	_____
crin/o	_____	phys/o	_____
dips/o	_____	pituitar/o	_____
estr/o	_____	somat/o	_____
gluc/o	_____	ster/o	_____
glyc/o	_____	thyr/o	_____
gonad/o	_____	thyroid/o	_____
home/o	_____	toc/o	_____
kal/i	_____	toxic/o	_____
hormon/o	_____	ur/o	_____

SUFFIXES

Suffix	Meaning	Suffix	Meaning
-agon	_____	-osis	_____
-ectomy	_____	-physis	_____
-emia	_____	-stasis	_____
-genic	_____	-tocin	_____
-in, -ine	_____	-tropin	_____
-megaly	_____	-uria	_____
-oid	_____		

PREFIXES

Prefix	Meaning	Prefix	Meaning
eu-	_____	pan-	_____
hyper-	_____	poly-	_____
hypo-	_____	tetra-	_____
oxy-	_____	tri-	_____

 Please refer to the enclosed CD for additional exercises and images related to this chapter.

chapter 19

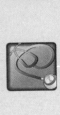

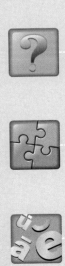

Cancer Medicine (Oncology)

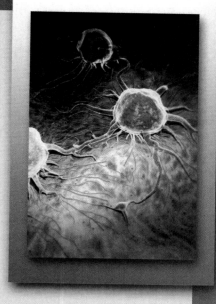

THIS CHAPTER IS DIVIDED INTO THE FOLLOWING SECTIONS

In this chapter you will

- Identify medical terms that describe the growth and spread of tumors.
- Recognize terms related to the causes, diagnosis, and treatment of cancer.
- Review how tumors are classified and described by pathologists.
- Describe x-ray studies, laboratory tests, and other procedures used by physicians for determining the presence and extent of spread (staging) of tumors.
- Apply your new knowledge to understanding medical terms in their usual contexts, such as medical reports and records.

Image Description: A microscopic conceptual visualization of breast cancer cells on the surface of breast tissue.

19

INTRODUCTION

Cancer is a disease caused by abnormal and excessive growth of cells in the body. It may occur in any tissue and at any time of life, although cancer occurs most frequently in older people. Cancer cells accumulate as growths called **malignant tumors,** which compress, invade, and ultimately destroy the surrounding normal tissue. In addition to their local growth, cancerous cells spread throughout the body by way of the bloodstream or lymphatic vessels. In some patients, the spread of cancers from their site of origin to distant organs occurs early in the course of tumor growth and ultimately results in death.

Although more than half of all patients who develop cancer are cured of their disease, it causes about one fifth of all deaths in the United States. Lung cancers, followed by breast and colorectal cancers, are the most common causes of cancer death for women, whereas lung, colorectal, and prostate cancers are the leading causes of death due to cancer in men. This chapter explores the terminology related to this common and often fatal group of diseases.

CHARACTERISTICS OF TUMORS

Tumors (also called **neoplasms**) are masses, or growths, that arise from normal tissue. They may be either **malignant** (capable of invasion and spread to other sites) or **benign** (noninvasive and not invading nearby tissues or spreading to other sites). There are several differences between benign and malignant tumors. Some of these differences are:

1. Benign tumors **grow slowly,** and malignant tumor cells **multiply rapidly.**
2. Benign tumors are often **encapsulated** (contained within a fibrous capsule or cover), so that the tumor cells do not invade the surrounding tissue. Malignant tumors characteristically are **invasive** and **infiltrative,** extending into neighboring normal tissue.
3. Benign tumors are composed of organized and specialized **(differentiated)** cells that closely resemble the normal, mature tissue from which they are derived. For example, benign tumors derived from cells that line the gastrointestinal tract or

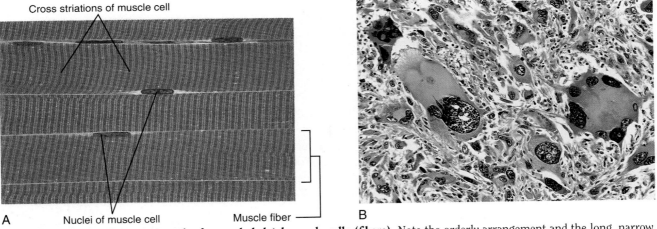

Cross striations of muscle cell

A Nuclei of muscle cell Muscle fiber B

FIGURE 19–1 **A, Photomicrograph of normal skeletal muscle cells (fibers).** Note the orderly arrangement and the long, narrow, threadlike shape of the cells. There are many nuclei per cell and many cross striations. **B, Anaplastic tumor cells of the skeletal muscle (rhabdomyosarcoma).** Note the variation in size and shape of the nuclei (pleomorphism; pleo = many, morph/o = shape), hyperchromatic nuclei, and tumor giant cells (which possess either one enormous nucleus or several nuclei). (**A** from Thibodeau GA, Patton KT: Anatomy & Physiology, 6th ed. St. Louis, Mosby, 2007, p. 176. **B** courtesy of Dr. Trace Worrell, Department of Pathology, University of Texas Southwestern Medical School, Dallas.)

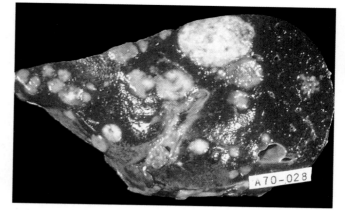

FIGURE 19–2 A liver studded with **metastatic cancer.** (From Kumar V, Cotran RS, Robbins SL: Robbins Basic Pathology, 7th ed. Philadelphia, WB Saunders, 2003, p. 172.)

glands look very much like gastrointestinal cells, their normal counterparts. Malignant tumors are composed of cancerous cells that resemble primitive cells and lack the capacity to perform mature cell functions. This characteristic of malignant tumors is called **anaplasia.** Anaplasia (ana- means backward and -plasia means growth) indicates that the cancerous cells are **dedifferentiated,** or **undifferentiated** (reverting to a less specialized state), in contrast to the normal, differentiated tissue of their origin. Anaplastic cells lack an orderly arrangement. Thus, tumor cells vary in size and shape and are piled one on top of the other in a disorganized fashion. The nuclei in these cells are large and **hyperchromatic** (stain excessively with dyes that recognize genetic material). Figure 19–1 shows normal skeletal muscle (in *A*) and anaplastic muscle tumor cells (in *B*).

4. Cells from benign tumors do not spread or **metastasize** to form secondary tumor masses in distant places in the body. Cells from malignant tumors, however, can detach themselves from the primary tumor site, penetrate a blood vessel or lymphatic vessel, travel through the bloodstream or lymphatic system, and establish a new tumor site at a distant tissue, such as the lung, liver, or bone marrow. The secondary growth is called a **metastasis.** Figure 19–2 shows metastatic cancer cells invading a liver.

Figure 19–3 reviews the differences between benign and malignant tumors.

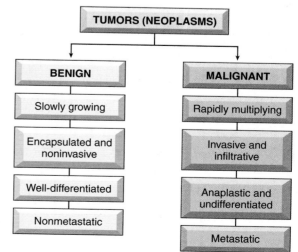

FIGURE 19–3 Differences between benign and malignant tumors.

CARCINOGENESIS

WHAT CAUSES CANCER?

The causes of transformation from a normal cell to a cancerous one **(carcinogenesis)** are only partially understood at the present time. What is clear is that malignant transformation results from damage to the genetic material, or **DNA (deoxyribonucleic acid),** of the cell. Strands of DNA in the cell nucleus form **chromosomes,** which become readily visible under a microscope when a cell is preparing to divide into two (daughter) cells. In order to understand what causes cancer, it is necessary to learn more about DNA and its functions in a normal cell.

DNA has two main functions in a normal cell. First, DNA controls the production of new cells (cell division). When a cell divides, the DNA material in each chromosome copies itself so that exactly the same DNA is passed to the two new daughter cells that are formed. This process of cell division is called **mitosis** (Fig. 19–4, *A*).

Second, DNA contains the master code for all proteins produced in the cell. Between cycles of mitosis, DNA controls the production of new proteins **(protein synthesis)** in the cell. DNA contains about 20,000 to 30,000 separate and distinct **genes** that direct the production of all proteins, which in turn control all aspects of cell function. Genes are composed of an arrangement of units called **nucleotides** (containing a sugar, phosphate, and a base, such as adenine, guanine, thymine, or cytosine). DNA (as a string of coded nucleotides) sends a molecular message outside the nucleus to the cytoplasm of the cell, directing the synthesis of specific proteins (such as hormones and enzymes) essential for normal cell function and growth. This message is transmitted in the following way. In the nucleus, the coded message with instructions for making a specific protein is copied from DNA onto another molecule called **RNA (ribonucleic acid).** Then RNA travels from the nucleus to the cytoplasm of the cell, carrying the coded message to direct the formation of specific proteins (see Fig. 19–4, *B*).

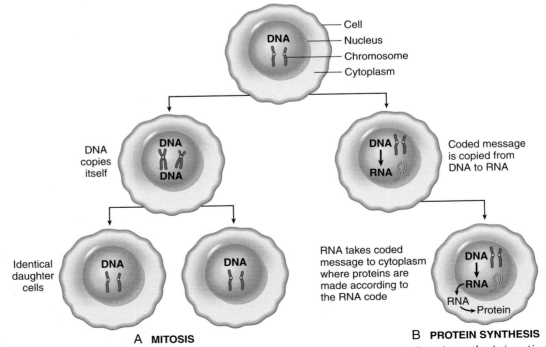

FIGURE 19–4 **Two functions of DNA. A,** Mitosis (the process of cell division). **B,** Protein synthesis (creating new proteins for cellular growth).

When a cell becomes malignant, however, the processes of mitosis and protein synthesis are disturbed. Cancer cells reproduce almost continuously, and abnormal proteins are made. Malignant cells are **anaplastic;** that is, their DNA stops making codes that allow the cells to carry on the function of mature cells. Instead, altered DNA and altered cellular programs make new signals that lead to cell proliferation, movement of cells, invasion of adjacent tissue, and metastasis.

Various kinds of damage to DNA results in malignancy; DNA damage may be caused by environmental factors, such as toxic chemicals, sunlight, tobacco smoke, and viruses. The specific damage usually involves chemical changes in the nucleotide components of DNA. These changes interfere with the accurate coding for new protein synthesis. Once these changes are established in a cell, they are passed on to daughter cells. Such an inheritable change in DNA is called a **mutation.** Mutations, particularly those that affect cell growth or DNA repair, lead to malignant growths.

Although most DNA changes, or mutations, lead to higher-than-normal rates of growth, some mutations found in cancer cells actually prevent the cells from dying. In recent years, scientists have recognized that in some types of cancers, the normal blueprints that direct aging or damaged cells to die are missing. Normal cells undergo spontaneous disintegration by a process known as **apoptosis,** or programmed cell death. Some cancer cells have lost elements of this program and thus can live indefinitely.

ENVIRONMENTAL AGENTS

Agents from the environment, such as chemicals, drugs, tobacco smoke, radiation, and viruses, can cause damage to DNA and thus produce cancer. These environmental agents are called **carcinogens.**

Chemical carcinogens are found in a variety of products and drugs, including **hydrocarbons** (in cigarette, cigar, and pipe smoke and automobile exhaust), insecticides, dyes, industrial chemicals, insulation, and hormones. For example, the hormone diethylstilbestrol (DES) causes a malignant tumor, carcinoma of the vagina, in daughters of women treated with DES during pregnancy. Drugs such as estrogens can cause cancer by stimulating the proliferation of cells in target organs such as the lining of the uterus.

Radiation, whatever its source—sunlight, x-rays, radioactive substances—is a wave of energy. When this energy interacts with DNA, it causes DNA damage and mutations that lead to cancer. Thus, leukemia (a cancerous condition of white blood cells) may be an occupational hazard of radiologists, who are routinely exposed to x-rays. There is a high incidence of leukemia and other cancers among survivors of atomic bomb explosions, as at Hiroshima and Nagasaki. Ultraviolet radiation given off by the sun can cause skin cancer, especially in persons with lightly pigmented, or fair, skin.

Some **viruses** are carcinogenic. For example, the human T cell leukemia virus (HTLV) causes a form of leukemia in adults. Kaposi sarcoma is caused by another virus, herpes type VIII. Other viruses are known to cause cervical cancer (papillomavirus) and a tumor of lymph nodes called Burkitt lymphoma (Epstein-Barr virus). These tumor-producing viruses, called **oncogenic viruses,** fall into two categories: **RNA viruses** (composed of RNA and known as retroviruses) and **DNA viruses** (composed of DNA).

In addition to transmission of cancer by whole viruses, pieces of normal DNA called **oncogenes** can cause normal cells to become malignant if they are activated by mutations. An oncogene (cancer-causing gene) is a piece of DNA whose activation is associated with the conversion of a normal cell into a cancerous cell. Some examples of oncogenes are *ras* (colon cancer), *myc* (lymphoma), and *abl* (chronic myelogenous leukemia).

In chronic myelogenous leukemia, the oncogene *abl* is activated when pieces from two different chromosomes switch locations. This genetic change (mutation) is called a

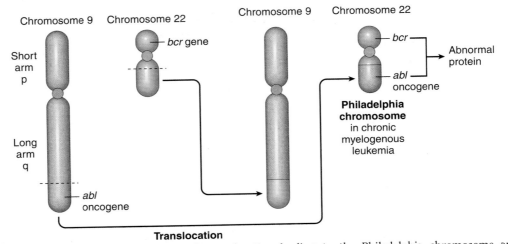

FIGURE 19–5 Chromosomal (oncogene) translocation leading to the Philadelphia chromosome and chronic myelogenous leukemia (CML). **A,** Normal chromosomes 9 and 22. **B,** Translocation of the *abl* oncogene from the long arm (q) of chromosome 9 to the long arm of chromosome 22 (next to the *bcr* gene). This forms a combination oncogene *bcr-abl* that produces an abnormal protein (tyrosine kinase), which leads to malignant transformation (CML).

translocation. The oncogene *abl* on chromosome 9 moves to a new location on the base of chromosome 22, in a chromosome region called **bcr** (**b**reakpoint **c**luster **r**egion). When these two genes are located near each other, they cause the production of an abnormal protein that makes the leukocyte divide and causes a malignancy (chronic myelogenous leukemia). The new chromosome formed from the translocation and containing the *bcr-abl* gene fragments is called the **Philadelphia chromosome** (it was discovered in 1970 in Philadelphia) (Fig. 19–5).

HEREDITY

Cancer may be caused not only by environmental factors, but also by inherited factors. Susceptibility to some forms of cancer is transmitted from parents to offspring through defects in the DNA of the egg or sperm cells. Examples of known inherited cancers are **retinoblastoma** (tumor of the retina of the eye), **polyposis coli syndrome** (polyps that grow in the colon and rectum), and certain other inherited forms of colon, breast, and kidney cancer.

Each of these diseases is caused by loss of a segment of DNA or by a change in the coding sequence of DNA. Detection of these changes in the DNA code is possible by analysis of genes on the chromosomes from any cell, such as a blood cell, taken from an affected individual. Such inherited defects are detected by DNA sequencing, a step-by-step analysis of the nucleotide sequence of the affected gene, or by small DNA probes that test the overall fit of a person's gene to a normal gene sequence.

In many cases, it is believed that these tumors arise because of inherited or acquired abnormalities in certain genes called **suppressor genes.** In normal individuals, these suppressor genes regulate growth, promote differentiation, and suppress oncogenes from causing cancer. Loss of a normal suppressor gene takes the brake off the process of cell division and leads to cancer. Examples of suppressor genes are the **retinoblastoma gene (Rb-1)** and the **p53** gene (named after the molecular weight of the protein for which it codes). A loss or mutation of the p53 (also called *TP53*) gene (located on chromosome 17) can lead to human cancers, such as brain tumors or breast cancer.

Table 19-1

Genes Implicated in Hereditary Cancers

Cancer	Gene	Chromosomal Location*
Breast; ovarian	BRCA1	7q21
Breast; ovarian	BRCA2	3q12-13
Polyposis coli syndrome	APC	5q21
Li-Fraumeni (multiple cancers)	p53	17p13
Retinoblastoma	Rb1	13q14
Wilms tumor	WT1	11p13
Renal cell carcinoma	VHL	3p21-26

*The first number is the chromosome; p is the short arm of the chromosome, and q is the long arm of the chromosome. The second number is the region (band) of the chromosome.

Because inherited changes can be detected in all tissues of the body, not simply cancerous cells, blood cells from family members may be tested to determine whether a person has inherited the cancer-causing gene. This is known as **genetic screening.** Affected individuals may be watched carefully to detect tumors at an early stage. Table 19-1 lists several hereditary cancers and the name of the responsible gene. Figure 19-6 reviews the role of environmental agents and heredity in carcinogenesis.

CLASSIFICATION OF CANCEROUS TUMORS

Almost half of all cancer deaths are caused by malignancies that originate in lung, breast, or colon; however, in all there are more than 100 distinct types of cancer, each having a unique set of symptoms and requiring a specific type of therapy. It is possible to divide these types of cancer into three broad groups on the basis of **histogenesis**—that is, by

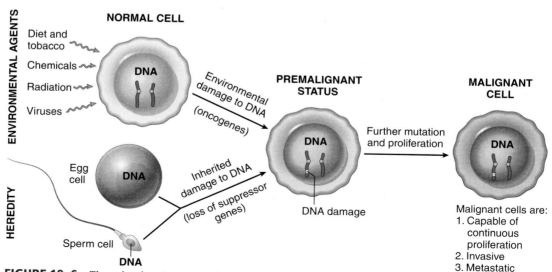

FIGURE 19-6 The role of environmental agents and heredity in carcinogenesis (transformation of a normal cell to a malignant cell).

identifying the particular type of tissue **(hist/o)** from which the tumor cells arise **(-genesis).** These major groups are **carcinomas, sarcomas,** and **mixed-tissue tumors.**

CARCINOMAS

Carcinomas, the largest group, are solid tumors that are derived from epithelial tissue that lines external and internal body surfaces, including skin, glands, and digestive, urinary, and reproductive organs. Approximately 90 percent of all malignancies are carcinomas.

Table 19–2 gives examples of specific carcinomas and the epithelial tissue from which they derive. Benign tumors of epithelial origin are usually designated by the term **adenoma,** which indicates that the tumor is of epithelial or glandular **(aden/o)** origin. For

Table 19–2

Carcinomas and the Epithelial Tissues from Which They Derive

Type of Epithelial Tissue	Malignant Tumor (Carcinomas)
GASTROINTESTINAL TRACT	
Colon	Adenocarcinoma of the colon
Esophagus	Esophageal carcinoma
Liver	Hepatocellular carcinoma (hepatoma)
Stomach	Gastric adenocarcinoma
GLANDULAR TISSUE	
Adrenal glands	Carcinoma of the adrenals
Breast	Carcinoma of the breast
Pancreas	Carcinoma of the pancreas (pancreatic adenocarcinoma)
Prostate	Carcinoma of the prostate
Salivary glands	Adenoid cystic carcinoma
Thyroid	Carcinoma of the thyroid
KIDNEY AND BLADDER	
	Renal cell carcinoma (hypernephroma)
	Transitional cell carcinoma of the bladder
LUNG	
	Adenocarcinoma (bronchioloalveolar)
	Large cell carcinoma
	Small (oat) cell carcinoma
	Squamous cell (epidermoid)
REPRODUCTIVE ORGANS	
	Adenocarcinoma of the uterus
	Carcinoma of the penis
	Choriocarcinoma of the uterus or testes
	Cystadenocarcinoma (mucinous or serous) of the ovaries
	Seminoma and embryonal cell carcinoma (testes)
	Squamous cell (epidermoid) carcinoma of the vagina or cervix
SKIN	
Basal cell layer	Basal cell carcinoma
Melanocyte	Malignant melanoma
Squamous cell layer	Squamous cell carcinoma

example, a gastric adenoma is a benign tumor of the glandular epithelial cells lining the stomach. Malignant tumors of epithelial origin are named by using the term **carcinoma** and adding the type of tissue in which the tumor occurs. Thus, a **gastric adenocarcinoma** is a cancerous tumor arising from glandular cells lining the stomach.

SARCOMAS

Sarcomas also are malignant tumors but are less common than carcinomas. They derive from connective tissues in the body, such as bone, fat, muscle, cartilage, and bone marrow and from cells of the lymphatic system. Often, the term **mesenchymal tissue** is used to describe embryonic connective tissue from which sarcomas are derived. The middle, or mesodermal, layer of the embryo gives rise to the connective tissues of the body as well as to blood and lymphatic vessels.

Table 19–3 gives examples of specific types of sarcomas and the connective tissues from which they derive. Benign tumors of connective tissue origin are named by adding the suffix **-oma** to the type of tissue in which the tumor occurs. For example, a benign tumor

Table 19–3

Sarcomas and the Connective Tissues from Which They Derive

Type of Connective Tissue	Malignant Tumor
BONE	
	Osteosarcoma (osteogenic sarcoma)
	Ewing sarcoma
MUSCLE	
Smooth (visceral) muscle	Leiomyosarcoma
Striated (skeletal) muscle	Rhabdomyosarcoma
CARTILAGE	
	Chondrosarcoma
FAT	
	Liposarcoma
FIBROUS TISSUE	
	Fibrosarcoma
BLOOD VESSEL TISSUE	
	Angiosarcoma
BLOOD-FORMING TISSUE	
All leukocytes	Leukemias
Lymphocytes	Hodgkin disease
	Non-Hodgkin lymphomas
	Burkitt lymphoma
Plasma cells (bone marrow)	Multiple myeloma
NERVE TISSUE	
Embryonic nerve tissue	Neuroblastoma
Glial tissue	Astrocytoma (tumor of glial cells called astrocytes)
	Glioblastoma multiforme
Nerve cells of the gastrointestinal tract	Gastrointestinal stromal tumor (GIST)

Table 19-4

Mixed-Tissue Tumors

Type of Tissue	Malignant Tumor
Kidney	Wilms tumor (embryonal adenosarcoma)
Ovaries and testes	Teratoma (tumor composed of bone, muscle, skin, gland cells, cartilage, etc.)

of bone is called an **osteoma.** Malignant tumors of connective tissue origin are frequently named by using the term **sarcoma** (**sarc/o** means flesh). For example, an **osteosarcoma** is a malignant tumor of bone.

In addition to the solid tumors of connective tissue origin, sarcomas include tumors arising from blood-forming tissue. **Leukemias** are tumors derived from bone marrow, and **lymphomas** are derived from immune cells of the lymphatic system. Connective tissue within the brain (glial cells) and embryonic tissue of the nervous system give rise to **gliomas** (such as astrocytomas of the brain) and **neuroblastomas.**

MIXED-TISSUE TUMORS

Mixed-tissue tumors are derived from tissue that is capable of differentiating into both epithelial and connective tissue. These uncommon tumors are thus composed of several different types of cells. Examples of mixed-tissue tumors (Table 19–4) are found in the kidney, ovaries, and testes.

PATHOLOGIC DESCRIPTIONS

The following terms are used to describe the appearance of a malignant tumor, on either gross (visual) or microscopic examination.

GROSS DESCRIPTIONS

cystic Forming large open spaces filled with fluid. **Mucinous** tumors are filled with mucus (thick, sticky fluid), and **serous** tumors are filled with a thin, watery fluid resembling serum. The most common site of cystic tumors is in ovaries. See Figure 19–7, *A.*

fungating Mushrooming pattern of growth in which tumor cells pile one on top of another and project from a tissue surface. Tumors found in the colon are often of this type.

inflammatory Having the features of inflammation; that is, redness, swelling, and heat. Inflammatory changes result from tumor blockage of the lymphatic drainage of the skin, as in breast cancer.

medullary Pertaining to large, soft, fleshy tumors. Thyroid and breast tumors may be medullary. See Figure 19–7, *B.*

necrotic Containing dead tissue. Any type of tumor can outgrow its blood supply and undergo necrosis.

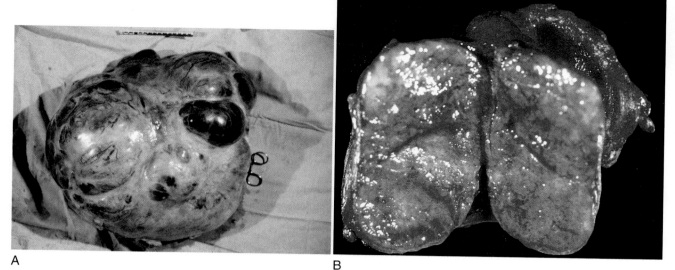

FIGURE 19–7   **A, Cystic ovarian adenocarcinoma. B, Medullary carcinoma** of the thyroid. Tumor shows a solid pattern of growth. (**A** courtesy of Dr. Annekathryn Goodman, Massachusetts General Hospital, Boston. **B** from Kumar V, Abbas AK, Fausto N: Robbins and Cotran Pathologic Basis of Disease, 7th ed. Philadelphia, 2007, WB Saunders, p. 1182.)

polypoid	**Growths that are like projections extending outward from a base.** **Sessile** polypoid tumors extend from a broad base, and **pedunculated** polypoid tumors extend from a stem or stalk. Both benign and malignant tumors of the colon may grow as polyps. See Figure 19–8, *A*.
ulcerating	**Characterized by an open, exposed surface resulting from the death of overlying tissue.** Ulcerating tumors often are found in the stomach, breast, colon, and skin. See Figure 19–8, *B*.

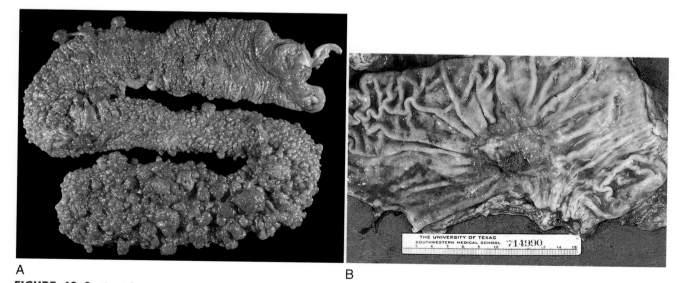

FIGURE 19–8   **A, Adenomatous polyposis** of the colon, These innumerable polypoid adenomas have a 100% frequency of progression to colon adenocarcinoma. **B, Gastric carcinoma** with a large irregular **ulcer.** (**A** from Kumar V, Abbas AK, Fausto N: Robbins and Cotran Pathologic Basis of Disease, 7th ed. Philadelphia, WB Saunders, 2007, p. 862. **B** from Kumar V, Cotran RS, Robbins SL: Robbins Basic Pathology, 7th ed. Philadelphia, WB Saunders, 2003, p. 562.)

19

verrucous	**Resembling a wart-like growth.** Tumors of the gingiva (gum) frequently are verrucous.

MICROSCOPIC DESCRIPTIONS

alveolar	**Tumor cells form patterns resembling small, microscopic sacs;** commonly found in tumors of muscle, bone, fat, and cartilage.
carcinoma in situ	**Referring to localized tumor cells that have not invaded adjacent structures.** (Latin *in situ* means in place.) Cancer of the cervix may begin as carcinoma in situ.
diffuse	**Spreading evenly throughout the affected tissue.** Malignant lymphomas may display diffuse involvement of lymph nodes.
dysplastic	**Abnormal appearing cells; not clearly cancerous.** Dysplastic nevi (moles on skin) are an example. They are often forerunners of skin cancers.
epidermoid	**Resembling squamous epithelial cells (thin, plate-like);** often occurring in the respiratory tract.
follicular	**Forming small, microscopic, gland-type sacs.** Thyroid gland cancer or lymphomas are examples. See Figure 19–9, *A*.
papillary	**Forming small, finger-like or nipple-like projections of cells.** Bladder or thyroid cancers are examples. See Figure 19–9, *B*.
pleomorphic	**Composed of a variety of types of cells.** Mixed-cell tumors are examples.
scirrhous	**Densely packed (scirrhous means hard) tumors, containing dense bands of fibrous tissue;** commonly found in breast or stomach cancers.
undifferentiated	**Lacking microscopic structures typical of normal mature cells.**

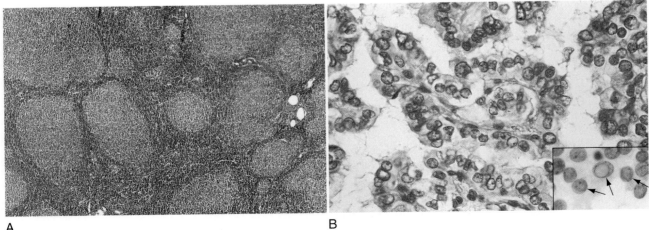

A   B

FIGURE 19–9   A, Follicular non-Hodgkin lymphoma involving a lymph node. **B, Papillary carcinoma** of the thyroid. (**A** from Kumar V, Abbas AK, Fausto N: Robbins and Cotran Pathologic Basis of Disease, 7th ed. Philadelphia, WB Saunders, 2007, p. 675. **B** from Cotran RS, Kumar V, Collin T: Robbins Pathologic Basis of Disease, 6th ed. Philadelphia, WB Saunders, 1999, p. 1143.)

GRADING AND STAGING SYSTEMS

Tumors are classified on the basis of their location, microscopic appearance, and extent of spread. Of particular importance are the tumor's **grade** (its degree of maturity or differentiation under the microscope) and its **stage** (its extent of spread within the body). These two properties influence the prognosis (the chances of successful treatment and survival) and determine the specific treatment to be used.

When **grading** a tumor, the pathologist is concerned with the microscopic appearance of the tumor cells, specifically with their degree of maturation or differentiation. Often, three or four grades are used. **Grade I** tumors are very well differentiated, so that they closely resemble cells from the normal parent tissue of their origin. **Grade IV** tumors are so undifferentiated or anaplastic that even recognition of the tumor's tissue of origin may be difficult. **Grades II** and **III** are intermediate in appearance, moderately or poorly differentiated, as opposed to well differentiated (grade I) and undifferentiated (grade IV).

Grading is often of value in determining the prognosis of certain types of cancers, such as cancer of the urinary bladder, prostate gland, ovary, and brain tumors (astrocytomas). Patients with grade I tumors have a high survival rate, and patients with grade II, III, and IV tumors have an increasingly poorer survival rate. Grading is also used in evaluating cells obtained from body fluids in preventive screening tests, such as **Papanicolaou (Pap) smears** of the uterine cervix, tracheal secretions, or stomach secretions.

The **staging** of cancerous tumors is based on the extent of spread of the tumor. An example of a staging system is the **TNM/International Staging System.** It has been applied to malignancies such as lung cancer, as well as to many other tumors. **T** refers to the size and degree of local extension of the **tumor; N** refers to the number of regional lymph **nodes** that have been invaded by tumor; and **M** refers to the presence or absence of **metastases** (spreads to distant sites) of the tumor cells. Numbers denote size and degree of involvement: For example, 0 indicates undetectable, and 1, 2, 3, and 4 a progressive increase in size or involvement. TNM may be based on clinical data (physical examination and radiologic assessment) or actual histopathologic evaluation of the tumor and adjacent lymph nodes. In some cases, bone marrow, liver, or other tissues are biopsied to confirm metastases. Table 19–5 presents the TNM staging system for lung cancer.

Table 19–5

International TNM Staging System for Lung Cancer

Stage	TNM Description	5-year Survival Rate (%)
I	T1-2, N0, M0	60–80
II	T1-2, N1, M0	25–50
III A	T3, N0-1, M0	25–40
	T1-3, N2, M0	10–30
III B	Any T4 or N3, M0	<5
IV	Any M1	<5

PRIMARY TUMOR (T)

T1	Tumor <3 cm diameter
T2	Tumor >3 cm diameter or has associated atelectasis-obstructive pneumonitis extending to the hilar region
T3	Tumor with direct extension into the chest wall, diaphragm, mediastinum, pleura, or pericardium
T4	Tumor invades the mediastinum or presence of a malignant pleural effusion

REGIONAL LYMPH NODES (N)

N0	No node involvement
N1	Metastasis to lymph nodes in the peribronchial and ipsilateral (same side as the primary tumor) hilar region
N2	Metastasis to ipsilateral hilar and subcarinal (under the bifurcation of the trachea into the lungs) lymph nodes
N3	Metastasis to contralateral mediastinal or hilar nodes or any nodes near the clavicular (collar) bone

DISTANT METASTASIS (M)

M0	No known metastasis
M1	Distant metastasis present with site specified (e.g., brain, liver)

TNM = tumor-node-metastases.
< = less than; > = more than.
Data from Harrison's Manual of Medicine, 15th ed. New York, McGraw-Hill Professional, 2002, p. 284.

CANCER TREATMENT

Four major approaches to cancer treatment are **surgery, radiation therapy, chemotherapy, and biological therapy.** Each method **(modality)** may be used alone, but often they are used together in combined-modality programs to improve the overall diagnosis and treatment result.

SURGERY

In many patients with cancer, the tumor is discovered before it has spread, and it may be cured by surgical excision. Some common cancers in which surgery may be curative are those of the stomach, breast, colon, lung, and uterus (endometrium). Often, surgical removal of the primary tumor prevents local spread or complications, even in the presence of distant disease. A **debulking procedure** may be used if the tumor is attached to a vital organ and cannot be completely removed. As much tissue as possible is removed and the patient receives **adjuvant** (assisting) radiation or chemotherapy.

The following is a list of terms that describe surgical procedures used in diagnosing and treating cancer.

cauterization	Process of burning tissue to destroy it. Examples are electrocauterization (using a needle or snare heated by electric current), laser, dry ice, and chemicals.
cryosurgery	Use of subfreezing temperature to destroy tissue.
en bloc resection	Tumor is removed along with a large area of surrounding tissue containing lymph nodes. Modified radical mastectomy, colectomy, and gastrectomy are examples.
excisional biopsy	Removal of tumor and a margin of normal tissue. This procedure provides a specimen for diagnosis and may be curative for small tumors.
exenteration	Wide resection involving removal of the tumor, its organ of origin, and all surrounding tissue in the body space. Pelvic exenteration may be performed to treat large primary tumors of the uterus.
fulguration	Destruction of tissue by electric sparks generated by a high-frequency current.
incisional biopsy	Piece of tumor is removed for examination to establish a diagnosis. More extensive surgical procedure or other forms of treatment, such as chemotherapy or x-ray therapy, then are used to treat the bulk of the tumor.

RADIATION THERAPY (RADIATION ONCOLOGY)

The goal of **radiation therapy (RT)** is to deliver a maximal dose of ionizing radiation **(irradiation)** to the tumor tissue and a minimal dose to the surrounding normal tissue. In reality, this goal is difficult to achieve, and usually one accepts a degree of residual normal cell damage **(morbidity)** as a side effect of the destruction of the tumor. High-dose radiation produces damage to DNA. Newer techniques of radiation utilize high-energy beams of **protons** (atomic particles) to improve the focus of the beam and limit damage to normal tissues.

19

Terms used in the field of radiation therapy for cancer are as follows:

brachytherapy
Implantation of small, sealed containers or seeds of radioactive material directly into the tumor (interstitial therapy); or in close proximity to the tumor (intracavitary therapy). An implant may be temporary (as in tumors of the head and neck or gynecologic malignancies) or permanent with prostatic implants (seeds) into tumors.

electron beams
Low-energy beams for treatment of skin or surface tumors.

external beam radiation (teletherapy)
Radiation therapy applied to a tumor from a distant source (linear accelerator).

fields
Dimensions of the size of radiation area used to treat a tumor from a specific angle.

fractionation
A method of dividing radiation into small, repeated doses rather than fewer large doses. Fractionation allows larger total doses to be given while causing less damage to normal tissue.

gray (Gy)
Unit of absorbed radiation dose. Historically, the term was **rad** (100 rads equals 1 Gy).

irradiation
Exposure to any form of radiant energy such as light, heat, or x-rays.

linear accelerator
Large electronic device that produces high-energy x-ray (or photon) beams for the treatment of deep-seated tumors. (See Figure 19–10.) Intraoperative radiation therapy (IORT) is direct application of radiation during surgery using a linear accelerator in the operating room. Sensitive structures can be moved from the field during the radiation.

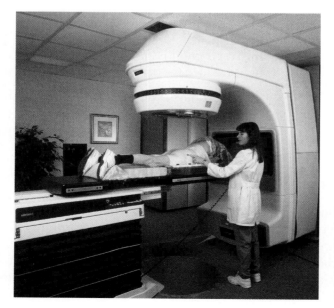

FIGURE 19–10 Linear accelerator. Radiation therapy (photon therapy) delivered to a patient positioned under a linear accelerator receiving treatment for a lesion in the posterior portion of his hip. (Courtesy of Dr. Arthur Brimberg, Riverhill Radiation Oncology, Yonkers, New York.)

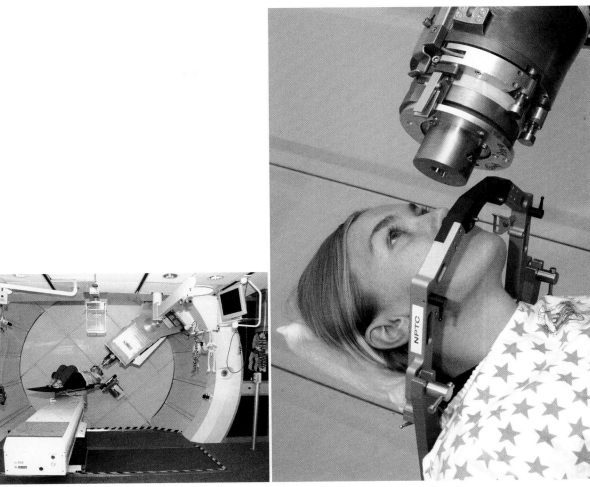

A   B

FIGURE 19–11 **A, Proton therapy machine.** Proton beam radiation therapy is useful in treating a variety of cancers including head and neck, brain, sarcomas, eye tumors, prostate, chest, and GI tumors. **B, Proton stereotactic radiosurgery.** A model poses to show how a proton beam device is brought near a patient in preparation for stereotactic radiosurgery. (Courtesy of Dr. Jay Loeffler, Massachusetts General Hospital Radiation Oncology Department, Boston.)

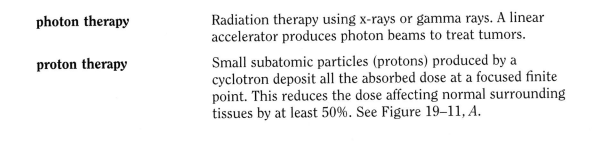

photon therapy — Radiation therapy using x-rays or gamma rays. A linear accelerator produces photon beams to treat tumors.

proton therapy — Small subatomic particles (protons) produced by a cyclotron deposit all the absorbed dose at a focused finite point. This reduces the dose affecting normal surrounding tissues by at least 50%. See Figure 19–11, *A*.

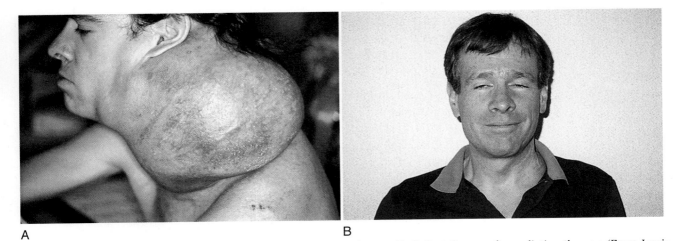

A   B

FIGURE 19–12   A, Patient with Hodgkin disease before radiation therapy. **B,** Patient 6 years after radiation therapy. (From Lewis SM, Heitkemper MM, Dirksen SR: Medical-Surgical Nursing: Assessment and Management of Clinical Problems, 5th ed. St. Louis, Mosby, 2000, p. 287.)

radiocurable tumor	Tumor that can be completely eradicated by radiation therapy. Usually, this is a localized tumor with no evidence of metastasis. Lymphomas and Hodgkin disease are examples. (See Figure 19–12.)
radioresistant tumor	Tumor that requires large doses of radiation to produce death of the cells. Connective tissue tumors are the most radioresistant.
radiosensitive tumor	Tumor in which irradiation can cause the death of cells without serious damage to surrounding tissue. Tumors of hematopoietic (blood-forming) and lymphatic origins are radiosensitive.
radiosensitizers	Drugs that increase the sensitivity of tumors to x-rays. Many cancer chemotherapy drugs, especially 5-fluorouracil and cisplatin, sensitize tumors and normal tissue to radiation, thereby improving the outcome of treatment.
simulation	Study prior to radiation therapy using CT scan or MRI to map treatment. Simulation is required for all patients undergoing RT.
stereotactic radiosurgery	A single large dose of radiation (gamma knife surgery) delivered under stereotactic (highly precise) guidance to destroy a vascular abnormality (arteriovenous malformation, which is a tangle of blood vessels in the brain) or to treat small intracranial tumors. See Figure 19–11, *B.*

Radiotherapy, although it may be either a **palliative** (relieving symptoms) or curative agent, can produce undesirable side effects on normal body tissues that are incidentally irradiated. Some complications are reversible with time, and recovery takes place soon after radiotherapy is completed. Side effects include the following:

Alopecia (baldness); usually permanent with radiation

Fibrosis (increase in connective tissue) in the lungs

Mucositis (inflammation and ulceration of mucous membranes); in the mouth, pharynx, vagina, bladder, large or small intestine

Myelosuppression (bone marrow depression); anemia, leukopenia, and thrombocytopenia

Nausea and vomiting; as reaction to radiation to the brain (vomiting center is located in the brain) or gastrointestinal tract (loss of epithelial lining tissue)

Pneumonitis (inflammation of the lungs)

Xerostomia (dryness of the mouth); occurs after radiation to the salivary glands

CHEMOTHERAPY, BIOLOGICAL THERAPY, AND DIFFERENTIATING AGENTS

Chemotherapy

Cancer chemotherapy is the treatment of cancer using chemicals (drugs). It is the standard treatment for many types of cancer, and it produces cures in most patients who have choriocarcinoma, testicular cancer, acute lymphocytic leukemia, and Hodgkin disease. Chemotherapy may be used alone or in combination with surgery and radiation to improve cure rates.

The field of **pharmacokinetics** (**-kinetic** means pertaining to movement) is concerned with measuring the amount of drug that is present over time in various body compartments (such as blood, urine, and spinal fluid). These measurements require specialized analytical equipment.

The ideal is to develop drugs that kill large numbers of tumor cells without harming normal cells. Because normal cells, such as bone marrow and gastrointestinal lining cells, have a rapidly dividing cell population, they suffer considerable damage from antitumor drugs. Scientists working in the field of pharmacokinetics measure the rate of disappearance of drugs from the bloodstream and tissues. They also use information from research to design better routes (oral, intravenous) and schedules of administration to achieve the greatest tumor kill with the least toxicity (harm) to normal cells.

Combination chemotherapy is the use of two or more antitumor drugs together to kill a specific type of malignant growth. In chemotherapy, drugs are given according to a written **protocol,** or plan, that details the route, schedule, and frequency of doses administered. Usually, drug therapy is continued until the patient achieves a complete **remission,** the absence of all signs of disease. At times, chemotherapy is an **adjuvant** (aid) to surgery. Drugs are used to kill possible hidden disease in patients who, after surgery, are otherwise free of any evidence of malignancy.

Drugs cause tumor cells to die by damaging their DNA. Tumor cells with damaged DNA undergo **apoptosis,** or self-destruction. They have impaired capacity to repair their DNA and, in general, are less able than normal cells to survive DNA damage due to drugs and radiation.

The following are categories of cancer chemotherapeutic agents. Table 19–6 lists the specific drugs in each of these categories and the particular cancers they are used to treat.

1. **Alkylating agents.** These are synthetic compounds containing one or two alkyl groups. The chemicals interfere with the process of DNA synthesis by attaching to DNA molecules. Toxic side effects include nausea and vomiting, diarrhea, bone marrow depression (myelosuppression), and alopecia (hair loss). These are common side effects because cells in the gastrointestinal tract, bone marrow, and scalp are rapidly dividing cells, which, along with tumor cells, are susceptible to the lethal effects of chemotherapeutic drugs. Most side effects disappear after treatment is suspended.

2. **Antibiotics.** These drugs are produced by bacteria or fungi. They act by binding to DNA in the cell, thus promoting DNA strand breaks and preventing the replication or copying of DNA. Toxic side effects include alopecia, stomatitis (inflammation of the mouth), myelosuppression, and gastrointestinal disturbances.

3. **Antimetabolites.** These drugs inhibit the synthesis of nucleotide components of DNA, or they may act as fraudulent copies of normal nucleotides and become incorporated into the DNA strand, where they directly block the replication of DNA. Toxic side effects are myelosuppression with leukopenia, thrombocytopenia, and anemia; and damage to cells that line the mouth and digestive tract leading to stomatitis, nausea, and vomiting.

4. **Antimitotics.** These chemicals are derived from bacteria, fungi, or plants or from animals found on coral reefs or in the ocean. **Taxol** and the vinca alkaloids are isolated from plants and block the function of the cell structural protein, the microtubule, which is essential for mitosis. They are used frequently in combination with other chemotherapeutic agents. Side effects include myelosuppression, alopecia, and nerve damage.

5. **Hormonal agents.** Hormones are a class of chemicals made by endocrine glands in the body. Examples are estrogens made in the ovaries and androgens made in the testes and adrenal glands. Hormones attach to receptor proteins in target tissues. The hormone-receptor complex stimulates certain normal tissues, such as breast or uterine lining cells, to divide and grow. Some tumors, such as prostate cancers, depend on the presence of a hormone (in this case, androgens) to grow, and hormone removal (orchiectomy) leads to tumor regression. Steroid (cholesterol-derived) hormones, such as prednisone, have growth-inhibiting effects on leukemias and breast cancer. Other compounds, called hormone antagonists, are designed to block the growth-promoting effects of estrogens or androgens, and are used in breast cancer and prostate cancer, respectively.

Breast cancers have **estrogen receptors.** These tumors respond to the removal of estrogen by oophorectomy or the use of antiestrogen drugs such as **tamoxifen,** which block estrogenic effects. **Flutamide** blocks androgen action and causes regression of prostate cancer. **Aromatase inhibitors**, such as anastrozole, prevent the conversion of androgen to estrogen, and starve breast tumors of their estrogen supply in postmenopausal women.

Table 19–6

Selected Cancer Chemotherapeutic Agents and the Cancers They Treat

Chemotherapeutic Agent	Type of Cancer
ALKYLATING AGENTS	
Carmustine (BCNU)	Brain
Carboplatin (Paraplatin)	Ovarian
Chlorambucil (Leukeran)	Chronic lymphocytic leukemia (CLL)
Cisplatin (Platinol)	Testicular; ovarian
Cyclophosphamide (Cytoxan)	Lymphoma
Dacarbazine (DTIC-Dome)	Hodgkin lymphoma
Mechlorethamine, nitrogen mustard (Mustargen)	Lymphoma
Melphalan (Alkeran)	Multiple myeloma
Temozolomide (Temodar)	Brain (glioma)
ANTIBIOTICS	
Capecitabine (Xeloda)	Breast and colon
Bleomycin (Blenoxane)	Testicular
Daunorubicin (Cerubidine)	Acute myelogenous leukemia (AML)
Doxorubicin (Adriamycin, Doxil)	Breast
Idarubicin (Idamycin)	Acute myelogenous leukemia (AML)
Mitomycin C (Mutamycin)	Lung
ANTIMETABOLITES	
Cladribine (Leustatin)	Hairy cell leukemia
Cytarabine (ara-C, Cytosar-U)	Acute myelogenous leukemia (AML)
Fludarabine (Fludara)	Chronic lymphocytic leukemia (CLL)
5-Fluorouracil, 5-FU (various)	Colon
Methotrexate, MTX (Folex, Mexate)	Acute lymphocytic leukemia (ALL)
Pentostatin, DCF (Nipent)	Hairy cell leukemia
ANTIMITOTICS	
Docetaxel (Taxotere)	Breast
Paclitaxel (Taxol)	Breast, ovary
Vinca alkaloids	Lymphoma
Vinblastine (Velban)	
Vincristine (Oncovin)	
Vinorelbine (Navelbine)	Breast
HORMONES AND HORMONE ANTAGONISTS	
Anastrozole (Arimidex)	Breast
Dexamethasone (Decadron)	Lymphoma
Flutamide (Eulexin)	Prostate
Letrozole (Femara)	Breast
Leuprolide (Lupron)	Prostate
Prednisone (various)	Acute lymphocytic leukemia (ALL)
Tamoxifen (Nolvadex)	Breast

Note: Brand names are in parentheses.

19

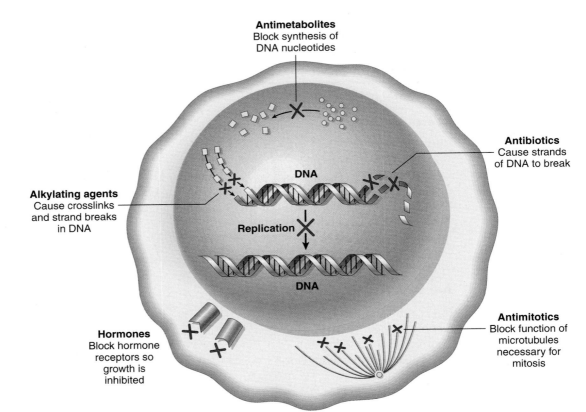

FIGURE 19–13 Mechanisms of action of cancer chemotherapeutic agents.

Figure 19–13 illustrates the mechanisms of action of cancer chemotherapeutic agents. Often, drugs are administered in combination, according to carefully planned regimens. Table 19–7 gives examples of drug combination regimens (protocols).

The newest class of anticancer drugs are **molecularly targeted drugs.** These drugs are designed to block the function of growth factors, their receptors, and signaling pathways

Table 19–7

Cancers and Chemotherapeutic Regimens

Type of Cancer	Combination	Regimen
Breast	**AC**	**A**driamycin (doxorubicin) **C**yclophosphamide
Bladder	**M-VAC**	**M**ethotrexate **V**inblastine **A**driamycin (doxorubicin) **C**isplatin
Hodgkin disease	**ABVD**	**A**driamycin (doxorubicin) **B**leomycin **V**inblastine **D**acarbazine
Ovarian	**Carbo-Tax**	**Carbo**platin **Tax**ol (paclitaxel)

Note: Generic names are in parentheses.

in tumor cells. **Gleevec** (imatinib mesylate), which blocks the *bcr-abl* tyrosine kinase in CML cells (see Figure 19–5), is the first drug of this type approved for use in cancer. **Tarceva** (erlotinib) is a new drug for lung cancer that blocks epidermal growth factor receptor (EGFR), which is overly active in many such tumors.

Tumor cells grow by establishing a new blood supply via **angiogenesis** (growth of new blood vessels). Tumors secrete specific proteins, such as vascular endothelial growth factor (VEGF), which stimulates the formation of new vessels. **Antiangiogenic drugs** interfere with angiogenesis. Examples of these drugs are **Avastin** (bevacizumab), a monoclonal antibody that destroys VEGF, and **Sutent** (sunitinib), a drug that blocks the VEGF receptor. These drugs prevent tumor growth by blocking the growth of new blood vessels. Thalomid (thalidomide) is believed to act as an antiangiogenic agent and is useful in treating multiple myeloma, a plasma cell tumor.

Biological Therapy

Another approach to cancer treatment is to use the body's own defenses to fight tumor cells. Investigators are exploring how the elements of the immune system can be restored, enhanced, mimicked, and manipulated to destroy cancer cells. Substances produced by normal cells that directly block tumor growth or that stimulate the immune system and other body defenses are called **biological response modifiers.** Examples of these substances are **interferons** (made by lymphocytes), **monoclonal antibodies** (made by mouse cells and capable of binding to human tumors), **colony-stimulating factors (CSFs)** that stimulate blood-forming cells to combat the myelosuppressive side effects of chemotherapy, and **interleukins** that stimulate the immune system to destroy tumors. Table 19–8 lists various biological agents and their modes of action.

Table 19–8

Biological Agents and Their Modes of Action

Biological Agent	Mode of Action
Bevacizumab (Avastin)	Monoclonal antibody that binds to VEGF
Cetuximab (Erbitux)	Monoclonal antibody that binds to EGFR
Darbepoetin alfa (Aranesp)	Long-acting erythropoietin
Erythropoietin (Epogen, Procrit)	Promotes growth of red blood cells
Filgrastim (Neupogen)	Colony-stimulating factor; promotes the growth of white blood cells (leukocytes)
Gemtuzumab ozogamicin (Mylotarg)	Monoclonal antibody with an attached toxin; binds specifically to leukemia cells and allows the toxin to enter and kill cells
Interferons (Roferon, Intron)	Promote broad immune response
Interleukin 2, or IL-2 (Interleukin-2)	Promotes immune response of T lymphocytes
Pegfilgrastim (Neulasta)	Long-acting filgrastim (Neupogen)
Rituximab (Rituxan)	Monoclonal antibody binding to cell surface receptor; induces apoptosis
Trastuzumab (Herceptin)	Monoclonal antibody binding to cell surface; blocks growth-signaling pathways within cell; induces apoptosis

Note: Brand names are in parentheses.

19

Table 19–9

Newest Anticancer Drugs and Their Modes of Action

Drug	Mode of Action
All-trans retinoic acid, or ATRA	Differentiating agent; useful in acute promyelocytic leukemia (APL)
Arsenic trioxide (Trisenox)	Differentiating agent; useful in acute promyelocytic leukemia (APL)
Erlotinib (Tarceva)	Binds to EGFR and prevents its signals from stimulating tumor cells to grow.
Imatinib mesylate (Gleevec)	Molecularly targeted drug; useful in chronic myelogenous leukemia (CML)
Thalidomide (Thalomid)	Antiangiogenic drug; useful in multiple myeloma

Note: Brand names are in parentheses.

Differentiating Agents

Some new drugs cause tumor cells to differentiate, stop growing, and die. These include ATRA (all-trans retinoic acid), a vitamin A derivative, which is highly active against acute promyelocytic leukemia (APL), and arsenic trioxide (Trisenox), which has similar effects on APL. Table 19–9 lists the newest anticancer drugs with their modes of action.

VOCABULARY

This list reviews many of the new terms introduced in the text. Short definitions reinforce your understanding of the terms. Refer to the Pronunciation of Terms section for help with unfamiliar or difficult words.

adjuvant therapy	Assisting primary treatment. Drugs are given early in the course of treatment, along with surgery or radiation to attack cancer cells that may be too small to be detected by diagnostic techniques.
alkylating agents	Synthetic chemicals containing alkyl groups that interfere with DNA synthesis.
anaplasia	Loss of differentiation of cells; reversion to a more primitive cell type.
angiogenesis	Process of forming new blood vessels.
antibiotics	Chemical substances, produced by bacteria or primitive plants. They inhibit the growth of cells and are used in cancer chemotherapy.
antimetabolites	Chemicals that prevent cell division by inhibiting formation of substances necessary to make DNA; used in cancer chemotherapy.
antimitotics	Drugs that block mitosis (cell division). Taxol is an antimitotic used to treat breast and ovarian cancers.
apoptosis	Programmed cell death. (Apo- means off, away; -ptosis means to fall.) Normal cells undergo apoptosis when damaged or aging. Some cancer cells have lost the ability to undergo apoptosis, and they live forever.

benign tumor	Noncancerous growth (neoplasm).
biological response modifiers	Substances produced by normal cells that either directly block tumor growth or stimulate the immune system to fight cancer.
biological therapy	Use of the body's own defenses to destroy tumor cells.
carcinogens	Agents that cause cancer; chemicals and drugs, radiation, and viruses.
carcinoma	Cancerous tumor made up of cells of epithelial origin.
cellular oncogenes	Pieces of DNA that, when broken or dislocated, can cause a normal cell to become malignant.
chemotherapy	Treatment with drugs.
combination chemotherapy	Use of several chemotherapeutic agents together for the treatment of tumors.
dedifferentiation	Loss of differentiation of cells; reversion to a more primitive, embryonic cell type; anaplasia or undifferentiation.
deoxyribonucleic acid (DNA)	Genetic material within the nucleus of a cell; controls cell division and protein synthesis.
differentiating agents	Drugs that promote tumor cells to differentiate, stop growing, and die.
differentiation	Specialization of cells; unspecialized cells are modified and altered to form specific and characteristic types and functions.
electron beams	Low-energy beams of radiation for treatment of skin or surface tumors.
encapsulated	Surrounded by a capsule; benign tumors are encapsulated.
external beam radiation	Radiation applied to a tumor from a distant source.
fields	Dimensions of the size of radiation used to treat a tumor from a specific angle.
fractionation	Giving radiation in small, repeated doses.
genetic screening	Family members are tested to determine whether they have inherited a cancer-causing gene.
grading of tumors	Evaluating the degree of maturity of tumor cells or indication of malignant transformation.
gray (Gy)	Unit of absorbed radiation dose.
gross description of tumors	Visual appearance of tumors to the naked eye: cystic, fungating, inflammatory, medullary, necrotic, polypoid, ulcerating, and verrucous tumors.
infiltrative	Extending beyond normal tissue boundaries.
invasive	Having the ability to enter and destroy surrounding tissue.
irradiation	Exposure to any form of radiant energy such as light, heat, or x-rays.
linear accelerator	Large electronic device that produces high-energy x-ray beams for treatment of deep-seated tumors.
malignant tumor	Tending to become worse and result in death; having the characteristics of invasiveness, anaplasia, and metastasis.

mesenchymal	Embryonic connective tissue; mes = middle, enchym/o = to pour. This is the tissue from which connective tissues (bone, muscle, fat, cartilage) arise.
metastasis	Spread of a malignant tumor to a secondary site; literally, beyond (meta-) control (-stasis).
microscopic description of tumors	Appearance of tumors when viewed under a microscope: alveolar, carcinoma in situ, diffuse, dysplastic, epidermoid, follicular, papillary, pleomorphic, scirrhous, undifferentiated.
mitosis	Replication of cells; a stage in a cell's life cycle involving the production of two identical cells from a parent cell.
mixed-tissue tumors	Tumors composed of different types of tissue (epithelial as well as connective tissue).
modality	Method of treatment, such as surgery, chemotherapy, or radiation.
molecularly targeted drugs	Anticancer drugs designed to block the function of growth factors, their receptors, and signaling pathways in specific tumor cells.
morbidity	Condition of being diseased; describing damage to normal tissues.
mucinous	Containing mucus.
mutation	Change in the genetic material (DNA) of a cell; may be caused by chemicals, radiation, or viruses or may occur spontaneously.
neoplasm	New growth; benign or malignant tumors.
nucleotide	Unit of DNA (gene) composed of a sugar, phosphate and a base. The sequence or arrangement of nucleotides on a gene is the genetic code.
oncogene	Region of DNA in tumor cells (cellular oncogene) or in viruses that cause cancer (viral oncogene). Oncogenes are designated by a three-letter word, such as *abl*, *erb*, *jun*, *myc*, *ras*, and *src*.
palliative	Relieving but not curing symptoms.
pedunculated	Possessing a stem or stalk (peduncle); characteristic of some polypoid tumors.
pharmacokinetics	Study of the distribution in and removal of drugs from the body over a period of time.
photon therapy	Radiation therapy using energy in the form of x-rays or gamma rays.
protocol	Detailed plan for treatment of an illness.
proton therapy	Subatomic particles (protons) produced by a cyclotron deposit an absorbed dose of radiation at a focused finite point in the body.
radiation	Energy carried by a stream of particles.
radiocurable tumor	Tumor cells that are destroyed by radiation therapy.
radioresistant tumor	Tumor cells that require large doses of radiation to be destroyed.
radiosensitive tumor	Tumor in which radiation can cause the death of cells without serious damage to surrounding tissue.
radiosensitizers	Drugs that increase the sensitivity of tumors to x-rays.
radiotherapy	Treatment of tumors using radiation; radiation oncology.
relapse	Return of symptoms of disease.

remission	Partial or complete disappearance of symptoms of disease.
ribonucleic acid (RNA)	Cellular substance that, along with DNA, plays an important role in protein synthesis.
sarcoma	Cancerous tumor derived from connective or flesh tissue.
serous	Pertaining to a thin, watery fluid (serum).
sessile	Having no stem; characteristic of some polypoid tumors.
simulation	Study using CT scan or MRI to map treatment before RT is given.
solid tumor	Tumor composed of a mass of cells.
staging of tumors	System of evaluating the extent of spread of tumors. An example is the TNM system (tumor-node-metastasis).
stereotactic radiosurgery	Dose of radiation delivered under stereotactic (highly precise) guidance (gamma knife surgery)
steroids	Complex, naturally occurring chemicals, such as hormones, that are used in cancer chemotherapy.
surgical procedures to treat cancer	Methods of removing cancerous tissue: cryosurgery, cauterization, en bloc resection, excisional biopsy, exenteration, fulguration, incisional biopsy.
viral oncogenes	Pieces of DNA from viruses that infect a normal cell and cause it to become malignant.
virus	An infectious agent that reproduces by entering a host cell and using the host's genetic material to make copies of itself.

COMBINING FORMS, SUFFIXES, PREFIXES, AND TERMINOLOGY

Write the meanings of the medical terms in the spaces provided.

COMBINING FORMS

Combining Form	Meaning	Terminology	Meaning
alveol/o	small sac	alveolar _____	
		Microscopic description of tumor cell arrangement (found in connective tissue tumors).	
cac/o	bad	cachexia _____	
		General ill health and malnutrition (wasting of muscle and emaciation) associated with chronic, severe disease (-hexia means habit).	
carcin/o	cancer, cancerous	carcinoma in situ _____	
		Localized cancer; confined to the site of origin.	

19

Combining Form	Meaning	Terminology	Meaning
cauter/o	burn, heat	electrocauterization _____	
chem/o	chemical, drug	chemotherapy _____	
cry/o	cold	cryosurgery _____	
cyst/o	sac of fluid	cystic tumor _____	
fibr/o	fibers	fibrosarcoma _____	
follicul/o	small glandular sacs	follicular _____ *A microscopic description of cellular arrangement in glandular tumors.*	
fung/i	fungus, mushroom	fungating tumor _____	
medull/o	soft, inner part	medullary tumor _____	
mucos/o	mucous membrane	mucositis _____	
mut/a	genetic change	mutation _____ *-ation means process.*	
mutagen/o	causing genetic change	mutagenic _____	
necr/o	death	necrotic _____	
onc/o	tumor	oncology _____	
papill/o	nipple-like	papillary _____ *A microscopic description of tumor cell growth.*	
pharmac/o	chemical, drug	pharmacokinetics _____ *The suffix -kinetic means pertaining to movement.*	
plas/o	formation	dysplastic _____ *Microscopic description of cells that are highly abnormal but not clearly cancerous. The suffix -tic means pertaining to.*	
ple/o	many, more	pleomorphic _____ *Microscopic description of tumors that are composed of a variety of cells.*	
polyp/o	polyp	polypoid tumor _____ *The suffix -oid means resembling.*	
radi/o	rays, x-rays	radiotherapy _____	
sarc/o	flesh, connective tissue	osteosarcoma _____	
scirrh/o	hard	scirrhous _____ *Microscopic description of densely packed, fibrous tumor cell composition.*	
xer/o	dry	xerostomia _____	

SUFFIXES

Suffix	Meaning	Terminology	Meaning
-blastoma	immature tumor	retinoblastoma _____	
		neuroblastoma _____	
		This sarcoma of nervous system origin affects infants and children up to the age of 10 years, usually arising in the autonomic nervous system or adrenal medulla.	
-genesis	formation	angiogenesis _____	
-oma	mass, tumor	adenocarcinoma _____	
-plasia	formation, growth	hyperplasia _____	
-plasm	formation, growth	neoplasm _____	
-suppression	to stop	myelosuppression _____	
-therapy	treatment	biological therapy _____	

PREFIXES

Prefix	Meaning	Terminology	Meaning
ana-	backward	anaplasia _____	
apo-	off, away	apoptosis _____	
brachy-	short (distance)	brachytherapy _____	
		Radiation delivered in close range to tumor site.	
epi-	upon	epidermoid _____	
		Microscopic description of tumor cells that resemble epidermal tissue.	
meta-	beyond; change	metastasis _____	
		metaplasia _____	
		The abnormal transformation of adult differentiated cells to differentiated tissue of another kind. This change is reversible. An example is the change (from columnar epithelial cells to squamous epithelial cells) that occurs in the respiratory epithelium of habitual cigarette smokers.	
prot/o	first	protocol _____	
		The ending –col, from Latin kolla, means glued page. A protocol is a written plan detailing the procedures to be followed in research or treatment.	
tele-	far	teletherapy _____	

LABORATORY TESTS

19

protein marker tests	**Measure the level of proteins in the blood or on the surface of tumor cells.**

These tests diagnose cancer or detect its recurrence after treatment. Examples are:

Protein	Where Measured	Type of Cancer
acid phosphatase	blood	prostate
alpha-fetoprotein (AFP)	blood	liver and testicular
beta-hCG	blood	choriocarcinoma and testicular
CA-125	blood	ovarian
CEA (carcinoembryonic antigen)	blood	colorectal and GI
estrogen receptor	tumor cells	breast
PSA (prostate-specific antigen)	blood	prostate
15.3 and 29.7	blood	breast
19.9	blood	pancreatic

CLINICAL PROCEDURES

The following are specialized procedures used to detect or treat malignancies. X-rays, CT scans, MRI, and ultrasound (described throughout the text and specifically in Chapter 20) also are important diagnostic procedures in oncology.

bone marrow biopsy	**Aspiration of bone marrow tissue and examination under a microscope for evidence of malignant cells.**

bone marrow or stem cell transplant	**Bone marrow or stem cells infused intravenously into a patient.**

In an **autologous transplant,** marrow previously obtained from the patient and stored is reinfused when needed. In an **allogeneic transplant** (all/o means other), marrow is obtained from a living donor other than the recipient. In a **stem cell transplant,** immature blood cells called stem cells are harvested from the peripheral blood of a patient instead of from the bone marrow. After receiving chemotherapy, the patient gets a reinfusion of the stem cells to repopulate the bone marrow with blood cells.

fiberoptic colonoscopy	**Visual examination of the colon using a fiberoptic instrument.**

This is an important screening procedure using an endoscope to detect cancer and remove premalignant polyps.

exfoliative cytology	**Cells are scraped from the region of suspected disease and examined under a microscope.** The Pap test (smear) to detect carcinoma of the cervix and vagina is an example (Fig. 19–14).
laparoscopy	**Visual examination of the abdominal cavity using small incisions and a laparoscope. Also known as peritoneoscopy.**
mammography	**X-ray examination of the breast to detect breast cancer.**
needle (core) biopsy	**Insertion of a needle into tissue to remove a core of cells for microscopic examination.** The physician uses needle aspiration to withdraw free cells from a fluid-filled cavity (cystic areas of the breast), or from a solid mass of tumor.
radionuclide scans	**Radioactive substances (radionuclides) are injected intravenously, and scans (images) of organs are obtained.** These tests detect tumor and metastases. Examples of radionuclides are gallium 67 (whole-body scan), rose Bengal (liver), and technetium 99m (liver and spleen).

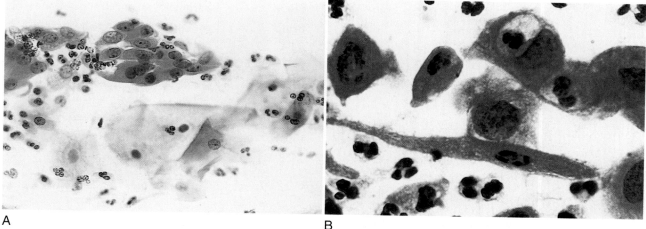

A   B

FIGURE 19–14   **A, Normal exfoliative cytologic smear (Pap smear) from the cervicovaginal region.** It shows flattened squamous cells and some neutrophils as well. **B, Abnormal cervicovaginal smear** shows numerous malignant cells that have pleomorphic (irregularly shaped) and hyperchromatic (stained) nuclei. (Courtesy of Dr. P. K. Gupta, Department of Pathology and Laboratory Medicine, University of Pennsylvania Medical Center, Philadelphia.)

ABBREVIATIONS

AFP	alpha-fetoprotein
BMT	bone marrow transplantation
bx	biopsy
CA	cancer
CEA	carcinoembryonic antigen
cGy	centigray (one hundredth of a gray) or rad
chemo	chemotherapy
CR	complete response—disappearance of all tumor
CSF	colony-stimulating factor—examples are G-CSF (granulocyte colony–stimulating factor) and GM-CSF (granulocyte-macrophage colony–stimulating factor)
DES	diethylstilbestrol
DNA	deoxyribonucleic acid
EGFR	epidermal growth factor receptor
ER	estrogen receptor
EPO	erythropoietin; promotes growth of red blood cells
5-FU	5-fluorouracil
Ga	gallium
GIST	gastrointestinal stromal tumor
Gy	gray—unit of absorbed radiation dose
H&E	hematoxylin and eosin—dyes used to stain pathology specimens
IGRT	intensity-modulated gated radiation therapy—use of imaging mechanism attached to linear accelerator is added to IMRT to gate (track) a tumor moving during respiration

IMRT	intensity-modulated radiation therapy—non-uniform intensities to tiny photon beams create a more specialized delivery than is possible with standard RT
IORT	intraoperative radiation therapy
mets	metastases
MoAb	monoclonal antibody
NED	no evidence of disease
NHL	non-Hodgkin lymphoma
Pap smear	Papanicolaou smear
PD	progressive disease—tumor increases in size
PR	partial response—tumor is one-half its original size
prot.	protocol
PSA	prostate-specific antigen
PSCT	peripheral stem cell transplant
PSRS	proton stereotactic radiosurgery
RNA	ribonucleic acid
RT	radiation therapy
SD	stable disease—tumor does not shrink but does not grow
TNM	tumor, nodes, metastases
VEGF	vascular endothelial growth factor
XRT, RT	radiation therapy

PRACTICAL APPLICATIONS

This section contains an FYI (for your information) exercise followed by an actual medical report and chart rounds using terms that you have studied in this and previous chapters. Answers to questions are on page 812.

FYI: MALIGNANT TUMORS WHOSE NAMES DO NOT CONTAIN THE COMBINING FORM CARCIN/O OR SARC/O

Malignant Tumor	Description
glioma	primary brain tumor
hepatoma	liver tumor (hepatocellular carcinoma)
hypernephroma	kidney tumor
lymphoma	lymph node tumor
melanoma	tumor of pigmented skin cells
mesothelioma	tumor of cells within the pleura
multiple myeloma	bone marrow cell tumor
thymoma	thymus gland tumor

Questions

1. Which tumor develops from a dysplastic nevus? _____

2. Which tumor arises from an organ located within the mediastinum?

   _____

3. Which tumor arises from an organ in the RUQ of the abdomen? _____

4. Which tumor has types called astrocytoma, ependymoma, glioblastoma multiforme?

   _____

5. Which tumor is also known as a renal cell carcinoma? _____

6. Which tumor is characterized by large numbers of plasma cells (bone marrow antibody-producing cells)? _____

7. Which tumor arises from membrane cells surrounding the lungs? _____

8. Which tumor has a type known as Hodgkin disease? _____

CASE REPORT

A 52-year-old married woman presented to her physician with a painless mass in her left breast. During breast examination a 1.0-cm, firm, nontender mass was palpated in the upper outer quadrant located at the 2 o'clock position, 3 cm from the areola. The mass was not fixed to the skin, and there was no cutaneous erythema or edema. No axillary or supraclavicular lymphadenopathy was noted.

An excisional biopsy of the mass was performed. The pathology report described a gross specimen of fatty breast tissue. Microscopic evaluation of the nodule revealed a scirrhous carcinoma. The margins of the excision were free of tumor. Sentinel node biopsy revealed no tumor involvement.

A portion of the specimen was sent for estrogen receptor assay and proved to be positive. The patient was informed of the diagnosis and underwent additional studies, including chest x-ray, liver chemistries, CBC, and bone scan; all results were negative.

The patient was staged as having a T1N0M0, stage I carcinoma of the left breast. She was referred to a radiation oncologist for primary radiation therapy. After completion of radiotherapy, she was treated with tamoxifen. Prognosis is excellent for cure.

Questions

1. Where was the primary breast lesion located?
   a. Under the pigmented area of the breast
   b. About an inch and a half to the upper left of the nipple and pigmented area
   c. Near the axilla and under the shoulder blade

2. Other associated findings were:
   a. Redness and swelling
   b. Enlarged lymph nodes under the armpit
   c. None of the above

3. The tumor was composed of:
   a. Dense connective tissue, giving it a hard structure
   b. Soft, glandular tissue
   c. Cells that had extended into the skin overlying the tumor

4. What procedure gave evidence that the tumor had not yet metastasized?
   a. Estrogen receptor assay
   b. Excisional biopsy of the mass
   c. Sentinel node biopsy

5. What additional therapy was undertaken?
   a. Bone scan, liver chemistries, CBC, and chest x-ray
   b. Radiation to the breast
   c. Radiation to the breast and hormonal treatment

6. Tamoxifen was prescribed because:
   a. The tumor was found to be nonresponsive to estrogen
   b. The tumor was found to be responsive to estrogen, and tamoxifen is an antiestrogen
   c. The tumor was a stage I carcinoma

CHART ROUNDS:
CENTER FOR RADIATION ONCOLOGY

(a) Patient has metastatic carcinoma and is being treated palliatively with 3000 cGy to the costovertebral junction.

(b) Patient is being treated for cervical esophageal carcinoma. Previously treated with a hockey field technique [XRT given covering the area in the shape of a hockey stick] for breast cancer and recurrent field is only being taken to 3000 cGy.

(c) Patient is being treated for a pathologic stage IIB Hodgkin disease on the mantle [upper chest and neck]-only protocol.

(d) The patient is being treated for a parietal GBM (glioblastoma multiforme). The plan needs to be signed. The films look fine.

Questions

1. Which patient is being treated for a brain tumor?_____
2. Which patient is being treated for lesions in the ribs? _____
3. Which patient has disease in cervical and thoracic lymph nodes? _____
4. Which patient is being treated for gastrointestinal cancer? _____

PATHOLOGY REPORT:
GROSS DESCRIPTION

The spleen weighs 127 grams, and measures 13.0×9.2 cm. External surface is smooth, leathery, homogeneous, and dark purplish-brown. There are no defects in the capsule. The blood vessels of the hilum of the spleen are patent, with no thrombi or other abnormalities. On section of the spleen at 2 to 3 mm intervals, there are three well-defined, pale gray nodules on the cut surface, ranging for 0.5 to 1.1 cm in greatest dimension. The remainder of the cut surface is homogeneous, dark purple, and firm. Possible diagnosis: Hodgkin disease

Question

Which information leads the pathologist to the diagnosis?
    a. Blood clots in patent blood vessels
    b. Capsular defects
    c. Uniform, smooth surface
    d. Pale gray nodules suggestive of invasive tumor

19

EXERCISES

Remember to check your answers carefully with those given in the Answers to Exercises, page 810.

A. Identify the following characteristics of malignant tumors based on their definitions as given below. Word parts are given as clues.

   1. loss of differentiation of cells and reversion to a more primitive cell type:

     ana_____

   2. extending beyond the normal tissue boundaries: in_____

   3. having the ability to enter and destroy surrounding tissue: in_____

   4. spreading to a secondary site: meta_____

B. Match the following terms or abbreviations with their meanings below.

chemical carcinogen	mitosis	RNA
DNA	mutation	ultraviolet radiation
ionizing radiation	oncogene	virus

   1. replication of cells; two identical cells are produced from a parent cell _____

   2. change in the genetic material of a cell _____

   3. genetic material within the nucleus that controls replication and protein synthesis

     _____

   4. cellular substance (ribonucleic acid) that is important in protein synthesis

     _____

   5. rays given off by the sun; can be carcinogenic _____

   6. energy carried by a stream of particles; can be carcinogenic _____

   7. infectious agent that reproduces by entering a host cell and using the host's genetic material to

     make copies of itself _____

   8. a region of genetic material found in tumor cells and in viruses that cause cancer

     _____

   9. an agent (hydrocarbon, insecticide, hormone) that causes cancer _____

C. Give the meanings of the following terms.

   1. solid tumor _____

   2. adenoma _____

   3. adenocarcinoma _____

   4. osteoma _____

   5. osteosarcoma _____

   6. mixed-tissue tumor _____

   7. neoplasm _____

   8. pharmacokinetics _____

   9. benign _____

  10. differentiation _____

D. Name the terms that describe microscopic tumor growth. Definitions and word parts are given.

   1. small nipple-like projections: pap_____

   2. abnormal formation of cells: dys_____

   3. localized growth of cells: carcin_____

   4. densely packed; containing fibrous tissue: _____ous

   5. patterns resembling small, microscopic sacs: alv_____

   6. small, gland-type sacs: foll_____

   7. variety of cell types: pleo_____

   8. lacking structures typical of mature cells: un_____

   9. spreading evenly throughout the tissue: di_____

  10. resembling epithelial cells: epiderm_____

E. Match the following gross descriptions of tumors with their meanings as given below.

cystic	medullary	ulcerating
fungating	necrotic	verrucous
inflammatory	polypoid	

   1. containing dead tissue _____

   2. mushrooming pattern of growth: tumor cells pile on top of each other _____

   3. characterized by large, open, exposed surfaces _____

   4. characterized by redness, swelling, and heat _____

   5. growths are projections from a base; sessile and pedunculated tumors are examples

     _____

   6. tumors from large, open spaces filled with fluid; serous and mucinous tumors are examples

     _____

   7. tumors resemble wart-like growths _____

   8. tumors are large, soft, and fleshy _____

19

F. Circle or supply the appropriate medical terms.

1. A **(carcinoma/sarcoma)** is a cancerous tumor composed of cells of epithelial tissue. An example of such a cancerous tumor is a/an _____.

2. A **(carcinoma/sarcoma)** is a cancerous tumor composed of connective tissue. An example of such a cancerous tumor is a/an _____.

3. Retinoblastoma and polyposis coli syndrome are examples of **(chemical carcinogens/inherited cancers)**.

4. The assessment of a tumor's degree of maturity or microscopic differentiation is **(grading/staging)** of the tumor.

5. The assessment of a tumor's extent of spread within the body is known as **(grading/staging)**.

6. In the TNM staging system, T stands for **(tissue/tumor)**, N stands for **(node/necrotic)**, and M stands for **(mitotic/metastasis)**.

7. The transformation of adult, differentiated tissue to differentiated tissue of another type is called **(metaplasia/anaplasia)**.

8. The formation of new blood vessels is known as **(apoptosis/angiogenesis)**.

G. Match the surgical procedure in Column I with its meaning in Column II. Write the letter of the meaning in the space provided.

Column I

1. fulguration _____
2. en bloc resection _____
3. incisional biopsy _____
4. excisional biopsy _____
5. cryosurgery _____
6. cauterization _____
7. exenteration _____

Column II

A. Removal of tumor and a margin of normal tissue for diagnosis and possible cure of small tumors
B. Burning a lesion to destroy tumor cells
C. Wide resection involving removal of tumor, its organ of origin, and surrounding tissue in the body space
D. Destruction of tissue by electric sparks generated by a high-frequency current
E. Removal of entire tumor and regional lymph nodes
F. Freezing a lesion to kill tumor cells
G. Cutting into a tumor and removing a piece to establish a diagnosis

H. Give medical terms for the following.

1. The method of treating cancer using high-energy radiation is _____.

2. If tumor tissue requires large doses of radiation to kill cells, it is a/an _____ tumor.

3. If radiation can cause loss of tumor cells without serious damage to surrounding regions, the tumor is _____.

4. A tumor that can be completely eradicated by RT is a/an _____ tumor.

5. The method of giving radiation in small, repeated doses is _____.

6. Drugs that increase the sensitivity of tumors to x-rays are _____.

7. Treatment of cancerous tumors with drugs is _____.

8. The study of the distribution and disappearance of drugs in the body is _____.

9. The use of two or more drugs to kill tumor cells is _____.

10. Large electronic device that produces high-energy x-ray or photon beams for treatment of

    deep-seated tumors is a/an_____.

11. Alkylating agents, antimetabolites, hormones, antibiotics, and antimitotics all are types of

    _____ agents.

12. Implantation of seeds of radioactive material directly into a tumor is _____.

13. The unit of absorbed radiation dose is _____.

14. Radiation applied to a tumor from a distant source is_____.

15. Technique in which subatomic particles produced by a cyclotron deposit a focused dose at a finite

    point is _____.

16. Dimension of the size of radiation area from a specific angle_____.

17. Study performed before RT using CT or MRI to map treatment is _____.

18. Technique in which a single large dose of radiation is delivered under precise 3D guidance to

    destroy vascular abnormalities and small brain tumors is _____.

I. **Match each of the following side effects of radiotherapy and chemotherapy with its description or treatment described below.**

alopecia   nausea   pneumonitis
fibrosis   oral mucositis   xerostomia
myelosuppression

1. Ulceration of lining cells in the mouth caused by radiation to the jaw: _____

2. Drug treatment for breast cancer destroys epithelial cells in the stomach and causes a sensation

   leading to vomiting: _____

3. Radiation to the lungs causes inflammation of the lungs: _____

4. Chemotherapy for ovarian cancer causes loss of hair on the head: _____

5. Bone marrow destruction with leukopenia, anemia, and thrombocytopenia:

   _____

6. Radiation to the lungs causes increase in connective tissue: _____

7. Radiation of salivary glands causes dryness of the mouth: _____

19

J. Give the meanings of the following medical terms.

1. modality _____

2. adjuvant therapy _____

3. protocol _____

4. remission _____

5. relapse _____

6. morbidity _____

7. biological therapy _____

8. biological response modifiers _____

9. interferon _____

10. monoclonal antibodies _____

11. apoptosis _____

12. cachexia _____

13. differentiating agents _____

14. molecularly targeted drugs _____

15. nucleotide _____

K. Match the test or procedure with its description below.

beta-HCG test	estrogen receptor assay	needle biopsy
bone marrow biopsy	exfoliative cytology	PSA test
CA-125	laparoscopy	stem cell transplant
CEA test		

1. test for the presence of a portion of human chorionic gonadotropin hormone (a marker for

   testicular cancer) _____

2. protein marker for ovarian cancer detected in the blood _____

3. visual examination of the abdominal cavity; peritoneoscopy _____

4. test for the presence of a hormone receptor on breast cancer cells _____

5. removal and microscopic examination of bone marrow tissue _____

6. aspiration of tissue for microscopic examination _____

7. blood test for the presence of an antigen related to prostate cancer _____

8. blood test for carcinoembryonic antigen (marker for GI cancer) _____

9. cells are scraped off tissue and microscopically examined _____

10. blood-forming cells are infused intravenously _____

L. Circle the correct term to complete each sentence.

1. Pauline was diagnosed with a meningioma, which is usually a (an) **(benign, anaplastic, necrotic)** tumor. The doctor told her that it was not malignant, but that it should be removed because of the pressure it was causing on the surrounding tissues.

2. Marlene underwent surgical resection of her breast mass. Dr. Smith recommended **(dedifferentiated, modality, adjuvant)** therapy because her tumor was large and she had one positive lymph node.

3. Unfortunately, at the time of diagnosis, the tumor had spread to distant sites because it was **(pleomorphic, metastatic, mutagenic)**. The oncologist recommended beginning chemotherapy as soon as possible.

4. The polyp in Lisa's colon was *not* pedunculated, and Dr. Sidney described it as flat and **(fungating, scirrhous, sessile)**.

5. Mr. Elder had difficulty urinating and had an elevated PSA test. Dr. Jones examined him and found a hard prostate gland. **(Laparoscopy, Electrocauterization, Biopsy)** demonstrated adenocarcinoma.

6. During the days following her chemotherapy for breast cancer, Doris experienced loss of appetite and **(fibrosis, nausea, xerostomia)**. Blood tests revealed low levels of blood cells, indicating **(hematopoiesis, myeloma, myelosuppression)**. Her physician prescribed **(EPO, VEGF, DES)** for anemia and **(Ca, cGy, G-CSF)** for leukopenia.

7. After being diagnosed with lung cancer, Mr. Smith's tumor was staged according to the **(DNA, RNA, TNM)** International Staging System. His stage was IIIA, indicating **(tumor <3 cm diameter, distant metastases, tumor with direct extension to the chest wall)**.

8. Mr. Smith's doctor told him he needed **(CA-125, XRT, PSA)** because his tumor was nonoperable and could not be **(resected, irradiated, electrocauterized)**.

19

MEDICAL SCRAMBLE

Unscramble the letters to form cancer-related terms from the clues. Use the letters in the squares to complete the bonus term. Answers are found on page 812.

1. *Clue:* Partial or complete disappearance of symptoms of disease.

   ___ ☐ ☐ ___ ___ ___ ___ ___ ☐   SNEMIIRSO

2. *Clue:* Spread of a cancerous tumor to another site or secondary location.

   ☐ ___ ___ ☐ ___ ___ ___ ___ ___ ☐   TTAEAISSSM

3. *Clue:* Pertaining to abnormal formation or development of cells; not clearly malignant.

   ___ ☐ ___ ___ ___ ___ ___ ___ ___ ☐   CLYASSPTID

4. *Clue:* Increased growth in numbers of normal cells.

   ☐ ___ ___ ☐ ___ ___ ☐ ___ ___ ___ ___   SPERIAYPHAL

BONUS TERM: *Clue:* Pertaining to embryonic connective tissue from which connective tissue tumors (sarcomas) arise.

☐ ☐ ☐ ☐ ☐ ☐ ☐ ☐ ☐ ☐

ANSWERS TO EXERCISES

A

1. anaplasia
2. infiltrative
3. invasive
4. metastasis

B

1. mitosis
2. mutation
3. DNA (deoxyribonucleic acid)
4. RNA
5. ultraviolet radiation
6. ionizing radiation
7. virus
8. oncogene
9. chemical carcinogen

C

1. tumor composed of a mass of cells
2. tumor of glandular tissue (benign)
3. cancerous (malignant) tumor of glandular tissue
4. tumor of bone (benign)
5. flesh (connective tissue) tumor of bone (malignant)
6. tumor composed of different types of tissue (both epithelial and connective tissues)
7. new formation (tumor)
8. study of the distribution and removal of drugs in the body over a period of time
9. noncancerous
10. specialization of cells

D

1. papillary
2. dysplastic
3. carcinoma in situ
4. scirrhous
5. alveolar
6. follicular
7. pleomorphic
8. undifferentiated
9. diffuse
10. epidermoid

E

1. necrotic
2. fungating
3. ulcerating
4. inflammatory
5. polypoid
6. cystic
7. verrucous
8. medullary

F

1. carcinoma; thyroid adenocarcinoma, squamous cell carcinoma
2. sarcoma; liposarcoma, chondrosarcoma, osteogenic sarcoma
3. inherited cancers
4. grading
5. staging
6. tumor; node; metastasis
7. metaplasia
8. angiogenesis

G

1. D
2. E
3. G
4. A
5. F
6. B
7. C

H

1. radiation therapy
2. radioresistant
3. radiosensitive
4. radiocurable
5. fractionation
6. radiosensitizers
7. chemotherapy
8. pharmacokinetics
9. combination chemotherapy
10. linear accelerator
11. chemotherapeutic agents
12. brachytherapy
13. gray
14. external beam radiation (teletherapy)
15. proton therapy
16. fields
17. simulation
18. stereotactic radiosurgery

I

1. oral mucositis
2. nausea
3. pneumonitis
4. alopecia
5. myelosuppression
6. fibrosis
7. xerostomia

J

1. method of treatment
2. assisting treatment
3. report or plan of steps taken in an experiment or disease case
4. absence of all signs of disease
5. symptoms of disease return
6. conditions of damage to normal tissue; disease
7. treatment that uses the body's own defense mechanisms to fight tumor cells
8. substances produced by normal cells that directly block tumor growth or that stimulate the immune system
9. a biological response modifier that is made by lymphocytes
10. biological response modifiers that are made by mouse cells and are able to bind to tumor cells
11. programmed cell death
12. malnutrition marked by weakness and emaciation; usually associated with later stages of cancer
13. drugs that promote tumor cells to differentiate (mature), stop growing, and die
14. anticancer drugs designed to block the function of growth factors, their receptors, and signaling pathways in tumor cells
15. unit of DNA composed of a sugar, phosphate, and base (adenine, cytosine, guanine, or thymine)

K

1. beta-hCG test
2. CA-125
3. laparoscopy
4. estrogen receptor assay
5. bone marrow biopsy
6. needle biopsy
7. PSA test
8. CEA test
9. exfoliative cytology
10. stem cell transplant

L

1. benign
2. adjuvant
3. metastatic
4. sessile
5. biopsy
6. nausea; myelosuppression; EPO; G-CSF
7. TNM; tumor with direct extension to the chest wall
8. XRT; resected

19

ANSWERS TO PRACTICAL APPLICATIONS

FYI: Malignant Tumors

1. melanoma (a nevus is a benign pigmented lesion or mole)
2. thymoma
3. hepatoma
4. glioma
5. hypernephroma
6. multiple myeloma
7. mesothelioma
8. lymphoma (previously known as lymphosarcoma)

Case Report

1. b
2. c
3. a
4. c
5. c
6. b

Chart Rounds

1. patient D
2. patient A
3. patient C
4. patient B

Pathology Report

1. d

ANSWERS TO MEDICAL SCRAMBLE

1. REMISSION 2. METASTASIS 3. DYSPLASTIC 4. HYPERPLASIA
BONUS TERM: MESENCHYMAL

PRONUNCIATION OF TERMS

PRONUNCIATION GUIDE

ā as in āpe   ă as in ăpple
ē as in ēven   ĕ as in ĕvery
ī as in īce   ĭ as in ĭnterest
ō as in ōpen   ŏ as in pŏt
ū as in ūnit   ŭ as in ŭnder

To test your understanding of the terminology in this chapter, write the meaning of each term in the space provided. In addition, you may wish to cover the terms and write them by looking at your definitions. Make sure your spelling is correct. The page number after each term indicates where it is defined or used in the book, so you can easily check your responses. You will find complete definitions for all of these terms and their audio pronunciations on the CD.

VOCABULARY AND TERMINOLOGY

Term	Pronunciation	Meaning
adenocarcinoma (797)	ăd-ĕ-nō-kăr-sĭ-NŌ-mă	
adjuvant therapy (792)	ĂD-jū-vănt THĔR-ă-pē	
alkylating agents (792)	ĂL-kĭ-lā-tĭng Ā-jents	
alopecia (787)	ăl-ō-PĒ-shē-ă	
alveolar (795)	ăl-vē-Ō-lăr *or* ăl-VĒ-ō-lăr	
anaplasia (792)	ăn-ă-PLĀ-zē-ă	
angiogenesis (797)	ăn-jē-ō-GĔN-ĕ-sĭs	
antibiotics (792)	ăn-tĭ-bī-ŎT-ĭks	
antimetabolites (792)	ăn-tĭ-mĕ-TĂB-ō-līts	
antimitotics (792)	ăn-tĭ-mī-TŎT-ĭks	

Term	Pronunciation	Meaning
apoptosis (797)	ăp-ō-TŌ-sĭs *or* ā-pŏp-TŌ-sĭs	
benign tumor (793)	bē-NĪN TOO-měr	
biological response modifier (793)	bī-ō-LŎJ-ĭ-kăl rě-SPŎNS MŎD-ĭ-fī-ěr	
biological therapy (793)	bī-ō-LŎJ-ĭ-kăl THĚR-ă-pē	
bone marrow biopsy (798)	bōn MĂ-rō BĪ-ŏp-sē	
bone marrow transplant (798)	bōn MĂ-rō TRĂNZ-plănt	
brachytherapy (797)	brā-kē-THĚ-ră-pē	
cachexia (795)	kă-KĔK-sē-ă	
carcinogen (793)	kăr-SĬN-ō-jěn	
carcinoma (793)	kăr-sĭ-NŌ-ma	
carcinoma in situ (795)	kăr-sĭ-NŌ-ma ĭn SĪ-too	
cauterization (783)	kăw-těr-ĭ-ZĀ-shŭn	
cellular oncogenes (793)	SĔL-ū-lăr ŎNGK-ō-jēnz	
chemotherapy (793)	kē-mō-THĚR-ă-pē	
combination chemotherapy (793)	KŎM-bĭ-NĀ-shŭn kē-mō-THĚR-ă-pē	
cryosurgery (796)	krī-ō-SŬR-jěr-ē	
cystic tumor (796)	SĬS-tĭk TOO-mŏr	
dedifferentiation (793)	dē-dĭf-ěr-ěn-shē-Ā-shŭn	
deoxyribonucleic acid (793)	dē-ŏx-ē-rī-bō-noo-KLĀ-ĭk ĂS-ĭd	
differentiating agents (793)	dĭf-ěr-ĔN-shē-ā-tĭng Ā-gěnts	
differentiation (793)	dĭf-ěr-ěn-shē-Ā-shŭn	
dysplastic (796)	dĭs-PLĂS-tĭk	
electron beams (793)	ē-LĔK-trŏn bēmz	
en bloc resection (783)	ěn blŏk rē-SĔK-shŭn	
encapsulated (793)	ěn-KĂP-sū-lāt-ěd	
epidermoid (797)	ěp-ĭ-DĚR-moyd	
excisional biopsy (783)	ek-SIZH-ŭn-ăl BĪ-ŏp-sē	
exenteration (783)	ěks-ěn-tě-RĀ-shŭn	
exfoliative cytology (799)	ěks-FŌ-lē-ā-tĭv sī-TŎL-ō-jē	
external beam radiation (793)	ěks-TĚR-năl bēm rā-dē-Ā-shŭn	
fiberoptic colonoscopy (798)	fī-běr-ŎP-tĭk kō-lōn-ŎS-kō-pē	
fibrosarcoma (796)	fī-brō-săr-KŌ-ma	
fibrosis (787)	fī-BRŌ-sĭs	

19

Term	Pronunciation	Meaning
follicular (796)	fō-LĬK-ū-lăr	
fractionation (793)	frăk-shă-NĀ-shŭn	
fulguration (783)	fŭl-gū-RĀ-shŭn	
fungating tumor (796)	fŭng-GĀ-tĭng *or* FŬNG-gā-tĭng TOO-mŏr	
genetic screening (793)	gĕ-NĚT-ĭk SCRĒ-nĭng	
grading of tumors (793)	GRĀ-dĭng ŏf TOO-mŏrz	
gray (793)	grā	
gross description of tumors (793)	GRŌS dĕ-SKRĬP-shŭn ŏf TOO-mŏrz	
hyperplasia (797)	hī-pĕr-PLĀ-zē-ă	
incisional biopsy (783)	ĭn-SĪZH-ŭn-ăl BĪ-ŏp-sē	
infiltrative (793)	ĬN-fĭl-trā-tĭv	
invasive (793)	ĭn-VĀ-sĭv	
irradiation (793)	ĭr-rā-dē-Ā-shŭn	
laparoscopy (799)	lă-păr-ŎS-kō-pē	
linear accelerator (793)	LĬN-ē-ăr ăk-sĕl-ĕ-RĀ-tŏr	
malignant tumor (793)	mă-LĬG-nănt TOO-mŏr	
mammography (799)	mă-MŎG-ră-fē	
medullary tumor (796)	MĚD-ū-lār-ē TOO-mŏr	
mesenchymal (794)	mĕs-ĕn-KĪ-măl	
metaplasia (797)	mĕ-tă-PLĀ-zē-ă	
metastasis (797)	mĕ-TĂS-tă-sĭs	
microscopic description of tumors (794)	mī-krō-SKŎP-ĭk dĕ-SKRĬP-shŭn ŏv TOO-mŏrz	
mitosis (794)	mī-TŌ-sĭs	
mixed-tissue tumors (794)	MĬKSD–TĬ-shū TOO-mŏrz	
modality (794)	mō-DĂL-ĭ-tē	
molecularly targeted drugs (794)	mō-LĚK-kū-lăr-lē TĂR-gĕt-ĕd drŭgz	
morbidity (794)	mŏr-BĬD-ĭ-tē	
mucinous (794)	MŪ-sĭ-nŭs	
mucositis (796)	mū-kō-SĪ-tĭs	
mutagenic (796)	mū-tă-JĚN-ĭk	
mutation (794)	mū-TĀ-shŭn	

Term	Pronunciation	Meaning
myelosuppression (797)	mī-ĕ-lō-sū-PRĔ-shŭn	_____
necrotic tumor (796)	nĕ-KRŎT-ĭk TOO-mŏr	_____
needle (core) biopsy (799)	NĒ-dl (kŏr) BĪ-ŏp-sē	_____
neoplasm (794)	NĒ-ō-plăzm	_____
neuroblastoma (797)	nŭ-rō-blăs-TŌ-mă	_____
nucleotide (794)	NŪ-klē-ō-tīd	_____
oncogene (794)	ŎNGK-ō-jēn	_____
oncology (796)	ŏn-KŎL-ō-jē	_____
osteosarcoma (796)	ŏs-tē-ō-săr-KŌ-mă	_____
palliative (794)	PĂL-ē-ă-tĭv	_____
papillary (796)	PĂP-ĭ-lăr-ē	_____
pedunculated (794)	pĕ-DŬNG-kū-lāt-ĕd	_____
pharmacokinetics (794)	făr-mă-kō-kĭ-NĔT-ĭks	_____
photon therapy (794)	FŌ-tŏn THĔR-ă-pē	_____
pleomorphic (796)	plē-ō-MŎR-fĭk	_____
pneumonitis (787)	noo-mō-NĪ-tĭs	_____
polypoid tumor (796)	PŎL-ĭ-poyd TOO-mŏr	_____
protein marker test (798)	PRŌ-tēn MĂRK-ĕr tĕst	_____
protocol (794)	PRŌ-tō-kŏl	_____
proton therapy (794)	PRŌ-tŏn THĔR-ă-pē	_____
radiation (794)	rā-dē-Ā-shŭn	_____
radiocurable tumor (794)	rā-dē-ō-KŪR-ă-b'l TOO-mŏr	_____
radionuclide scans (799)	rā-dē-ō-NŪ-klīd skănz	_____
radioresistant tumor (794)	rā-dē-ō-rĕ-ZĬS-tănt TOO-mŏr	_____
radiosensitive tumor (794)	rā-dē-ō-SĔN-sĭ-tĭv TOO-mŏr	_____
radiosensitizers (794)	rā-dē-ō-SĔN-sĭ-tī-zĕrz	_____
radiotherapy (794)	rā-dē-ō-THĔR-ă-pē	_____
relapse (794)	rē-LĂPS	_____
remission (795)	rē-MĬSH-ŭn	_____
retinoblastoma (797)	rĕt-ĭ-nō-blăs-TŌ-mă	_____
ribonucleic acid (795)	rī-bō-noo-KLĒ-ik ĂS-ĭd	_____
sarcoma (795)	săr-KŌ-mă	_____
scirrhous (796)	SKĬR-ŭs	_____
serous (795)	SĒ-rŭs	_____

Term	Pronunciation	Meaning
sessile (795)	SĔS-ĭl	_____
simulation (795)	sĭm-ū-LĀ-shŭn	_____
solid tumor (795)	SŎL-ĭd TOO-mŏr	_____
staging of tumors (795)	STĀ-jĭng ŏv TOO-mŏrz	_____
stem cell transplant (798)	stĕm sĕl TRĂNZ-plănt	_____
stereotactic radiosurgery (795)	stĕ-rē-ō-TĂK-tĭc rā-dē-ō-SŬR-jĕr-ē	_____
steroids (795)	STĔR-oydz	_____
teletherapy (797)	tĕl-ē-THĔ-ră-pē	_____
ulcerating tumor (779)	ŬL-sĕ-rā-tĭng TOO-mŏr	_____
verrucous tumor (780)	vĕ-ROO-kŭs TOO-mŏr	_____
viral oncogenes (795)	VĪ-răl ŎNGK-ō-jēnz	_____
virus (795)	VĪ-rŭs	_____
xerostomia (796)	zĕr-ō-STŌ-mē-ă	_____

REVIEW SHEET

Write the meanings of the combining forms in the spaces provided and test yourself. Check your answers with the information in the chapter or in the glossary (Medical Word Parts—English) at the back of the book.

COMBINING FORMS

Combining Form	Meaning	Combining Form	Meaning
aden/o	_____	mut/a	_____
alveol/o	_____	mutagen/o	_____
cac/o	_____	necr/o	_____
carcin/o	_____	onc/o	_____
cauter/o	_____	papill/o	_____
chem/o	_____	pharmac/o	_____
cry/o	_____	plas/o	_____
cyst/o	_____	ple/o	_____
fibr/o	_____	polyp/o	_____
follicul/o	_____	radi/o	_____
fung/i	_____	sarc/o	_____
medull/o	_____	scirrh/o	_____
mucos/o	_____	xer/o	_____

19

SUFFIXES

Suffix	Meaning	Suffix	Meaning
-ary	_____	-ptosis	_____
-blastoma	_____	-stasis	_____
-oid	_____	-stomia	_____
-oma	_____	-suppression	_____
-plasia	_____	-therapy	_____
-plasm	_____		

PREFIXES

Prefix	Meaning	Prefix	Meaning
ana-	_____	epi-	_____
anti-	_____	hyper-	_____
apo-	_____	meta-	_____
brachy-	_____	tele-	_____
dys-	_____		

 Please refer to the enclosed CD for additional exercises and images related to this chapter.

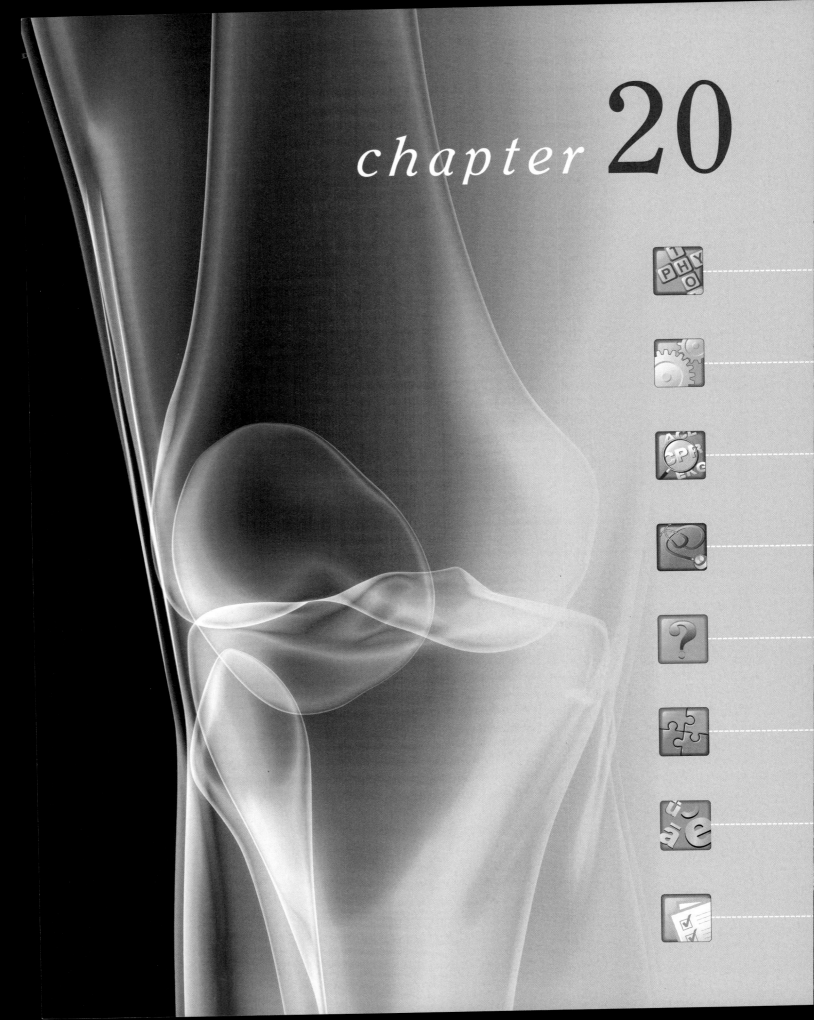

chapter 20

Radiology and Nuclear Medicine

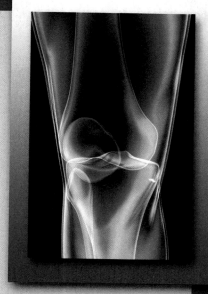

THIS CHAPTER IS DIVIDED INTO THE FOLLOWING SECTIONS

In this chapter you will

- List the physical properties of x-rays.
- Identify diagnostic techniques used by radiologists and nuclear physicians.
- Name the x-ray views and patient positions used in x-ray examinations.
- Describe the role of radioactivity in the diagnosis of disease.
- Recognize medical terms used in the specialties of radiology and nuclear medicine.
- Apply your new knowledge to understanding medical terms in their proper contexts, such as medical reports and records.

Image Description: Vertical x-ray image of the knee joint.

INTRODUCTION

Radiology (also called **roentgenology** after its discoverer, Wilhelm Konrad Roentgen) is the medical specialty concerned with the study of x-rays. **X-rays** are invisible waves of energy that are produced by an energy source (x-ray machine, cathode ray tube) and are useful in the diagnosis and treatment of disease.

Nuclear medicine is the medical specialty that studies the characteristics and uses of **radioactive substances** in the diagnosis of disease. Radioactive substances are materials that emit high-speed particles and energy-containing rays from the interior of their matter. The emitted particles and rays are called **radioactivity** and can be of three types: **alpha particles, beta particles,** and **gamma rays. Gamma rays** are used effectively as a diagnostic label to trace the path and uptake of chemical substances in the body.

The professionals involved in these medical fields are varied. A **radiologist** is a physician who specializes in the practice of diagnostic radiology. A **nuclear medicine physician** specializes in diagnostic nuclear medicine procedures.

Allied health care professionals who work with physicians in the fields of radiology and nuclear medicine are **radiologic technologists.** Different radiologic technologists are **radiographers** (aid physicians in administering diagnostic x-ray procedures), **nuclear medicine technologists** (attend to patients undergoing nuclear medicine procedures and operate devices under the direction of a nuclear physician), and **sonographers** (aid physicians in performing ultrasound procedures).

RADIOLOGY

CHARACTERISTICS OF X-RAYS

Several characteristics of x-rays are useful to physicians in the diagnosis and treatment of disease. Some of these characteristics are the following:

1. **Ability to cause exposure of a photographic plate.** If a photographic plate is placed in front of a beam of x-rays, the x-rays, traveling unimpeded through the air, will expose the silver coating of the plate and cause it to blacken.
2. **Ability to penetrate different substances to varying degrees.** X-rays pass through the different types of substances in the human body (air in the lungs, water in blood vessels and lymph, fat around muscles, and metal such as calcium in bones) with varying ease. Air is the least dense substance and exhibits the greatest transmission. Fat is denser, water is next, followed by metal, which is the densest and transmits least. If the x-rays are absorbed (stopped) by the denser body substance (e.g., calcium in bones), they do not reach the photographic plate held behind the patient, and white areas are left in the x-ray film (plate). Figure 20–1 is an example of an x-ray photograph.

   A substance is said to be **radiolucent** if it permits passage of most of the x-rays. Lung tissue (containing air) is an example of a radiolucent substance, and it appears black on an x-ray image. **Radiopaque** substances (bones) are those that absorb most of the x-rays they are exposed to, allowing only a small fraction of the x-rays to reach the x-ray plate. Thus, normally radiopaque, calcium-containing bone appears white on an x-ray image.
3. **Invisibility.** X-rays cannot be detected by sight, sound, or touch. Workers exposed to x-rays must wear a **film badge** to detect and record the amount of radiation to which they have been exposed. The film badge contains a special film that is exposed

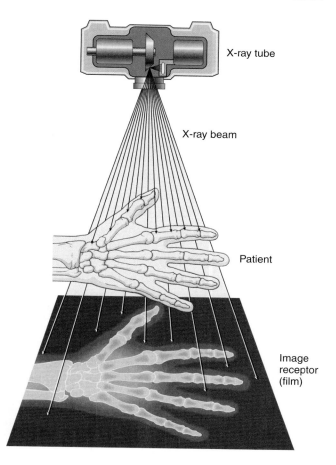

X-ray tube

X-ray beam

Patient

Image
receptor
(film)

FIGURE 20–1 X-ray photograph (radiograph) of the hand. Relative position of x-ray tube, patient (hand), and film necessary to make the x-ray photograph is shown. Bones tend to stop diagnostic x-rays, but soft tissue does not. This results in the light and dark regions that form the image.

by x-rays. The amount of blackness on the film is an indication of the amount of x-rays or gamma rays received by the wearer.

4. **Travel in straight lines.** This property allows the formation of precise shadow images on the x-ray plate and also permits x-ray beams to be directed accurately at a tissue site during radiotherapy.

5. **Scattering of radiation.** Scattering occurs when x-rays come in contact with any material. Greater scatter occurs with dense objects and less scatter with those substances that are radiolucent. In addition, because scatter can cause fog (density that serves no useful purpose) on images, a grid (containing thin lead strips arranged parallel to the x-ray beams) is placed in front of the film to absorb scattered radiation before it strikes the x-ray film. In digital imaging an image receptor replaces film.

6. **Ionization.** X-rays have the ability to ionize substances through which they pass. Ionization is a chemical process in which the energy of an x-ray beam causes rearrangement and disruption within a substance, so that previously neutral particles are changed to charged particles called **ions.** This strongly ionizing ability of x-rays is a double-edged sword. In x-ray therapy, the ionizing effect of x-rays can help kill cancerous cells and stop tumor growth; however, ionizing x-rays in even small doses can affect normal body cells, leading to tissue damage and malignant changes. Thus, persons exposed to high doses of x-rays are at risk of developing leukemia, thyroid tumors, breast cancer, or other malignancies.

DIAGNOSTIC TECHNIQUES

X-Ray Studies

X-ray imaging is used in a variety of ways to detect pathologic conditions. The most common use of diagnostic x-ray studies is in dental practice, to locate cavities (caries) in teeth. Other areas examined include the digestive, nervous, reproductive, and endocrine systems and the chest and bones. Some special diagnostic x-ray techniques are described next.

Computed Tomography (CT). Machines called **CT scanners** beam x-rays at multiple angles through a section of the patient's body. The absorption of all of these x-rays, after they pass through the body, is detected and used by a computer to create multiple views, especially cross-sectional images (Fig. 20–2). The ability of the CT scanner to detect abnormalities (the sensitivity of the scanner) is increased by the use of iodine-containing contrast agents, which outline blood vessels.

The CT scanners are highly sensitive in detecting disease in bones and can actually provide images of internal organs that are impossible to visualize with ordinary x-ray technique. Figure 20–3 shows a series of CT scans through various regions of the body. New ultrafast CT scanners can produce a three-dimensional (3D) image of a beating heart and surrounding blood vessels. They are called "64-slice" CT scanners, and the process is **CT angiography.**

Contrast Studies. In x-ray film, the natural differences in the density of body tissues (e.g., air in lung, calcium in bone) produce contrasting shadow images on the x-ray film; however, when x-rays pass through two adjacent body parts composed of substances of the same density (e.g., different digestive organs in the abdomen), their images cannot be distinguished from one another on the film or on the screen. It is necessary, then, to inject a **contrast medium** into the structure or fluid to be visualized so that a specific part, organ, tube, or liquid can be visualized as a negative imprint on the dense contrast agent.

The following are artificial contrast materials used in diagnostic radiologic studies:

Barium Sulfate. Barium sulfate is a radiopaque medium that is mixed in water and used for examination of the upper and lower GI (gastrointestinal) tract. An **upper GI series (UGI)** involves oral ingestion of barium sulfate so that the esophagus, stomach, and duodenum can be visualized. A **small bowel follow-through (SBFT)** traces the passage of barium in a sequential manner as it passes through the small intestine. A **barium enema (BE)** is a lower gastrointestinal series that opacifies the lumen (passageway) of the large intestine using an enema containing barium sulfate.

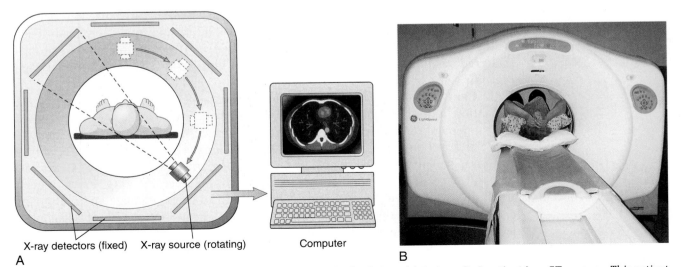

X-ray detectors (fixed)   X-ray source (rotating)   Computer

A   B

FIGURE 20–2   **A, A CT scanner** has a rotating x-ray source and a fixed ring of detectors. **B, A patient in a CT scanner.** This patient has her arms above her head during a chest CT examination.

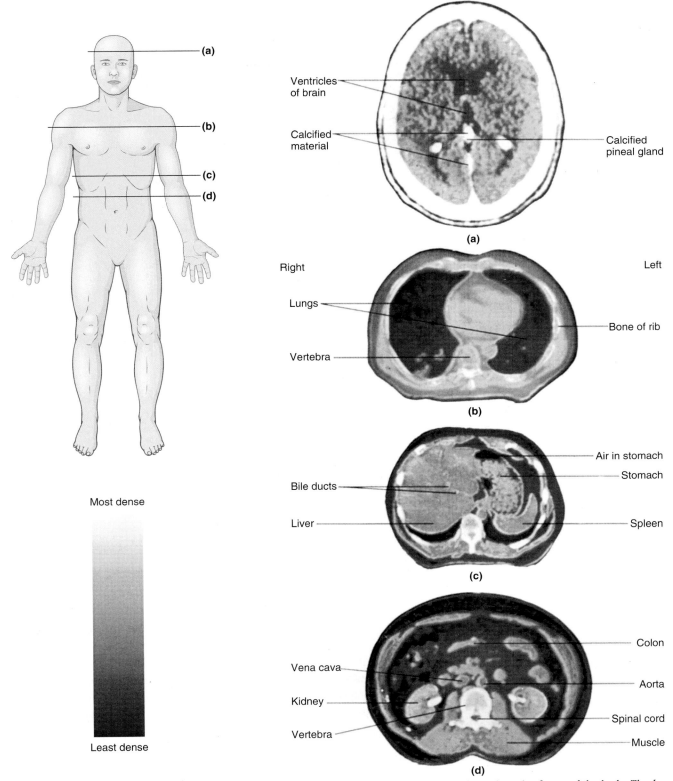

Most dense

Least dense

FIGURE 20–3   CT scans through various regions of the body. The level of the scan is indicated on the figure of the body. The *bar* below the figure indicates the gradient of structure density as represented by black (least dense, such as air) and white (most dense, such as bone). (CT scan courtesy of Professor Jan H. Ehringer.)

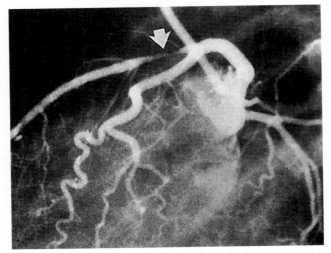

FIGURE 20–4 **Coronary angiography** shows stenosis (see *arrow*) of the left anterior descending coronary artery. (From Braunwald E: Heart Disease: A Textbook of Cardiovascular Medicine, 4th ed. Philadelphia, WB Saunders, 1992.)

A **double-contrast study** uses both a radiopaque and a radiolucent contrast medium. For example, the walls of the stomach or intestine are coated with barium and the lumen is filled with air. The radiographs show the pattern of mucosal ridges.

Iodine Compounds. Radiopaque fluids containing up to 50 percent iodine are used in the following tests:

angiography	**X-ray image (angiogram) of blood vessels and heart chambers is obtained after contrast is injected through a catheter into the appropriate blood vessel or heart chamber.** In clinical practice, the terms angiogram and arteriogram are used interchangeably. Figure 20–4 shows **coronary angiography,** which determines the degree of obstruction of the arteries that supply blood to the heart. Figure 20–5, *A* and *B*, shows coronary angiograms before and after stenting of the artery.
arthrography	**Contrast or air or both are injected into a joint, and x-ray images of the joint are obtained.**
cholangiography	**X-ray imaging after injection of contrast into bile ducts.** This is typically accomplished by injecting contrast directly into the common bile duct via a procedure called **endoscopic retrograde cholangiopancreatography (ERCP)** or after surgery of the gallbladder or biliary tract **(intraoperative cholangiography).** An alternative route for injection of contrast is via a needle through the skin and into the liver. This is **percutaneous transhepatic cholangiography** (Fig. 20–6).

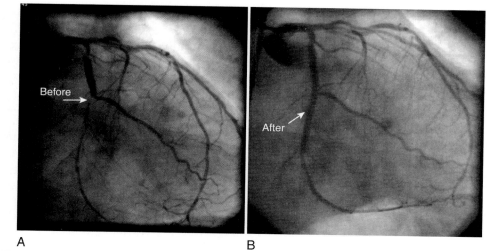

A   B

FIGURE 20–5 **Coronary angiograms before and after stenting. A,** Coronary angiogram before stenting shows narrowed coronary artery preventing blood flow to heart muscle. **B,** Coronary angiogram after stenting shows opening of coronary artery *(arrow)* and increased blood flow to heart muscle. (Courtesy of Dr. Daniel Simon and Mr. Paul Zambino.)

digital subtraction angiography (DSA)	X-ray image of contrast-injected blood vessels is produced by taking two x-ray pictures (the first without contrast) and using a computer to subtract obscuring shadows from the second image.
hysterosalpingography	X-ray record of the endometrial cavity and fallopian tubes is obtained after injection of contrast material through the vagina and into the endocervical canal. This procedure determines the patency of the fallopian tubes.

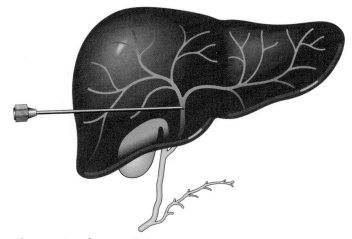

FIGURE 20–6 **Percutaneous transhepatic cholangiography.** Under fluoroscopic visualization, the aspirating needle is passed through the skin and liver tissue until the tip penetrates the hepatic duct. Contrast medium is then introduced, and x-ray pictures are taken to visualize the biliary tree.

myelography	**X-ray imaging of the spinal cord (myel/o) after injection of contrast agent into the subarachnoid space surrounding the spinal cord.** It usually is performed in patients who cannot undergo MRI (magnetic resonance imaging). After injection of contrast, x-ray films and a CT scan are obtained. This procedure is CT myelography.
pyelography	**X-ray imaging of the renal pelvis and urinary tract.** Contrast is injected into a vein (intravenous pyelogram) or through a catheter placed through the urethra, bladder, or ureter and into the renal pelvis **(retrograde pyelogram).** **Urography** also describes the process of recording x-ray images of the urinary tract after the introduction of contrast.

Patients may experience side effects caused by iodine-containing contrast substances. These effects can range from mild reactions such as flushing, nausea, warmth, or tingling sensations to severe, life-threatening reactions characterized by airway spasm, hives, laryngeal edema (swelling of the larynx), vasodilation, and tachycardia. Treatment involves immediate establishment of an airway and ventilation followed by injections of epinephrine (adrenaline), corticosteroids, or antihistamines.

Fluoroscopy. This x-ray procedure uses an image intensifier (fluorescent screen) instead of a photographic plate to derive a visual image from the x-rays that pass through the patient. The fact that ionizing radiation produces **fluorescence** (rays of light energy emitted as a result of exposure to and absorption of radiation from x-rays) is the basis for fluoroscopy. The fluorescent screen glows when it is struck by the x-rays. Opaque tissue such as bone appears as a dark shadow image on the fluorescent screen.

A major advantage of fluoroscopy over normal radiography is that internal organs, such as the heart and digestive tract organs, can be observed in motion. In addition, the patient's position can be changed constantly to provide the right view at the right time so that the most useful diagnostic information can be obtained.

Digital imaging techniques can be used to enhance conventional and fluoroscopic x-ray images. A lower dose of x-ray is used to achieve higher quality images, and digital images can be sent via networks to other locations and computer monitors so that many people can share information and assist in diagnoses.

Image-intensifier systems for fluoroscopy brighten fluoroscopic images and are combined with television and movie cameras and videotape recorders to obtain a permanent record of either a fluoroscopic or an x-ray examination. This procedure is **cineradiography** (cine- means motion).

Interventional Radiology. Interventional radiologists perform invasive procedures (therapeutic or diagnostic) under fluoroscopic, CT, and MR (magnetic resonance) guidance. Procedures include percutaneous biopsies, placement of drainage catheters, drainage of abscesses, occlusion of bleeding vessels, and catheter instillation of antibiotics or chemotherapy. In addition, interventional radiologists perform **radiofrequency ablation** (removal) of tumors and tissues (liver, kidney, adrenals). Neurointerventional radiologists are involved in vertebroplasty, whereas vascular interventional radiologists perform laser treatments for varicose veins and uterine fibroid embolization.

Ultrasound Imaging

Ultrasound imaging, or **ultrasonography,** uses high-frequency, inaudible sound waves that bounce off body tissues and are then recorded to give information about the anatomy of an internal organ. An instrument called a **transducer** or **probe** is placed near or on the skin, which is covered with a thin coating of gel to ensure good transmission of sound waves. The transducer emits sound waves in short, repetitive pulses. The ultrasound waves move with different speeds through body tissues and detect interfaces between tissues of different densities. An echo reflection of the sound waves is formed as the waves hit the various body tissues and pass back to the transducer.

These ultrasonic echoes are then recorded as a composite picture of the area of the body over which the instrument has passed. The record produced by ultrasound is called a **sonogram.**

Ultrasound imaging is used as a diagnostic tool not only by radiologists but also by neurosurgeons and ophthalmologists to detect intracranial and ophthalmic lesions, by cardiologists to detect heart valve and blood vessel disorders **(echocardiography),** by gastroenterologists to locate abdominal masses outside the digestive organs, and by obstetricians and gynecologists to differentiate single from multiple pregnancies, as well as to help in performing amniocentesis and in locating tumors or cysts. Fetal size and age also can be measured using ultrasound techniques. The measurements are made of the head, abdomen, and femur based on ultrasound images obtained in various fetal planes (Fig. 20–7).

Ultrasound imaging has several advantages in that the sound waves are nonionizing and noninjurious to tissues at the energy ranges utilized for diagnostic purposes. Because water is an excellent conductor of the ultrasonic beams, patients are requested to drink large quantities of water before examination so that the urinary bladder will be distended, allowing better viewing of pelvic and abdominal organs.

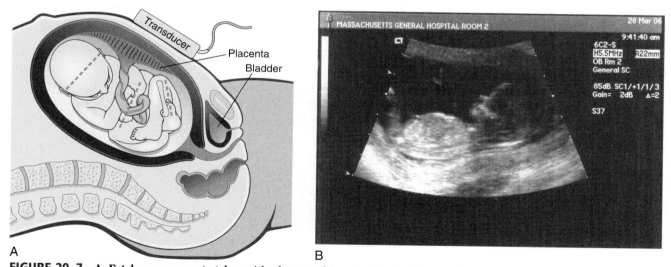

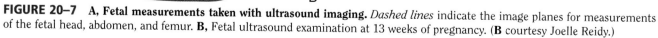

FIGURE 20–7   A, Fetal measurements taken with ultrasound imaging. *Dashed lines* indicate the image planes for measurements of the fetal head, abdomen, and femur. **B,** Fetal ultrasound examination at 13 weeks of pregnancy. (**B** courtesy Joelle Reidy.)

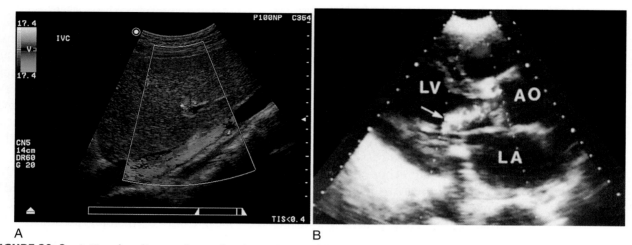

FIGURE 20–8 **A, Doppler ultrasound scan** showing an image of the vena cava *(blue color)*. **B, Color-flow imaging in a patient with aortic regurgitation.** The brightly colored, high-velocity jet *(arrow)* can be seen passing from the aorta (AO) to the left ventricle (LV). The center of the jet is *white*, and the edges are shades of *blue*. (**A** from Gill KA: Abdominal Ultrasound: A Practitioner's Guide. Philadelphia, WB Saunders, 2001. **B** from Braunwald E: Heart Disease: A Textbook of Cardiovascular Medicine, 5th ed. Philadelphia, WB Saunders, 1997.)

Two ultrasound techniques, **Doppler ultrasound** and **color-flow imaging,** make it possible to record blood flow velocity (in diagnosing vascular disease) and to image major blood vessels in patients at risk for stroke. Figure 20–8, *A* and *B,* shows Doppler ultrasound scanning and color-flow imaging.

Ultrasonography, like fluoroscopy, is used in interventional radiology to guide needle biopsies for the puncture of cysts and for the placement of needles for amniocentesis and seeds for radiotherapy.

Magnetic Resonance Imaging

Magnetic resonance imaging (MRI) uses electromagnetic energy rather than x-rays. This technique produces sagittal, coronal (frontal), and axial (cross-sectional) images and is based on the fact that the nuclei of some atoms behave like little magnets when a larger magnetic field is applied—this is the phenomenon of magnetic resonance (MR). The nuclei in tissue spin and emit radio waves that create an image as the nuclei move back to an equilibrium position. Hydrogen nuclei, present in water and abundant in living tissue, are the nuclei used to create the image.

MRI examinations are performed with and without contrast. The contrast agent most commonly used is **gadolinium (Gd).** As iodine contrast does with CT, gadolinium enhances vessels and tissues, increases the sensitivity for lesion detection, and helps differentiate between normal and abnormal tissues and structures. MRI provides excellent soft-tissue images, detecting edema in the brain, providing direct image of the spinal cord, detecting tumors in the chest and abdomen, and visualizing the cardiovascular system. Figure 20–9 shows three different MR images (coronal, axial, and sagittal).

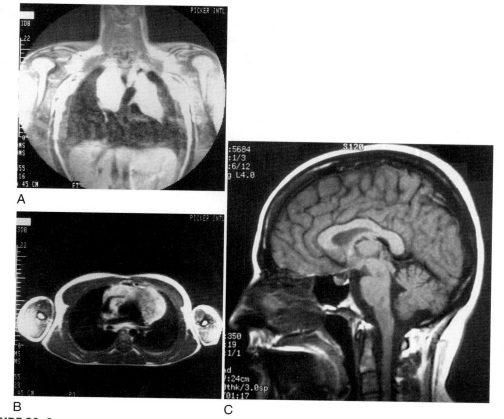

FIGURE 20–9 **Magnetic resonance images. A,** Frontal (coronal) view of the upper body. White masses in the chest are Hodgkin disease lesions. **B,** Transverse view of the upper body in the same patient, who had a chest mass. **C,** Image obtained in the sagittal plane of the head (the usual MRI view) showing cerebrum, ventricles, cerebellum, and medulla oblongata. (**C** from Black JM, Hawks JH, Keene AM: Medical-Surgical Nursing: Clinical Management for Positive Outcomes, 6th ed. Philadelphia, WB Saunders, 2001, p. 1895.)

MRI is not used for patients with pacemakers or metallic implants because the powerful MR magnet can alter position and functioning of such devices. The sounds (loud tapping) heard during the test are caused by the pulsing of the magnetic field as it scans the body.

Figure 20–10 summarizes radiologic diagnostic techniques.

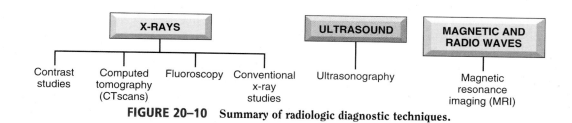

FIGURE 20–10   **Summary of radiologic diagnostic techniques.**

20

X-RAY POSITIONING

In order to take the best view of the part of the body being radiographed, the patient, film, and x-ray tube must be positioned in the most favorable alignment possible. Radiologists use special terms to refer to the direction of travel of the x-ray through the patient. X-ray terms describing the direction of the x-ray beam follow and are illustrated in Figure 20–11:

1. **Posteroanterior (PA) view.** In this most commonly requested chest x-ray view, x-rays travel from a posteriorly placed source to an anteriorly placed detector.
2. **Anteroposterior (AP) view.** X-rays travel from an anteriorly placed source to a posteriorly placed detector.
3. **Lateral view.** In a left lateral view, x-rays travel from a source located to the right of the patient to a detector placed to the left of the patient.
4. **Oblique view.** X-rays travel in a slanting direction at an angle from the perpendicular plane. Oblique views show regions or structures ordinarily hidden and superimposed in routine PA and AP views.

The following terms are used to describe the position of the patient or part of the body in the x-ray examination:

abduction	Movement away from the midline of the body.
adduction	Movement toward the midline of the body.
eversion	Turning outward.

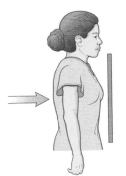 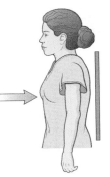

1. Posteroanterior (PA) view   2. Anteroposterior (AP) view

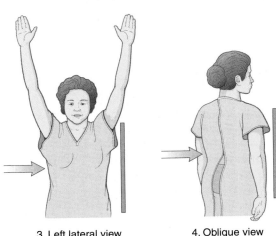

3. Left lateral view   4. Oblique view

FIGURE 20–11 **Positions for x-ray views.** The *arrow* denotes the direction of the x-ray beam through the patient.

extension	Lengthening or straightening a flexed limb.
flexion	Bending a part of the body.
inversion	Turning inward.
lateral decubitus	Lying down on the side (with the x-ray beam horizontally positioned).
prone	Lying on the belly (face down).
recumbent	Lying down (may be prone or supine).
supine	Lying on the back (face up).

NUCLEAR MEDICINE

RADIOACTIVITY AND RADIONUCLIDES

The emission of energy in the form of particles or rays coming from the interior of a substance is called **radioactivity.** A **radionuclide** (or **radioisotope**) is a substance that gives off high-energy particles or rays as it disintegrates. Radionuclides are produced in either a nuclear reactor or a charged-particle accelerator (cyclotron) or by irradiating stable substances, causing disruption and instability. **Half-life** is the time required for a radioactive substance (radionuclide) to lose half of its radioactivity by disintegration. Knowledge of a radionuclide's half-life is important in determining how long the radioactive substance will emit radioactivity when in the body. The half-life must be long enough to allow for diagnostic imaging but as short as possible to minimize patient exposure to radiation.

Radionuclides emit three types of radioactivity: **alpha particles, beta particles,** and **gamma rays.** Gamma rays, which have greater penetrating ability than alpha and beta particles, and more ionizing power, are especially useful to physicians in both the diagnosis and the treatment of disease. **Technetium-99m** (^{99m}Tc) is essentially a pure gamma emitter with a half-life of 6 hours. Its properties make it the most frequently used radionuclide in diagnostic imaging.

NUCLEAR MEDICINE TESTS: IN VITRO AND IN VIVO PROCEDURES

Nuclear medicine physicians use two types of tests in the diagnosis of disease: **in vitro** (in the test tube) procedures and **in vivo** (in the body) procedures. **In vitro** procedures involve analysis of blood and urine specimens using radioactive chemicals. For example, a **radioimmunoassay (RIA)** is an in vitro procedure that combines the use of radioactive chemicals and antibodies to detect hormones and drugs in a patient's blood. The test allows the detection of minute amounts of substances or compounds. RIA is used to monitor the amount of digitalis, a drug used to treat heart disease, in a patient's bloodstream and can detect hypothyroidism in newborn infants.

In vivo tests trace the amounts of radioactive substances within the body. They are given directly to the patient to evaluate the function of an organ or to image it. For example, in **tracer studies** a specific radionuclide is incorporated into a chemical substance and administered to a patient. The combination of the radionuclide and a drug or chemical is called a **radiopharmaceutical** (or **radiolabeled compound**). Each radiopharmaceutical is designed to concentrate in a certain organ. The organ can then be imaged using the radiation given off by the radionuclide.

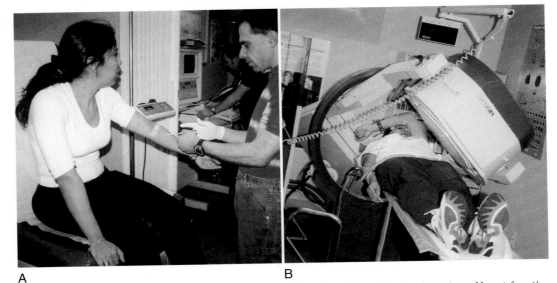

FIGURE 20–12   A, Patient receiving intravenous injection of a radionuclide for detection of heart function. **B,** Gamma camera moves around the patient, detecting radioactivity in heart muscle.

A sensitive, external detection instrument called a **gamma camera** is used to determine the distribution and localization of the radiopharmaceutical in various organs, tissues, and fluids. See Figure 20–12. The amount of radiopharmaceutical at a given location is proportional to the rate at which the gamma rays are emitted. Nuclear medicine studies depict the physiologic behavior (how the organ works) rather than the specific anatomy of an organ.

The procedure of making an image to track the distribution of radioactive substance in the body is **radionuclide scanning. Uptake** refers to the rate of absorption of the radiopharmaceutical into an organ or tissue.

Radiopharmaceuticals are administered by different routes to obtain a scan of a specific organ in the body. For example, in the case of a **lung scan,** the radiopharmaceutical is given intravenously (for **perfusion studies,** which rely on passage of the radioactive compound through the capillaries of the lungs) or by inhalation of a gas or aerosol (for **ventilation studies**), which fills the air sacs (alveoli). The combination of these tests permits sensitive and specific diagnosis of clots in the lung (pulmonary emboli).

Other examples of diagnostic procedures that utilize radionuclides are as follows:

1. **Bone scan.** ^{99m}Tc (technetium) is used to label phosphate substances and then is injected intravenously. The phosphate compound is taken up preferentially by bone, and the skeleton is imaged in 2 or 3 hours. Waiting 2 to 3 hours allows much of the radiopharmaceutical to be excreted in urine and allows for better visualization of the skeleton. The scan detects infection, inflammation, or tumors involving the skeleton, which appear as areas of high uptake ("hot spots") on the scan. See Figure 15–31, *B,* page 598.
2. **Gallium scan.** The radioisotope gallium 67 is injected intravenously and has an affinity for tumors and non-neoplastic lesions such as abscesses. Gallium also has an affinity for areas of inflammation as occurs in pneumonitis.
3. **Liver and spleen scans.** To visualize the liver and spleen, a radiopharmaceutical (^{99m}Tc and sulfur colloid) is injected intravenously, and images are taken with a

gamma camera. Areas of tumor or abscess are shown as **photopenic** areas (regions of reduced uptake). Abnormalities such as cirrhosis, abscesses, tumor, hepatomegaly, and hepatitis can be detected by liver scanning, and splenomegaly due to tumor, cyst, abscess, or rupture can be diagnosed with spleen scanning.

4. **Positron emission tomography (PET scan).** This radionuclide technique produces images of the distribution of radioactivity (through emission of positrons) in a region of the body. It is similar to the CT scan, but radioisotopes are used instead of contrast and x-rays. The radionuclides are incorporated (by intravenous injection) into the tissues to be scanned, and an image is made showing where the radionuclide (most often ^{18}F-FDG, a radioactive glucose molecule) is or is not being metabolized. For example, PET scanning has determined that schizophrenics do not metabolize glucose equally in all parts of the brain and that drug treatment can bring improvement to these regions. Thus, areas of metabolic deficiency can be pinpointed by PET, making it helpful in diagnosing and treating other neurologic disorders such as stroke, epilepsy, Alzheimer disease, and brain tumors, as well as abdominal and pulmonary malignancies. See Figure 20–13.

5. **Single photon emission computed tomography (SPECT).** This technique involves an intravenous injection of radioactive tracer (such as technetium-99m) and the computer reconstruction of a 3D image based on a composite of many views. Clinical applications include detecting liver tumors, detecting cardiac ischemia, and evaluating bone disease of the spine.

6. **Technetium Tc-99m sestamibi (Cardiolite) scan.** This radiopharmaceutical is injected intravenously and traced to heart muscle. An exercise tolerance test (ETT) is used with it for an ETT-MIBI scan. In a **mu**ltiple **g**ated **a**cquisition **(MUGA)** scan, ^{99m}Tc is injected intravenously to study the motion of the heart wall muscle and the ventricle's ability to eject blood (ejection fraction).

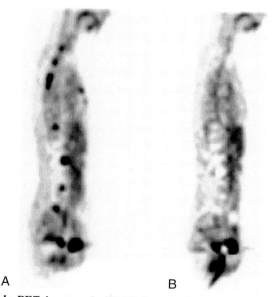

A   B

FIGURE 20–13   Whole-body PET images. A, ^{18}F-FDG **sagittal image** obtained in a patient with breast cancer metastases. Numerous tumors *(dark spots)* are seen along the spine and sternum. **B, Image obtained after chemotherapy** shows regression of the cancer. (From Ballinger PW, Frank ED: Merrill's Atlas of Radiographic Positions and Radiologic Procedures, 10th ed, vol. 3. St. Louis, Mosby, 2003, p. 549.)

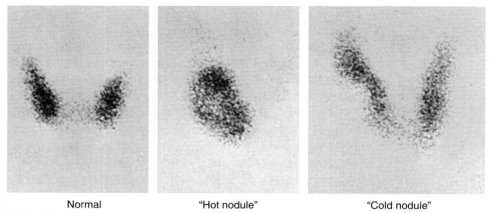

Normal   "Hot nodule"   "Cold nodule"

FIGURE 20–14   **Thyroid scans.** The scan of a "hot nodule" shows a darkened area of increased uptake, which indicates a diseased thyroid gland. The scan of a "cold nodule" shows an area of decreased uptake, which indicates a non-functioning region, a common occurrence when normal tissue is replaced by malignancy. (From Beare PG, Myers JL: Adult Health Nursing, 3rd ed. St. Louis, Mosby, 1998.)

7. **Thallium (Tl) scan.** Thallium-201 (^{201}Tl) is injected intravenously to evaluate myocardial perfusion. A high concentration of ^{201}Tl is present in well-perfused heart muscle cells, but infarcted or scarred myocardium does not extract any thallium, showing up as "cold spots." If the defective area is ischemic, the cold spots fill in (become "warm") on delayed images (obtained later).

8. **Thyroid scan.** An iodine radionuclide, usually iodine-131 (^{131}I), is administered intravenously, and the scan reveals the size and shape of the thyroid gland. Hyperfunctioning thyroid nodules (adenomas) accumulate higher amounts of ^{131}I radioactivity and are termed "hot." Thyroid carcinoma does not concentrate radioiodine well and is seen as a "cold" spot on the scan. Figure 20–14 shows thyroid scans.

Figure 20–15 reviews in vitro and in vivo nuclear medicine diagnostic tests.

NUCLEAR MEDICINE TESTS

IN VITRO	Radioimmunoassay

IN VIVO	Tracer Studies:
	Bone scan
	Gallium scan
	Liver/spleen scan
	Lung scan (ventilation/perfusion)
	Positron emission tomography (PET)
	Single-photon emission computed tomography (SPECT)
	^{99m}Technetium-sestamibi scan
	^{201}Thallium scan
	Thyroid scan

FIGURE 20–15   In vitro and in vivo nuclear medicine diagnostic tests.

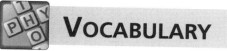

VOCABULARY

This list reviews many of the new terms introduced in the text. Short definitions reinforce your understanding of the terms. Refer to the Pronunciation of Terms section for help with unfamiliar or difficult words.

cineradiography	Use of motion picture techniques to record a series of x-ray images during fluoroscopy.
computed tomography (CT)	Diagnostic x-ray procedure whereby a cross-sectional image of a specific body segment is produced. Newer CT scanners can create 3D images as well.
contrast studies	Materials (contrast media) are injected to obtain contrast with surrounding tissue when shown on the x-ray film.
fluorescence	Emission of glowing light results from exposure to and absorption of radiation from x-rays.
fluoroscopy	X-ray technique that produces a fluorescent image on an image intensifier.
gamma camera	Machine to detect gamma rays emitted from radiopharmaceuticals during scanning for diagnostic purposes.
gamma rays	High-energy rays emitted by radioactive substances in tracer studies.
half-life	Time required for a radioactive substance to lose half its radioactivity by disintegration.
interventional radiology	Therapeutic procedures performed by a radiologist.
in vitro	Process, test, or procedure is performed, measured, or observed *outside* a living organism.
in vivo	Process, test, or procedure is performed, measured, or observed *within* a living organism.
ionization	Transformation of electrically neutral substances into electrically charged particles. X-rays cause ionization of particles within tissues.
labeled compound	Radiopharmaceutical; used in nuclear medicine studies.
magnetic resonance imaging (MRI)	Magnetic field and radio waves produce sagittal, coronal, and axial images of the body.
nuclear medicine	Medical specialty that studies the uses of radioactive substances (radionuclides) in diagnosis of disease.
positron emission tomography (PET)	Positron-emitting radioactive substances given intravenously create a cross-sectional image of cellular metabolism based on local concentration of the radioactive substance. PET scans give information about organ function.
radioimmunoassay	Test combines radioactive chemicals and antibodies to detect minute quantities of substances in a patient's blood.
radioisotope	Radioactive form of an element substance; radionuclide.

radiology	Medical specialty concerned with the study of x-rays and their use in the diagnosis of disease; includes other forms of energy, such as ultrasound and magnetic waves. Also called diagnostic radiology.
radiolucent	Permitting the passage of x-rays. Radiolucent structures appear black on x-ray film.
radionuclide	Radioactive form of an element that gives off energy in the form of radiation; radioisotope.
radiopaque	Obstructing the passage of x-rays. Radiopaque structures appear white on the x-ray film.
radiopharmaceutical	Radioactive drug (radionuclide plus chemical) that is administered safely for diagnostic and therapeutic purposes.
roentgenology	Study of x-rays; radiology.
scan	Image of an area, organ or tissue of the body obtained from ultrasound, radioactive tracer studies, computed tomography, or magnetic resonance imaging.
single photon emission computed tomography (SPECT)	Radioactive tracer is injected intravenously and a computer reconstructs a 3D image based on a composite of many views.
tagging	Attaching a radionuclide to a chemical and following its path in the body.
tracer studies	Radionuclides are used as tags, or labels, attached to chemicals and followed as they travel through the body.
transducer	Handheld device that sends and receives ultrasound signals.
ultrasonography (US, U/S)	Diagnostic technique that projects and retrieves high-frequency sound waves as they echo off parts of the body.
uptake	Rate of absorption of a radionuclide into an organ or tissue.
ventilation-perfusion studies	Radiopharmaceutical is inhaled (ventilation) and injected intravenously (perfusion) followed by imaging its passage through the respiratory tract.

COMBINING FORMS, SUFFIXES, PREFIXES, AND TERMINOLOGY

Write the meanings of the medical terms in the spaces provided.

COMBINING FORMS

Combining Form	Meaning	Terminology	Meaning
fluor/o	luminous, fluorescence	fluoroscopy _____ _In this term, -scopy does not refer to visual examination with an endoscope. In fluoroscopy, x-rays can be viewed directly, without taking and developing x-ray photographs. Light is emitted from the image intensifier when it is exposed to x-rays._	

Combining Form	Meaning	Terminology	Meaning
is/o	same	radioisotope _____	
		Top/o means place; radioisotopes of an element have similar structures but different weights and electric charges. A radioisotope (radionuclide) is an unstable form of an element that emits radioactivity.	
pharmaceut/o	drug	radiopharmaceutical _____	
		In this term, radi/o stands for radioactive.	
radi/o	x-rays	radiographer _____	
roentgen/o	x-rays	roentgenology _____	
son/o	sound	hysterosonogram _____	
		Saline solution is injected through a catheter inserted through the vagina and into the endocervical canal to distend the uterine cavity, which is then examined by ultrasound.	
therapeut/o	treatment	therapeutic _____	
vitr/o	glass	in vitro _____	
viv/o	life	in vivo _____	

SUFFIXES

Suffix	Meaning	Terminology	Meaning
-gram	record	angiogram _____	
		hysterosalpingogram _____	
		pyelogram _____	
-graphy	process of recording	computed tomography _____	
		Tom/o means to cut, as in viewing in slices.	
-lucent	to shine	radiolucent _____	
		Radiolucent (indicating that x-rays pass through easily) areas on x-ray film appear dark on exposed film.	
-opaque	obscure	radiopaque _____	
		Radiopaque (indicating that x-rays do not penetrate) areas on x-ray film appear white or light on exposed film.	

PREFIXES

Prefix	Meaning	Terminology	Meaning
cine-	movement	cineradiography _____	
echo-	a repeated sound	echocardiography _____	
ultra-	beyond	ultrasonography _____	
		Sound waves are beyond the normal range of those that a human can hear.	

ABBREVIATIONS

Angio	angiography
AP	anteroposterior
Ba	barium
BE	barium enema
C-spine	cervical spine films
CT	computed tomography
CXR	chest x-ray (film)
Decub	decubitus—lying down
DICOM	digital image communication in medicine—standard protocol for transmission between imaging devices (e.g., CT scans and PACS workstations)
DI	diagnostic imaging
DSA	digital subtraction angiography
FDG	fluorodeoxyglucose—radiopharmaceutical used in PET scanning
^{67}Ga	radioactive gallium—used in whole-body scans
Gd	gadolinium—MRI contrast agent
^{131}I	radioactive iodine—used in thyroid, liver, and kidney scans and for treatment of malignant and nonmalignant conditions of the thyroid
IVP	intravenous pyelogram
KUB	kidneys, ureters, bladder—x-ray imaging of these organs without contrast medium
LAT	lateral
LS films	lumbosacral spine films
L-spine	lumbar spine films
MR, MRI	magnetic resonance, magnetic resonance imaging

MRA	magnetic resonance angiography
MRV	magnetic resonance venography
MUGA	multiple-gated acquisitions (scan)—radioactive test to show heart function
PA	posteroanterior
PACS	picture archival and communications system—replacement of traditional films with digital equivalents that can be accessed from several places and retrieved more rapidly
PET	positron emission tomography
PET/CT	positron emission tomography/computed tomography—both studies are performed using a single machine
RFA	radiofrequency ablation
SBFT	small bowel follow-through
SPECT	single photon emission computed tomography; radioactive substances and a computer are used to create 3D images
^{99m}Tc	radioactive technetium—used in heart, brain, skull, thyroid, liver, spleen, bone, and lung scans
^{201}Tl	thallium-201—radioisotope used in scanning heart muscle
T-spine	thoracic spine
UGI	upper gastrointestinal (series)
US, U/S	ultrasound; ultrasonography
V/Q scan	ventilation-perfusion scan of the lungs (Q stands for rate of blood flow or blood volume)

20

PRACTICAL APPLICATIONS

Answers to the questions are found on page 847.

CASE STUDY

Bill Smith, a 51-year-old sales representative, was initially diagnosed with stage III melanoma 4 years ago. He underwent surgery and interferon treatment at that time. At his 3-month follow-up CT scan last year, Mr. Smith received bad news. The CT scan indicated a small 1-cm nodule, which could be a melanoma metastasis. To confirm the diagnosis, Mr. Smith underwent a PET scan.

He was admitted to the nuclear medicine unit of the hospital on the morning of the scan. He had been informed to fast (no food or beverage 12 hours before the scan). The nuclear physician had told him especially not to eat any type of sugar, which would compete with the radiopharmaceutical ^{18}F-FDG (fluorodeoxyglucose), which is a radioactive glucose molecule that travels to every cell in the body.

The PET scan began with an injection of a trace amount of ^{18}F-FDG by the physician. Bill was asked to lie still for about an hour in a dark, quiet room and to avoid talking to prevent the compound from concentrating in the tongue and vocal cords. The waiting time allowed the ^{18}F-FDG to be absorbed and released from normal tissue. After emptying his bladder, Bill reclined on a bed that moved slowly and quietly through a PET scanner, a tube similar to a CT scanner. The radioactive glucose emits charged particles called positrons, which interact with electrons, producing gamma rays that are in turn detected by the scanner. Color-coded images indicate the intensity of metabolic activity throughout the body. Cancerous cells absorb more radioactive glucose than noncancerous cells. The malignant cells show up brighter on the PET scan.

Bill's PET scan proved the CT wrong. His melanoma had not metastasized. He returned home quite relieved.

Questions

1. In CT scanning
   a. A radioactive tracer is used
   b. Magnetic images reveal images in all three planes of the body
   c. A nuclear physician performs the ultrasound procedure
   d. X-rays and a computer produce images in the axial plane

2. In PET scanning
   a. A radioactive tracer is used
   b. X-ray images reveal images in all three planes of the body
   c. A nuclear physician performs the ultrasound procedure
   d. Doppler ultrasound is used

3. Bill's case showed that
   a. CT scanning and PET scanning are equally effective in diagnosis of metastases
   b. PET scanning is useful in cancer diagnosis and staging
   c. Melanoma never progresses to stage IV
   d. A diet high in glucose helps concentrate the radioactive ^{18}F-DFG before the PET scan

GENERAL HOSPITAL: NUCLEAR MEDICINE DEPARTMENT

Available Radionuclides

Radionuclide	Radiopharmaceutical	Admission Route	Target Organ
^{133}Xe	xenon gas	inhaled	lungs
^{99m}Tc	albumin microspheres	IV	lungs
^{87m}Sr (strontium)	solution	IV	bone
^{99m}Tc	diphosphonate	IV	bone
^{99m}Tc	pertechnetate	IV	brain
^{99m}Tc	sulfur colloid	IV	liver/spleen
^{99m}Tc	HIDA*	IV	gallbladder
^{131}I	rose bengal	IV	colon
^{99m}Tc	DTPA†	IV	kidney
^{99m}Tc	DMSA‡	IV	kidney
^{131}I	iodide	IV	thyroid
^{201}Tl (thallium)	thallium chloride	IV	heart
^{99m}Tc	sestamibi	IV	heart
^{67}Ga (gallium)	gallium citrate	IV	tumors and abscesses

*HIDA = N-(2,6-dimethyl)iminodiacetic acid.
†DTPA = diethylenetriamine penta-acetic acid.
‡DMSA = dimercaptosuccinic acid.

Questions

1. Which radionuclide is used with sestamibi in an ETT of heart function?
   a. Thallium-201
   b. Iodine-131
   c. Gallium-67
   d. Technetium-99m

2. Which radionuclide would be used to diagnose disease in an endocrine gland?
   a. ^{99m}Tc
   b. ^{131}I
   c. ^{199}Au
   d. ^{87m}Sr

? EXERCISES

Remember to check your answers carefully with those given in the Answers to Exercises, page 846.

A. Complete the medical terms based on the definitions and word parts given.

1. obstructing the passage of x-rays: radio_____

2. permitting the passage of x-rays: radio_____

3. aids physicians in performing ultrasound procedures: _____grapher

4. transformation of stable substances into charged particles: _____ization

5. radioactive drug administered for diagnostic purposes: radio_____

6. radioactive chemical that gives off energy in the form of radiation: radio_____

7. a physician who specializes in diagnostic radiology: radi_____

8. study of the uses of radioactive substances in the diagnosis of disease: _____

B. Match the special diagnostic techniques below with their definitions.

cineradiography	fluoroscopy	magnetic resonance imaging
computed tomography	interventional radiology	ultrasonography
contrast studies		

1. radiopaque substances are given and conventional x-rays taken _____

2. use of motion picture techniques to record x-ray images _____

3. use of echoes of high-frequency sound waves to diagnose disease _____

4. x-ray beams are focused onto an image intensifier that glows as a result of the ionizing effect of x-rays _____

5. a magnetic field and radio waves are used to form images of the body _____

6. x-ray pictures are taken circularly around an area of the body, and a computer synthesizes the information into composite images _____

7. therapeutic procedures are performed by a radiologist under the guidance of fluoroscopy, CT, MRI, or ultrasonography _____

20

C. Match the diagnostic x-ray test in Column I with the part of the body that is imaged in Column II.

Column I

1. myelography   _____
2. retrograde pyelography   _____
3. angiography   _____
4. arthrography   _____
5. upper GI series   _____
6. cholangiography   _____
7. barium enema   _____
8. hysterosalpingography _____

Column II

A. joints
B. spinal cord
C. uterus and fallopian tubes
D. blood vessels
E. esophagus, stomach, and small intestine
F. lower gastrointestinal tract
G. urinary tract
H. bile vessels (ducts)

D. Match the x-ray views or positions in column I with their meanings in column II. Write the letter of the answer in the space provided.

Column I

1. PA   _____
2. supine   _____
3. prone   _____
4. AP   _____
5. lateral   _____
6. oblique   _____
7. lateral decubitus _____
8. adduction   _____
9. inversion   _____
10. abduction   _____
11. recumbent   _____
12. eversion   _____
13. flexion   _____
14. extension   _____

Column II

A. on the side
B. turned inward
C. movement away from the midline
D. lying on the belly
E. x-ray tube positioned on an angle
F. bending a part
G. straightening a limb
H. lying on the back
I. lying down on the side
J. lying down; prone or supine
K. anteroposterior view (front to back)
L. turning outward
M. posteroanterior view (back to front)
N. movement toward the midline

E. Give the meanings of the following medical terms.

1. in vitro _____

2. in vivo _____

3. radiopharmaceutical _____

4. tracer studies _____

5. uptake _____

6. perfusion lung scan _____

7. ventilation lung scan _____

8. bone scan _____

9. gallium scan _____

10. thyroid scan _____

11. technetium Tc-99m sestamibi scan _____

F. Give the meanings of the following terms.

1. gamma camera _____

2. positron emission tomography (PET) _____

3. radioisotope _____

4. transducer _____

5. uptake _____

6. echocardiography _____

7. roentgenology _____

G. Give the meanings of the following word parts.

1. -gram _____   6. pharmaceut/o _____

2. ultra- _____   7. son/o _____

3. fluor/o _____   8. cine- _____

4. vitr/o _____   9. therapeut/o _____

5. viv/o _____

H. Give the meanings of the abbreviations and then select from column II the best association for each.

Column I

1. MRI _____ _____
2. SPECT _____ _____
3. PACS _____ _____
4. UGI _____ _____
5. CXR _____ _____
6. DSA _____ _____
7. IVP _____ _____
8. LAT _____ _____
9. U/S _____ _____
10. ^{99m}Tc _____ _____

Column II

A. X-ray examination of the kidney after injection of contrast.
B. Diagnostic procedure frequently used to assess fetal size and development.
C. X-ray examination of the esophagus, stomach, and intestines.
D. X-ray of blood vessels made by taking two images (with and without contrast) and subtracting the digitized data for one from the data for the other.
E. Radioisotope used in nuclear medicine (tracer studies).
F. Radioactive substances and a computer are used to create 3D images.
G. Diagnostic procedure produces magnetic resonance images of all three planes of the body and visualizes soft tissue in the nervous and musculoskeletal systems.
H. Replacement of traditional films with digital equivalents.
I. X-ray view from the side.
J. Diagnostic procedure (x-rays are used) necessary to investigate thoracic disease.

I. Circle the correct term to complete each sentence.

1. Mr. Jones was scheduled for ultrasound-guided thoracentesis. He was sent to the **(interventional radiology, radiation oncology, nuclear medicine)** department for the procedure.

2. In order to better visualize Mr. Smith's colon, Dr. Wong ordered a **(perfusion study, hysterosalpingography, barium enema)**. She hoped to determine why he was having blood in his stools.

3. After the head-on collision, Sam was taken to the emergency room in an unconscious state. The paramedics suspected head trauma, and the doctors ordered an emergency **(PET scan, U/S, CT scan)** of his head.

4. In light of Sue's symptoms of fever, cough, and malaise, the doctors thought that the consolidated, hazy **(radioisotope, radiolucent, radiopaque)** area on the chest x-ray represented a pneumonia.

5. Fred, a lung cancer patient, experienced a seizure recently. His oncologist ordered a brain **(ultrasound, pulmonary angiogram, MRI)** that showed a tumor involving the left frontal lobe of the brain. Fred was treated with **(gamma camera, gamma knife, gallium)** irradiation, and the tumor decreased in size. He has had no further seizures.

6. Tom recently developed a cough and fever. A chest x-ray and **(CT, myelogram, IVP)** of the chest show that a **(pelvic, spinal, mediastinal)** mass is present. **(Mediastinoscopy, Cystoscopy, Lumbar puncture)** and biopsy of the mass reveal Hodgkin disease on histopathologic examination. He is treated with chemotherapy, and his symptoms disappear. A repeat x-ray shows that the mass has decreased remarkably, and a **(SPECT, MR, PET)** scan shows no uptake of ^{18}F-FDG in the chest, indicating that the mass is fibrosis and not tumor.

7. Paola, a 50-year-old woman with diabetes, experiences chest pain during a stress test, and her **(U/S, ECG, EEG)** shows evidence of ischemia. A **(contrast agent, transducer, radiopharmaceutical)** called technetium Tc-99m sestamibi (Cardiolite) is injected IV, and uptake is assessed with a **(probe, CT scanner, gamma camera)**, which shows an area of poor perfusion in the left ventricle.

8. Sally has a routine pelvic examination, and her **(neurologist, gynecologist, urologist)** feels an irregular area of enlargement in the anterior wall of the uterus. A pelvic **(angiogram, U/S study, PET scan)** is performed, which demonstrates the presence of fibroids in the uterine wall. The examination involves placing a gel over her abdominopelvic area and applying a **(transducer, radionuclide, probe)** to send/receive sound vibrations to/from the pelvic region.

MEDICAL SCRAMBLE

Unscramble the letters to form radiology and nuclear medicine terms from the clues. Use the letters in the squares to complete the bonus term. Answers are found on page 847.

1. *Clue:* Movement toward the midline of the body.

   __ ☐ __ __ __ ☐ __ __ __   CIDTNOUDA

2. *Clue:* Obstructing the passage of x-rays.

   __ ☐ __ __ __ __ __ __ ☐ __   PURDOQEIAA

3. *Clue:* Lying on one's back.

   ☐ __ __ __ __ ☐   NESIPU

4. *Clue:* X-ray image of blood vessels after injecting contrast material into the vessels.

   __ ☐ __ __ __ __ ☐ __ __   MAGAGORNI

5. *Clue:* Permitting the passage of x-rays.

   ☐ __ __ __ __ __ __ ☐ __ __ __   CUTLEDAIRON

BONUS TERM: *Clue:* Handheld device that sends and receives ultrasound signals.

☐ ☐ ☐ ☐ ☐ ☐ ☐ ☐ ☐

ANSWERS TO EXERCISES

A

1. radiopaque
2. radiolucent
3. sonographer

4. ionization
5. radiopharmaceutical
6. radioisotope or radionuclide

7. radiologist
8. nuclear medicine

B

1. contrast studies
2. cineradiography; a type of fluoroscopy
3. ultrasonography

4. fluoroscopy
5. magnetic resonance imaging

6. computed tomography
7. interventional radiology

C

1. B
2. G
3. D

4. A
5. E
6. H

7. F
8. C

D

1. M	6. E	11. J
2. H	7. I	12. L
3. D	8. N	13. F
4. K	9. B	14. G
5. A	10. C	

E

1. process, test, or procedure in which something is measured or observed outside a living organism
2. process, test, or procedure in which something is measured or observed in a living organism
3. radioactive drug (radionuclide plus chemical) that is given for diagnostic or therapeutic purposes
4. tests in which radioactive substance (radioisotopes) are used with chemicals and followed as they travel throughout the body
5. the rate of absorption of a radionuclide into an organ or tissue
6. imaging technique in which a radiopharmaceutical is injected intravenously and traced within the blood vessels of the lung
7. imaging technique in which a radiopharmaceutical is inhaled and its passage through the respiratory tract is traced on a scan
8. imaging technique in which a radiopharmaceutical is given intravenously and taken up by bone tissue, followed by scanning to detect the amount of the radioactive substance in the bone
9. imaging technique in which the radioisotope gallium-67 is injected intravenously and the body is scanned
10. imaging technique in which a radioactive substance is given intravenously and a scan (image) is made to assess its uptake in the thyroid gland
11. test of heart muscle function

F

1. machine that detects rays emitted by radioactive substances
2. radioactive glucose is injected and traced to body cells
3. a radioactive form (radionuclide) of a substance; gives off radiation
4. handheld device that sends and receives ultrasound signals
5. rate of absorption of a radionuclide into an organ or tissue
6. ultrasound used to create an image of the heart
7. study of x-rays; radiology

G

1. record	4. glass	7. sound
2. beyond	5. life	8. motion
3. luminous, fluorescence	6. drug	9. treatment

H

1. magnetic resonance imaging: G
2. single-photon emission computed tomography: F
3. picture archival and communications system: H
4. upper gastrointestinal (series): C
5. chest x-ray: J
6. digital subtraction angiography; D
7. intravenous pyelogram: A
8. lateral: I
9. ultrasound: B
10. radioactive technetium: E

I

1. interventional radiology
2. barium enema
3. CT scan
4. radiopaque
5. MRI, gamma knife
6. CT, mediastinal, mediastinoscopy, PET
7. ECG, radiopharmaceutical, gamma
8. gynecologist, U/S, transducer

ANSWERS TO PRACTICAL APPLICATIONS

Case Study
1. d
2. a
3. b

General Hospital
1. d
2. b

ANSWERS TO MEDICAL SCRAMBLE

1. ADDUCTION   2. RADIOPAQUE   3. SUPINE   4. ANGIOGRAM   5. RADIOLUCENT
BONUS TERM: TRANSDUCER

PRONUNCIATION OF TERMS

To test your understanding of the terminology in this chapter, write the meaning of each term in the space provided. In addition, you may wish to cover the terms and write them by looking at your definitions. Make sure your spelling is correct. The page number after each term indicates where it is defined or used in the book, so you can easily check your responses. You will find complete definitions for all of these terms and their audio pronunciations on the CD.

Term	Pronunciation	Meaning
abduction (830)	ăb-DŬK-shŭn	_____
adduction (830)	ă-DŬK-shŭn	_____
angiogram (837)	ĂN-jē-ō-grăm	_____
anteroposterior (830)	ăn-tĕr-ō-pōs-TĔ-rē-ŏr	_____
arthrography (824)	ăr-THRŎG-ră-fē	_____
bone scan (832)	bōn skăn	_____
cholangiography (824)	kō-lăn-jē-ŎG-ră-fē	_____
cineradiography (835)	sĭn-ĕ-rā-dē-ŎG-ră-fē	_____
computed tomography (835)	kŏm-PŪ-tĕd tō-MŎG-ră-fē	_____
contrast studies (835)	KŎN-trăst STŬD-ēz	_____
echocardiography (837)	ĕk-ō-kăr-dē-ŎG-ră-fē	_____
eversion (830)	ē-VĔR-zhŭn	_____
extension (831)	ĕk-STĔN-shŭn	_____
flexion (831)	FLĔK-shŭn	_____
fluorescence (835)	floo-RĔS-ĕns	_____
fluoroscopy (835)	floo-RŎS-kō-pē	_____
gallium scan (832)	GĂ-lē-ŭm skăn	_____
gamma camera (835)	GĂ-mă KĂM-ĕr-ă	_____
gamma rays (835)	GĂ-mă rāz	_____
half-life (835)	hăf līf	_____
hysterosalpingogram (837)	hĭs-tĕr-ō-săl-PĬNG-gō-grăm	_____
hysterosonogram (837)	hĭs-tĕr-ō-SŎN-ō-grăm	_____
interventional radiology (835)	ĭn-tĕr-VĔN-shŭn-ăl rā-dē-ŎL-ō-jē	_____
inversion (831)	ĭn-VĔR-zhŭn	_____
in vitro (835)	ĭn VĒ-trō	_____

Term	Pronunciation	Meaning
in vivo (835)	ĭn VĒ-vō	_____
ionization (835)	ī-ŏn-ĭ-ZĀ-shŭn	_____
labeled compound (835)	LĀ-bĕld KŎM-pŏwnd	_____
lateral decubitus (831)	LĂ-tĕr-ăl dĕ-KŪ-bĭ-tŭs	_____
magnetic resonance imaging (835)	măg-NĔT-ĭk RĔZ-ō-năns ĬM-ă-jĭng	_____
myelography (826)	mī-ĕ-LŎG-ră-fē	_____
nuclear medicine (835)	NOO-klē-ăr MĔD-ĭ-sĭn	_____
oblique (830)	ŏ-BLĒK	_____
positron emission tomography (835)	PŎS-ĭ-trŏn ē-MĬSH-ŭn tō-MŎG-ră-fē	_____
posteroanterior (830)	pōs-tĕr-ō-ăn-TĒ-rē-ŏr	_____
prone (831)	prōn	_____
pyelogram (837)	PĪ-ē-lō-grăm	_____
radiographer (837)	rā-dē-ŎG-ră-fĕr	_____
radioimmunoassay (835)	rā-dē-ō-ĭ-mū-nō-ĂS-ā	_____
radioisotope (835)	rā-dē-ō-Ī-sō-tōp	_____
radiology (836)	rā-dē-ŎL-ō-gē	_____
radiolucent (836)	rā-dē-ō-LŪ-sĕnt	_____
radionuclide (836)	rā-dē-ō-NŪ-klīd	_____
radiopaque (836)	rā-dē-ō-PĀK	_____
radiopharmaceutical (836)	rā-dē-ō-făr-mă-SŪ-tĭ-kăl	_____
recumbent (831)	rē-KŬM-bĕnt	_____
roentgenology (836)	rĕnt-gĕ-NŎL-ō-jē	_____
scan (836)	scăn	_____
single photon emission computed tomography (836)	SĬNG-'l PHŌ-tŏn ē-MĬ-shŭn kŏm-PŪ-tĕd tō-MŎG-ră-fē	_____
sonogram (827)	SŎN-ō-grăm	_____
supine (831)	SOO-pīn	_____
tagging (836)	TĂG-ĭng	_____
technetium Tc-99m sestamibi scan (831)	tĕk-NĒ-shē-ŭm 99m sĕs-tă-MĬ-bē skăn	_____
thallium scan (834)	THĂL-ē-ŭm skăn	_____
therapeutic (837)	thĕr-ă-PŪ-tik	_____

Term	Pronunciation	Meaning
thyroid scan (834)	THĪ-rŏyd skăn	_____
tomography (837)	tō-MŎG-ră-fē	_____
tracer studies (836)	TRĀ-sĕr STŪ-dēz	_____
transducer (836)	trănz-DOO-sĕr	_____
ultrasonography (837)	ŭl-tră-sō-NŎG-ră-fē	_____
uptake (836)	ŬP-tāk	_____
urography (826)	ū-RŎG-ră-fē	_____
ventilation-perfusion studies (836)	vĕn-tĭ-LĀ-shŭn-pĕr-FŪ-shŭn STŪ-dēz	_____

REVIEW SHEET

Write the meanings of the combining forms in the spaces provided and test yourself. Check your answers with the information in the text or in the glossary (Medical Word Parts—English) at the back of the book.

COMBINING FORMS

Combining Form	Meaning	Combining Form	Meaning
fluor/o	_____	roentgen/o	_____
ion/o	_____	son/o	_____
is/o	_____	therapeut/o	_____
myel/o	_____	vitr/o	_____
pharmaceut/o	_____	viv/o	_____
radi/o	_____		

SUFFIXES

Suffix	Meaning	Suffix	Meaning
-gram	_____	-lucent	_____
-graphy	_____	-opaque	_____

PREFIXES

Prefix	Meaning	Prefix	Meaning
cine-	_____	ultra-	_____
echo-	_____		

 Please refer to the enclosed CD for additional exercises and images related to this chapter.

INTRODUCTION

Drugs (medicines) are substances used to prevent or treat a condition or disease. Some drugs are obtained from parts of **plants,** such as the roots, leaves, and fruit. An example of a plant-derived drug is a cardiac medicine, digitalis (from the foxglove plant). Other drugs (antibiotics such as penicillin) are obtained from yeast, molds, and fungi. Drugs also are obtained from **animals;** for example, hormones are secretions from the glands of animals. Some drugs are **synthesized** in a laboratory. Anticancer drugs, such as methotrexate and prednisone, are laboratory-synthesized drugs. **Vitamins** are drugs that are isolated from plant or animal sources and are contained in foods.

A **pharmacist** prepares and dispenses drugs through a **pharmacy** (drugstore) on written orders from a physician. Currently, most schools/colleges of pharmacy offer a PharmD (Doctor of Pharmacy) degree after six or seven years of study. As a health care professional, a pharmacist cooperates with, consults with, and sometimes advises licensed practitioners concerning drugs. In addition, the pharmacist answers patients' questions concerning their prescription needs.

Pharmacology is the study of the preparation, properties, uses, and actions of drugs. A **pharmacologist** is either an MD (Doctor of Medicine) or a PhD (Doctor of Philosophy) who specializes in pharmacology. Pharmacology contains many subdivisions of study: **medicinal chemistry, pharmacodynamics, pharmacokinetics, molecular pharmacology, chemotherapy,** and **toxicology.**

Medicinal chemistry is the study of new drug synthesis and the relationship between chemical structure and biological effects. **Pharmacodynamics** involves the study of drug effects in the body. Other scientists study processes of drug absorption (how drugs pass into the bloodstream), distribution into body compartments, metabolism (changes that drugs undergo within the body), and excretion (removal of the drug from the body). The mathematical description of drug disposition (appearance and disappearance) in the body over time is **pharmacokinetics.**

Molecular pharmacology involves the interaction of drugs and subcellular entities, such as DNA, RNA, and enzymes. It provides important information about the mechanism of action of drugs.

Chemotherapy is the study of drugs that destroy microorganisms, parasites, or malignant cells within the body. Chemotherapy includes treatment of infectious diseases and cancer.

Toxicology is the study of the harmful effects of drugs and chemicals on the body. Toxicologic studies in animals are required by law before new drugs can be tested in humans. A toxicologist also is interested in finding proper **antidotes** to any harmful effects of drugs. Antidotes are substances given to neutralize unwanted effects of drugs.

Figure 21–1 reviews the subspecialty areas of pharmacology.

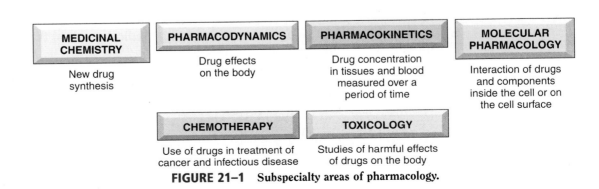

FIGURE 21–1 Subspecialty areas of pharmacology.

INTRODUCTION

Drugs (medicines) are substances used to prevent or treat a condition or disease. Some drugs are obtained from parts of **plants,** such as the roots, leaves, and fruit. An example of a plant-derived drug is a cardiac medicine, digitalis (from the foxglove plant). Other drugs (antibiotics such as penicillin) are obtained from yeast, molds, and fungi. Drugs also are obtained from **animals;** for example, hormones are secretions from the glands of animals. Some drugs are **synthesized** in a laboratory. Anticancer drugs, such as methotrexate and prednisone, are laboratory-synthesized drugs. **Vitamins** are drugs that are isolated from plant or animal sources and are contained in foods.

A **pharmacist** prepares and dispenses drugs through a **pharmacy** (drugstore) on written orders from a physician. Currently, most schools/colleges of pharmacy offer a PharmD (Doctor of Pharmacy) degree after six or seven years of study. As a health care professional, a pharmacist cooperates with, consults with, and sometimes advises licensed practitioners concerning drugs. In addition, the pharmacist answers patients' questions concerning their prescription needs.

Pharmacology is the study of the preparation, properties, uses, and actions of drugs. A **pharmacologist** is either an MD (Doctor of Medicine) or a PhD (Doctor of Philosophy) who specializes in pharmacology. Pharmacology contains many subdivisions of study: **medicinal chemistry, pharmacodynamics, pharmacokinetics, molecular pharmacology, chemotherapy,** and **toxicology.**

Medicinal chemistry is the study of new drug synthesis and the relationship between chemical structure and biological effects. **Pharmacodynamics** involves the study of drug effects in the body. Other scientists study processes of drug absorption (how drugs pass into the bloodstream), distribution into body compartments, metabolism (changes that drugs undergo within the body), and excretion (removal of the drug from the body). The mathematical description of drug disposition (appearance and disappearance) in the body over time is **pharmacokinetics.**

Molecular pharmacology involves the interaction of drugs and subcellular entities, such as DNA, RNA, and enzymes. It provides important information about the mechanism of action of drugs.

Chemotherapy is the study of drugs that destroy microorganisms, parasites, or malignant cells within the body. Chemotherapy includes treatment of infectious diseases and cancer.

Toxicology is the study of the harmful effects of drugs and chemicals on the body. Toxicologic studies in animals are required by law before new drugs can be tested in humans. A toxicologist also is interested in finding proper **antidotes** to any harmful effects of drugs. Antidotes are substances given to neutralize unwanted effects of drugs.

Figure 21–1 reviews the subspecialty areas of pharmacology.

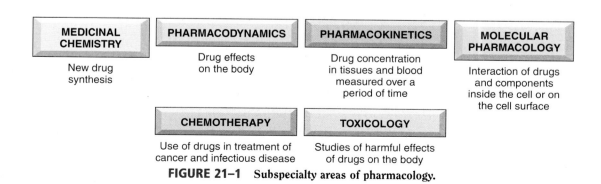

FIGURE 21–1   **Subspecialty areas of pharmacology.**

Pharmacology

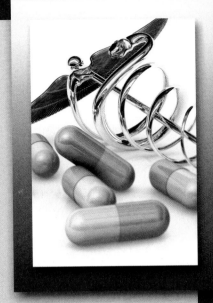

THIS CHAPTER IS DIVIDED INTO THE FOLLOWING SECTIONS

In this chapter you will

- Describe the various subspecialty areas of pharmacology.
- Identify the various routes of drug administration.
- Differentiate among the various classes of drugs and name their actions and side effects.
- Define medical terms using combining forms, prefixes, and suffixes that relate to pharmacology.
- Apply your new knowledge to understanding medical terms in their proper contexts, such as medical reports and records.

Image Description: A caduceus with medicinal capsules. Note the caduceus is a medical insignia bearing a representation of a staff with two entwined snakes and two wings at the top.

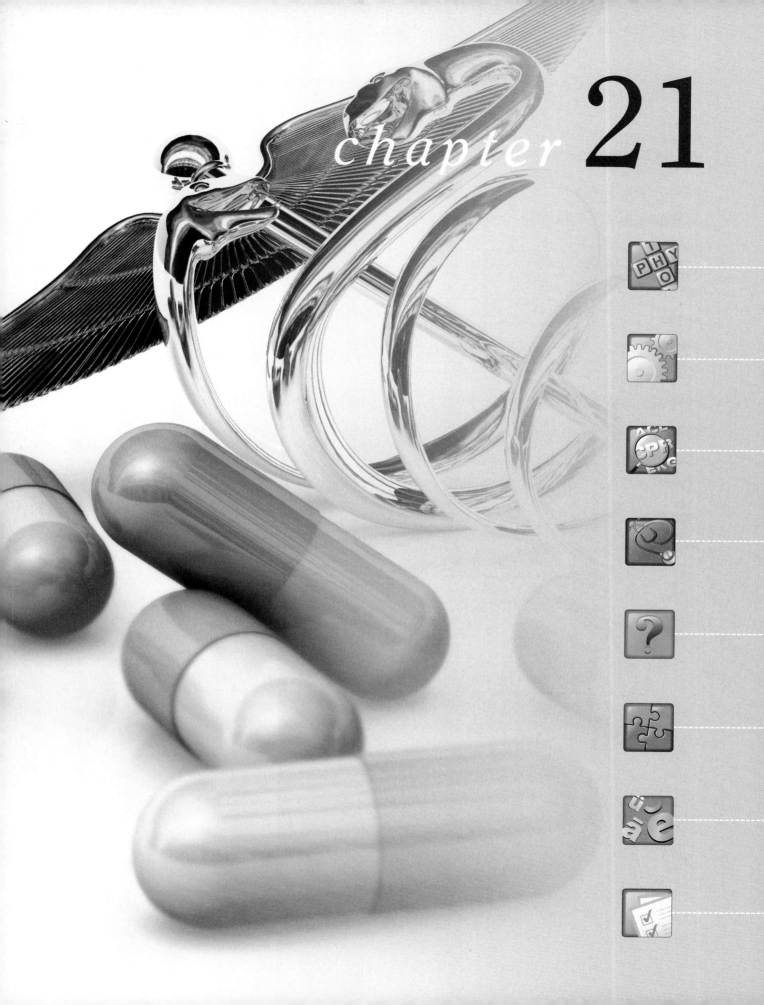

chapter 21

REVIEW SHEET

Write the meanings of the combining forms in the spaces provided and test yourself. Check your answers with the information in the text or in the glossary (Medical Word Parts—English) at the back of the book.

20

COMBINING FORMS

Combining Form	Meaning	Combining Form	Meaning
fluor/o	_____	roentgen/o	_____
ion/o	_____	son/o	_____
is/o	_____	therapeut/o	_____
myel/o	_____	vitr/o	_____
pharmaceut/o	_____	viv/o	_____
radi/o	_____		

SUFFIXES

Suffix	Meaning	Suffix	Meaning
-gram	_____	-lucent	_____
-graphy	_____	-opaque	_____

PREFIXES

Prefix	Meaning	Prefix	Meaning
cine-	_____	ultra-	_____
echo-	_____		

 Please refer to the enclosed CD for additional exercises and images related to this chapter.

DRUG NAMES, STANDARDS, AND REFERENCES

NAMES

A drug can have three different names. The **chemical name** specifies the chemical makeup of the drug. This name often is long and complicated.

The **generic name,** typically shorter and less complicated, identifies the drug legally and scientifically. The generic name becomes public property after 17 years of use by the original manufacturer, and any drug manufacturer may use it thereafter. There is only one generic name for each drug.

The **brand name** or trademark is the private property of the individual drug manufacturer, and no competitor may use it. A brand name (also called trade name) often has the superscript ® after or before the name, indicating that it is a registered brand name. Drugs can have several brand names because each manufacturer producing the drug gives it a different name. When a specific brand name is ordered on a prescription by a physician, it must be dispensed by the pharmacist; no other brand name may be substituted. It is usual practice to capitalize the first letter of a brand name.

The following list shows the chemical, generic, and brand names of the antibiotic drug ampicillin; note that the drug has several brand names but only one generic, or official, name:

Chemical Name	Generic Name	Brand Name
derivative of 6-aminopenicillanic acid	ampicillin	Omnipen
		Polycillin
		Principen
		Totacillin

STANDARDS

The U.S. **Food and Drug Administration (FDA)** has the legal responsibility for deciding whether a drug may be distributed and sold. It sets rigorous standards for efficacy (effectiveness) and purity and requires extensive experimental testing in animals and people before it approves a new drug for sale in the United States. An independent committee of physicians, pharmacologists, pharmacists, and manufacturers, called the **United States Pharmacopeia (USP),** reviews the available commercial drugs and continually reappraises their effectiveness. Three important standards of the USP are that the drug must be safe, clinically useful (effective for patients) and available in pure form (made by good manufacturing methods). If a drug has USP after its name, it has met with the standards of the Pharmacopeia.

REFERENCES

Two large reference listings of drugs are available at libraries and hospitals. The most complete and up-to-date listing is the **Hospital Formulary,** which gives information about the characteristics of drugs and their clinical usage (application to patient care) as approved by that particular hospital.

The **Physicians' Desk Reference (PDR)** is published by a private firm, and drug manufacturers pay to have their products listed. The PDR is a useful reference with several different indices to identify drugs, along with precautions, warnings about side effects, and information about the recommended dosage and administration of each drug.

21

ADMINISTRATION OF DRUGS

The route of administration of a drug (how it is introduced into the body) determines its rate and completeness of absorption into the blood, and its speed and duration of action.

Various methods of administering drugs are:

Oral Administration. Drugs given by mouth are slowly absorbed into the bloodstream through the stomach or intestinal wall. This method, although convenient for the patient, has several disadvantages. If the drug is destroyed in the digestive tract by digestive juices, or if the drug is unable to pass through the intestinal mucosa, it will be ineffective. Oral administration is also disadvantageous if time is a factor in therapy in that it takes several hours to be absorbed into the bloodstream.

Sublingual Administration. Drugs placed under the tongue dissolve in the saliva. For some agents, absorption may be rapid. Nitroglycerin tablets are administered in this way to treat attacks of angina (chest pain).

Rectal Administration. Suppositories (cone-shaped objects containing drugs) and aqueous solutions are inserted into the rectum. Drugs are given by rectum when oral administration presents difficulties, as when the patient is nauseated and vomiting.

Parenteral Administration. Injection of drug from a **syringe** (tube) through a hollow needle placed under the skin, into a muscle, vein, or body cavity. There are several types of parenteral injections and instillations:

1. **Intracavitary instillation.** This injection is made into a body cavity, such as the peritoneal or pleural cavity. For example, drugs may be introduced into the pleural cavity in people who have pleural effusions due to malignant disease. The drug causes the pleural surfaces to adhere, thereby obliterating the pleural space and preventing the accumulation of fluid. This procedure is known as **pleurodesis.**
2. **Intradermal injection.** This shallow injection is made into the upper layers of the skin and is used chiefly in skin testing for allergic reactions.
3. **Subcutaneous (hypodermic) injection (SC).** A hypodermic needle is introduced into the subcutaneous tissue under the skin, usually on the upper arm, thigh, or abdomen.
4. **Intramuscular injection (IM).** The buttock or upper arm is the usual site for this injection into muscle. When drugs are irritating to the skin or when a large volume of solution must be administered, IM injections are used.
5. **Intrathecal instillation.** This instillation occurs in the space under the membranes (meninges) surrounding the spinal cord and brain. Methotrexate (a cancer chemotherapeutic drug) is introduced intrathecally for treatment of leukemia involving the spinal canal.
6. **Intravenous injection (IV).** This injection is given directly into a vein. It is used when an immediate effect from the drug is desired or when the drug cannot be safely introduced into other tissues. Good technical skill is needed with intravenous injections because leakage of a drug into surrounding tissues may result in irritation and inflammation.

Inhalation. Vapors, or gases, taken into the nose or mouth are absorbed into the bloodstream through the thin walls of air sacs in the lungs. **Aerosols** (particles of drug suspended in air) are administered by inhalation, as are many anesthetics. Examples of aerosols are pentamidine, used to treat a form of pneumonia associated with acquired immunodeficiency syndrome (AIDS), and various aerosolized medicines used to treat asthma (spasm of the lung airways).

Topical Application. Drugs are applied locally on the skin or mucous membranes of the body. **Antiseptics** (against infection) and **antipruritics** (against itching) commonly are used

Table 21–1

Routes of Drug Administration

Oral	Sublingual	Rectal	Parenteral	Inhalation	Topical
Caplets Capsules Tablets	Tablets	Suppositories	Injections and instillations Intracavitary Intradermal Intramuscular Intrathecal Intravenous Subcutaneous	Aerosols	Lotions Creams Ointments Transdermal patches

as ointments, creams, and lotions. **Transdermal patches** are used to deliver drugs (such as estrogen for hormone replacement therapy, pain medications, and nicotine for smoking cessation programs) continuously through the skin.

Table 21–1 summarizes the various routes of drug administration. Figure 21–2 illustrates examples of vehicles for drug administration.

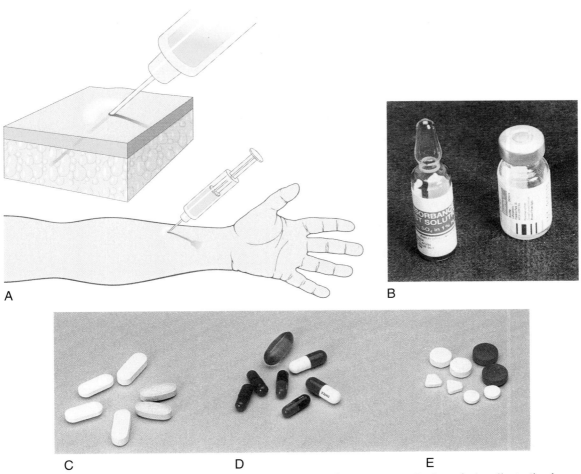

FIGURE 21–2   **Examples of vehicles for drug administration. A, Hypodermic syringe. B, Ampule** (small, sterile glass or plastic container containing a single dose of drug) and **vial** (glass container with a metal-enclosed rubber seal). **C, Caplets** (coated like a capsule, but solid like a tablet). **D, Capsules** (small soluble container, usually made of gelatin, used for a dose of medication for swallowing). **E, Tablets** (small solid pill containing a dose of medication). (**A** from Chabner DE: Medical Terminology: A Short Course, 4th ed. Philadelphia, WB Saunders, 2005, p. 18. **B–E** from Young AP, Kennedy DB: Kinn's The Medical Assistant, 9th ed. Philadelphia, WB Saunders, 2003, pp. 601, 606.)

TERMINOLOGY OF DRUG ACTION

When a drug enters the body, the target substance with which the drug interacts to produce its effects is called a **receptor.** A drug may cross the cell membrane to reach its intracellular receptor or may react with a receptor on the cell's surface.

The following terms describe the action and interaction of drugs in the body after they have been absorbed into the bloodstream:

Additive Action. If the combination of two similar drugs is equal to the **sum** of the effects of each, then the drugs are called additive. For example, if drug A gives 10 percent tumor kill as a chemotherapeutic agent and drug B gives 20 percent tumor kill, using A and B together would give 30 percent tumor kill.

If two drugs give less than an additive effect, they are called **antagonistic.** If they produce greater than additive effects, they are **synergistic** (see **Synergism,** next).

Synergism. A combination of two drugs sometimes can cause an effect that is **greater** than the sum of the individual effects of each drug given alone. For example, penicillin and streptomycin, two antibiotic drugs, are given together in the treatment of bacterial endocarditis because of their synergistic effect.

Tolerance. The effects of a given dose diminish as treatment goes on, and increasing amounts are needed to produce the same effect. Tolerance is a feature of addiction to drugs such as morphine and meperidine hydrochloride (Demerol). **Addiction** is the physical and psychological **dependence** on and craving for a drug and the presence of clear effects when that drug or other agent is withdrawn.

Controlled substances are drugs that produce tolerance and dependence and have potential for abuse or addiction. See page 876 in the Practical Applications section for information about these drugs.

DRUG TOXICITY

Drug toxicity is the poisonous and potentially dangerous effects of some drugs. **Idiosyncrasy** is an example of an unpredictable type of drug toxicity. This is any unexpected effect that appears in the patient after administration of a drug. For example, in some individuals penicillin causes an idiosyncratic reaction, such as **anaphylaxis** (acute hypersensitivity with asthma and shock). Anaphylaxis occurs as a result of exposure to a previously encountered drug or foreign protein (antigen).

Other types of drug toxicity are more predictable and are based on the dosage of the drug given. Physicians are trained to be aware of the potential toxic effects of all drugs that they prescribe. **Iatrogenic** (produced by treatment) disorders can occur, however, as a result of mistakes in drug use or because of unrecognized individual sensitivity to a given agent.

Side effects are toxic effects that routinely result from the use of a drug. They often occur with the usual therapeutic dosage of a drug and generally are tolerable or are considered acceptable. For example, nausea, vomiting, and alopecia are common side effects of the chemotherapeutic drugs used to treat cancer.

Contraindications are factors in a patient's condition that make the use of a drug dangerous and ill advised. For example, in the presence of renal failure, it is unwise to administer a drug that is normally eliminated by the kidneys because excess drug will accumulate in the body and cause side effects.

CLASSES OF DRUGS

The following are major classes of drugs with indications for their use in the body. Specific drugs are included in tables for your reference (brand names are capitalized; generic names begin with a small letter). Appendix IV is a complete list of these drugs and their class or type. Notice that many drug types end with the adjectival suffix -ic, meaning pertaining to, although they are used as nouns.

ANALGESICS

An analgesic (alges/o means sensitivity to pain) is a drug that lessens pain. Mild analgesics relieve mild to moderate pain, such as myalgias, headaches, and toothaches. More potent analgesics are **narcotics** or **opioids,** which contain or are derived from opium. These drugs may induce stupor (a condition of near-unconsciousness and reduced mental and physical activity). They are used only to relieve severe pain because they may produce dependence and tolerance.

Some non-narcotic analgesics reduce fever, pain, and inflammation and are used for joint disorders (osteoarthritis and rheumatoid arthritis), painful menstruation, and acute pain. These agents are not steroid hormones (such as cortisone) and are known as **nonsteroidal anti-inflammatory drugs (NSAIDs).** NSAIDs act on tissues to inhibit prostaglandins (hormone-like substances that sensitize peripheral pain receptors). A newer class of NSAIDs are COX-2 (cyclooxygenase-2) inhibitors. They block the effects of an enzyme that activates prostaglandins. They relieve pain and inflammation as do traditional NSAIDs, but produce fewer gastrointestinal side effects. They may increase the risk of clots and heart attacks. Examples are Celebrex and Aleve, which are listed in Table 21–2 with other analgesics.

Table 21–2

Analgesics and Anesthetics

ANALGESICS	ANESTHETICS
Mild acetaminophen (Tylenol) aspirin tramadol (Ultram)	**General** ether halothane (Fluothane) nitrous oxide thiopental (Pentothal)
Narcotic (Opioid) codeine hydrocodone w/APAP* hydromorphone (Dilaudid) meperidine (Demerol) morphine oxycodone (Oxycontin) propoxyphene HC (Darvon)	**Local** lidocaine (Xylocaine) lidocaine-prilocaine (EMLA—eutectic mixture of local anesthetics) procaine (Novocaine)
Nonsteroidal Anti-inflammatory Drug [NSAID] celecoxib (Celebrex) diclofenac (Voltaren) ibuprofen (Motrin, Advil) naproxen (Naprosyn, Aleve)	

*APAP = acetyl-*p*-aminophenol—acetaminophen (Tylenol, others).
Note: Brand names are in parentheses.

21

ANESTHETICS

An anesthetic is an agent that reduces or eliminates sensation. This effect may occur in all tissues of the body **(general anesthetic)** or may be limited to a particular region **(local anesthetic).** General anesthetics are used for surgical procedures; they depress the activity of the central nervous system, producing loss of consciousness. Local anesthetics inhibit the conduction of impulses in sensory nerves in the region in which they are injected or applied.

Table 21–2 gives examples of specific anesthetics.

ANTIBIOTICS AND ANTIVIRALS

An antibiotic is a chemical substance produced by a microorganism (bacterium, yeast, or mold) that inhibits **(bacteriostatic)** or kills **(bactericidal)** bacteria, fungi, or parasites. The use of antibiotics (penicillin was first in general use in 1945) has largely controlled many conditions such as pneumonia, urinary tract infection, and streptococcal pharyngitis. Caution about the use of antibiotics is warranted because they are powerful agents. With indiscriminate use, pathogenic organisms can develop resistance to the antibiotic, thereby destroying the antibiotic's disease-fighting capability.

Table 21–3

Antibiotics and Antivirals

ANTIFUNGALS

fluconazole (Diflucan)
itraconazole (Sporanox)
miconazole (Monistat)
nystatin (Nilstat)
terbinafine (Lamisil)

ANTITUBERCULARS

isoniazid [INH] (Nydrazid)
rifampin (Rifadin)

ANTIVIRALS

acyclovir (Zovirax)
efavirenz (Sustiva)‡
indinavir (Crixivan)*
interferon alfa-n1 (Wellferon)
lamivudine (Epivir)†
zidovudine *or* azidothymidine [AZT] (Retrovir)†
zidovudine plus lamivudine (Combivir)†

CEPHALOSPORINS—*bactericidal and similar to penicillins*

cefprozil (Cefzil)
ceftazidime (Fortaz)
cephalexin (Keflex)
cefuroxime axetil (Ceftin)

ERYTHROMYCINS—*bacteriostatic*

azithromycin (Zithromax)
clarithromycin (Biaxin)
erythromycin (Ery-Tab)

PENICILLINS—*bactericidal*

amoxicillin trihydrate (Amoxil, Trimox)
amoxicillin with clavulanate (Augmentin)
nafcillin (Unipen)
oxacillin (Bactocill)

QUINOLONES—*bactericidal and wide-spectrum*

ciprofloxacin (Cipro)
levofloxacin (Levaquin)
ofloxacin (Floxin)

SULFONAMIDES OR SULFA DRUGS—*bactericidal*

sulfamethoxazole with trimethoprim (Bactrim)
sulfisoxazole (Gantrisin)

TETRACYCLINES—*bacteriostatic*

doxycycline
tetracycline

*Anti-HIV: protease inhibitor.
†Anti-HIV: nucleoside reverse transcriptase inhibitor (NRTI).
‡Anti-HIV: non-nucleoside reverse transcriptase inhibitor (NNRTI).
Note: Brand names are in parentheses.

Antifungal medications treat fungal infections of the skin (ringworm), vagina, mouth, central nervous system, bloodstream, and other organs. Antituberculosis drugs treat tuberculosis. Antiviral drugs are used against viruses, such as herpesviruses, Epstein-Barr virus, cytomegalovirus (CMV), and human immunodeficiency virus (HIV).

Table 21–3 lists types of antibiotics, antifungals, antituberculars, and antiviral drugs and gives specific examples of each.

ANTICOAGULANTS AND ANTIPLATELET DRUGS

Anticoagulants prevent clotting (coagulation) of blood. They prevent formation of clots or break up clots in blood vessels in conditions such as thrombosis and embolism. They also are used to prevent coagulation in preserved blood used for transfusions. **Heparin** is a natural anticoagulant produced by liver cells and some white blood cells. Other anticoagulants, including **warfarin (Coumadin),** are manufactured. **Tissue-type plasminogen activator (tPA)** dissolves clots and is used to open vessels after myocardial infarction.

Antiplatelet drugs reduce the tendency of platelets to stick together. Aspirin is an example of an antiplatelet drug; it is recommended for patients with coronary artery disease and for those who have had heart attacks. Plavix inhibits the aggregation of platelets and is used to prevent clotting in stents after angioplasty.

Table 21–4 lists anticoagulants and antiplatelet drugs.

Table 21–4

Anticoagulants, Anticonvulsants, Antidepressants, and Antidiabetics

ANTICOAGULANTS AND ANTIPLATELET DRUGS

argatroban (Novastan)
aspirin
clopidogrel bisulfate (Plavix)
dalteparin (Fragmin)
enoxaparin sodium (Lovenox) [injection of low-molecular-weight heparin]
tissue plasminogen activator [tPA]
warfarin (Coumadin)

ANTICONVULSANTS

carbamazepine (Tegretol)
felbamate (Felbatol)
gabapentin (Neurontin)
phenobarbital
phenytoin sodium (Dilantin)
valproic acid (Depakote)

ANTIDEPRESSANTS AND ANTI-ALZHEIMER DRUGS

amitriptyline (Elavil)*
bupropion (Wellbutrin SR)
citalopram hydrobromide (Celexa)‡
donepezil (Aricept)†
fluoxetine (Prozac)‡

memantine (Namenda)
nortriptyline (Pamelor)*
paroxetine (Paxil)‡
sertraline (Zoloft)‡
trazodone (Desyrel)

ANTIDIABETICS

Insulins
Short-acting
human insulin (Humalog)
Intermediate-acting
human insulin NPH (Humulin N)
insulin zinc suspension (Lente)
Long-acting
protamine zinc suspension (PZI)
extended insulin zinc suspension (Ultralente)

Oral Drugs
acarbose (Precose): alpha-glucosidase inhibitor
glipizide (Glucotrol XL): sulfonylurea
glyburide: sulfonylurea
metformin (Glucophage): biguanide
pioglitazone (Actos): thiazolidinedione
repaglinide (Prandin): meglitinide
rosiglitazone (Avandia): thiazolidinedione

*Tricyclic drug.
†Anti-Alzheimer drug.
‡Selective serotonin reuptake inhibitor (SSRI).
Note: Brand names are in parentheses.

ANTICONVULSANTS

An anticonvulsant prevents or reduces the frequency of convulsions in various types of epilepsy. Ideally, anticonvulsants depress abnormal spontaneous activity of the brain arising from areas of scar or tumor, without affecting normal brain function. Table 21–4 lists examples of anticonvulsants.

ANTIDEPRESSANTS AND ANTI-ALZHEIMER DRUGS

Antidepressants treat symptoms of depression. They can elevate mood, increase physical activity and mental alertness, and improve appetite and sleep patterns. Many antidepressants also are mild sedatives and treat mild forms of depression associated with anxiety.

The largest class of antidepressants increases the action of neurotransmitters by blocking their removal (reuptake) from the synapses (spaces between nerve cells). These drugs include **tricyclic antidepressants (TCAs)**, and **selective serotonin reuptake inhibitors (SSRIs).** Other antidepressants are **monoamine oxidase inhibitors (MAOIs)**, which increase the length of time neurotransmitters work by blocking monoamine oxidase, an enzyme that normally inactivates neurotransmitters.

Lithium is a drug that is used to stabilize the mood swings and unpredictable behavior of people with bipolar disorder (manic-depressive illness).

Drugs used to treat symptoms of Alzheimer disease act by aiding brain neurotransmitters or shielding brain cells from glutamate, a neurotransmitter that at high levels contributes to death of brain cells. Table 21–4 gives examples of antidepressants and **anti-Alzheimer drugs**.

ANTIDIABETICS

Antidiabetics are used to treat diabetes mellitus (a condition in which the hormone insulin either is not produced by the pancreas or is not effective in the body). Patients with type 1 (insulin-dependent) diabetes must receive daily injections of **insulin.** Human insulin produced by recombinant DNA research (biosynthesis) has replaced animal-derived insulin in the management of diabetes. Rapid or short-acting insulin starts to work 30 to 60 minutes and lasts 12 to 16 hours. Intermediate-acting insulins start working 1 to 2½ hours after injection and last for 24 hours. Long-acting insulins begin working in 4 to 8 hours and last for 36 hours or more.

Patients with type 2 (non–insulin-dependent) diabetes are given **oral antidiabetic drugs.** These include **sulfonylureas** (lower the levels of glucose in the blood by stimulating the production of insulin), **biguanides** (increase the body's sensitivity to insulin and reduce the production of glucose by the liver), **alpha-glucosidase inhibitors** (temporarily block enzymes that digest sugars), **thiazolidinediones** (enhance glucose uptake into tissues), and **meglitinides** (stimulate the beta cells in the pancreas to produce insulin).

An **insulin pump** is a device strapped to the patient's waist that periodically delivers (via needle) the desired amount of insulin.

Table 21–4 lists antidiabetic drugs.

ANTIHISTAMINES

These drugs block the action of histamine, which is normally released in the body in allergic reactions. Histamine causes allergic symptoms such as hives, bronchial asthma, hay fever, and in severe cases **anaphylactic shock** (dyspnea, hypotension, and loss of consciousness). Antihistamines cannot cure the allergic reaction, but they relieve its symptoms. Many antihistamines have strong **antiemetic** (prevention of nausea) activity and are used to prevent motion sickness. The most common side effects of antihistamines are drowsiness, blurred vision, tremors, digestive upset, and lack of motor coordination. Table 21–5 lists common antihistamines.

ANTIOSTEOPOROSIS DRUGS

Osteoporosis is a disorder marked by abnormal loss of bone density. Calcium, vitamin D, and estrogen are prescribed to increase calcium deposition in bone. Several different drugs are used to treat osteoporosis. **Bisphosphonates** prevent bone loss, and hormone-like drugs called selective estrogen receptor modulators **(SERMs)** increase bone formation. See Table 21–5.

CARDIOVASCULAR DRUGS

Cardiovascular drugs act on the heart or the blood vessels to treat hypertension, angina (pain due to decreased oxygen delivery to heart muscle), myocardial infarction (heart attack), congestive heart failure, and arrhythmias. Often, before other drugs are used, daily aspirin therapy (to prevent clots in blood vessels) and sublingual **nitroglycerin** (to dilate coronary blood vessels) are prescribed. **Digoxin (Lanoxin)** helps the heart pump more forcefully in heart failure. Other cardiovascular drugs include:

Angiotensin-converting enzyme (ACE) inhibitors—dilate blood vessels to lower blood pressure, improve the performance of the heart, and reduce its workload. They prevent the conversion of angiotensin I into angiotensin II, which is a powerful vasopressor (vasoconstrictor). ACE inhibitors reduce the risk of future heart attack, stroke, and death even if a patient is not hypertensive.

Angiotensin II receptor blockers (ARBs)—lower blood pressure by preventing angiotensin from acting on receptors in blood vessels. They are used in patients who do not tolerate ACE inhibitors because of cough or angioedema (swelling of tissues).

Antiarrhythmics—reverse abnormal heart rhythms. They slow the response of heart muscle to nervous system stimulation or slow the rate at which nervous system impulses are carried through the heart.

Beta-blockers—decrease muscular tone in blood vessels (vasodilation), decrease output of the heart, and reduce blood pressure by blocking the action of epinephrine at receptor sites in the heart muscle and in blood vessels. Beta-blockers are prescribed for angina, hypertension, and arrhythmias and prevention of a second heart attack.

Table 21–5

Antihistamines and Antiosteoporosis Drugs

ANTIHISTAMINES	ANTIOSTEOPOROSIS DRUGS
cetirizine (Zyrtec)	*Bisphosphonates*
chlorpheniramine maleate (Chlor-Trimeton)	alendronate (Fosamax)
diphenhydramine (Benadryl)	ibandronate sodium (Boniva)
fexofenadine (Allegra)	pamidronate disodium (Aredia)
loratadine (Claritin)	zoledronic acid (Zometa)
meclizine (Antivert)	*Selective Estrogen Receptor Modulator (SERM)*
promethazine (Phenergan)	raloxifene (Evista)

Note: Brand names are in parentheses.

21

Table 21–6

Cardiovascular Drugs

ANGIOTENSIN-CONVERTING ENZYME (ACE) INHIBITORS	CALCIUM CHANNEL BLOCKERS
enalapril maleate (Vasotec) lisinopril (Prinivil, Zestril) quinapril (Accupril) ramipril (Altace)	amlodipine amlodipine besylate (Norvasc) diltiazem (Cardizem CD) nifedipine (Adalat CC, Procardia)
ANGIOTENSIN II RECEPTOR BLOCKERS	**CHOLESTEROL-LOWERING DRUGS (STATINS)**
irbesartan (Avapro) losartan (Cozaar) valsartan (Diovan)	atorvastatin calcium (Lipitor) lovastatin (Mevacor) pravastatin (Pravachol) rosuvastatin calcium (Crestor) simvastatin sodium (Zocor)
ANTIARRHYTHMICS	**DIURETICS**
amiodarone (Cordarone) ibutilide (Corvert) sotalol (Betapace)	furosemide (Lasix) hydrochlorothiazide (Hydrodiuril, Diuril) spironolactone (Aldactone) triamterene (Dyazide)
BETA-BLOCKERS	
atenolol (Tenormin) carvedilol (Coreg) metoprolol (Lopressor, Toprol-XL) propranolol (Inderal)	

Note: Brand names are in parentheses.

Calcium channel blockers—dilate blood vessels and lower blood pressure and are used to treat angina and arrhythmias. They inhibit the entry of calcium (necessary for blood vessel contraction) into the muscles of the heart and blood vessels.

Cholesterol-lowering drugs (statins)—control hypercholesterolemia (high levels of cholesterol in the blood), which is a major factor in the development of heart disease. Also called **statins,** these drugs lower cholesterol by reducing its production in the liver.

Diuretics—reduce the volume of blood in the body by promoting the kidney to remove water and salt through urine. They treat hypertension (high blood pressure) and congestive heart failure.

Table 21–6 reviews and gives examples of cardiovascular drugs.

ENDOCRINE DRUGS

Endocrine preparations act in much the same manner as the naturally occurring (endogenous) hormones discussed in Chapter 18. **Androgens,** normally made by the testes and adrenal glands, are used for male hormone replacement and to treat endometriosis and breast cancer in women. **Antiandrogens** slow the uptake of androgens or interfere with their binding in tissues. They are prescribed for prostate cancer. **Estrogens** are female hormones, normally produced by the ovaries, that are used for symptoms associated with menopause (estrogen replacement therapy) and to prevent postmenopausal osteoporosis. They also are used for chemotherapy in some types of cancer (e.g., prostate cancer). An important **antiestrogen** drug is **tamoxifen (Nolvadex),** which is used to prevent recurrence of breast cancer and to treat metastatic breast cancer. **Aromatase inhibitors** also reduce the amount of estrogen (estradiol) in the blood.

21

A **selective estrogen receptor modulator (SERM)** has estrogen-like effects on bone (increase in bone mineral density) and on lipid (decrease in cholesterol levels) metabolism; however, it lacks estrogenic effects on uterus and breast tissue. **Progestins** are prescribed for abnormal uterine bleeding caused by hormonal imbalance and, together with estrogen, in hormone replacement therapy and oral contraceptives.

Thyroid hormone is administered when there is a low output of hormone from the thyroid gland. **Glucocorticoids** (adrenal corticosteroids) are prescribed for reduction of inflammation and a wide range of other disorders, including arthritis, severe skin and allergic conditions, respiratory and blood disorders, gastrointestinal ailments, and malignant conditions.

Table 21–7 gives examples of endocrine drugs.

GASTROINTESTINAL DRUGS

Gastrointestinal drugs often are used to relieve uncomfortable and potentially dangerous symptoms, rather than as cures for specific diseases. **Antacids** neutralize the hydrochloric acid in the stomach to relieve symptoms of peptic ulcer, esophagitis, and epigastric discomfort. **Antiulcer** drugs block secretion of acid by cells in the lining of the stomach and are prescribed for patients with gastric and duodenal ulcers and gastroesophageal reflux disease **(GERD).** Histamine H_2 receptor antagonists such as **ranitidine (Zantac)** and **cimetidine (Tagamet)** turn off the system (histamine) that produces stomach acid. Another drug, **omeprazole (Prilosec),** works by stopping acid production by a different method (proton pump inhibition).

Antidiarrheal drugs relieve diarrhea and decrease the rapid movement (peristalsis) in the walls of the colon. **Cathartics** relieve constipation and promote defecation for diagnostic and operative procedures and are used to treat disorders of the gastrointestinal tract. Some cathartics increase the intestinal salt content to cause fluid to fill the intestines; others increase the bulk of the feces to promote peristalsis. Another type of

Table 21–7

Endocrine Drugs

ANDROGEN	GLUCOCORTICOID
fluoxymesterone (Halotestin) methyltestosterone (Virilon)	dexamethasone (Decadron) prednisone (Deltasone)
ANTIANDROGEN	**PROGESTIN**
flutamide (Eulexin) nilutamide (Casodex)	medroxyprogesterone acetate (Cycrin, Provera) megestrol (Megace)
ESTROGEN	
estrogens (Premarin, Prempro, Estradiol)	**SERM**
ANTIESTROGEN	raloxifene (Evista)
tamoxifen (Nolvadex)	**THYROID HORMONE**
AROMATASE INHIBITOR	levothyroxine (Levothroid, Levoxyl, Synthroid)
anastrozole (Arimidex) exemestane (Aromasin) fulvestrant (Faslodex) letrozole (Femara)	liothyronine (Cytomel) liotrix (Thyrolar)

Note: Brand names are in parentheses.

Table 21–8

Gastrointestinal Drugs

ANTACID	ANTIULCER AND ANTI-GASTROINTESTINAL REFLUX DISEASE (GERD) DRUGS
aluminum and magnesium antacid (Gaviscon) magnesium antacid (milk of magnesia) aluminum antacid (Rolaids)	cimetidine (Tagamet) esomeprazole (Nexium) famotidine (Pepcid) lansoprazole (Prevacid) omeprazole (Prilosec) ranitidine (Zantac)
ANTIDIARRHEAL	
diphenoxylate and atropine (Lomotil) loperamide (Imodium) paregoric	**CATHARTIC**
ANTINAUSEANT (ANTIEMETIC)	casanthranol plus docusate sodium (Peri-Colace)
metoclopramide (Reglan) ondansetron (Zofran) promethazine (Phenergan) prochlorperazine maleate (Compazine)	

Note: Brand names are in parentheses.

cathartic lubricates the intestinal tract to produce soft stools. **Laxatives** are mild cathartics, and **purgatives** are strong cathartics.

Antinauseants (antiemetics) relieve nausea and vomiting and also overcome vertigo, dizziness, motion sickness, and symptoms due to labyrinthitis (inflammation of the inner ear).

Table 21–8 lists the various types of gastrointestinal drugs and examples of each.

RESPIRATORY DRUGS

Respiratory drugs are prescribed for the treatment of asthma, emphysema, chronic bronchitis, and bronchospasm. **Bronchodilators** open bronchial tubes and are administered by injection or aerosol inhalers. **Steroid drugs** are inhaled or given

Table 21–9

Respiratory Drugs

BRONCHODILATORS	STEROIDS: INHALERS
albuterol (Proventil) epinephrine (Primatene) ipratropium bromide (Atrovent) ipratropium plus albuterol (Combivent) metaproterenol (Alupent) salbutamol (Ventolin) salmeterol (Serevent) tiotropium (Spiriva)	beclomethasone (Vanceril) flunisolide (AeroBid) fluticasone propionate (Flovent) triamcinolone (Azmacort)
	STEROIDS: IV OR ORAL
LEUKOTRIENE MODIFIERS	methylprednisolone (Medrol) prednisone
montelukast (Singulair) zafirlukast (Accolate) zileuton (Zyflo Filmtab)	

Note: Brand names are in parentheses.

intravenously and orally to reduce chronic inflammation in respiratory passageways. **Leukotriene modifiers** are recent additions to the anti-inflammatory therapy of asthma. They prevent asthma attacks by blocking leukotriene (a bronchoconstrictor) from binding to receptors in respiratory tissues. Table 21–9 gives examples of respiratory drugs.

SEDATIVE-HYPNOTICS

Sedative-hypnotics are medications that depress the central nervous system and promote drowsiness (sedatives) and sleep (hypnotics). They are prescribed for insomnia and sleep disorders. These products have a very high abuse potential and should be used only for short periods of time and under close supervision. **Barbiturates** and **benzodiazepines** are the two major categories of sedative-hypnotics.

Low doses of **benzodiazepines** (which influence the part of the brain responsible for emotions) may act as sedatives and, in higher doses, as hypnotics (to promote sleep).

Table 21–10 gives examples of sedative-hypnotics.

STIMULANTS

Stimulants are drugs that act on the brain to speed up vital processes (heart and respiration) in cases of shock and collapse. They also increase alertness and inhibit hyperactive behavior in children. High doses can produce restlessness, insomnia, and hypertension. Examples of stimulants are **amphetamines**—used to prevent narcolepsy (seizures of sleep), to suppress appetite, and to calm hyperkinetic children. **Caffeine** also is a cerebral stimulant. It is used in drugs to relieve certain types of headache by constricting cerebral blood vessels. Table 21–10 lists examples of stimulants.

TRANQUILIZERS

Tranquilizers are useful for controlling anxiety. Minor tranquilizers **(benzodiazepines)** control minor symptoms of anxiety. Major tranquilizers **(phenothiazines)** control more severe disturbances of behavior. Table 21–10 lists examples of minor and major tranquilizers.

Table 21–10

Sedative-Hypnotics, Stimulants, Tranquilizers

SEDATIVE-HYPNOTICS	TRANQUILIZERS
butabarbital (Butisol)	*Minor*
phenobarbital	alprazolam (Xanax)*
temazepam (Restoril)*	buspirone (BuSpar)
triazolam (Halcion)*	diazepam (Valium)*
zolpidem tartrate (Ambien)	lorazepam (Ativan)*
STIMULANTS	*Major*
caffeine	chlorpromazine (Thorazine)†
dextroamphetamine sulfate (Dexedrine)	lithium carbonate (Eskalith)
methylphenidate (Ritalin)	olanzapine (Zyprexa)
modafinil (Provigil)	thioridazine (Mellaril)†
	trifluoperazine (Stelazine)†

*Benzodiazepine.
†Phenothiazine.
Note: Brand names are in parentheses.

VOCABULARY

21

This list reviews many of the new terms introduced in the text. Short definitions reinforce your understanding of the terms. Refer to the Pronunciation of Terms section for help with unfamiliar or difficult words.

GENERAL TERMS	
addiction	Physical and psychological dependence on and craving for a drug.
additive action	Drug action in which the combination of two similar drugs is equal to the sum of the effects of each.
aerosol	Particles of drug suspended in air.
anaphylaxis	Exaggerated hypersensitivity reaction to a previously encountered drug or foreign protein.
antagonistic action	Combination of two drugs gives less than an additive effect (action).
antidote	Agent given to counteract an unwanted effect of a drug.
brand name	Commercial name for a drug; trademark or trade name.
chemical name	Chemical formula for a drug.
contraindications	Factors in the patient's condition that prevent the use of a particular drug or treatment.
controlled substances	Drugs that produce tolerance and dependence and have potential for abuse or addiction.
Food and Drug Administration (FDA)	Governmental agency having the legal responsibility for enforcing proper drug manufacture and clinical use.
generic name	Legal noncommercial name for a drug.
iatrogenic	Condition caused by treatment (drugs or procedures) given by physicians or medical personnel.
idiosyncrasy	Unexpected effect produced in a particularly sensitive individual but not seen in most patients.
inhalation	Administration of drugs in gaseous or vapor form through the nose or mouth.
medicinal chemistry	Study of new drug synthesis; relationship between chemical structure and biological effects.
molecular pharmacology	Study of interaction of drugs and their target molecules such as enzymes, or cell surface receptors.
oral administration	Drugs are given by mouth.
parenteral administration	Drugs are given by injection into the skin, muscles, or veins (any route other than through the digestive tract). Examples are subcutaneous, intradermal, intramuscular, intravenous, intrathecal, and intracavitary injections.
pharmacist	Specialist in preparing and dispensing drugs.
pharmacy	Location for preparing and dispensing drugs; also the study of preparing and dispensing drugs.
pharmacodynamics	Study of the effects and strength of a drug within the body.

pharmacokinetics	Calculation of drug concentration in tissues and body fluids over a period of time.
pharmacologist	Specialist in the study of the properties, uses, and actions of drugs.
pharmacology	Study of the preparation, properties, uses, and actions of drugs.
Physicians' Desk Reference (PDR)	Reference book that lists drug products.
receptor	Target substance with which a drug interacts in the body.
rectal administration	Drugs are inserted through the anus into the rectum.
side effect	Adverse reaction that routinely results from the use of a drug.
sublingual administration	Drugs are given by placement under the tongue.
synergism	Combination of two drugs causes an effect that is greater than the sum of the individual effects of each drug alone.
syringe	Instrument (tube) for introducing or withdrawing fluids from the body.
tolerance	Larger and larger drug doses must be given to achieve the desired effect. The patient becomes resistant to the action of a drug as treatment progresses.
topical application	Drugs are applied locally on the skin or mucous membranes of the body; ointments, creams, and lotions are applied topically.
toxicity	Harmful effects of a drug.
toxicology	Study of harmful chemicals and their effects on the body.
transport	Movement of a drug across a cell membrane into body cells.
United States Pharmacopeia (USP)	Authoritative list of drugs, formulas, and preparations that sets a standard for drug manufacturing and dispensing.
vitamin	Substance found in foods and essential in small quantities for growth and good health.

CLASSES OF DRUGS AND RELATED TERMS

ACE inhibitor	Lowers blood pressure. Angiotensin-converting enzyme (ACE) inhibitors block the conversion of angiotensin I to angiotensin II (a powerful vasoconstrictor).
amphetamine	Central nervous system stimulant.
analgesic	Relieves pain.
androgen	Male hormone.
anesthetic	Reduces or eliminates sensation; general and local.
angiotensin II receptor antagonist	Lowers blood pressure by preventing angiotensin from acting on receptors in blood vessels.
antacid	Neutralizes acid in the stomach.
antiandrogen	Slows the uptake of androgens or interferes with their effect in tissues.
antiarrhythmic	Treats abnormal heart rhythms.

21

antibiotic	Chemical substance, produced by a plant or microorganism, that has the ability to inhibit or destroy foreign organisms in the body. Examples are antifungals, cephalosporins, erythromycin, tetracycline, antituberculars, penicillins, quinolones, and sulfonamides.
anticoagulant	Prevents blood clotting.
anticonvulsant	Prevents convulsions (abnormal brain activity).
antidepressant	Relieves symptoms of depression.
antidiabetic	Drug given to prevent or treat diabetes mellitus.
antidiarrheal	Prevents diarrhea.
antiemetic	Prevents nausea and vomiting.
antihistamine	Blocks the action of histamine and helps prevent symptoms of allergy.
antinauseant	Relieves nausea and vomiting; antiemetic.
antiplatelet	Reduces the tendency of platelets to stick together and form a clot.
antiulcer	Inhibits the secretion of acid by cells lining the stomach.
antiviral	Acts against viruses such as herpesviruses and HIV.
aromatase inhibitor	Reduces estrogen in the blood by blocking the enzyme aromatase.
bactericidal	Kills bacteria (-cidal means able to kill).
bacteriostatic	Inhibits bacterial growth (-static means stopping or controlling).
beta-blocker	Blocks the action of epinephrine at sites on receptors of heart muscle cells, the muscle lining of blood vessels, and bronchial tubes; antiarrhythmic, antianginal, and antihypertensive.
bisphosphonate	Prevents bone loss in osteoporosis and osteopenia.
caffeine	Central nervous system stimulant.
calcium channel blocker	Blocks the entrance of calcium into heart muscle and muscle lining of blood vessels; used as an antiarrhythmic, antianginal, and antihypertensive; also called **calcium antagonist.**
cardiovascular drug	Acts on the heart and blood vessels. This category of drug includes ACE inhibitors, beta-blockers, calcium channel blockers, cholesterol-lowering drugs or statins, and diuretics.
cathartic	Relieves constipation.
diuretic	Increases the production of urine and thus reduces the volume of fluid in the body; antihypertensive.
emetic	Promotes vomiting.
endocrine	A hormone or hormone-like drug. Examples are androgens, estrogens, progestins, SERMs, thyroid hormone, and glucocorticoids.
estrogen	Female hormone that promotes development of secondary sex characteristics and supports reproductive tissues.
gastrointestinal	Relieves symptoms of diseases in the gastrointestinal tract. Examples are antacids, antiulcer drugs, antidiarrheal drugs, cathartics, laxatives, purgatives, and antinauseants (antiemetics).

glucocorticoid	Hormone from the adrenal cortex that raises blood sugar and reduces inflammation.
hypnotic	Produces sleep or a trance-like state.
laxative	Weak cathartic.
narcotic	Habit-forming drug (potent analgesic) that relieves pain by producing stupor or insensibility; morphine and opium are examples.
progestin	Female hormone that stimulates the uterine lining during pregnancy and is also used in treatment of abnormal uterine bleeding and for hormone replacement therapy.
purgative	Relieves constipation; strong cathartic.
respiratory drug	Treats asthma, emphysema, and infections of the respiratory system. Bronchodilators are examples.
sedative	A mildly hypnotic drug that relaxes without necessarily producing sleep. Benzodiazepines are examples.
stimulant	Excites and promotes activity. Caffeine and amphetamines are examples.
thyroid hormone	Stimulates cellular metabolism.
tranquilizer	Controls anxiety and severe disturbances of behavior.

COMBINING FORMS, PREFIXES, AND TERMINOLOGY

Write the meaning of the medical term in the space provided.

COMBINING FORMS

Combining Form	Meaning	Terminology	Meaning
aer/o	air	aerosol _____ *The suffix -sol means solution.*	
alges/o	sensitivity to pain	analgesic _____	
bronch/o	bronchial tube	bronchodilator _____ *Theophylline is a smooth muscle relaxant used to treat asthma, emphysema, and chronic bronchitis.*	
chem/o	drug	chemotherapy _____	
cras/o	mixture	idiosyncrasy _____ *Idi/o means individual, peculiar; syn- means together. An idiosyncrasy is an abnormal, unexpected effect of a drug that is peculiar to an individual.*	
cutane/o	skin	subcutaneous _____	
derm/o	skin	hypodermic _____	

21

Combining Form	Meaning	Terminology	Meaning
erg/o	work	synergism _____	
esthes/o	feeling, sensation	anesthesia _____	
hist/o	tissue	antihistamine _____	

The suffix -amine indicates a nitrogen-containing compound. Histamine is a substance found in all body tissues (it causes capillary dilation and gastric acid secretion and constricts bronchial tube smooth muscle); an excess of histamine is released when the body comes in contact with substances to which it is sensitive.

Combining Form	Meaning	Terminology	Meaning
hypn/o	sleep	hypnotic _____	
iatr/o	treatment	iatrogenic _____	
lingu/o	tongue	sublingual _____	
myc/o	mold, fungus	erythromycin _____	
narc/o	stupor	narcotic _____	
or/o	mouth	oral _____	
pharmac/o	drug	pharmacology _____	
prurit/o	itching	antipruritic _____	
pyret/o	fever	antipyretic _____	
thec/o	sheath (of brain and spinal cord)	intrathecal _____	
tox/o	poison	toxic _____	
toxic/o	poison	toxicology _____	
vas/o	vessel	vasodilator _____	
ven/o	vein	intravenous _____	
vit/o	life	vitamin _____	

The first vitamins discovered were nitrogen-containing substances called amines. Table 21–11 lists vitamins, their medical names, and foods that are a major source of each.

Table 21–11

Vitamins

Vitamin	Chemical Name(s)	Food Sources
vitamin A	retinol; dehydroretinol	green, leafy and yellow vegetables; liver, eggs, cod liver oil
vitamin B_1	thiamine	yeast, ham, liver, peanuts, milk
vitamin B_2	riboflavin	milk, liver, green vegetables
niacin	nicotinic acid	yeast, liver, peanuts, fish, poultry
vitamin B_6	pyridoxine	liver, fish, yeast
vitamin B_{12}	cyanocobalamin	milk, eggs, liver
vitamin C	ascorbic acid	citrus fruits, vegetables
vitamin D	calciferol	cod liver oil, milk, egg yolk
vitamin E	α-tocopherol	wheat germ oil, cereals, egg yolk
vitamin K	phytonadione; menaquinone; menadione	alfalfa, spinach, cabbage

PREFIXES

Prefix	Meaning	Terminology	Meaning
ana-	upward, excessive, again	anaphylaxis _____ *The suffix -phylaxis means protection.*	
anti-	against	antidote _____ *The suffix -dote comes from Greek, meaning what is given.*	
		antibiotic _____	
contra-	against, opposite	contraindication _____ *Alternatively, drug **indications** are reasons to prescribe a medication; a bacterial infection may be an indication to prescribe a specific antibiotic.*	
par-	other than, apart from	parenteral _____ *Enter/o means intestine.*	
syn-	together, with	synergistic _____	

21

ABBREVIATIONS

Many of the notations used by physicians in writing prescriptions are abbreviations for Latin phrases, which appear in italics.

a.c., ac	before meals *(ante cibum)*	**PCA**	patient-controlled analgesia
ACE	angiotensin-converting enzyme	**PDR**	Physicians' Desk Reference
ad lib	freely, as desired *(ad libitum)*	**p.o., po, PO**	by mouth *(per os)*
APAP	acetaminophen (Tylenol)	**p.r.n., prn**	as needed; as necessary *(pro re nata, as the occasion arises)*
b.i.d., bid	two times a day *(bis in die)*		
c̄	with	**Pt**	patient
Caps	capsules	**q**	every *(quaque)*
cc	cubic centimeter	**q.h., qh**	every hour *(quaque hora)*
FDA	Food and Drug Administration	**q2h**	every 2 hours
gm, g	gram	**q.i.d., qid**	four times a day *(quater in die)*
gtt	drops *(guttae)*	**q.s., qs**	sufficient quantity *(quantum satis)*
h	hour *(hora)*	**qAM**	every morning
h.s., hs	at bedtime	**qPM**	every evening
H₂ blocker	histamine H_2 receptor antagonist	**Rx**	prescription
HRT	hormone replacement therapy	**s̄**	without *(sine)*
IM	intramuscular	**SERM**	selective estrogen receptor modulator
INH	isoniazid—antituberculosis agent	**Sig.**	directions—how to take medication
IV	intravenous	**SL**	sublingual
MAOI	monoamine oxidase inhibitor—an antidepressant	**s.o.s.**	if it is necessary *(si opus sit)*
		SSRI	selective serotonin reuptake inhibitor—an antidepressant
mg	milligram		
ml, mL	milliliter	**SQ**	subcutaneous
NPO	nothing by mouth *(nil per os)*	**tab**	tablet
NSAID	nonsteroidal anti-inflammatory drug	**TCA**	tricyclic antidepressant
p̄	after *(post)*	**t.i.d., tid**	three times daily *(ter in die)*
p.c., pc	after meals *(post cibum)*		

PRACTICAL APPLICATIONS

Relevant material presented here includes a list of frequently prescribed drugs, some actual patient prescriptions, and a table of controlled substances. Answers to the Prescriptions exercise are on page 887.

TOP 30 PRESCRIPTION DRUGS—2005

The following are the top 30 prescription drugs for 2005. Data from the Rx List Internet Dry Index NDC Health Pharmaceutical. The top 200 are listed at www.rxlist.com/top200.htm.

Trade Name	Drug Generic Name	Type/Use
1. Hydrocodone w/APAP	hydrocodone w/APAP	analgesic (narcotic)
2. Lipitor	atorvastatin	cholesterol-lowering statin
3. Amoxicillin	amoxicillin	antibiotic (penicillin-type)
4. Lisinopril	lisinopril	antihypertensive (diuretic)
5. Hydrochlorothiazide	hydrochlorothiazide	antihypertensive (diuretic)
6. Atenolol	atenolol	antihypertensive (beta-blocker)
7. Zithromax Z-Pk	azithromycin	antibiotic (erythromycin-type)
8. Furosemide	furosemide (oral)	antihypertensive (diuretic)
9. Xanax	alprazolam	antianxiety
10. Toprol XL	metoprolol succinate	antihypertensive (beta-blocker)
11. Albuterol aerosol	albuterol	bronchodilator
12. Norvasc	amlodipine	antihypertensive (calcium channel blocker)
13. Synthroid	levothyroxine	hormone (thyroid gland)
14. Metformin HCL	metformin	antidiabetic
15. Zoloft	sertraline	antidepressant (SSRI)
16. Lexapro	escitalopram oxalate	antidepressant
17. Ibuprofen	ibuprofen	analgesic/NSAID
18. Cephalexin	cephalexin	antibiotic (cephalosporin)
19. Ambien	zolpidem	sedative-hypnotic
20. Prednisone oral	prednisone oral	steroid/anti-inflammatory
21. Nexium	esomeprazole magnesium	antiulcer/antiGERD
22. Triamterene w/HCTZ	triamterene w/HCTZ	antihypertensive (diuretic)
23. Propoxyphene-N	acetaminophen	analgesic
24. Zocor	simvastatin	cholesterol-lowering statin
25. Singulair	montelukast	antiallergy drug
26. Prevacid	lansoprazole	antiulcer/antiGERD
27. Metoprolol	metoprolol	antihypertensive (beta-blocker)
28. Prozac	fluoxetine	antidepressant
29. Ativan	lorazepam	antianxiety
30. Plavix	clopidogrel bisulfate	ADP inhibitor

21

PRESCRIPTIONS

The usual order of drug prescription information is as follows: name of the drug, dosage, route of administration, time of administration. Frequently, the physician will include a qualifying phrase to indicate why the prescription is being written. Not all information is listed with every prescription.

Exercise

Match the following prescriptions with their explanations below.

a. Fluoxetine (Prozac) 20 mg p.o. b.i.d.
b. Lisinopril (Zestril) 20 mg 1 cap qAM.
c. Ondansetron (Zofran) 4 mg 1 tab/cap t.i.d. p.r.n. for nausea
d. Ranitidine (Zantac) 300 mg 1 tab p.c. t.i.d
e. Olanzapine (Zyprexa) 5 mg 1 tab qPM
f. Acetaminophen (300 mg) & codeine (30 mg) 1 tab q.i.d. p.r.n. for pain

1. anti-GERD drug taken after meals 3 times a day   _____

2. Tylenol with a narcotic taken 4 times a day as needed   _____

3. antidepressant taken by mouth twice a day   _____

4. antiemetic taken 3 times a day as needed   _____

5. antihypertensive taken every morning   _____

6. antipsychotic, one tablet every evening   _____

CONTROLLED SUBSTANCES

Controlled substances are drugs regulated under existing federal law. The substances are divided into five classes (schedules) based on the substance's medicinal value, harmfulness, and potential for abuse or addiction. Schedule I includes the most dangerous drugs that have no recognized medicinal use, while Schedule V includes the least dangerous drugs. The following table lists examples of drugs in each class with their type, trade and/or "street" names, and medical uses.

Drug	Type	Trade or other name	Medical use
Class (Schedule) I			
heroin	narcotic	Diacetylmorphine, horse, smack	none
LSD	hallucinogen	acid, microdot	none
mescaline, peyote	hallucinogen	mesc, buttons, cactus	none
marijuana	cannabis	pot, Acapulco, grass, reefer	under investigation
Class (Schedule) II			
hydromorphine	narcotic	Dilaudid	analgesic
meperidine	narcotic	Demerol	analgesic
methaqualone	depressant	Quaalude, Sopor	sedative-hypnotic
cocaine	stimulant	coke, flake, snow	local anesthetic
methylphenidate	stimulant	Ritalin	hyperkinesis
phencyclidine	hallucinogen	PCP, angel dust, hog	veterinary anesthetic
Class (Schedule) III			
opium	narcotic	Dover's powder, paregoric	analgesic, antidiarrheal
morphine	narcotic	morphine, pectoral syrup	analgesic, antitussive
codeine	narcotic	codeine	analgesic, antitussive
barbiturates	depressants	phenobarbital, Butisol, Secobarbital	anesthetic, anticonvulsant, sedative-hypnotic
amphetamines	stimulants	Dexedrine, Desoxyn	weight control, narcolepsy
Class (Schedule) IV			
benzodiazepines	depressants	Ativan, diazepam, Librium, Valium, clonopin	antianxiety, sedative-hypnotic, anti-convulsant

Class (Schedule) V

This class includes narcotics such as Percodan and Darvon (analgesics), Lomotil (antidiarrheal), and Robitussin A-C (antitussive).

? EXERCISES

21 Remember to check your answers carefully with those given in the Answers to Exercises, page 885.

A. Name the pharmacologic specialty based on its description below.

1. use of drugs in the treatment of disease _____

2. study of new drug synthesis _____

3. study of how drugs interact with their target molecules _____

4. study of the harmful effects of drugs _____

5. study of drug effects in the body _____

6. measurement of drug concentrations in tissues and in blood over a period of time

_____

B. Match the following terms with their meanings below.

antidote	pharmacist	toxicologist
chemical name	pharmacologist	trade (brand) name
Food and Drug Administration	Physicians' Desk Reference	United States Pharmacopeia
generic name		

1. Specialist in the study of the harmful effects of drugs on the body is a/n _____.

2. Agent given to counteract harmful effects of a drug is a/an _____.

3. Governmental agency with legal responsibility for enforcing proper drug manufacture and clinical

   use is _____.

4. The _____ is the commercial name for a drug.

5. The _____ is the complicated chemical formula for a drug.

6. The _____ is the legal noncommercial name for a drug.

7. Professional who prepares and dispenses drugs is a/an _____.

8. Specialist (MD or PhD) who studies the properties, uses, and actions of drugs is a/an

   _____.

9. Reference book listing drug products is _____.

10. Authoritative list of drugs, formulas, and preparations that sets a standard for drug manufacturing

    and dispensing is _____.

C. Name the route of drug administration based on its description as given below.

1. administered via suppository or fluid into the anus _____

2. administered via vapor or gas into the nose or mouth _____

3. administered under the tongue _____

4. applied locally on skin or mucous membrane_____

5. injected via syringe under the skin or into a vein, muscle, or body cavity _____

6. given by mouth and absorbed through the stomach or intestinal wall _____

D. Give the meanings of the following terms.

1. intravenous _____

2. intrathecal _____

3. antiseptic _____

4. antipruritic _____

5. aerosol _____

6. intramuscular _____

7. subcutaneous_____

8. intracavitary_____

9. addiction _____

E. Match the routes of drug administration in Column I with the medications or procedures in Column II. Write the letter of the answer in the space provided.

Column I

1. intravenous _____

2. rectal _____

3. oral _____

4. topical _____

5. inhalation _____

6. intrathecal _____

7. intramuscular _____

8. intradermal _____

Column II

A. Lotions, creams, ointments
B. Tablets and capsules
C. Skin testing for allergy
D. Lumbar puncture
E. Deep injection, usually in buttock
F. Suppositories
G. Blood transfusions
H. Aerosol medications

21

F. The following are descriptions of drug actions. Supply the word that fits the description.

1. combination of two drugs is greater than the total effects of each drug by itself

_____

2. combination of two drugs that is equal to the sum of the effects of each _____

3. effects of a given drug dose become less as treatment continues, and larger and larger doses must

be given to achieve the desired effect _____

4. an unexpected effect that may appear in a patient following administration of a drug

_____

5. two drugs give less than an additive effect (action) _____

G. Give the meanings of the following terms that describe classes of drugs.

1. antibiotic _____

2. antidepressant _____

3. antihistamine_____

4. analgesic _____

5. anticoagulant_____

6. anesthetic _____

7. antidiabetic _____

8. sedative _____

9. stimulant _____

10. tranquilizer _____

H. Match the term in Column I with the associated term in Column II. Write the letter of the answer in the space provided.

Column I

1. antihistamine   _____
2. analgesic   _____
3. antidiabetic   _____
4. anticoagulant   _____
5. antibiotic   _____
6. stimulant   _____
7. sedative/hypnotic   _____
8. tranquilizer   _____

Column II

A. Caffeine or amphetamines
B. Penicillin or erythromycin
C. Insulin
D. Benzodiazepine
E. Heparin
F. Nonsteroidal anti-inflammatory drug
G. Phenothiazine
H. Anaphylactic shock

21

I. Give the meanings of the following terms.

1. beta-blocker _____

2. androgen _____

3. glucocorticoid _____

4. calcium channel blocker _____

5. estrogen _____

6. antacid _____

7. cathartic _____

8. antiemetic _____

9. bronchodilator _____

10. hypnotic _____

11. diuretic _____

12. cholesterol-lowering drug _____

J. Match the type of drug in Column I with the condition it treats in Column II. Write the letter of the answer in the space provided.

Column I		Column II
1. anticonvulsant	_____	A. Abnormal uterine bleeding caused by hormonal imbalance
2. anticoagulant	_____	B. Severe behavior disturbances and anxiety
3. antacid	_____	C. Epilepsy
4. progestins	_____	D. Congestive heart failure and hypertension
5. antibiotic	_____	E. Epigastric discomfort
6. ACE inhibitor	_____	F. Myalgia and neuralgia
7. bronchodilator	_____	G. Anaphylactic shock
8. antihistamine	_____	H. Thrombosis and embolism
9. tranquilizer	_____	I. Streptococcal pharyngitis
10. analgesic	_____	J. Asthma

21

K. Complete the following terms based on definitions given.

1. agent that reduces fever: anti_____

2. agent that reduces itching: anti_____

3. habit-forming analgesic: _____tic

4. two drugs cause an effect greater than the sum of each alone: syn_____

5. antibiotic derived from a red mold: _____mycin

6. legal nonproprietary name of a drug: _____name

7. factor in a patient's condition that prevents the use of a particular drug:

   contra_____

8. drug that produces an absence of sensation or feeling: an_____

L. Using the terms listed below, complete the following sentences.

ACE inhibitor   antidepressant   diuretic
anesthetic   antiestrogen   NSAID
antibiotic   antihistamine   oral antidiabetic
anticonvulsant   antiviral   SERM

1. Cephalosporins (such as cefuroxime and cefprozil) and penicillins are examples of a/an

   _____ drug.

2. Advil (ibuprofen) is an example of a/an _____.

3. Tegretol (carbamazepine) and phenytoin (Dilantin) are examples of a/an

   _____ drug.

4. Zovirax (acyclovir) and Crixivan (indinavir) are both types of a/an _____ drug.

5. Nolvadex (tamoxifen), used to treat estrogen receptor positive breast cancer in women, is an

   example of a/an _____ drug.

6. Patients with high blood pressure may need Vasotec (enalapril) or Zestril (lisinopril). Both of these

   are examples of a/an _____.

7. Glucophage (metformin) and rosiglitazone (Avandia) are two types of _____
   drugs.

8. Evista (raloxifene), used to treat osteoporosis in postmenopausal women, is an example of a

   selective estrogen receptor modulator or _____.

9. Elavil (amitriptyline) and fluoxetine (Prozac) are two types of a/an _____
   drug.

PHARMACOLOGY   **883**

21

10. If you have an allergy, your doctor may prescribe Allegra (fexofenadine), which is a/an

    _____ drug.

11. Two agents that reduce the amount of fluid in the blood and thus lower blood pressure are Lasix

    (furosemide) and Aldactone (spironolactone). These are _____ drugs.

12. Xylocaine (lidocaine) and Pentothal (thiopental) are examples of a/an _____
    drug.

M. Give the meanings of the following abbreviations.

1. NSAID _____

2. p.r.n. _____

3. q.i.d. _____

4. ad lib _____

5. t.i.d. _____

6. mg _____

7. c̄ _____

8. s̄ _____

9. NPO _____

10. p.c. _____

11. b.i.d. _____

12. q.h. _____

13. p.o. _____

14. q _____

N. Translate the following prescription orders.

1. 1 tab p.o. q.i.d. p.c. and h.s. _____

2. 15-60 mg IM q4-6h _____

3. 2 caps p.o. h.s. _____

4. 1 tab SL p.r.n. _____

5. Apply topically qhs prn _____

21

O. Circle the term that best completes the meaning of the sentence.

1. After his heart attack, Bernie was supposed to take many drugs, including diuretics and a(an) **(progestin, laxative, anticoagulant)** to prevent blood clots.

2. Estelle was always anxious and had a hard time sleeping. Dr. Max felt that a mild **(antacid, anticonvulsant, tranquilizer)** would help her relax and concentrate on her work.

3. During chemotherapy Helen was very nauseated. Dr. Cohen prescribed an **(antihypertensive, antiemetic, antianginal)** to relieve her symptoms of queasy stomach.

4. The two antibiotics worked together and were therefore **(idiosyncratic, generic, synergistic)** in killing the bacteria in Susan's bloodstream.

5. The label warned that the drug might impair fine motor skills. It listed the **(side effects, antidote, pharmacodynamics)** of the sedative.

6. After receiving the results of Judy's sputum culture, her physician, an expert in **(endocrinology, cardiology, infectious disease)**, recommended Biaxin and other **(antihistamines, antibiotics, antidepressants)** to combat the *Mycobacterium avium* complex disease in her **(heart, thyroid gland, lungs)**.

7. Our dog, Eli, has had seizures since he was hit by a car last year. The veterinarian currently prescribes phenobarbital, an **(anticoagulant, antinauseant, anticonvulsant)**, 45 mg b.i.d. **(every other day, twice a day, every evening)**.

8. To control his type 1 **(heart disease, asthma, diabetes)**, David gives himself daily injections of **(oral drugs, insulin, aromatase inhibitors)**.

9. Many students who want to stay awake to study are taking **(stimulants, sedatives, tranquilizers)** containing **(lithium, caffeine, butabarbital)**.

10. Shelly's wheezing, coughing, and shortness of breath when she is stressed and exposed to animal dander all pointed to a diagnosis of **(pneumonia, asthma, heart disease)**, which required treatment with steroids and **(antivirals, diuretics, bronchodilators)**.

MEDICAL SCRAMBLE

Unscramble the letters to form pharmacology terms from the clues. Use the letters in the squares to complete the bonus term. Answers are found on page 887.

1. *Clue:* Drug that acts against viruses such as the herpes virus and HIV.

___ ☐ ___ ___ ___ ___ ☐ ___   RATVALINI

2. *Clue:* Movement of a drug across a cell membrane into body cells.

___ ___ ☐ ___ ___ ___ ___ ___ ___   PONRRTTAS

3. *Clue:* Pertaining to under the skin.

___ ___ ___ ___ ☐ ___ ___ ___ ☐   MYOPRICHED

4. *Clue:* Pertaining to a condition that is produced by a physician or treatment.

☐ ___ ___ ___ ☐ ___ ___ ___ ___   CANIETORIG

5. *Clue:* Pertaining to under the tongue.

☐ ___ ___ ___ ___ ___ ___ ___ ☐   BUGINLLUSA

BONUS TERM: *Clue:* Drug that relieves pain.

☐ ☐ ☐ ☐ ☐ ☐ ☐ ☐ ☐

ANSWERS TO EXERCISES

A

1. chemotherapy
2. medicinal chemistry
3. molecular pharmacology
4. toxicology
5. pharmacodynamics
6. pharmacokinetics

B

1. toxicologist
2. antidote
3. Food and Drug Administration
4. trade (brand) name
5. chemical name
6. generic name
7. pharmacist
8. pharmacologist
9. Physicians' Desk Reference
10. United States Pharmacopeia

C

1. rectal
2. inhalation
3. sublingual
4. topical
5. parenteral
6. oral

D

1. within a vein
2. within a sheath (membranes around the spinal cord or brain)
3. an agent that works against infection

4. an agent that works against itching
5. a solution of particles (drug) in air (vapor or gas)
6. within a muscle

7. under the skin
8. within a cavity
9. physical and psychological dependence on a drug

E

1. G
2. F
3. B

4. A
5. H
6. D

7. E
8. C

F

1. synergism (potentiation)
2. additive action
3. tolerance

4. idiosyncrasy
5. antagonistic

G

1. an agent that inhibits or kills germ life (microorganisms)
2. an agent that relieves the symptoms of depression
3. an agent that blocks the action of histamine and relieves allergic symptoms

4. an agent that relieves pain
5. an agent that prevents blood clotting
6. an agent that reduces or eliminates sensation
7. an agent used to prevent diabetes mellitus

8. an agent (mildly hypnotic) that relaxes and calms nervousness
9. an agent that excites and promotes activity
10. a drug used to control anxiety and severe disturbances of behavior

H

1. H
2. F
3. C

4. E
5. B
6. A

7. D
8. G

I

1. drug that blocks the action of epinephrine at sites of receptors of heart muscles, blood vessels, and bronchial tubes (antihypertensive, antianginal, and antiarrhythmic)
2. a drug that produces male sexual characteristics
3. a hormone from the adrenal glands that reduces inflammation and raises blood sugar

4. a drug that blocks the entrance of calcium into heart muscle and blood vessel walls (antianginal, antiarrhythmic, and antihypertensive)
5. a hormone that produces female sexual characteristics
6. a drug that neutralizes acid in the stomach

7. a drug that relieves constipation
8. a drug that prevents nausea and vomiting
9. a drug that opens air passages
10. an agent that produces sleep
11. a drug that reduces the volume of blood and lowers blood pressure
12. a drug that reduces hypercholesterolemia

J

1. C
2. H
3. E
4. A

5. I
6. D
7. J

8. G
9. B
10. F

K

1. antipyretic
2. antipruritic
3. narcotic

4. synergism
5. erythromycin
6. generic

7. contraindication
8. anesthetic

L

1. antibiotic
2. NSAID
3. anticonvulsant
4. antiviral

5. antiestrogen
6. ACE inhibitor
7. oral antidiabetic for type 2 diabetes
8. SERM

9. antidepressant
10. antihistamine
11. diuretic
12. anesthetic

M

1. nonsteroidal anti-inflammatory drug
2. as needed
3. four times a day
4. freely as desired
5. three times a day
6. milligram
7. with
8. without
9. nothing by mouth
10. after meals
11. twice a day
12. every hour
13. by mouth
14. every

N

1. take one tablet by mouth, 4 times a day, after meals and at bedtime
2. administer 15-60 milligrams intramuscularly, every 4-6 hours
3. take 2 capsules by mouth at bedtime
4. place one tablet under the tongue, as needed
5. apply to the skin, at bedtime as needed

O

1. anticoagulant
2. tranquilizer
3. antiemetic
4. synergistic
5. side effects
6. infectious disease, antibiotics, lungs
7. anticonvulsant, twice a day
8. diabetes, insulin
9. stimulants, caffeine
10. asthma, bronchodilators

ANSWERS TO PRACTICAL APPLICATIONS

Prescriptions

1. d
2. f
3. a
4. c
5. b
6. e

ANSWERS TO MEDICAL SCRAMBLE

1. ANTIVIRAL 2. TRANSPORT 3. HYPODERMIC 4. IATROGENIC 5. SUBLINGUAL
BONUS TERM: ANALGESIC

PRONUNCIATION OF TERMS

PRONUNCIATION GUIDE

ā as in āpe   ă as in ăpple
ē as in ēven   ĕ as in ĕvery
ī as in īce   ĭ as in ĭnterest
ō as in ōpen   ŏ as in pŏt
ū as in ūnit   ŭ as in ŭnder

To test your understanding of the terminology in this chapter, write the meaning of each term in the space provided. In addition, you may wish to cover the terms and write them by looking at your definitions. Make sure your spelling is correct. The page number after each term indicates where it is defined or used in the book, so you can easily check your responses. You will find complete definitions for all of these terms and their audio pronunciations on the CD.

Term	Pronunciation	Meaning
ACE inhibitor (869)	ĀCE ĭn-HĬB-ĭ-tŏr	_____
addiction (868)	ă-DĬK-shŭn	_____
additive action (868)	ĂD-ĭ-tĭv ĂK-shŭn	_____
aerosol (868)	ĀR-ō-sōl	_____
amphetamine (869)	ăm-FĔT-ă-mēn	_____
analgesic (869)	ăn-ăl-JĒ-zĭk	_____
anaphylaxis (868)	ăn-ă-fĭ-LĂK-sĭs	_____

21

Term	Pronunciation	Meaning
androgen (869)	ĂN-drō-jĕn	_____
anesthesia (872)	ăn-ĕs-THĒ-zē-ă	_____
anesthetic (869)	ăn-ĕs-THĔ-tĭk	_____
angiotensin II receptor antagonist (869)	ăn-jē-ō-TĔN-sĭn II rē-SĔP-tŏr ăn-TĂG-ō-nĭst	_____
antacid (869)	ănt-ĂS-ĭd	_____
antagonistic action (868)	ăn-tă-gŏn-NĬS-tĭk ĂK-shŭn	_____
antiandrogen (869)	ăn-tē-ĂN-drō-jĕn	_____
antiarrhythmic (869)	ăn-tē-ā-RĬTH-mĭk	_____
antibiotic (870)	ăn-tĭ-bī-ŎT-ĭk	_____
anticoagulant (870)	ăn-tĭ-kō-ĂG-ū-lănt	_____
anticonvulsant (870)	ăn-tĭ-kŏn-VŬL-sănt	_____
antidepressant (870)	ăn-tĭ-dĕ-PRĔS-ănt	_____
antidiabetic (870)	ăn-tĭ-dī-ă-BĔT-ĭk	_____
antidiarrheal (870)	ăn-tĭ-dī-ă-RĒ-ăl	_____
antidote (868)	ĂN-tĭ-dōt	_____
antiemetic (870)	ăn-tĭ-ĕ-MĔ-tĭk	_____
antihistamine (870)	ăn-tĭ-HĬS-tă-mēn	_____
antinauseant (870)	ăn-tĭ-NAW-zē-ănt	_____
antiplatelet (870)	ăn-tĭ-PLĀT-lĕt	_____
antipruritic (872)	ăn-tĭ-proo-RĬT-ĭk	_____
antipyretic (872)	ăn-tĭ-pĭ-RĔT-ĭk	_____
antiulcer (870)	ăn-tĭ-ŬL-sĕr	_____
antiviral (870)	ăn-tē-VĪ-răl	_____
aromatase inhibitor (870)	ă-RŌ-mă-tās ĭn-HĬB-ĭ-tŏr	_____
bactericidal (870)	băk-tĕ-rĭ-SĪ-dăl	_____
bacteriostatic (870)	băk-tĕ-rē-ō-STĂ-tĭk	_____
beta-blocker (870)	BĀ-tă-BLŎK-ĕr	_____
bronchodilator (871)	brŏng-kō-DĪ-lā-tŏr	_____
bisphosphonate (870)	bĭs-FŎS-fō-nāt	_____
brand name (868)	brănd nām	_____
caffeine (870)	kăf-ĒN	_____
calcium channel blocker (870)	KĂL-sē-ŭm CHĂN-ĕl BLŎK-ĕr	_____

Term	Pronunciation	Meaning
cardiovascular drug (870)	kăr-dē-ō-VĂS-kū-lăr drŭg	_____
cathartic (870)	kă-THĂR-tĭk	_____
chemical name (868)	KĔM-ĭ-kal năm	_____
chemotherapy (871)	kē-mō-THĔR-ă-pē	_____
contraindication (868)	kŏn-tră-ĭn-dĭ-KĀ-shŭn	_____
controlled substances (868)	kŏn-TRŌLD SŬB-stăn-sĕz	_____
diuretic (870)	dī-ū-RĔT-ĭk	_____
emetic (870)	ĕ-MĔT-ĭk	_____
erythromycin (872)	ă-rīth-rō-MĪ-sĭn	_____
endocrine drug (870)	ĔN-dō-krĭn drŭg	_____
estrogen (870)	ĔS-trō-jĕn	_____
gastrointestinal drug (870)	găs-trō-ĭn-TĔS-tĭ-năl drŭg	_____
generic name (868)	jĕ-NĔR-ĭk năm	_____
glucocorticoid (871)	gloo-kō-KŎR-tĭ-koyd	_____
hypnotic (871)	hĭp-NŎT-ĭk	_____
hypodermic (871)	hī-pō-DĔR-mĭk	_____
iatrogenic (868)	ī-ăt-rō-JĔN-ĭk	_____
idiosyncrasy (868)	ĭd-ē-ō-SĬN-kră-sē	_____
inhalation (868)	ĭn-hă-LĀ-shŭn	_____
intrathecal (857)	ĭn-tră-THĒ-kăl	_____
laxative (871)	LĂK-să-tĭv	_____
medicinal chemistry (868)	mĕ-DĬ-sĭ-năl KĔM-ĭs-trē	_____
molecular pharmacology (868)	mō-LĔK-ū-lăr făr-mă-KŎL-ō-jē	_____
narcotic (871)	năr-KŎT-ĭk	_____
oral administration (868)	ŎR-ăl ăd-mĭn-ĭs-TRĀ-shŭn	_____
parenteral administration (868)	pă-RĔN-tĕr-ăl ăd-mĭn-ĭs-TRĀ-shŭn	_____
pharmacist (868)	FĂR-mă-sĭst	_____
pharmacy (868)	FĂR-mă-sē	_____
pharmacodynamics (868)	făr-mă-kō-dī-NĂM-ĭks	_____
pharmacokinetics (869)	făr-mă-kō-kĭ-NĔT-ĭks	_____
pharmacologist (869)	făr-mă-KŎL-ō-gĭst	_____
pharmacology (869)	făr-mă-KŎL-ō-gē	_____

Term	Pronunciation	Meaning
progestin (871)	prō-JĔS-tĭn	_____
purgative (871)	PŬR-gă-tĭv	_____
receptor (869)	rē-SĔP-tŏr	_____
rectal administration (869)	RĔK-tăl ăd-mĭn-ĭs-TRĀ-shŭn	_____
respiratory drug (871)	rĕs-pĭr-ă-TŎR-ē drŭg	_____
sedative (871)	SĔD-ă-tĭv	_____
side effect (869)	sīd ĕ-FĔKT	_____
stimulant (871)	STĬM-ū-lănt	_____
subcutaneous (871)	sŭb-KŪ-tā-nē-ŭs	_____
sublingual (869)	sŭb-LĬNG-wăl	_____
synergism (869)	SĬN-ĕr-jĭzm	_____
synergistic (873)	sĭn-ĕr-JĬS-tĭk	_____
syringe (869)	sĭ-RĬNJ	_____
thyroid hormone (871)	THĪ-royd HŎR-mōn	_____
tolerance (869)	TŎL-ĕr-ănz	_____
topical application (869)	TŎP-ĭ-k'l ăp-lĭ-KĀ-shŭn	_____
toxicity (869)	tŏk-SĬS-ĭ-tē	_____
toxicology (869)	tŏk-sĭ-KŎL-ō-jē	_____
tranquilizer (871)	TRĂN-kwĭ-lī-zĕr	_____
transport (869)	TRĂNZ-pŏrt	_____
vasodilator (872)	văz-ō-DĪ-lā-tŏr	_____
vitamin (869)	VĪ-tă-mĭn	_____

REVIEW SHEET

Write the meanings of the word parts in the spaces provided and test yourself. Check your answers with the information in the chapter or in the glossary (Medical Word Parts—English) at the back of the book.

COMBINING FORMS

Combining Form	Meaning	Combining Form	Meaning
aer/o	_____	lingu/o	_____
alges/o	_____	myc/o	_____
bronch/o	_____	narc/o	_____
chem/o	_____	or/o	_____
cras/o	_____	pharmac/o	_____
cutane/o	_____	prurit/o	_____
derm/o	_____	pyret/o	_____
enter/o	_____	thec/o	_____
erg/o	_____	tox/o	_____
esthes/o	_____	toxic/o	_____
hist/o	_____	vas/o	_____
hypn/o	_____	ven/o	_____
iatr/o	_____	vit/o	_____

SUFFIXES

Suffix	Meaning	Suffix	Meaning
-amine	_____	-in	_____
-dote	_____	-phylaxis	_____
-genic	_____	-sol	_____

PREFIXES

Prefix	Meaning	Prefix	Meaning
ana-	_____	par-	_____
anti-	_____	syn-	_____
contra-	_____		

 Please refer to the enclosed CD for additional exercises and images related to this chapter.

chapter 22

Psychiatry

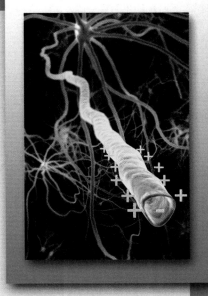

In this chapter you will

- Differentiate among a psychiatrist, a psychologist, and other mental health specialists.
- Describe tests used by clinical psychologists to evaluate a patient's mental health and intelligence.
- Define terms that describe major psychiatric disorders.
- Identify terms that describe psychiatric symptoms.
- Compare different types of therapy for psychiatric disorders.
- Identify the categories of psychiatric drugs, and name commonly used drugs in each category.
- Define combining forms, suffixes, prefixes, and abbreviations related to psychiatry.
- Apply your new knowledge to understanding medical terms in their proper contexts, such as medical reports and records.

Image Description: Stylized image of an axon (portion of a nerve cell).

INTRODUCTION

You will find this chapter different from others in the book. Most psychiatric disorders are not readily explainable in terms of abnormalities in the structure or chemistry of an organ or tissue, as are other illnesses. In addition, the causes of mental disorders are complex and include significant psychological and social as well as chemical and structural elements. This chapter provides a simple outline and definitions of major psychiatric terms. For more extensive and detailed information, you may wish to consult the **Diagnostic and Statistical Manual of Mental Disorders,** 4th edition revised **(DSM-IV-TR),** published by the American Psychiatric Association (Washington, DC), as well as other textbooks of psychiatry.

Psychiatry (psych/o means mind, **iatr/o** means treatment) is the branch of medicine that deals with the diagnosis, treatment, and prevention of mental illness. It is a specialty of clinical medicine comparable to surgery, internal medicine, pediatrics, and obstetrics.

Psychiatrists complete the same medical training (4 years of medical school) as other physicians and receive an MD (doctor of medicine) degree. Then they spend a variable number of years training in the methods and practice of **psychotherapy** (psychological techniques for treating mental disorders) and **psychopharmacology** (drug therapy). Psychiatrists complete four years of residency training and then extra years of fellowship training to specialize in various aspects of psychiatry. **Child psychiatrists** specialize in the treatment of children; **forensic psychiatrists** specialize in the legal aspects of psychiatry, such as the determination of mental competence in criminal cases. **Psychoanalysts** complete 3 to 5 years of training in a special psychotherapeutic technique called **psychoanalysis** in which the patient freely relates her or his thoughts to the analyst, who does not interfere in the flow of thoughts.

A **psychologist** is a nonmedical professional who is trained in methods of psychotherapy, analysis, and research and completes a doctor of philosophy (PhD) or doctor of education (EdD) degree program in a specific field of interest, such as **clinical** (patient-oriented) **psychology, experimental research,** or **social psychology** (focusing on social interaction and the ways the actions of others influence the behavior of the individual). A **clinical psychologist,** like a psychiatrist, can use various methods of psychotherapy to treat patients but, unlike a psychiatrist, cannot prescribe drugs or electroconvulsive therapy. Other nonphysicians trained in the treatment of mental illness are licensed clinical social workers, psychiatric nurses, and licensed mental health clinicians (LMHCs).

Clinical psychologists also are trained in the use of tests to evaluate various aspects of a patient's mental health and intelligence. Examples are **intelligence (IQ) tests** such as the **Wechsler Adult Intelligence Scale (WAIS)** and the **Stanford-Binet Intelligence Scale. Projective (personality) tests** are the use of **Rorschach technique,** in which inkblots, as shown in Figure 22–1, are used to bring out associations, and the **Thematic Apperception**

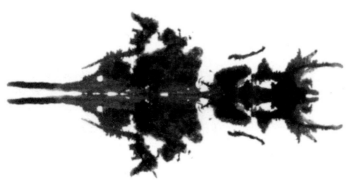

FIGURE 22–1 **Inkblots** like this one are presented on 10 cards in the Rorschach test. The patient describes images seen in the blot.

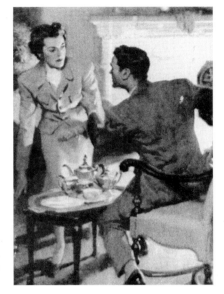

FIGURE 22–2   A sample picture from the **Thematic Apperception Test.** The patient is asked to tell the story that the picture illustrates. (From the New York Public Library/Art Resource, NY.)

Test (TAT), in which pictures are used as stimuli for making up stories (Fig. 22–2). Both tests are revealing of personality structure. **Graphomotor projection tests** are the **Draw a Person Test,** in which the patient is asked to copy a body, and the **Bender-Gestalt Test,** in which the patient is asked to draw certain geometric designs. The Bender-Gestalt Test picks up deficits in mental processing and memory caused by brain damage and is used to screen children for developmental delays. The **Minnesota Multiphasic Personality Inventory (MMPI)** contains true-false questions that reveal aspects of personality, such as sense of duty or responsibility, ability to relate to others, and dominance. This test is widely used as an objective measure of psychological health in adolescents and adults. A patient's responses to questions are compared with responses made by patients with diagnoses of schizophrenia, depression, and so on.

PSYCHIATRIC CLINICAL SYMPTOMS

These terms describe abnormalities that are evident to an examining mental health professional. Familiarity with these terms will help you to understand the next section, Psychiatric Disorders.

amnesia	Loss of memory.
anxiety	Varying degrees of uneasiness, apprehension, or dread often accompanied by palpitations, tightness in the chest, breathlessness, and choking sensations.
apathy	Absence of emotions; lack of interest or emotional involvement.
autistic thought	Thinking is internally stimulated and ideas have a private meaning. (Auto- means self). Fantasy life may be thought of as reality; often a symptom of schizophrenia.
compulsion	Uncontrollable urge to perform an act repeatedly.

conversion	Anxiety becomes a bodily symptom, such as blindness, deafness, or paralysis, that does not have an organic basis.
delusion	A fixed, false belief that cannot be changed by logical reasoning or evidence.
dissociation	Uncomfortable feelings are separated from their real object. In order to avoid mental distress, the feelings are redirected toward a second object or behavior pattern.
dysphoria	Sadness, hopelessness; depressive mood, or feeling "low."
euphoria	Exaggerated feeling of well-being ("high").
hallucination	False or unreal sensory perception as, for example, hearing voices when none are present; an **illusion** is a false perception of an actual sensory stimulus.
labile	Unstable; undergoing rapid emotional change.
mania	State of excessive excitability; hyperactive elation.
mutism	Nonreactive state; stupor.
obsession	An involuntary, persistent idea or emotion; the suffix -mania indicates a strong obsession with something (e.g., pyromania is an obsession with fire)
paranoia	Overly suspicious system of thinking; fixed delusion that one is being harassed, persecuted, or unfairly treated.

PSYCHIATRIC DISORDERS

Sigmund Freud's ideas of personality structure play an important role in the understanding of many types of psychiatric disorders. Freud believed that personality is made up of three major parts: the **id,** the **ego,** and the **superego.** The **id** represents the unconscious instincts and psychic energy present from birth. The id contains basic drives that, operating according to the pleasure principle, seek immediate gratification regardless of the reality of the situation.

The **ego** is the central coordinating branch of the personality. It is the mediator between the id and the outside world. It is the part of the personality that evaluates and assesses the reality of a situation **(reality testing)** and, if necessary, postpones the gratification of a need or drive (id) until a satisfactory object or situation arises. The ego is perceived as being "self" by the individual.

The **superego** is the internalized conscience and moral part of the personality. It encompasses the sense of discipline derived from parental authority and society. Guilt feelings, for example, arise from behavior and thoughts that do not conform to the standards of the superego.

Freud believed that certain psychological disorders occur when conflicts arise between two or more of these aspects of the personality. **Defense mechanisms,** such as denial, are techniques people employ to ward off the anxiety produced by these conflicts. For example, a person afflicted with a serious illness may avoid confronting his or her present or future problems by denial. Thus, he or she may refuse to believe the diagnosis, may miss appointments, may neglect medication, or may ignore symptoms. All individuals utilize defense mechanisms to cope with difficult problems. The use of these mechanisms may be regarded as abnormal or normal according to whether that use makes a constructive or destructive contribution to the individual's personality.

The term **psychosis** is frequently used to describe mental illness. A **psychosis** involves significant impairment of reality testing, with symptoms such as **delusions** (false beliefs), **hallucinations** (false sensory perceptions), and bizarre behavior. Schizophrenic disorders are examples of psychoses. Patients exhibit a disturbed sense of self, inappropriate affect (emotional reactions), and withdrawal from the external world.

Psychiatric disorders that are discussed in this section are **anxiety disorders, delirium** and **dementia, dissociative disorders, eating disorders, mood disorders, personality disorders, pervasive developmental disorders, schizophrenia, sexual** and **gender identity disorders, somatoform disorders,** and **substance-related disorders.**

ANXIETY DISORDERS

These disorders are characterized by anxiety—the experience of unpleasant tension, distress, troubled feelings, and avoidance behavior. A **panic attack (disorder),** marked by intense fear or discomfort and symptoms such as palpitations, sweating, trembling, and dizziness, can occur on its own with no symbolic meaning for the patient (i.e., it occurs "out of the blue"), or it can occur in the context of the following anxiety disorders: **phobic disorders, obsessive-compulsive disorder,** and **post-traumatic stress disorder.**

Phobic disorders are characterized by irrational or debilitating fears associated with a specific object or situation. The patient with a phobic disorder goes to extreme lengths to avoid the object of her or his fear. The object that is feared often is symbolic of an unconscious conflict that is the cause of the phobia and thus diverts the patient's attention from the conflict, keeping it unconscious. Panic attacks (periods of intense apprehension and fear) can occur in anticipation of the phobic situation.

Agoraphobia (agora- means marketplace) is the fear of being alone or in open, crowded, public places from which escape would be difficult or in which help might not be available. Persons with agoraphobia limit their normal activities to avoid situations that trigger their anxiety. Thus, they may feel comfortable only by remaining at home or in the company of a friend or relative.

A **social phobia (social anxiety disorder)** is the fear of situations in which the individual is open to public scrutiny, which could result in possible embarrassment and humiliation. Fear of speaking in public, using public lavatories, or eating in public are examples of social phobias.

Other specific phobias are **claustrophobia** (fear of closed-in places; **claustr/o** means barrier), **acrophobia** (fear of heights; **acr/o** means extremity), and **zoophobia** (fear of animals; **zo/o** means animals).

Obsessive-compulsive disorder (OCD) involves recurrent thoughts **(obsessions)** and repetitive acts **(compulsions)** that dominate the patient's life. The patient experiences anxiety if he or she is prevented from performing special rituals. Often the OCD consumes time and interferes with the individual's social or occupational functioning. Several antidepressant drugs, including clomipramine, have been used to treat OCD with considerable success, particularly when combined with cognitive behavioral therapy.

Post-traumatic stress disorder is the development of symptoms (intense fear, helplessness, insomnia, nightmares, and diminished responsiveness to the external world) following exposure to a traumatic event. Many survivors of the September 11, 2001, attack on the World Trade Center towers and the Pentagon experienced post-traumatic stress disorder.

DELIRIUM AND DEMENTIA

Delirium and **dementia** are both disorders of abnormal **cognition** (mental processes of thinking, perception, reasoning, judgment).

Delirium is an acute, temporary disturbance of consciousness characterized by mental confusion and often psychotic symptoms. The affected person usually presents with rambling, irrelevant, or incoherent speech, sensory misperceptions, and disorientation as to time, place, or person and with memory impairment. Delirium is caused by a variety of conditions, including drug intoxication or withdrawal, seizures or head trauma, and metabolic disturbances such as hypoxia, hypoglycemia, electrolyte imbalances, or hepatic or renal failure. **Delirium tremens** is brought on by withdrawal after prolonged periods of heavy alcohol ingestion.

Dementia is a general, more gradual loss of intellectual abilities that involves impairment of judgment, memory, and abstract thinking as well as changes in personality. Dementia may be caused by conditions, some reversible and some progressive, involving damage to the brain. The most common cause is Alzheimer disease, but others are cerebrovascular disease (stroke), central nervous system (CNS) infection, medications and drugs, brain trauma, tumors, and Parkinson and Huntington diseases. Depression also can present as (pseudo)dementia.

DISSOCIATIVE DISORDERS

Dissociative disorders are chronic or sudden disturbances of memory, identity, consciousness, or perception of the environment that are not caused by the direct effects of brain damage or drug abuse. Examples of dissociative disorders are **dissociative identity disorder**, which is the existence within the individual of two or more distinct personalities that take hold of the affected person's behavior (illustrated in literature by Dr. Jekyll and Mr. Hyde); **dissociative amnesia** (inability to remember important personal information that is too extensive to be explained by ordinary forgetfulness); and **dissociative fugue** (sudden, unexpected travel away from home or customary work locale). The fugue (Latin *fuga* means flight) disorder includes the assumption of a new identity and an inability to recall one's previous identity.

EATING DISORDERS

Eating disorders are severe disturbances in eating behavior. Examples are **anorexia nervosa** and **bulimia nervosa.** Anorexia nervosa is a refusal to maintain a minimally normal body weight. An individual is intensely afraid of gaining weight and has a disturbance in the perception of the shape or size of her or his body. (The term **anorexia**, meaning "lack of appetite," is a misnomer because lack of appetite is rare.) The condition predominantly affects adolescent females, and its principal symptom is a conscious, relentless attempt to diet along with excessive, compulsive overactivity, such as exercise, running, or gymnastics. Most postmenarchal females with this disorder are amenorrheic.

Bulimia nervosa (**bulimia** means abnormal increase in hunger) is characterized by binge eating (uncontrolled indulgence in food) followed by purging (eliminating food from the body). Persons with bulimia maintain normal or nearly normal weight because after binging they engage in inappropriate purging. Examples are self-induced vomiting and the misuse of laxatives or enemas.

MOOD DISORDERS

A mood disorder is prolonged emotion such as depression or mania (elation) that dominates a patient's entire mental life. Examples of mood disorders are **bipolar disorders** and **depressive disorders.**

Bipolar disorders (**bi**- means two; **pol/o** means extreme) are characterized by one or more **manic** episodes alternating with depressive episodes. A manic episode is a period during which the predominant mood is excessively elevated (euphoria), expansive, or irritable. Associated symptoms include inflated self-esteem, or grandiosity, decreased need for sleep, a nearly continuous flow of rapid speech with quick changes of topic, distractibility, an increase in goal-directed activity, and excessive involvement in pleasurable activities that have a high potential for painful consequences. Often there is increased sociability and participation in multiple activities marked by intrusive, domineering, and demanding behavior. **Hypomania** (in this term, **hypo**- means decrease) describes a mood resembling mania, but of lesser intensity. **Bipolar disorder I** is one or more manic episodes, often alternating with major depressive episodes. **Bipolar disorder II** is recurrent major depressive episodes alternating with hypomanic episodes.

Cyclothymic disorder (**cycl/o** means cycle, **thym/o** means mind) is a mild form of bipolar disorder characterized by at least 2 years of hypomania and numerous depressive episodes that do not meet the criteria that define a major depressive episode.

Depressive disorders are marked by one or more major depressive episodes without a history of mania or hypomania. **Major depression** involves episodes of severe **dysphoria** (sadness, hopelessness, worry, discouragement). Other symptoms are appetite disturbances and changes in weight, sleep disorders such as insomnia or hypersomnia, fatigue or low energy, feelings of worthlessness, hopelessness, or excessive or inappropriate guilt, difficulty thinking or concentrating, and recurrent thoughts of death or suicide. **Dysthymia** (or **dysthymic disorder**) is a depressive disorder involving depressed mood (feeling sad or "down in the dumps") that persists over a 2-year period but is not as severe as major depression. Also, there are no psychotic features (delusions, hallucinations, incoherent thinking) as are sometimes found in major depression. Dysthymic disorder can be very impairing but commonly responds well to medication.

Physicians have noted a relationship between the onset of an episode of depressive disorder and a particular period of the year. A regular appearance of depression may occur for approximately 60 days, between the beginning of October and the end of November, every year. This is referred to as **seasonal affective** (mood) **disorder (SAD).** A change from depression to mania or hypomania also may occur within a 60-day period from mid-February to mid-April.

PERSONALITY DISORDERS

Personality traits are established patterns of thinking and ways of relating to and perceiving the environment and the self; however, when these traits become inflexible and rigid, causing impairment of functioning, distress, and conflict with others, they constitute personality disorders. Examples of personality disorders are as follows:

antisocial	No loyalty to or concern for others, and without moral standards; acts only in response to desires and impulses; cannot tolerate frustration and blames others when he or she is at fault.
borderline	Instability in interpersonal relationships and sense of self; characterized by alternating involvement with and

	rejection of people. Frantic efforts are made to avoid real or imagined abandonment.
histrionic	Emotional, attention-seeking, immature, and dependent; irrational outbursts and tantrums; flamboyant and theatrical; having general dissatisfaction with the self and angry feelings about the world.
narcissistic	Grandiose sense of self-importance or uniqueness and preoccupation with fantasies of success and power. **Narcissism** is a pervasive interest in the self with a lack of empathy for others.
paranoid	Continually suspicious and mistrustful of other people but not to a psychotic or delusional degree; jealous and overly concerned with hidden motives of others; quick to take offense.
schizoid	Emotionally cold and aloof; indifferent to praise or criticism or to the feelings of others; few friendships and rarely appears to experience strong emotions, such as anger or joy.

PERVASIVE DEVELOPMENTAL DISORDERS

These are a group of childhood disorders characterized by delays in the development of socialization and communication skills. Examples are **autism** and **Asperger syndrome.** **Autism,** commonly appearing during the first 3 years of life, is marked by difficulties in verbal and nonverbal communication and in social and play interactions. It is a spectrum disorder, affecting each individual differently and at varying degrees. Persons with autism may exhibit some of the following traits:

Resistance to change; insistence on sameness
Using gestures or pointing instead of words to communicate needs
Repeating words or phrases
Preference for being alone; aloof in manner
Tantrums
Difficulty in interacting with others
Not wanting to be touched
Little or no eye contact
Uneven gross/fine motor skills
Sensitivity to sound
Obsessive attachment to objects

Symptoms of autism may lessen as the child develops and receives treatment.

Asperger syndrome is often referred to as a less severe type of autism. Children with Asperger syndrome frequently have normal language skills and normal intelligence. They usually want to interact with others but don't know how to do it. They may have fine rote memory skills but have difficulty with abstract concepts. Repetitive and restricted patterns of behavior may occur as well.

SCHIZOPHRENIA

Schizophrenia is characterized by withdrawal from reality into an inner world of disorganized thinking and conflict. There is mental deterioration from a previous level of function in areas such as work, social relations, and self-care. Some characteristic symptoms of schizophrenia are:

Delusions such as thought broadcasting (the affected person believes that his or her thoughts, as they occur, are broadcast from his or her head to the external world so that others can hear them).

Hallucinations, which may involve many voices the person perceives as coming from outside her or his head.

Disorganized thinking such as loosening of associations (ideas shift from one subject to another, completely unrelated or only obliquely connected). This may result in incoherent, incomprehensible speech.

Flat affect marked by monotonous voice, immobile face, and no signs of expression. Affect (external expression of emotion) also may be inappropriate (giggling and laughing when talking about torture and illness).

Impaired interpersonal functioning and relationship to the external world such as emotional detachment and social withdrawal. **Autistic thought** (preoccupation with self-centered, illogical ideas and fantasies that exclude the external world) often is a feature of schizophrenia.

Psychiatrists describe several types of schizophrenia, such as **catatonic type** (characterized by **catatonia** in which the patient is mute and does not move or react to the outside environment); **disorganized type** (disorganized speech and behavior and flat or inappropriate affect); and **paranoid type** (presence of prominent delusions of grandeur or persecution and auditory hallucinations).

SEXUAL AND GENDER IDENTITY DISORDERS

Sexual disorders are divided into two types: **paraphilias** and **sexual dysfunctions.** **Paraphilias** (**para-** means abnormal, **-philia** means attraction to or love) are characterized by recurrent intense sexual urges, fantasies, or behaviors that involve unusual objects, activities, or situations. Sexual dysfunctions are disturbances in sexual desire or psychosexual changes in sexual response, such as premature ejaculation and dyspareunia (painful sexual intercourse) that are not the result of a general medical condition.

Examples of paraphilias are:

exhibitionism	Compulsive need to expose one's body, particularly the genitals, to an unsuspecting stranger.
fetishism	The use of nonliving objects (articles of clothing) as substitutes for a human sexual love object.
pedophilia	Sexual urges and fantasies involving sexual activity with a prepubescent child (age 13 or younger).
sexual masochism	Sexual gratification is gained by being humiliated, beaten, bound, or otherwise made to suffer by another person.
sexual sadism	Sexual gratification is gained by inflicting physical or psychological pain or humiliation on others.

transvestic fetishism	Cross-dressing; wearing clothing of the opposite sex. This disorder has been described only in heterosexual males who have intense sexually arousing fantasies, urges, or behaviors involving cross-dressing.
voyeurism	Sexual excitement is achieved by observing unsuspecting people who are naked, undressing, or engaging in sexual activity.

A **gender identity disorder** is a strong and persistent cross-gender identification with the opposite sex. This transsexual identification is manifested in preference for cross-dressing and cross-gender roles in make-believe play or in persistent fantasies of being the other sex.

SOMATOFORM DISORDERS

These are a group of disorders in which the patient's mental conflicts are expressed as physical symptoms. The physical symptoms, such as abdominal or chest pain, nausea, vomiting, diarrhea, palpitations, deafness, blindness, and paralysis, are not adequately explained by a physical or other mental disorder or by injury and are not side effects of medication, drugs, or alcohol. There is no diagnosable medical condition such as depression that fully accounts for a physical symptom.

Examples of somatoform (**somat/o** means body) disorders are **conversion disorder** and **hypochondriasis.**

Conversion disorder is a loss of physical functioning that suggests a physical disorder but that instead is an expression of a psychological conflict or need. The patient usually has a feared or unconscious conflict that threatens to escape from **repression** (a defense mechanism in which a person removes unacceptable ideas or impulses from consciousness), but the energies associated with this conflict are experienced as a physical symptom. The conversion symptom (examples are paralysis, blindness, seizures, paresthesias, and dyskinesia) enables the individual to avoid the conflict and get support from the surrounding environment. For example, a person with repressed anger and desire to physically harm a family member may suddenly develop paralysis of the arm (conversion symptom). Another example of conversion disorder is shell shock or combat fatigue, in which a soldier becomes paralyzed and cannot participate in battle.

Hypochondriasis is a preoccupation with bodily aches, pains, and discomforts in the absence of real illness. Appropriate physical evaluation does not support the diagnosis of any physical disorder that can account for the symptoms or the person's interpretation of them. Ruling out a physical abnormality does not reassure the person with hypochondriasis.

SUBSTANCE-RELATED DISORDERS

Substance-related disorders are characterized by symptoms and behavioral changes associated with regular use of substances that affect the central nervous system. Continued or periodic use of certain drugs produces a state of dependence. **Psychological dependence** is a compulsion to continue taking a drug despite adverse consequences, and **physical dependence** is characterized by the onset of withdrawal symptoms when the drug is discontinued abruptly. A significant feature of dependence is **tolerance.** Tolerance is the declining effect of the drug so that the dose must be increased to give the same effect.

Examples of substances that are associated with drug abuse (use of a drug for purposes other than those for which it is prescribed) and dependence are:

Alcohol. Alcohol dependence often is associated with the use and abuse of other psychoactive drugs (cannabis, cocaine, heroin, amphetamines). Signs of alcohol dependence and intoxication include slurred speech, incoordination, unsteady gait, nystagmus (rapid, rhythmic movement of the eyeball), impairment in attention or memory, stupor or coma. It also is associated with depression, as either a cause or a consequence of the drinking.

Amphetamines. These central nervous system stimulants are taken orally or intravenously. Examples are amphetamine (Benzedrine), dextroamphetamine (Dexedrine), and methamphetamine (Desoxyn, or "speed"). Appetite suppressants (diet pills) are amphetamine-like drugs. Psychological and behavioral changes associated with amphetamine dependence include anger, tension or anxiety, impaired judgment, inability to enjoy what was previously pleasurable, and social isolation. Physical signs and symptoms include tachycardia or bradycardia, pupillary dilation, nausea, elevated or low blood pressure, and muscular weakness. Serious depression can occur during withdrawal.

Cannabis. This class of drugs includes all substances with psychoactive properties derived from the cannabis plant plus chemically similar synthetic substances. Examples are **marijuana,** hashish, and purified delta-9-tetrahydrocannabinol (THC), the major psychoactive ingredient in these substances. Psychological and physical signs and symptoms following the smoking of cannabis include euphoria, impaired motor coordination, anxiety, sensation of slowed time, social withdrawal, and impaired memory and judgment. Other signs of cannabis intoxication are increased appetite, dry mouth, tachycardia, and paranoia.

Cocaine. Cocaine is a stimulant drug that produces euphoria as well as vasoconstriction, tachycardia, and hypertension. It comes from the leaves of the coca tree, which grows in Central and South America. The form of cocaine most commonly used in the United States is cocaine hydrochloride powder, which is inhaled through the nostrils and then absorbed into the bloodstream through mucous membranes. It also can be injected intravenously, either alone or mixed with heroin (speedball). This mixture is particularly dangerous because cocaine and heroin act synergistically to depress respiratory function. If the cocaine is separated from its powdered salt form and combined with ether, ammonia, or baking soda, the resulting cocaine alkaloid is commonly called freebase. This form can be smoked and is known as crack or rock. Often, the user of cocaine also is dependent on alcohol or sedatives, which are taken in an attempt to alleviate the unpleasant aftereffects (anxiety, depression, and fatigue) of cocaine intoxication.

Hallucinogens. These drugs produce a state of central nervous system excitement, hyperactivity, hallucinations, delusions, hypertension, and mood changes. Examples of hallucinogens are **lysergic acid diethylamide (LSD), mescaline (peyote),** and **phencyclidine (PCP).** The use of hallucinogens generally is episodic because their psychoactive effects are so potent; frequent use may lead to marked tolerance.

Opioids. This group of drugs includes **heroin** and **morphine** and synthetic drugs with morphine-like action, such as **codeine** and meperidine (Demerol) and OxyContin. These compounds are prescribed as analgesics (painkillers), anesthetics, or cough suppressants. Typical signs and symptoms of opioid intoxication are pupillary constriction, euphoria, slowness in movement, drowsiness, and slurred speech. Effects of overdose are slow and shallow breathing, convulsions, coma, and possible death. Signs and symptoms of opioid withdrawal are watery eyes, rhinorrhea (runny nose), pupillary dilation, abdominal cramps and diarrhea, and muscle and joint pain.

Sedatives, hypnotics, or anxiolytics. These drugs have a soothing, relaxing, euphoric effect and also can produce sleep (hypnotics). Sleeping pills include **barbiturates** such as phenobarbital and secobarbital. Other drugs that produce a barbiturate-like effect are **benzodiazepines,** including temazepam (Restoril), clonazepam (Klonopin), alprazolam

22

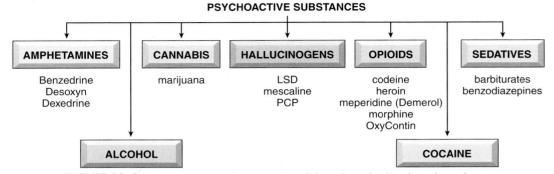

FIGURE 22–3 **Psychoactive substances** that if abused can lead to drug dependence.

(Xanax), and diazepam (Valium). Intoxication is characterized by slurred speech and disorientation. Effects of overdose are shallow respiration, cold and clammy skin, dilated pupils, weak and rapid pulse, coma, and possibly death. Sudden cessation of these drugs can result in seizures.

Figure 22–3 reviews the types of psychoactive substances that lead to drug dependence and abuse.

Table 22–1 reviews psychiatric disorders and gives examples of each type.

THERAPEUTIC TERMINOLOGY

Some major therapeutic techniques that are used to treat psychiatric disorders are **psychotherapy, electroconvulsive therapy,** and **drug therapy (psychopharmacology).**

PSYCHOTHERAPY

This is the treatment of emotional problems by using psychological techniques. The following are psychotherapeutic techniques used by psychiatrists, psychologists, and other mental health professionals.

Cognitive Behavioral Therapy (CBT). Conditioning (changing behavior patterns and responses by training and repetition) is used to relieve anxiety and treat phobias and other disorders. In CBT, the affected person learns how certain thinking patterns can cause symptoms, creating anxiety, depression, or anger for no good reason. Then, therapy helps the person take action to weaken connections between difficult situations and habitual reactions to them.

Family Therapy. Treatment of an entire family can help the members resolve and understand their conflicts and problems.

Group Therapy. In a group with a health professional leader as a neutral moderator, patients with similar problems gain insight into their own personalities through discussions and interaction with each other. In **psychodrama,** patients express their feelings by acting out family and social roles along with other patient-actors on a stage. After a scene has been presented, the audience (composed of other patients) is asked to make comments and offer interpretations about what they have observed.

Hypnosis. A **trance** (state of altered consciousness) is created to increase the speed of psychotherapy or to help recovery of deeply repressed memories.

Insight-Oriented Psychotherapy. Face-to-face discussion of life problems and associated feelings; **psychodynamic therapy**. This therapy aims to increase understanding of underlying themes, thoughts, and behavior patterns to improve mood (depressive feelings).

Table 22–1

Psychiatric Disorders

Category	Example(s)
Anxiety disorders	Panic disorder Phobic disorders Obsessive-compulsive disorder Post-traumatic stress disorder
Delirium and dementia	Delirium tremens
Dissociative disorders	Dissociative identity disorder Dissociative amnesia Dissociative fugue
Eating disorders	Anorexia nervosa Bulimia nervosa
Mood disorders	Bipolar I Bipolar II Cyclothymic disorder Depressive disorders Seasonal affective disorder (SAD)
Personality disorders	Antisocial, borderline, histrionic, narcissistic, paranoid, schizoid
Pervasive developmental disorders	Autism, Asperger syndrome
Schizophrenia	Catatonic, disorganized, and paranoid types
Sexual and gender identity disorders	Paraphilias Sexual dysfunction Gender identity disorder
Somatoform disorders	Conversion disorder Hypochondriasis
Substance-related disorders	Alcohol, amphetamines, cannabis, cocaine, hallucinogens, opioids, sedatives

Play Therapy. In this form of therapy, the child uses play with toys to express conflicts and feelings that he or she is unable to communicate in a direct manner.

Psychoanalysis. This long-term and intense form of psychotherapy seeks to influence behavior and resolve internal conflicts by allowing patients to bring their unconscious emotions to the surface. Through techniques such as **free association** (the patient speaks his or her thoughts one after another without censorship), **transference** (the patient relates to the therapist as to a person who figured prominently in early childhood, such as a parent or sibling), and **dream interpretation,** the patient is able to bring unconscious emotional conflicts to awareness and thus can overcome these problems.

Sex Therapy. This form of therapy helps individuals overcome sexual dysfunctions such as **frigidity** (inhibited sexual response in women), **impotence** (inability of a man to achieve and/or maintain an erection), and **premature ejaculation** (release of semen before coitus can be achieved).

Supportive Psychotherapy. The therapist offers encouragement, support, and hope to patients facing difficult life transitions and events.

ELECTROCONVULSIVE THERAPY

In electroconvulsive therapy (ECT), an electric current is applied to the brain while the patient is anesthetized, with assisted ventilation as needed. The current produces changes in brain wave patterns that result in convulsions (involuntary muscular contractions) and loss of consciousness. With modern techniques, the convulsions usually are observable only in the form of a twitching of the toe. This therapy is used chiefly for serious depression and the depressive phase of bipolar (manic-depressive) disorder. With the introduction of antidepressant drugs, there are fewer indications for electroconvulsive therapy, although it can be life-saving when a rapid response is needed.

DRUG THERAPY

The following are categories of drugs used to treat psychiatric disorders. Figure 22–4 reviews these groups and lists specific drugs in each category.

- **Antianxiety and antipanic agents.** These drugs lessen anxiety, tension, and agitation, especially when they are associated with panic attacks. Examples are **benzodiazepines (BZDs),** which act as antianxiety agents, sedatives, or anticonvulsants (clonazepam). Benzodiazepines directly affect the brain to slow down the transmission of nerve impulses. Other antianxiety and antipanic agents are **selective serotonin reuptake inhibitors (SSRIs).** These agents prevent the reuptake of serotonin (a neurotransmitter) into nerve endings, allowing it to remain in the space between it and the next nerve cell.
- **Antidepressants.** These drugs gradually reverse depressive symptoms and produce feelings of well-being. The basis of depression is thought to be an imbalance in the levels of neurotransmitters in the brain. Several groups of drugs are used as antidepressants. These include:
  1. **SSRIs (selective serotonin reuptake inhibitors)** such as fluoxetine (Prozac). They improve mood, mental alertness, physical activity, and sleep patterns.
  2. **Monoamine oxidase (MAO) inhibitors.** These drugs suppress an enzyme, monoamine oxidase, that normally degrades neurotransmitters. MAO inhibitors are not as widely prescribed as other antidepressants because serious cardiovascular and liver complications can occur with their use.
  3. **Tricyclic antidepressants.** These drugs contain three fused rings (tricyclic) in their chemical structure. They block the reuptake of neurotransmitters at nerve endings.
  4. **Atypical antidepressants.** These are antidepressants that do not fit in the previous categories.
- **Anti–obsessive-compulsive disorder (OCD) agents.** These drugs are prescribed to relieve the symptoms of obsessive-compulsive disorder. Tricyclic antidepressants and SSRIs are examples of these agents.
- **Antipsychotics (neuroleptics).** These drugs modify psychotic symptoms and behavior. **Atypical antipsychotics** are the major examples. They are used to treat schizophrenia, bipolar disorder, and other mental illness. They reduce the anxiety, tension, agitation, and aggressiveness associated with psychoses and modify psychotic symptoms such as delusions and hallucinations. Other drugs, such as **phenothiazines** and haloperidol (Haldol), are still commonly used as well. An important side effect of taking neuroleptic drugs is **tardive dyskinesia (TD);** tardive means late and dyskinesias are abnormal movements. This is a potentially irreversible condition marked by involuntary movements. Early detection is

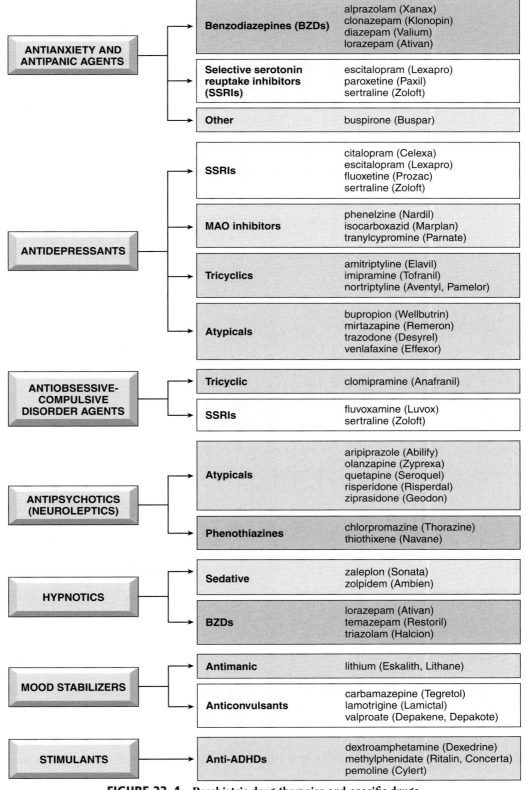

FIGURE 22–4 Psychiatric drug therapies and specific drugs.

important. The AIMS (Abnormal Involuntary Movement Scale) is used to monitor patients for signs of TD. Weight gain and increased risk for developing diabetes also are important side effects of atypical antipsychotics.

- **Hypnotics.** These drugs are used to produce sleep (hypn/o = sleep) and relieve insomnia. Examples are sedatives and benzodiazepines.
- **Mood stabilizers.** These drugs are used primarily to treat patients with mania-predominant form of bipolar disease. **Lithium** (Eskalith, Lithane) is commonly used to reduce the levels of manic symptoms, such as rapid speech, hyperactive movements, grandiose ideas, agitation and irritability, and decreased need for sleep. It also is used as an adjunct in the treatment of depression. Lithium is a simple salt that is thought to stabilize nerve membranes. **Anticonvulsant drugs** also are used as mood stabilizers.
- **Stimulants.** These drugs **(amphetamines)** are prescribed for **attention-deficit hyperactivity disorder (ADHD)** in children. Common symptoms of ADHD are having a short attention span and being easily distracted, emotionally unstable, impulsive, and moderately to severely hyperactive.

 # VOCABULARY

This list reviews many of the new terms introduced in the text. Short definitions reinforce your understanding of the terms. Refer to the Pronunciation of Terms section for help with unfamiliar or difficult words.

GENERAL TERMS, SYMPTOMS, AND DISORDERS	
affect	External expression of emotion, or emotional response.
amnesia	Loss of memory.
anorexia nervosa	Eating disorder with excessive dieting and refusal to maintain a normal body weight.
anxiety disorders	Characterized by unpleasant tension, distress, and avoidance behavior; examples are phobias, obsessive-compulsive disorder, and post-traumatic stress disorder.
apathy	Absence of emotions; lack of interest or emotional involvement.
autistic thought	Thinking is internally stimulated and ideas have a private meaning; fantasy thought of as reality.
bipolar disorder	Mood disorder with alternating periods of mania and depression.
bulimia nervosa	Eating disorder with binge eating followed by vomiting, purging, and depression.
cannabis	Active substance in marijuana; THC.
compulsion	Uncontrollable urge to perform an act repeatedly.
conversion disorder	Condition marked by physical symptoms with no organic basis, appearing as a result of anxiety and unconscious inner conflict.
defense mechanism	Unconscious technique (coping mechanism) a person uses to resolve or conceal conflicts and anxiety. It protects the individual against anxiety and stress; examples are acting out and denial.
delirium	Confusion in thinking; faulty perceptions and irrational behavior. **Delirium tremens** is associated with alcohol withdrawal.

delusion	Fixed, false belief that cannot be changed by logical reasoning or evidence.
dementia	Loss of intellectual abilities with impairment of memory, judgment, and reasoning as well as changes in personality.
depression	Major mood disorder with chronic sadness, loss of energy, hopelessness, worry, and discouragement and, commonly, suicidal impulses and thoughts.
dissociative disorder	Chronic or sudden disturbance in memory, identity, or consciousness; examples are multiple personality disorder, psychogenic disorders, amnesia, and fugue.
ego	Central coordinating branch of the personality or mind.
fugue	Flight from customary surroundings; dissociative disorder.
gender identity disorder	Strong and persistent cross-gender identification with the opposite sex.
hallucination	False sensory perception (hearing voices and seeing things).
id	Major unconscious part of the personality; energy from instinctual drives and desires.
labile	Unstable; undergoing rapid emotional change.
mania	Extreme excitement, hyperactive elation, and agitation. Don't confuse with the suffix -mania (see page 912), meaning obsession.
mood disorders	Prolonged emotion dominates a person's life; examples are bipolar and depressive disorders.
mutism	Nonreactive state; stupor.
neurosis	Repressed conflicts lead to mental symptoms such as anxiety and fears that disturb ability to function; less severe than a psychosis.
obsessive-compulsive disorder	Anxiety disorder in which recurrent thoughts and repetitive acts dominate behavior.
paranoia	Overly suspicious system of thinking; fixed delusions that one is being harassed, persecuted, or unfairly treated.
paraphilia	Recurrent intense sexual urge, fantasy, or behavior that involves unusual objects, activities, or situations.
personality disorders	Lifelong personality patterns marked by inflexibility and impairment of social functioning.
pervasive developmental disorders	Group of childhood disorders characterized by delays in socialization and communication skills; autism and Asperger syndrome are examples.
phobia	Irrational or disabling fear (avoidance) of an object or situation.
post-traumatic stress disorder	Anxiety-related symptoms appear after personal experience of a traumatic event.
projective (personality) test	Diagnostic personality test using unstructured stimuli (inkblots, pictures, abstract patterns, incomplete sentences) to evoke responses that reflect aspects of an individual's personality.

22

psychiatrist	Physician (MD) with medical training in the diagnosis, prevention, and treatment of mental disorders. Examples are a **child psychiatrist** (diagnosing and treating children) and a **forensic psychiatrist** (specializing in legal aspects such as criminal responsibility, guardianship, and competence to stand trial). Forensic comes from the Latin *forum*, meaning public place.
psychologist	Nonmedical professional (often a PhD or an EdD) specializing in mental processes and how the brain functions in health and disease. Areas of interest are **clinical psychology** (providing testing and counseling services to patients with mental and emotional disorders), **experimental psychology** (performing laboratory tests and experiments in a controlled environment to study mental processes), and **social psychology** (study of the effects of group membership on behavior and attitudes of individuals).
psychosis	A disorder marked by loss of contact with reality; often with delusions and hallucinations.
reality testing	Ability to perceive fact from fantasy; severely impaired in psychoses.
repression	Defense mechanism by which unacceptable thoughts, feelings, and impulses are automatically pushed into the unconscious.
schizophrenia	A psychosis marked by withdrawal (split) from reality into an inner world of disorganized thinking and conflict.
sexual disorders	Disorders of paraphilias and sexual dysfunctions.
somatoform disorders	Having physical symptoms that cannot be explained by any actual physical disorder or other well-described mental disorder such as depression.
substance-related disorders	Regular overuse of psychoactive substances (alcohol, amphetamines, cannabis, cocaine, hallucinogens, opioids, and sedatives) that affect the central nervous system.
superego	Internalized conscience and moral part of the personality.
THERAPY	
amphetamines	Central nervous system stimulants that may be used to treat depression and attention-deficit hyperactivity disorder.
atypical antipsychotics	Drugs that treat psychotic symptoms and behavior (schizophrenia, bipolar disease, and other mental illness).
benzodiazepines	Drugs that lessen anxiety, tension, agitation, and panic attacks.
cognitive behavioral therapy	Conditioning (changing behavior patterns by training and repetition) is used to relieve anxiety and improve symptoms of illness.
electroconvulsive therapy	Electric current is used to produce changes in brain wave patterns with resulting convulsions and loss of consciousness; effective in the treatment of major depression. Modern techniques use anesthesia, so the convulsion is not observable.
family therapy	Treatment of an entire family to resolve and shed light on conflicts.
free association	Psychoanalytic technique in which the patient verbalizes, without censorship, the passing contents of his or her mind.

group therapy	Group of patients with similar problems gain insight into their personalities through discussion and interaction with each other.
hypnosis	Trance (state of altered consciousness) is used to increase the pace of psychotherapy.
insight-oriented therapy	Face-to-face discussion of life problems and associated feelings.
lithium	Medication used to treat the manic stage of manic-depressive illness.
neuroleptic drug	Any drug that favorably modifies psychotic symptoms. Examples are atypical antipsychotics.
phenothiazines	Antipsychotic drugs.
play therapy	Treatment in which a child, through use of toys in a playroom setting, expresses conflicts and feelings unable to be communicated in a direct manner.
psychoanalysis	Treatment that allows the patient to explore inner emotions and conflicts so as to understand and change current behavior.
psychodrama	Group therapy in which a patient expresses feelings by acting out family and social roles with other patients.
psychopharmacology	Treatment of psychiatric disorders with drugs.
sedatives	Drugs that lessen anxiety.
supportive psychotherapy	Offering encouragement, support, and hope to patients facing difficult life transitions and events.
transference	Psychoanalytic process in which the patient relates to the therapist as though the therapist were a prominent childhood figure.
tricyclic antidepressants	Drugs used to treat severe depression; three-ringed fused structure.

COMBINING FORMS, SUFFIXES, PREFIXES, AND TERMINOLOGY

Write the meanings of the medical terms in the spaces provided.

COMBINING FORMS

Combining Form	Meaning	Terminology	Meaning
anxi/o	uneasy, anxious, distressed	anxiolytic _____ *This type of drug relieves anxiety.*	
aut/o	self	autism _____	
hallucin/o	hallucination, to wander in the mind	hallucinogen _____ *A **hallucination** is a sensory perception in the absence of any external stimuli, and an **illusion** is an error in perception in which sensory stimuli are present but incorrectly interpreted.*	

22

Combining Form	Meaning	Terminology	Meaning
hypn/o	sleep	hypnosis _____	
		The Greek god of sleep (Hypnos) put people to sleep by touching them with his magic wand or by fanning them with his dark wings.	
iatr/o	treatment	psychiatrist _____	
ment/o	mind	mental _____	
neur/o	nerve	neurosis _____	
		Describes mental disorder in which repressed conflicts lead to mental symptoms such as anxieties and fears that disturb ability to function. Reality testing is not impaired (as in psychosis).	
phil/o	attraction to, love	paraphilia _____	
		Para- means abnormal.	
phren/o	mind	schizophrenia _____	
		Schiz/o means split.	
psych/o	mind	psychosis _____	
		Loss of contact with reality with symptoms such as delusions, hallucinations, and bizarre behavior.	
		psychopharmacology _____	
		psychotherapy _____	
schiz/o	split	schizoid _____	
		Used to describe a mild form of schizophrenia or a withdrawn, introverted personality.	
somat/o	body	psychosomatic _____	
		somatoform disorder _____	
		The suffix -form means resembling. Symptoms of these disorders resemble those of actual physical disease, but the origins are in the mind (psychogenic).	

SUFFIXES

Suffix	Meaning	Terminology	Meaning
-genic	produced by	psychogenic _____	
-leptic	to seize hold of	neuroleptic drugs _____	
-mania	obsessive preoccupation	kleptomania _____	
		Klept/o means to steal.	
		pyromania _____	
		Pyr/o means fire, heat.	

Suffix	Meaning	Terminology	Meaning
-phobia	fear (irrational and often disabling)	agoraphobia _____ *Agora-* means marketplace. Agoraphobics fear leaving home or a safe place.	
		xenophobia _____ *Xen/o* means stranger. Table 22–2 lists other phobias.	
-phoria	feeling, bearing	euphoria _____	
		dysphoria _____	
-thymia	mind	cyclothymia _____ *cycl/o* means circle, recurring. Alternating periods of hypomania and depression; lesser intensity than in bipolar disorder.	
		dysthymia _____ *Depressed mood that is not as severe as major depression.*	

Table 22–2

Phobias

Source of Fear/Anxiety	Medical Term	Source of Fear/Anxiety	Medical Term
Air	Aerophobia	Heights	Acrophobia
Animals	Zoophobia	Insects	Entomophobia
Bees	Apiphobia, melissophobia	Light	Photophobia
		Marriage	Gamophobia
Blood or bleeding	Hematophobia, hemophobia	Men	Androphobia
		Needles	Belonephobia
Books	Bibliophobia	Pain	Algophobia
Cats	Ailurophobia		
Corpses	Necrophobia	Sexual intercourse	Coitophobia, cypridophobia
Crossing a bridge	Gephyrophobia	Sleep	Hypnophobia
Darkness	Nyctophobia, scotophobia	Snakes	Ophidiophobia
		Spiders	Arachnophobia
Death	Thanatophobia	Traveling	Hodophobia
Dogs	Cynophobia	Vomiting	Emetophobia
Drugs	Pharmacophobia	Women	Gynephobia; gynophobia
Eating	Phagophobia		
Enclosed places	Claustrophobia	Worms	Helminthophobia
Hair	Trichophobia, trichopathophobia	Writing	Graphophobia

22

PREFIXES

Prefix	Meaning	Terminology	Meaning
a-, an-	no, not	apathy _____	
cata-	down	catatonia _____ *Ton/o means tension. A state of psychologically induced immobility with muscular rigidity.*	
hypo-	deficient, less than, below	hypomania _____	
		hypochondriasis _____ *Chondr/o means cartilage. The Greeks believed that the liver and spleen (under the cartilage of the ribs) were the seat of melancholy or sadness.*	
para-	abnormal	paranoia _____ *The no- in this term comes from the Greek word* nous, *meaning mind.*	

ABBREVIATIONS

AD	Alzheimer disease—a form of dementia	**MAO**	monoamine oxidase
ADHD	attention-deficit hyperactivity disorder	**MDD**	major depressive disorder
		MMPI	Minnesota Multiphasic Personality Inventory
ADL	activities of daily living	**MR**	mental retardation
AIMS	abnormal involuntary movement scale	**OCD**	obsessive-compulsive disorder
ASD	autism spectrum disorder	**PDD**	pervasive developmental disorder—includes autism and Asperger syndrome
CA	chronologic age		
CBT	cognitive behavior therapy		
CNS	central nervous system	**PTSD**	post-traumatic stress disorder
DSM-IV-TR	Diagnostic and Statistical Manual of Mental Disorders, 4th edition, revised	**Rx**	therapy
		SAD	seasonal affective disorder
		SSRI	selective serotonin reuptake inhibitor—examples: fluoxetine (Prozac), paroxetine (Paxil), sertraline (Zoloft)
DT	delirium tremens		
ECT	electroconvulsive therapy		
IQ	intelligence quotient	**TAT**	Thematic Apperception Test
	An IQ test is a standardized test to determine mental age of an individual. The average person is considered to have an IQ of between 90 and 110. Those who score below 70 are considered mentally retarded.	**TD**	tardive dyskinesia
		THC	delta-9-tetrahydrocannabinol—active ingredient in marijuana
		WAIS	Wechsler Adult Intelligence Scale
		WISC	Wechsler Intelligence Scale for Children
LSD	lysergic acid diethylamide—a hallucinogen	**Ψ**	symbol for psych-
MA	mental age—as determined by psychological tests	**ΨRx**	psychotherapy

PRACTICAL APPLICATIONS

CASE REPORT 1: MAJOR DEPRESSION

Mrs. Carr, a 58-year-old widow, was brought to an emergency ward by her daughter, who found her at home in bed in the middle of the day. For a period of months, Mrs. Carr had become increasingly withdrawn and dysphoric, without any precipitating events. She had become progressively less active and even required encouragement to eat and perform her daily tasks. Her daughter and son-in-law became alarmed but did not know what to do. Mrs. Carr's medical history was unremarkable, but her psychiatric history revealed an episode of postpartum depression following the birth of one of her children.

On examination, the ER physician noted that Mrs. Carr was withdrawn and negativistic, refusing to cooperate with the examination, and even refusing to open her mouth. There were signs of acute dehydration and decline in personal hygiene and grooming.

Further questioning of Mrs. Carr's daughter revealed that Mrs. Carr had become increasingly paranoid and had delusions of sinfulness and guilt. Recently, she had shown signs of increasing mutism.

The physician recognized signs of major depression and arranged for immediate hospitalization. Mrs. Carr responded favorably to combined use of an antipsychotic and an antidepressant drug. An alternative treatment would have been a course of electroconvulsive therapy, which also produces favorable results.

CASE REPORT 2: SOMATOFORM DISORDER

A 35-year-old man presented with a 6-year history of abdominal pain that he was convinced was cancer. For most of his life, the patient had been dominated by a tyrannical father who never gave him the love he craved. When the patient was 29, his father died of carcinoma of the colon, and soon afterward, the patient developed abdominal pain. His complaints gradually increased as his identification with his father, as well as his unconscious hostility toward him, increased. The patient began to present to the clinic almost daily with complaints of bloody stools (the feces were found to be free of blood) and the belief that he had cancer. He felt that none of the clinic doctors listened to him, just as his father had not.

Treatment included development of a long-standing, trusting, positive relationship with one of the clinic physicians, who allowed the patient time to talk about the illness. His hypochondriasis gradually subsided during a 12-month period of a supportive physician-patient relationship.

ⓘ EXERCISES

22   Remember to check your answers carefully with those given in the Answers to Exercises, page 923.

A. Give the terms for the following definitions.

1. physician specializing in treating mental illness: _____

2. nonphysician trained in the treatment of mental illness: _____

3. therapist who practices psychoanalysis: _____

4. branch of psychiatry dealing with legal matters: _____ psychiatry

5. unconscious part of the personality: _____

6. conscious, coordinating part of the personality: _____

7. conscience or moral part of the personality: _____

8. the ability to perceive fact from fantasy: _____ testing

9. unconscious technique used to resolve or conceal conflicts and anxiety:

    _____ mechanism

10. branch of psychology dealing with patient care: _____ psychology

B. Match the following psychiatric symptoms with their meanings as given below.

amnesia	compulsion	hallucination
anxiety	conversion	mania
apathy	delusion	mutism
autistic thought	dissociation	obsession

1. a nonreactive state; stupor _____

2. state of excessive excitability; agitation _____

3. loss of memory _____

4. uncontrollable urge to perform an act repeatedly _____

5. persistent idea, emotion, or urge _____

6. feelings of apprehension, uneasiness, dread _____

7. uncomfortable feelings are separated from their real object and redirected toward a second object

    or behavior pattern _____

8. anxiety becomes a bodily symptom that has no organic basis _____

9. thinking is internally stimulated; ideas have a private meaning _____

10. absence of emotions _____

22

11. fixed false belief that cannot be changed by logical reasoning or evidence

   _____

12. false or unreal sensory perception _____

C. Give the meanings of the following terms.

1. dysphoria _____

2. euphoria_____

3. amnesia _____

4. paranoia _____

5. psychosis _____

6. neurosis _____

7. phobia _____

8. agoraphobia _____

9. labile _____

10. affect _____

D. Select from the following terms to complete the sentences below.

anxiety disorder   eating disorder   sexual disorder
delirium   mood disorder   somatoform disorder
dementia   personality disorder   substance-related disorder
dissociative disorder

1. Disturbance of memory and identity that hides the anxiety of unconscious conflicts is

   _____.

2. Troubled feelings, unpleasant tension, distress, and avoidance behavior describe a/an

   _____.

3. An illness related to regular use of drugs and alcohol is a/an _____.

4. Bulimia nervosa is an example of a/an _____.

5. A disorder involving paraphilias is a/an _____.

6. An illness marked by prolonged emotions (mania and depression) is a/an

   _____.

7. A mental disorder in which physical symptoms cannot be explained by an actual physical disorder

   is a/an _____.

22

8. A lifelong personality pattern that is inflexible and causes distress, conflict, and impairment of social functioning is a/an _____.

9. Loss of intellectual abilities with impairment of memory, judgment, and reasoning is

_____.

10. Confusion in thinking with faulty perceptions and irrational behavior is

_____.

E. Give the meanings of the following terms.

1. obsessive-compulsive disorder _____

2. post-traumatic stress disorder _____

3. bipolar disorder _____

4. fugue _____

5. paranoia _____

6. amphetamines _____

7. cannabis _____

8. schizophrenia _____

9. sexual sadism _____

10. hypochondriasis _____

F. Match the general psychiatric disorder in Column I with its example in Column II. Write the letter of the answer in the space provided.

Column I

1. somatoform disorder _____

2. sexual disorder _____

3. anxiety disorder _____

4. mood disorder _____

5. substance-related disorder _____

6. schizophrenia _____

7. dissociative disorder _____

8. personality disorder _____

9. pervasive developmental disorder _____

Column II

A. Conversion disorder
B. Cocaine abuse
C. Phobia
D. Catatonia
E. Pedophilia
F. Autism
G. Bipolar I and II
H. Narcissism
I. Fugue

22

G. Give the meanings of the following terms.

1. anorexia nervosa _____

2. bulimia nervosa _____

3. repression _____

4. dementia _____

5. hypomania _____

6. hallucinogen _____

7. opioids _____

8. cocaine _____

9. cyclothymic disorder _____

10. dysthymia _____

H. Identify the personality disorder based on its description as given below.

1. flamboyant, theatrical, emotionally immature _____

2. no loyalty or concern for others; does not tolerate frustration and blames others when he or she is

   at fault _____

3. fantasies of success and power and a grandiose sense of self-importance _____

4. pervasive, unwarranted suspiciousness and mistrust of people _____

5. emotionally cold, aloof, indifferent to praise or criticism or to the feelings of others

   _____

6. instability in personal relationships and sense of self; alternating overinvolvement with and rejection

   of people _____

I. Identify the psychotherapeutic technique based on its description as given below.

1. patients express feelings by acting out roles with other patients _____

2. a trance helps patients recover deeply repressed feelings _____

3. long-term and intense exploration of unconscious feelings uses techniques such as transference

   and free association _____

4. toys help a child express conflicts and feelings _____

5. conditioning changes actual behavior patterns rather than focusing on subconscious thoughts and

   feelings _____

22

6. techniques help patients overcome sexual dysfunctions _____

7. electric current is applied to the brain to reverse major depression _____

8. agents (chemicals) relieve symptoms of psychiatric disorders _____

9. face-to-face discussion of life's problems and associated feelings _____

10. offering encouragement, support, and hope to patients facing difficult life transitions and events

_____

J. Match the following terms with their meanings below.

agoraphobia	dysthymia	phenothiazines
amphetamines	kleptomania	pyromania
benzodiazepines	lithium	tricyclic antidepressants
cyclothymia	MAO inhibitors	xenophobia

1. Fear of strangers is _____.

2. Obsessive preoccupation with stealing is _____.

3. Antidepressant agents that work by blocking the action of a specific enzyme are

_____.

4. Mood disorder marked by depressive periods milder than major depression is

_____.

5. Antipsychotic (neuroleptic) tranquilizers such as Thorazine are _____.

6. Fear of being left alone in unfamiliar surroundings is _____.

7. Stimulants used as therapy for mood disorders or for treatment of children with attention-deficit

hyperactivity disorder are _____.

8. Mild form of bipolar disorder in which hypomanic episodes alternate with depression is

_____.

9. Obsessive preoccupation with fire is _____.

10. Drugs (containing three fused rings) used to elevate mood and increase physical activity and

mental alertness are _____.

11. Anxiolytic agents that lessen the anxiety associated with panic attacks are

_____.

12. Drug that treats the manic episodes of bipolar disorder is _____.

22

K. Give the meanings of the following word parts.

1. phren/o _____   8. -phobia _____

2. hypn/o _____   9. -thymia _____

3. somat/o _____   10. -tropic _____

4. phil/o _____   11. -genic _____

5. iatr/o _____   12. para- _____

6. schiz/o _____   13. hypo- _____

7. -mania _____   14. cata- _____

L. Match the following psychiatric drugs with their type and the conditions they treat (consult Figure 22–4).

alprazolam (Xanax)   lamotrigine (Lamictal)   thiothixene (Navane)
amitriptyline (Elavil)   methylphenidate (Ritalin,   zolpidem (Ambien)
aripiprazole (Abilify)   Concerta)
escitalopram (Lexapro)

1. SSRI; treats anxiety and depression _____

2. atypical antipsychotic; treats schizophrenia and bipolar disorder _____

3. stimulant; treats attention-deficit hyperactivity disorder _____

4. tricyclic antidepressant; treats depression _____

5. benzodiazepine; treats anxiety and panic attacks _____

6. sedative; treats insomnia _____

7. anticonvulsant; treats mood disorders (bipolar illness) _____

8. phenothiazine; treats schizophrenia _____

22

M. Circle the term that best completes the meaning of the sentence.

1. Robin fluctuated between bouts of depression and mania and finally was diagnosed as having a **(xenophobic, histrionic, bipolar)** disorder.

2. Although the root of Jon's problems could hardly be addressed simply with medication, his personality disorder and his depression were treated with a selective serotonin reuptake inhibitor (SSRI) called **(lithium, Prozac, Valium)**.

3. Hillary had an enormous fear of open-air markets, shopping malls, and stadiums. She was diagnosed as having **(agoraphobia, xenophobia, pyromania)**.

4. When Sam was admitted to the hospital after his automobile accident, his physicians were told of his alcoholism. They needed to know Sam's history so that they could prevent **(dementia, dysthymia, delirium tremens)**.

5. Hanna was afraid of everyone she met. She had the **(paranoid, narcissistic, schizoid)** delusion that everyone was out to get her.

6. Bill was told that an important potential side effect of taking neuroleptic drugs such as phenothiazines was **(amnesia, gender identity disorder, tardive dyskinesia)**.

7. Ever since she was trapped in an elevator for 3 hours, Lil experienced a **(social phobia, panic attack, somatoform disorder)** marked by palpitations, sweating, and trembling when she was unable to get out of an enclosed space.

8. The few survivors of the nightclub fire were diagnosed with **(OCD, dissociative fugue, post-traumatic stress disorder)**. They regularly experienced insomnia, nightmares, and feelings of helplessness.

9. Sarah couldn't stop herself from eating a gallon of ice cream and box of cookies every evening. She would then feel very anxious and guilty about overeating and induce vomiting. Her mother took her to a/an **(endocrinologist, psychiatrist, gastroenterologist)**, who diagnosed her condition as **(anorexia nervosa, hypochondriasis, bulimia nervosa)** and prescribed **(sex therapy, ECT, psychotherapy)**.

10. Bill felt depressed during the months of November through February. In March his **(OCD, ADHD, SAD)** changed and his mood was characterized by **(hypomania, dysphoria, paranoia)**.

MEDICAL SCRAMBLE

Unscramble the letters to form psychiatry terms from the clues. Use the letters in the squares to complete the bonus term. Answers are found on page 925.

1. *Clue:* Unstable; undergoing rapid emotional change.

   ___ ___ ☐ ___ ___ ☐   L E L A I B

2. *Clue:* Strong impulse (obsessive urge) to set objects on fire.

   ☐ ___ ___ ☐ ___ ___ ___ ☐ ___ ___   M Y A I O R A N P

3. *Clue:* Sadness, hopelessness, and depressive mood; feeling "low."

   ___ ___ ___ ___ ☐ ___ ___ ___ ☐   R I Y H S O P D A

4. *Clue:* Drug that relieves anxiety and produces a relaxing effect.

   ___ ___ ☐ ___ ___ ___ ___ ___ ☐ ___   X Y N T A C I L I O

BONUS TERM: *Clue:* Fear of strangers.

☐ ☐ ☐ ☐ ☐ ☐ ☐ ☐ ☐ ☐

ANSWERS TO EXERCISES

A

1. psychiatrist
2. psychologist, psychiatric nurse, licensed clinical social worker
3. psychoanalyst
4. forensic psychiatry
5. id
6. ego
7. superego
8. reality
9. defense
10. clinical

B

1. mutism
2. mania
3. amnesia
4. compulsion
5. obsession
6. anxiety
7. dissociation
8. conversion
9. autism
10. apathy
11. delusion
12. hallucination

C

1. sadness, hopelessness, unpleasant feeling
2. exaggerated feeling of well-being ("high")
3. loss of memory
4. suspicious system of thinking; fixed delusion that one is being treated unfairly or harassed
5. loss of contact with reality; often delusions and hallucinations.
6. repressed conflicts lead to mental symptoms such as anxiety and fears that disturb ability to function
7. irrational fear (avoidance) of an object or a situation
8. fear of leaving one's home or a safe place
9. unstable; undergoing rapid emotional change; fluctuating
10. expression of emotion

22

D
1. dissociative disorder
2. anxiety disorder
3. substance-related disorder
4. eating disorder
5. sexual disorder
6. mood disorder
7. somatoform disorder
8. personality disorder
9. dementia
10. delirium

E
1. recurrent thoughts and repetitive acts that dominate a person's behavior
2. anxiety-related symptoms appear following exposure to personal experience of a traumatic event
3. alternating periods of mania and depression
4. amnesia with flight from customary surroundings
5. delusions of persecution or grandeur
6. CNS stimulants
7. marijuana, hashish; active substance in marijuana; THC
8. psychosis marked by a split from reality; disorganized thinking and behavior
9. achievement of sexual gratification by inflicting physical or psychological pain
10. preoccupation with bodily aches, pains, and discomforts (in the absence of real illness)

F
1. A
2. E
3. C
4. G
5. B
6. D
7. I
8. H
9. F

G
1. eating disorder marked by excessive dieting because of emotional factors
2. eating disorder characterized by binge eating followed by vomiting, purging, and depression
3. a defense mechanism by which unacceptable thoughts, feelings, and impulses are pushed into the unconscious
4. loss of higher mental functioning, memory, judgment, and reasoning
5. mood disorder resembling mania (exaggerated excitement, hyperactivity) but of lesser intensity
6. drug that produces hallucinations (false sensory perceptions)
7. drugs that are derived from opium (morphine and heroin)
8. stimulant drug that causes euphoria and hallucinations
9. alternating periods of hypomania and depressive episodes of lesser intensity than bipolar illness
10. depressed mood persisting over a 2-year period but not as severe as a major depression

H
1. histrionic
2. antisocial
3. narcissistic
4. paranoid
5. schizoid
6. borderline

I
1. psychodrama
2. hypnosis
3. psychoanalysis
4. play therapy
5. behavioral therapy
6. sexual therapy
7. electroconvulsive therapy
8. psychopharmacology, or drug therapy
9. insight-oriented therapy
10. supportive psychotherapy

J
1. xenophobia
2. kleptomania
3. MAO inhibitors
4. dysthymia
5. phenothiazines
6. agoraphobia
7. amphetamines
8. cyclothymia
9. pyromania
10. tricyclic antidepressants
11. benzodiazepines
12. lithium

K
1. mind
2. sleep
3. body
4. love, attraction to
5. treatment
6. split
7. obsessive preoccupation
8. fear
9. mind
10. to influence, turn
11. produced by
12. abnormal
13. deficient, less than, below
14. down

L

1. escitalopram (Lexapro)
2. aripiprazole (Abilify)
3. methylphenidate (Ritalin, Concerta)
4. amitriptyline (Elavil)
5. alprazolam (Xanax)
6. zolpidem (Ambien)
7. lamotrigine (Lamictal)
8. thiothixene (Navane)

22

M

1. bipolar
2. Prozac
3. agoraphobia
4. delirium tremens
5. paranoid
6. tardive dyskinesia
7. panic attack
8. post-traumatic stress disorder
9. psychiatrist; bulimia nervosa; psychotherapy
10. SAD; hypomania

ANSWERS TO MEDICAL SCRAMBLE

1. LABILE   2. PYROMANIA   3. DYSPHORIA   4. ANXIOLYTIC
BONUS TERM: XENOPHOBIA

PRONUNCIATION OF TERMS

PRONUNCIATION GUIDE

ā as in āpe	ă as in ăpple
ē as in ēven	ĕ as in ĕvery
ī as in īce	ĭ as in ĭnterest
ō as in ōpen	ŏ as in pŏt
ū as in ūnit	ŭ as in ŭnder

To test your understanding of the terminology in this chapter, write the meaning of each term in the space provided. In addition, you may wish to cover the terms and write them by looking at your definitions. Make sure your spelling is correct. The page number after each term indicates where it is defined or used in the book, so you can easily check your responses. You will find complete definitions for all of these terms and their audio pronunciations on the CD.

Term	Pronunciation	Meaning
affect (908)	ĂF-fĕkt	_____
agoraphobia (913)	ăg-ŏ-ră-FŌ-bē-ă	_____
amnesia (908)	ăm-NĒ-zē-ă	_____
amphetamines (910)	ăm-FĔT-ă-mēnz	_____
anorexia nervosa (908)	ăn-ō-RĔK-sē-ă nĕr-VŌ-să	_____
antisocial personality (899)	ăn-tē-SŌ-shăl pĕr-sŏ-NĂL-ĭ-tē	_____
anxiety disorders (895)	ăng-ZĪ-ĕ-tē dĭs-ŎR-dĕrz	_____
anxiolytic (911)	ăng-zī-ō-LĬT-ik	_____
apathy (908)	ĂP-ă-thē	_____
Asperger syndrome (900)	ĂS-pĕr-gĕr SĬN-drōm	_____
atypical antipsychotics (910)	ā-TĬP-ĭ-kăl ăn-tĭ-sī-KŎT-ĭks	_____
autism (900)	AW-tĭzm	_____
autistic thought (908)	aw-TĬS-tĭk thawt	_____
benzodiazepines (910)	bĕn-zō-dī-ĂZ-ĕ-pēnz	_____
bipolar disorder (908)	bī-PŌ-lăr dĭs-ŎR-der	_____

22

Term	Pronunciation	Meaning
borderline personality (899)	BŎR-děr-līn pěr-sŏ-NĂL-ĭ-tē	_____
bulimia nervosa (908)	bū-LĒ-mē-ă něr-VŌ-să	_____
cannabis (908)	KĂ-nă-bis	_____
catatonia (914)	kăt-ă-TŎN-ē-ă	_____
claustrophobia (897)	klaws-trō-FŌ-bē-ă	_____
cognitive behavioral therapy (910)	KŎG-nĭ-tĭv bē-HĀV-yŏr-ăl THĔR-ă-pē	_____
compulsion (908)	kŏm-PŬL-shŭn	_____
conversion disorder (908)	kŏn-VĔR-zhŭn dĭs-ŎR-děr	_____
cyclothymia (913)	sī-klō-THĪ-mē-ă	_____
defense mechanism (908)	dē-FĔNS mě-kăn-NĬ-zm	_____
delirium (908)	dě-LĬR-ē-ŭm	_____
delirium tremens (908)	dě-LĬR-ē-ŭm TRĔ-měnz	_____
delusion (909)	dě-LŪ-zhŭn	_____
dementia (909)	dē-MĔN-shē-ă	_____
depression (909)	dē-PRĔ-shŭn	_____
dissociative disorder (909)	dĭs-SŌ-shē-ă-tĭv dĭs-ŎR-der	_____
dysphoria (896)	dĭs-FŎR-ē-ă	_____
dysthymia (913)	dĭs-THĪ-mē-ă	_____
ego (909)	Ē-gō	_____
electroconvulsive therapy (910)	ē-lěk-trō-kŏn-VŬL-sĭv THĔR-ă-pē	_____
euphoria (896)	ū-FŎR-ē-ă	_____
exhibitionism (901)	ěk-sĭ-BĬSH-ŭ-nĭzm	_____
family therapy (910)	FĂM-ĭ-lē THĔR-ă-pē	_____
fetishism (901)	FĔT-ĭsh-ĭzm	_____
free association (910)	frē ă-sō-shē-Ā-shŭn	_____
fugue (909)	fūg	_____
gender identity disorder (909)	GĔN-děr ī-DĔN-tĭ-tē dĭs-ŎR-děr	_____
group therapy (911)	groop THĔR-ă-pē	_____
hallucination (909)	hă-lū-sĭ-NĀ-shŭn	_____
hallucinogen (911)	hă-LŪ-sĭ-nō-jěn	_____
histrionic personality (900)	hĭs-trē-ŎN-ĭk pěr-sŏn-ĂL-ĭ-tē	_____
hypnosis (911)	hĭp-NŌ-sĭs	_____

Term	Pronunciation	Meaning
hypochondriasis (902)	hī-pō-kŏn-DRĪ-ă-sĭs	_____
hypomania (914)	hī-pō-MĀ-nē-ă	_____
id (909)	ĭd	_____
insight-oriented therapy (911)	ĬN-sīt ŎR-ē-ĕn-tĕd THĔR-ă-pē	_____
kleptomania (912)	klĕp-tō-MĀ-nē-ă	_____
labile (909)	LĀ-bĭl	_____
lithium (911)	LĬTH-ē-ŭm	_____
mania (909)	MĀ-nē-ă	_____
mental (912)	MĔN-tăl	_____
mood disorders (909)	mood dĭs-ŎR-dĕrz	_____
mutism (909)	MŪ-tĭzm	_____
narcissistic personality (900)	năr-sĭ-SĬS-tĭk pĕr-sŏ-NĂL-ĭ-tē	_____
neuroleptic drug (911)	nū-rō-LĔP-tĭk drŭg	_____
neurosis (909)	nū-RŌ-sĭs	_____
obsession (896)	ŏb-SĔSH-ŭn	_____
obsessive-compulsive disorder (909)	ŏb-SĔS-ĭv cŏm-PŬL-sĭv dĭs-ŎR-dĕr	_____
opioid (903)	Ō-pē-ŏyd	_____
paranoia (909)	păr-ă-NŎY-ă	_____
paranoid personality (900)	PĂR-ă-nŏyd pĕr-sŏ-NĂL-ĭ-tē	_____
paraphilia (909)	păr-ă-FĬL-ē-ă	_____
pedophilia (901)	pē-dō-FĬL-ē-ă	_____
personality disorders (909)	pĕr-sŏ-NĂL-ĭ-tē dĭs-ŎR-dĕrz	_____
pervasive developmental disorders (909)	pĕr-VĀS-ĭv dĕ-VĔL-ŏp-mĕnt-ăl dĭs-ŎR-dĕrz	_____
phenothiazines (911)	fē-nō-THĪ-ă-zēnz	_____
phobia (909)	FŌ-bē-ă	_____
play therapy (911)	plā THĔR-ă-pē	_____
post-traumatic stress disorder (909)	pōst-traw-MĂT-ĭk strĕs dĭs-ŎR-dĕr	_____
projective test (909)	prō-JĔK-tĭv tĕst	_____
psychiatrist (910)	sī-KĪ-ă-trĭst	_____
psychiatry (894)	sī-KĪ-ă-trē	_____
psychoanalysis (911)	sī-kō-ă-NĂL-ĭ-sĭs	_____

Term	Pronunciation	Meaning
psychodrama (911)	sī-kō-DRĂ-mă	_____
psychogenic (912)	sī-kō-JĔN-ĭk	_____
psychologist (910)	sī-KŎL-ō-jĭst	_____
psychopharmacology (911)	sī-kō-făr-mă-KŎL-ō-jē	_____
psychosis (910)	sī-KŌ-sĭs	_____
psychosomatic (912)	sī-kō-sō-MĂT-ĭk	_____
psychotherapy (904)	sī-kō-THĔR-ă-pē	_____
pyromania (912)	pī-rō-MĀ-nē-ă	_____
reality testing (910)	rē-ĂL-ĭ-tē TĔS-tĭng	_____
repression (910)	rē-PRĔ-shŭn	_____
schizoid personality (900)	SKĬZ-ŏyd or SKĬT-sŏyd pĕr-sŏ-NĂL-ĭ-tē	_____
schizophrenia (910)	skĭz-ō-FRĔ-nē-ă	_____
sedatives (911)	SĔD-ă-tĭvz	_____
sexual disorders (910)	SĔX-ū-ăl dĭs-ŎR-dĕrz	_____
sexual masochism (901)	SĔX-ū-ăl MĂS-ō-kĭzm	_____
sexual sadism (901)	SĔX-ŭ-ăl SĀ-dĭzm	_____
somatoform disorders (910)	sō-MĂT-ō-fŏrm dĭs-ŎR-dĕrz	_____
substance-related disorders (910)	SŬB-stăns—rē-LĀ-tĕd dīs-ŎR-dĕrz	_____
superego (910)	sū-pĕr-Ē-gō	_____
supportive psychotherapy (911)	sū-PŎR-tĭv sī-kō-THĔR-ă-pē	_____
tolerance (902)	TŎL-ĕr-ăns	_____
transference (911)	trăns-FŬR-ĕns	_____
transvestic fetishism (902)	trăns-VĔS-tĭk FĔT-ĭsh-ĭzm	_____
tricyclic antidepressants (911)	trī-SĬK-lĭk ăn-tĭ-dĕ-PRĔ-săntz	_____
voyeurism (902)	VŎY-yĕr-ĭzm	_____
xenophobia (913)	zĕn-ō-FŌ-bē-ă	_____

Review Sheet

Write the meanings of the word parts in the spaces provided and test yourself. Check your answers with the information in the chapter or in the glossary (Medical Word Parts—English) at the back of the book.

COMBINING FORMS

Combining Form	Meaning	Combining Form	Meaning
anxi/o	_____	phil/o	_____
aut/o	_____	phren/o	_____
cycl/o	_____	psych/o	_____
hallucin/o	_____	pyr/o	_____
hypn/o	_____	schiz/o	_____
iatr/o	_____	somat/o	_____
klept/o	_____	ton/o	_____
ment/o	_____	xen/o	_____
neur/o	_____		

SUFFIXES

Suffix	Meaning	Suffix	Meaning
-form	_____	-pathy	_____
-genic	_____	-phobia	_____
-kinesia	_____	-phoria	_____
-leptic	_____	-somnia	_____
-mania	_____	-thymia	_____
-oid	_____	-tropic	_____

PREFIXES

Prefix	Meaning	Prefix	Meaning
a-, an-	_____	dys-	_____
agora-	_____	hypo-	_____
cata-	_____	para-	_____

 Please refer to the enclosed CD for additional exercises and images related to this chapter.

Glossary

MEDICAL WORD PARTS—ENGLISH

Combining Form, Suffix, or Prefix	Meaning	Combining Form, Suffix, or Prefix	Meaning
a-, an-	no; not; without	amyl/o	starch
ab-	away from	an/o	anus
abdomin/o	abdomen	-an	pertaining to
-ac	pertaining to	ana-	up; apart; backward; again, anew
acanth/o	spiny; thorny	andr/o	male
acetabul/o	acetabulum (hip socket)	aneurysm/o	aneurysm (widened blood vessel)
acous/o	hearing	angi/o	vessel (blood)
acr/o	extremities; top; extreme point	anis/o	unequal
acromi/o	acromion (extension of shoulder bone)	ankyl/o	stiff
		ante-	before; forward
actin/o	light	anter/o	front
acu/o	sharp; severe; sudden	anthrac/o	coal
-acusis	hearing	anthr/o	antrum of the stomach
ad-	toward	anti-	against
-ad	toward	anxi/o	uneasy; anxious
aden/o	gland	aort/o	aorta (largest artery)
adenoid/o	adenoids	-apheresis	removal
adip/o	fat	aphth/o	ulcer
adren/o	adrenal gland	apo-	off, away
adrenal/o	adrenal gland	aponeur/o	aponeurosis (type of tendon)
aer/o	air	append/o	appendix
af-	toward	appendic/o	appendix
agglutin/o	clumping; sticking together	aque/o	water
-agon	to assemble, gather	-ar	pertaining to
agora-	marketplace	-arche	beginning
-agra	excessive pain	arter/o	artery
-al	pertaining to	arteri/o	artery
alb/o	white	arteriol/o	arteriole (small artery)
albin/o	white	arthr/o	joint
albumin/o	albumin (protein)	-arthria	articulate (speak distinctly)
alges/o	sensitivity to pain	articul/o	joint
-algesia	sensitivity to pain	-ary	pertaining to
-algia	pain	asbest/o	asbestos
all/o	other	-ase	enzyme
alveol/o	alveolus; air sac; small sac	-asthenia	lack of strength
ambly/o	dim; dull	atel/o	incomplete
-amine	nitrogen compound	ather/o	plaque (fatty substance)
amni/o	amnion (sac surrounding the embryo)	-ation	process; condition
		atri/o	atrium (upper heart chamber)

Combining Form, Suffix, or Prefix	Meaning
audi/o	hearing
audit/o	hearing
aur/o	ear
auricul/o	ear
aut/o	self, own
aut-, auto-	self, own
axill/o	armpit
azot/o	urea; nitrogen
bacill/o	bacilli (bacteria)
bacteri/o	bacteria
balan/o	glans penis
bar/o	pressure; weight
bartholin/o	Bartholin glands
bas/o	base; opposite of acid
bi-	two
bi/o	life
bil/i	bile; gall
bilirubin/o	bilirubin
-blast	embryonic; immature cell
-blastoma	immature tumor (cells)
blephar/o	eyelid
bol/o	cast; throw
brachi/o	arm
brachy-	short
brady-	slow
bronch/o	bronchial tube
bronchi/o	bronchial tube
bronchiol/o	bronchiole
bucc/o	cheek
bunion/o	bunion
burs/o	bursa (sac of fluid near joints)
byssin/o	cotton dust
cac/o	bad
calc/o	calcium
calcane/o	calcaneus (heel bone)
calci/o	calcium
cali/o	calyx
calic/o	calyx
capillar/o	capillary (tiniest blood vessel)
capn/o	carbon dioxide
-capnia	carbon dioxide
carcin/o	cancerous; cancer
cardi/o	heart
carp/o	wrist bones (carpals)
cata-	down
caud/o	tail; lower part of body
caus/o	burn; burning
cauter/o	heat; burn
cec/o	cecum (first part of the colon)
-cele	hernia
celi/o	belly; abdomen
-centesis	surgical puncture to remove fluid
cephal/o	head

Combining Form, Suffix, or Prefix	Meaning
cerebell/o	cerebellum (posterior part of the brain)
cerebr/o	cerebrum (largest part of the brain)
cerumin/o	cerumen
cervic/o	neck; cervix (neck of uterus)
-chalasia	relaxation
-chalasis	relaxation
cheil/o	lip
chem/o	drug; chemical
-chezia	defecation; elimination of wastes
chir/o	hand
chlor/o	green
chlorhydr/o	hydrochloric acid
chol/e	bile; gall
cholangi/o	bile vessel
cholecyst/o	gallbladder
choledoch/o	common bile duct
cholesterol/o	cholesterol
chondr/o	cartilage
chore/o	dance
chori/o	chorion (outermost membrane of the fetus)
chorion/o	chorion
choroid/o	choroid layer of eye
chrom/o	color
chron/o	time
chym/o	to pour
cib/o	meal
-cide	killing
-cidal	pertaining to killing
cine/o	movement
cirrh/o	orange-yellow
cis/o	to cut
-clasis	to break
-clast	to break
claustr/o	enclosed space
clavicul/o	clavicle (collar bone)
-clysis	irrigation; washing
coagul/o	coagulation (clotting)
-coccus (-cocci, pl.)	berry-shaped bacterium
coccyg/o	coccyx (tailbone)
cochle/o	cochlea (inner part of ear)
col/o	colon (large intestine)
coll/a	glue
colon/o	colon (large intestine)
colp/o	vagina
comat/o	deep sleep
comi/o	to care for
con-	together, with
coni/o	dust
conjunctiv/o	conjunctiva (lines the eyelids)
-constriction	narrowing

Combining Form, Suffix, or Prefix	Meaning	Combining Form, Suffix, or Prefix	Meaning
contra-	against; opposite	-eal	pertaining to
cor/o	pupil	ec-	out; outside
core/o	pupil	echo-	reflected sound
corne/o	cornea	-ectasia	dilation; dilatation; widening
coron/o	heart	-ectasis	dilation; dilatation; widening
corpor/o	body	ecto-	out; outside
cortic/o	cortex, outer region	-ectomy	removal; excision; resection
cost/o	rib	-edema	swelling
crani/o	skull	-elasma	flat plate
cras/o	mixture; temperament	electr/o	electricity
crin/o	secrete	em-	in
-crine	to secrete; separate	-ema	condition
-crit	to separate	-emesis	vomiting
cry/o	cold	-emia	blood condition
crypt/o	hidden	-emic	pertaining to blood condition
culd/o	cul-de-sac	emmetr/o	in due measure
-cusis	hearing	en-	in; within
cutane/o	skin	encephal/o	brain
cyan/o	blue	end-	in; within
cycl/o	ciliary body of eye; cycle; circle	endo-	in; within
-cyesis	pregnancy	enter/o	intestines (usually small intestine)
cyst/o	urinary bladder; cyst; sac of fluid	eosin/o	red; rosy; dawn-colored
cyt/o	cell	epi-	above; upon; on
-cyte	cell	epididym/o	epididymis
-cytosis	condition of cells; slight increase in numbers	epiglott/o	epiglottis
dacry/o	tear	episi/o	vulva (external female genitalia)
dacryoaden/o	tear gland	epitheli/o	skin; epithelium
dacryocyst/o	tear sac; lacrimal sac	equin/o	horse
dactyl/o	fingers; toes	-er	one who
de-	lack of; down; less; removal of	erg/o	work
dem/o	people	erythem/o	flushed; redness
dent/i	tooth	erythr/o	red
derm/o	skin	-esis	action; condition; state of
-derma	skin	eso-	inward
dermat/o	skin	esophag/o	esophagus
desicc/o	drying	esthes/o	nervous sensation (feeling)
-desis	to bind, tie together	esthesi/o	nervous sensation
dia-	complete; through	-esthesia	nervous sensation
diaphor/o	sweat	estr/o	female
-dilation	widening; stretching; expanding	ethm/o	sieve
dipl/o	double	eti/o	cause
dips/o	thirst	eu-	good; normal
dist/o	far; distant	-eurysm	widening
dors/o	back (of body)	ex-	out; away from
dorsi-	back	exanthemat/o	rash
-dote	to give	exo-	out; away from
-drome	to run	extra-	outside
duct/o	to lead, carry	faci/o	face
duoden/o	duodenum	fasci/o	fascia (membrane supporting muscles)
dur/o	dura mater	femor/o	femur (thigh bone)
-dynia	pain	-ferent	to carry
dys-	bad; painful; difficult; abnormal		

Combining Form, Suffix, or Prefix	Meaning
fibr/o	fiber
fibros/o	fibrous connective tissue
fibul/o	fibula
-fication	process of making
-fida	split
flex/o	to bend
fluor/o	luminous
follicul/o	follicle; small sac
-form	resembling; in the shape of
fung/i	fungus; mushroom (organism lacking chlorophyll)
furc/o	forking; branching
-fusion	to pour; to come together
galact/o	milk
ganglion/o	ganglion; collection of nerve cell bodies
gastr/o	stomach
-gen	substance that produces
-genesis	producing; forming
-genic	produced by or in
ger/o	old age
geront/o	old age
gest/o	pregnancy
gester/o	pregnancy
gingiv/o	gum
glauc/o	gray
gli/o	glial cells; neuroglial cells (supportive tissue of nervous system)
-globin	protein
-globulin	protein
glomerul/o	glomerulus
gloss/o	tongue
gluc/o	glucose; sugar
glyc/o	glucose; sugar
glycogen/o	glycogen; animal starch
glycos/o	glucose; sugar
gnos/o	knowledge
gon/o	seed
gonad/o	sex glands
goni/o	angle
-grade	to go
-gram	record
granul/o	granule(s)
-graph	instrument for recording
-graphy	process of recording
gravid/o	pregnancy
-gravida	pregnant woman
gynec/o	woman; female
hallucin/o	hallucination
hem/o	blood
hemat/o	blood
hemi-	half

Combining Form, Suffix, or Prefix	Meaning
hemoglobin/o	hemoglobin
hepat/o	liver
herni/o	hernia
-hexia	habit
hidr/o	sweat
hist/o	tissue
histi/o	tissue
home/o	sameness; unchanging; constant
hormon/o	hormone
humer/o	humerus (upper arm bone)
hydr/o	water
hyper-	above; excessive
hypn/o	sleep
hypo-	deficient; below; under; less than normal
hypophys/o	pituitary gland
hyster/o	uterus; womb
-ia	condition
-iac	pertaining to
-iasis	abnormal condition
iatr/o	physician; treatment
-ic	pertaining to
-ical	pertaining to
ichthy/o	dry; scaly
-icle	small
idi/o	unknown; individual; distinct
ile/o	ileum
ili/o	ilium
immun/o	immune; protection; safe
in-	in; into; not
-in, -ine	a substance
-ine	pertaining to
infra-	below; inferior to; beneath
inguin/o	groin
insulin/o	insulin (pancreatic hormone)
inter-	between
intra-	within; into
iod/o	iodine
ion/o	ion; to wander
-ion	process
-ior	pertaining to
ipsi-	same
ir-	in
ir/o	iris (colored portion of eye)
irid/o	iris (colored portion of eye)
is/o	same; equal
isch/o	to hold back; back
ischi/o	ischium (part of hip bone)
-ism	process; condition
-ist	specialist
-itis	inflammation
-ium	structure; tissue
jaund/o	yellow

Combining Form, Suffix, or Prefix	Meaning	Combining Form, Suffix, or Prefix	Meaning
jejun/o	jejunum	macro-	large
kal/i	potassium	mal-	bad
kary/o	nucleus	-malacia	softening
kerat/o	cornea; hard, horny tissue	malleol/o	malleolus
kern-	nucleus (collection of nerve cells in the brain)	mamm/o	breast
		mandibul/o	mandible (lower jaw bone)
ket/o	ketones; acetones	-mania	obsessive preoccupation
keton/o	ketones; acetones	mast/o	breast
kines/o	movement	mastoid/o	mastoid process (behind the ear)
kinesi/o	movement	maxill/o	maxilla (upper jaw bone)
-kinesia	movement	meat/o	meatus (opening)
-kinesis	movement	medi/o	middle
klept/o	to steal	mediastin/o	mediastinum
kyph/o	humpback	medull/o	medulla (inner section); middle; soft, marrow
labi/o	lip		
lacrim/o	tear; tear duct; lacrimal duct	mega-	large
lact/o	milk	-megaly	enlargement
lamin/o	lamina (part of vertebral arch)	melan/o	black
lapar/o	abdominal wall; abdomen	men/o	menses; menstruation
-lapse	to slide, fall, sag	mening/o	meninges (membranes covering the spinal cord and brain)
laryng/o	larynx (voice box)		
later/o	side	meningi/o	meninges
leiomy/o	smooth (visceral) muscle	ment/o	mind; chin
-lemma	sheath, covering	meso-	middle
-lepsy	seizure	meta-	change; beyond
lept/o	thin, slender	metacarp/o	metacarpals (hand bones)
-leptic	to seize, take hold of	metatars/o	metatarsals (foot bones)
leth/o	death	-meter	measure
leuk/o	white	metr/o	uterus (womb); measure
lex/o	word; phrase	metri/o	uterus (womb)
-lexia	word; phrase	mi/o	smaller; less
ligament/o	ligament	micro-	small
lingu/o	tongue	-mimetic	mimic; copy
lip/o	fat; lipid	-mission	to send
-listhesis	slipping	mon/o	one; single
lith/o	stone; calculus	morph/o	shape; form
-lithiasis	condition of stones	mort/o	death
-lithotomy	incision (for removal) of a stone	-mortem	death
lob/o	lobe	-motor	movement
log/o	study	muc/o	mucus
-logy	study (process of)	mucos/o	mucous membrane (mucosa)
lord/o	curve; swayback	multi-	many
-lucent	to shine	mut/a	genetic change
lumb/o	lower back; loin	mutagen/o	causing genetic change
lute/o	yellow	my/o	muscle
lux/o	to slide	myc/o	fungus
lymph/o	lymph	mydr/o	wide
lymphaden/o	lymph gland (node)	myel/o	spinal cord; bone marrow
lymphangi/o	lymph vessel	myocardi/o	myocardium (heart muscle)
-lysis	breakdown; separation; destruction; loosening	myom/o	muscle tumor
		myos/o	muscle
-lytic	to reduce, destroy; separate; breakdown	myring/o	tympanic membrane (eardrum)
		myx/o	mucus

Combining Form, Suffix, or Prefix	Meaning
narc/o	numbness; stupor; sleep
nas/o	nose
nat/i	birth
natr/o	sodium
necr/o	death
nect/o	to bind, tie, connect
neo-	new
nephr/o	kidney
neur/o	nerve
neutr/o	neither; neutral; neutrophil
nid/o	nest
noct/o	night
norm/o	rule; order
nos/o	disease
nucle/o	nucleus
nulli-	none
nyct/o	night
obstetr/o	pregnancy; childbirth
ocul/o	eye
odont/o	tooth
odyn/o	pain
-oid	resembling; derived from
-ole	little; small
olecran/o	olecranon (elbow)
olig/o	scanty
om/o	shoulder
-oma	tumor; mass; fluid collection
omphal/o	umbilicus (navel)
onc/o	tumor
-one	hormone
onych/o	nail (of fingers or toes)
o/o	egg
oophor/o	ovary
-opaque	obscure
ophthalm/o	eye
-opia	vision condition
-opsia	vision condition
-opsy	view of
opt/o	eye; vision
optic/o	eye; vision
-or	one who
or/o	mouth
orch/o	testis
orchi/o	testis
orchid/o	testis
-orexia	appetite
orth/o	straight
-ose	full of; pertaining to; sugar
-osis	condition, usually abnormal
-osmia	smell
ossicul/o	ossicle (small bone)
oste/o	bone
-ostosis	condition of bone

Combining Form, Suffix, or Prefix	Meaning
ot/o	ear
-otia	ear condition
-ous	pertaining to
ov/o	egg
ovari/o	ovary
ovul/o	egg
ox/o	oxygen
-oxia	oxygen
oxy-	swift; sharp; acid
oxysm/o	sudden
pachy-	heavy; thick
palat/o	palate (roof of the mouth)
palpebr/o	eyelid
pan-	all
pancreat/o	pancreas
papill/o	nipple-like; optic disc (disk)
par-	other than; abnormal
para-	near; beside; abnormal; apart from; along the side of
-para	to bear, bring forth (live births)
-parous	to bear, bring forth
parathyroid/o	parathyroid glands
-paresis	weakness
-pareunia	sexual intercourse
-partum	birth; labor
patell/a	patella
patell/o	patella
path/o	disease
-pathy	disease; emotion
pector/o	chest
ped/o	child; foot
pelv/i	pelvis; hip region
pelv/o	pelvis; hip region
pend/o	to hang
-penia	deficiency
-pepsia	digestion
per-	through
peri-	surrounding
perine/o	perineum
peritone/o	peritoneum
perone/o	fibula
-pexy	fixation; to put in place
phac/o	lens of eye
phag/o	eat; swallow
-phage	eat; swallow
-phagia	eating; swallowing
phak/o	lens of eye
phalang/o	phalanges (of fingers and toes)
phall/o	penis
pharmac/o	drug
pharmaceut/o	drug
pharyng/o	throat (pharynx)
phas/o	speech

Combining Form, Suffix, or Prefix	Meaning
-phasia	speech
phe/o	dusky; dark
-pheresis	removal
phil/o	like; love; attraction to
-phil	attraction for
-philia	attraction for
phim/o	muzzle
phleb/o	vein
phob/o	fear
-phobia	fear
phon/o	voice; sound
-phonia	voice; sound
-phor/o	to bear
-phoresis	carrying; transmission
-phoria	to bear, carry; feeling (mental state)
phot/o	light
phren/o	diaphragm; mind
-phthisis	wasting away
-phylaxis	protection
physi/o	nature; function
-physis	to grow
phyt/o	plant
-phyte	plant
pil/o	hair
pineal/o	pineal gland
pituitar/o	pituitary gland
-plakia	plaque
plant/o	sole of the foot
plas/o	development; formation
-plasia	development; formation; growth
-plasm	formation; structure
-plastic	pertaining to formation
-plasty	surgical repair
ple/o	more; many
-plegia	paralysis; palsy
-plegic	paralysis; palsy
pleur/o	pleura
plex/o	plexus; network (of nerves)
-pnea	breathing
pneum/o	lung; air; gas
pneumon/o	lung; air; gas
pod/o	foot
-poiesis	formation
-poietin	substance that forms
poikil/o	varied; irregular
pol/o	extreme
polio-	gray matter (of brain or spinal cord)
poly-	many; much
polyp/o	polyp; small growth
pont/o	pons (a part of the brain)
-porosis	condition of pores (spaces)

Combining Form, Suffix, or Prefix	Meaning
post-	after; behind
poster/o	back (of body); behind
-prandial	meal
-praxia	action
pre-	before; in front of
presby/o	old age
primi-	first
pro-	before; forward
proct/o	anus and rectum
pros-	before; forward
prostat/o	prostate gland
prot/o	first
prote/o	protein
proxim/o	near
prurit/o	itching
pseudo-	false
psych/o	mind
-ptosis	droop; sag; prolapse; protrude
-ptysis	spitting
pub/o	pubis (anterior part of hip bone)
pulmon/o	lung
pupill/o	pupil (dark center of the eye)
purul/o	pus
py/o	pus
pyel/o	renal pelvis
pylor/o	pylorus; pyloric sphincter
pyr/o	fever; fire
pyret/o	fever
pyrex/o	fever
quadri-	four
rachi/o	spinal column; vertebrae
radi/o	x-rays; radioactivity; radius (lateral lower arm bone)
radicul/o	nerve root
re-	back; again; backward
rect/o	rectum
ren/o	kidney
reticul/o	network
retin/o	retina
retro-	behind; back; backward
rhabdomy/o	striated (skeletal) muscle
rheumat/o	watery flow
rhin/o	nose
rhytid/o	wrinkle
roentgen/o	x-rays
-rrhage	bursting forth (of blood)
-rrhagia	bursting forth (of blood)
-rrhaphy	suture
-rrhea	flow; discharge
-rrhexis	rupture
rrhythm/o	rhythm
sacr/o	sacrum

Combining Form, Suffix, or Prefix	Meaning
salping/o	fallopian tube; auditory (eustachian) tube
-salpinx	fallopian tube; oviduct
sarc/o	flesh (connective tissue)
scapul/o	scapula; shoulder blade
-schisis	to split
schiz/o	split
scint/i	spark
scirrh/o	hard
scler/o	sclera (white of eye)
-sclerosis	hardening
scoli/o	crooked; bent
-scope	instrument for visual examination
-scopy	visual examination
scot/o	darkness
seb/o	sebum
sebace/o	sebum
sect/o	to cut
semi-	half
semin/i	semen; seed
seps/o	infection
sial/o	saliva
sialaden/o	salivary gland
sider/o	iron
sigmoid/o	sigmoid colon
silic/o	glass
sinus/o	sinus
-sis	state of; condition
-sol	solution
somat/o	body
-some	body
somn/o	sleep
-somnia	sleep
son/o	sound
-spadia	to tear, cut
-spasm	sudden contraction of muscles
sperm/o	spermatozoa; sperm cells
spermat/o	spermatozoa; sperm cells
sphen/o	wedge; sphenoid bone
spher/o	globe-shaped; round
sphygm/o	pulse
-sphyxia	pulse
splanchn/o	viscera (internal organs)
spin/o	spine (backbone)
spir/o	to breathe
splen/o	spleen
spondyl/o	vertebra (backbone)
squam/o	scale
-stalsis	contraction
staped/o	stapes (middle ear bone)
staphyl/o	clusters; uvula
-stasis	to stop; control; place

Combining Form, Suffix, or Prefix	Meaning
-static	pertaining to stopping; controlling
steat/o	fat, sebum
-stenosis	tightening; stricture
ster/o	solid structure; steroid
stere/o	solid; three-dimensional
stern/o	sternum (breastbone)
steth/o	chest
-sthenia	strength
-stitial	to set; pertaining to standing or positioned
stomat/o	mouth
-stomia	condition of the mouth
-stomy	new opening (to form a mouth)
strept/o	twisted chains
styl/o	pole or stake
sub-	under; below
submaxill/o	mandible (lower jaw bone)
-suppression	to stop
supra-	above, upper
sym-	together; with
syn-	together; with
syncop/o	to cut off, cut short; faint
syndesm/o	ligament
synov/o	synovia; synovial membrane; sheath around a tendon
syring/o	tube
tachy-	fast
tars/o	tarsus; hindfoot or ankle (7 bones between the foot and the leg)
tax/o	order; coordination
tel/o	complete
tele/o	distant
ten/o	tendon
tendin/o	tendon
-tension	pressure
terat/o	monster; malformed fetus
test/o	testis (testicle)
tetra-	four
thalam/o	thalamus
thalass/o	sea
the/o	put; place
thec/o	sheath
thel/o	nipple
therapeut/o	treatment
-therapy	treatment
therm/o	heat
thorac/o	chest
-thorax	chest; pleural cavity
thromb/o	clot
thym/o	thymus gland
-thymia	mind (condition of)
-thymic	pertaining to mind

Combining Form, Suffix, or Prefix	Meaning
thyr/o	thyroid gland; shield
thyroid/o	thyroid gland
tibi/o	tibia (shin bone)
-tic	pertaining to
toc/o	labor; birth
-tocia	labor; birth (condition of)
-tocin	labor; birth (a substance for)
tom/o	to cut
-tome	instrument to cut
-tomy	process of cutting
ton/o	tension
tone/o	to stretch
tonsill/o	tonsil
top/o	place; position; location
tox/o	poison
toxic/o	poison
trache/o	trachea (windpipe)
trans-	across; through
-tresia	opening
tri-	three
trich/o	hair
trigon/o	trigone (area within the bladder)
-tripsy	to crush
troph/o	nourishment; development
-trophy	nourishment; development (condition of)
-tropia	to turn
-tropic	turning
-tropin	stimulate; act on
tympan/o	tympanic membrane (eardrum); middle ear
-type	classification; picture
-ule	little; small
uln/o	ulna (medial lower arm bone)
ultra-	beyond; excess
-um	structure; tissue; thing
umbilic/o	umbilicus (navel)
ungu/o	nail
uni-	one
ur/o	urine; urinary tract

Combining Form, Suffix, or Prefix	Meaning
ureter/o	ureter
urethr/o	urethra
-uria	urination; condition of urine
urin/o	urine
-us	structure; thing
uter/o	uterus (womb)
uve/o	uvea, vascular layer of eye (iris, choroid, ciliary body)
uvul/o	uvula
vag/o	vagus nerve
vagin/o	vagina
valv/o	valve
valvul/o	valve
varic/o	varicose veins
vas/o	vessel; duct; vas deferens
vascul/o	vessel (blood)
ven/o, ven/i	vein
vener/o	venereal (sexual contact)
ventr/o	belly side of body
ventricul/o	ventricle (of heart or brain)
venul/o	venule (small vein)
-verse	to turn
-version	to turn
vertebr/o	vertebra (backbone)
vesic/o	urinary bladder
vesicul/o	seminal vesicle
vestibul/o	vestibule of the inner ear
viscer/o	internal organs
vit/o	life
vitr/o	vitreous body (of the eye)
vitre/o	glass
viv/o	life
vol/o	to roll
vulv/o	vulva (female external genitalia)
xanth/o	yellow
xen/o	stranger
xer/o	dry
xiph/o	sword
-y	condition; process
zo/o	animal life

ENGLISH—MEDICAL WORD PARTS

Meaning	Combining Form, Suffix, or Prefix	Meaning	Combining Form, Suffix, or Prefix
abdomen	abdomin/o (use with -al, -centesis)	appetite	-orexia
		arm	brachi/o
	celi/o (use with -ac)	arm bone, lower, lateral	radi/o
	lapar/o (use with -scope, -scopy, -tomy)	arm bone, lower, medial	uln/o
abdominal wall	lapar/o	arm bone, upper	humer/o
abnormal	dys-	armpit	axill/o
	par-	arteriole	arteriol/o
	para-	artery	arter/o
abnormal condition	-iasis		arteri/o
	-osis	articulate (speak distinctly)	-arthria
above	epi-	asbestos	asbest/o
	hyper-	assemble	-agon
	supra-	atrium	atri/o
acetabulum	acetabul/o	attraction for	-phil
acetones	ket/o		-philia
	keton/o	attraction to	phil/o
acid	oxy-	auditory tube	salping/o
acromion	acromi/o	away from	ab-
across	trans-		apo-
action	-praxia		ex-
act on	-tropin		exo-
adrenal glands	adren/o	back	re-
	adrenal/o		retro-
after	post-	back, lower	lumb/o
again	ana-, re-	back portion of body	dorsi-
against	anti-		dors/o
	contra-		poster/o
air	aer/o	backbone	spin/o (use with -al)
	pneum/o		spondyl/o (use with -itis, -listhesis, -osis, -pathy)
	pneumon/o		vertebr/o (use with -al)
air sac	alveol/o	backward	ana-
albumin	albumin/o		retro-
all	pan-	bacteria	bacteri/o
along the side of	para-	bacterium (berry-shaped)	-coccus (-cocci, pl.)
alveolus	alveol/o		
anew	ana-	bacilli (rod-shaped bacteria)	bacill/o
amnion	amni/o		
aneurysm	aneurysm/o	bad	cac/o
angle	goni/o		dys-
animal life	zo/o		mal-
animal starch	glycogen/o	barrier	claustr/o
ankle	tars/o	base (not acidic)	bas/o
antrum (of stomach)	antr/o	bear, to	-para
anus	an/o		-parous
anus and rectum	proct/o		-phoria
anxiety	anxi/o		phor/o
apart	ana-		
apart from	para-		
appendix	append/o (use with -ectomy) appendic/o (use with -itis)		

Meaning	Combining Form, Suffix, or Prefix	Meaning	Combining Form, Suffix, or Prefix
before	ante-	**bone**	oste/o
	pre-	**bone condition**	-ostosis
	pro-	**bone marrow**	myel/o
	pros-	**brain**	encephal/o
beginning	-arche		cerebr/o
behind	post-	**branching**	furc/o
	poster/o	**break**	-clasis
	retro-		-clast
belly	celi/o	**breakdown**	-lysis
belly side of body	ventr/o	**breast**	mamm/o (use with -ary, -gram, -graphy, -plasty)
below, beneath	hypo-		
	infra-		mast/o (use with -algia, -dynia, -ectomy, -itis)
	sub-		
bend, to	flex/o	**breastbone**	stern/o
bent	scoli/o	**breathe**	spir/o
beside	para-	**breathing**	-pnea
between	inter-	**bring forth**	-para
beyond	hyper-		-parous
	meta-	**bronchial tube**	bronch/o
	ultra-	(bronchus)	bronchi/o
bile	bil/i	**bronchiole**	bronchiol/o
	chol/e	**bunion**	bunion/o
bile vessel	cholangi/o	**burn**	caus/o
bilirubin	bilirubin/o		cauter/o
bind	-desis	**bursa**	burs/o
	nect/o	**bursting forth**	-rrhage
birth	nat/i	(of blood)	-rrhagia
	-partum	**calcaneus**	calcane/o
	toc/o	**calcium**	calc/o
	-tocia		calci/o
birth, substance for	-tocin	**calculus**	lith/o
births, live	-para	**calyx**	cali/o
black	anthrac/o		calic/o
	melan/o	**cancerous**	carcin/o
bladder (urinary)	cyst/o (use with -ic, -itis, -cele, -gram, -scopy, -stomy, -tomy)	**capillary**	capillar/o
		carbon dioxide	capn/o
	vesic/o (use with -al)		-capnia
blood	hem/o (use with -dialysis, -globin, -lysis, -philia, -ptysis, -rrhage, -stasis, -stat)	**care for, to**	comi/o
		carry	duct/o
			-ferent
	hemat/o (use with -crit, -emesis, -logist, -logy, -oma, -poiesis, -uria)		-phoria
		carrying	-phoresis
		cartilage	chondr/o
blood condition	-emia	**cast; throw**	bol/o
	-emic	**cause**	eti/o
blood vessel	angi/o (use with -ectomy, -genesis, -gram, -graphy, -oma, -plasty, -spasm)	**cecum**	cec/o
		cell	cyt/o
			-cyte
	vas/o (use with -constriction, -dilation, -motor)	**cells, condition of**	-cytosis
		cerebellum	cerebell/o
	vascul/o (use with -ar, -itis)	**cerebrum**	cerebr/o
blue	cyan/o	**cerumen**	cerumin/o
body	corpor/o	**cervix**	cervic/o
	somat/o	**change**	meta-
	-some	**cheek**	bucc/o

Meaning	Combining Form, Suffix, or Prefix	Meaning	Combining Form, Suffix, or Prefix
chemical	chem/o	cortex	cortic/o
chest	pector/o	cotton dust	byssin/o
	steth/o	crooked	scoli/o
	thorac/o	crush, procedure to	-tripsy
	-thorax	curve	lord/o
child	ped/o	cut	cis/o
childbirth	obstetr/o		sect/o, -section
chin	ment/o		tom/o
cholesterol	cholesterol/o	cut off	syncop/o
chorion	chori/o	cutting, process of	-tomy
	chorion/o	cycle	cycl/o
choroid layer	choroid/o	cyst (sac of fluid)	cyst/o
(of the eye)		dance	chore/o
ciliary body (of	cycl/o	dark	phe/o
the eye)		darkness	scot/o
circle *or* cycle	cycl/o	dawn-colored	eosin/o
clavicle (collar bone)	clavicul/o	death	leth/o
clot	thromb/o		mort/o, -mortem
clumping	agglutin/o		necr/o
clusters	staphyl/o	defecation	-chezia
coagulation	coagul/o	deficiency	-penia
coal dust	anthrac/o	deficient	hypo-
coccyx	coccyg/o	derived from	-oid
cochlea	cochle/o	destroy	-lytic
cold	cry/o	destruction	-lysis
collar bone	clavicul/o	development	plas/o
colon	col/o (use with -ectomy, -itis,		-plasia
	-pexy, -stomy)		troph/o
	colon/o (use with -ic, -pathy,		-trophy
	-scope, -scopy)	diaphragm	phren/o
color	chrom/o	difficult	dys-
come together	-fusion	digestion	-pepsia
common bile duct	choledoch/o	dilation	-ectasia
complete	dia-		-ectasis
	tel/o	dim	ambly/o
condition	-ation	discharge	-rrhea
	-ema	disease	nos/o
	-esis		path/o
	-ia		-pathy
	-ism	distant	dist/o
	-sis		tele/o
	-y	distinct	idi/o
condition, abnormal	-iasis	double	dipl/o
	-osis	down	cata-
connect	nect/o		de-
connective tissue	sarc/o	droop	-ptosis
constant	home/o	drug	chem/o
control	-stasis, -stat		pharmac/o
contraction	-stalsis		pharmaceut/o
contraction of	-spasm	dry	ichthy/o
muscles, sudden			xer/o
coordination	tax/o	drying	desicc/o
copy	-mimetic	duct	vas/o
cornea (of the eye)	corne/o	dull	ambly/o
	kerat/o	duodenum	duoden/o

Meaning	Combining Form, Suffix, or Prefix	Meaning	Combining Form, Suffix, or Prefix
dura mater	dur/o	**far**	dist/o
dusky	phe/o	**fascia**	fasci/o
dust	coni/o	**fast**	tachy-
ear	aur/o (use with -al, -icle)	**fat**	adip/o (use with -ose, -osis)
	auricul/o (use with -ar)		lip/o (use with -ase, -cyte,
	ot/o (use with -algia, -ic, -itis,		-genesis, -oid, -oma)
	-logy, -mycosis, -rrhea,		steat/o (use with -oma, -rrhea)
	-sclerosis, -scope, -scopy)	**fear**	phob/o
ear, condition of	-otia		-phobia
eardrum	myring/o (use with -ectomy, -itis,	**feeling**	esthesi/o
	-tomy)		-phoria
	tympan/o (use with -ic, -metry,	**female**	estr/o (use with -gen, -genic)
	-plasty)		gynec/o (use with -logist, -logy,
eat	phag/o		-mastia)
	-phage	**femur**	femor/o
eating	-phagia	**fever**	pyr/o
egg cell	o/o		pyret/o
	ov/o		pyrex/o
	ovul/o	**fiber**	fibr/o
elbow	olecran/o	**fibrous connective**	fibros/o
electricity	electr/o	**tissue**	
elimination of	-chezia	**fibula**	fibul/o (use with -ar)
wastes			perone/o (use with -al)
embryonic	-blast	**finger and toe bones**	phalang/o
enlargement	-megaly	**fingers**	dactyl/o
enzyme	-ase	**fire**	pyr/o
epididymis	epididym/o	**first**	prot/o
epiglottis	epiglott/o	**fixation**	-pexy
equal	is/o	**flat plate**	-elasma
esophagus	esophag/o	**flesh**	sarc/o
eustachian tube	salping/o	**flow**	-rrhea
excess	ultra-	**fluid collection**	-oma
excessive	hyper-	**flushed**	erythem/o
excision	-ectomy	**foot**	pod/o
expansion	-ectasia	**foot bones**	metatars/o
	-ectasis	**forking**	furc/o
extreme	pol/o	**form**	morph/o
extreme point	acr/o	**formation**	plas/o
extremities	acr/o		-plasia
eye	ocul/o (use with -ar, -facial,		-plasm
	-motor)		-poiesis
	ophthalm/o (use with -ia, -ic,	**forming**	-genesis
	-logist, -logy, -pathy, -plasty,	**forward**	ante-, pro-, pros-
	-plegia, -scope, -scopy)	**four**	quadri-
	opt/o (use with -ic, -metrist)	**front**	anter/o
	optic/o (use with -al, -ian)	**full of**	-ose
eyelid	blephar/o (use with -chalasis, -itis,	**fungus**	fung/i (use with -cide, -oid, -ous,
	-plasty, -plegia, -ptosis, -tomy)		-stasis)
	palpebr/o (use with -al)		myc/o (use with -logist, -logy,
face	faci/o		-osis, -tic)
faint	syncop/o	**gall**	bil/i (use with -ary)
fall	-ptosis		chol/e (use with -lithiasis)
fallopian tube	salping/o	**gallbladder**	cholecyst/o
	-salpinx	**ganglion**	gangli/o
false	pseudo-		ganglion/o

Meaning	Combining Form, Suffix, or Prefix	Meaning	Combining Form, Suffix, or Prefix
gas	pneum/o	heavy	pachy-
	pneumon/o	heel bone	calcane/o
gather	-agon	hemoglobin	hemoglobin/o
genetic change	mut/a	hernia	-cele
	mutagen/o		herni/o
give, to	-dote	hidden	crypt/o
given, what is	-dote	hip region	pelv/i, pelv/o
gland	aden/o	hold back	isch/o
glans penis	balan/o	hormone	hormon/o
glass	silic/o		-one
	vitre/o	horny	kerat/o
glial cells	gli/o	horse	equin/o
globe-shaped	spher/o	humerus	humer/o
glomerulus	glomerul/o	humpback	kyph/o
glucose	gluc/o	hydrochloric acid	chlorhydr/o
	glyc/o	ileum	ile/o
	glycos/o	ilium	ili/o
glue	coll/a	immature cell	-blast
	gli/o	immature tumor	-blastoma
glycogen	glycogen/o	(cells)	
go, to	-grade	immune	immun/o
good	eu-	in, into, within	em-
granule(s)	granul/o		en-
gray	glauc/o		endo-
gray matter	poli/o		in-, intra-
green	chlor/o		ir-
groin	inguin/o	in due measure	emmetr/o
grow	-physis	in front of	pre-
growth	-plasia	incomplete	atel/o
gum	gingiv/o	increase in cell	-cytosis
habit	-hexia	numbers (blood	
hair	pil/o	cells)	
	trich/o	individual	idi/o
half	hemi-	infection	seps/o
	semi-	inferior to	infra-
hallucination	hallucin/o	inflammation	-itis
hand	chir/o	instrument for	-graph
hand bones	metacarp/o	recording	
hang, to	pend/o	instrument for	-scope
hard	kerat/o	visual	
	scirrh/o	examination	
hardening	-sclerosis	instrument to cut	-tome
head	cephal/o	insulin	insulin/o
hearing	acous/o	internal organs	splanchn/o
	audi/o		viscer/o
	audit/o	intestine, large	col/o
	-acusis	intestine, small	enter/o
	-cusis	iodine	iod/o
heart	cardi/o (use with -ac, -graphy,	ion	ion/o
	-logy, -logist, -megaly, -pathy,	iris	ir/o
	-vascular)		irid/o
	coron/o (use with -ary)	iron	sider/o
heart muscle	myocardi/o	irregular	poikil/o
heat	cauter/o	irrigation	-clysis
	therm/o	ischium	ischi/o

Meaning	Combining Form, Suffix, or Prefix	Meaning	Combining Form, Suffix, or Prefix
itching	prurit/o	**lung**	pneum/o (use with -coccus, -coniosis, -thorax)
jaw, lower	mandibul/o		pneumon/o (use with -ectomy, -ia, -ic, -itis, -lysis)
	submaxill/o		pulmon/o (use with -ary)
jaw, upper	maxill/o	**lymph**	lymph/o
joint	arthr/o	**lymph gland**	lymphaden/o
	articul/o	**lymph vessel**	lymphangi/o
ketones	ket/o	**make, to**	-fication
	keton/o	**male**	andr/o
kidney	nephr/o (use with -algia, -ectomy, -ic, -itis, -lith, -megaly, -oma, -osis, -pathy, -ptosis, -sclerosis, -stomy, -tomy)	**malformed fetus**	terat/o
		malleolus	malleol/o
		mandible	mandibul/o
			submaxill/o
	ren/o (use with -al, -gram, -vascular)	**many**	multi-
			ple/o
killing	-cidal		poly-
	-cide	**marketplace**	agora-
knowledge	gnos/o, gno/o	**marrow**	medull/o
labor	-partum	**mass**	-oma
	toc/o	**mastoid process**	mastoid/o
	-tocia	**maxilla**	maxill/o
labor, substance for	-tocin	**meal**	cib/o
lack of	de-		-prandial
lack of strength	-asthenia	**measure**	-meter
lacrimal duct	dacry/o		metr/o
	lacrim/o	**meatus**	meat/o
lacrimal sac	dacryocyst/o	**mediastinum**	mediastin/o
lamina	lamin/o	**medulla oblongata**	medull/o
large	macro-	**meninges**	mening/o
	mega-		meningi/o
larynx	laryng/o	**menstruation; menses**	men/o
lead	duct/o		
lens of eye	phac/o	**metacarpals**	metacarp/o
	phak/o	**metatarsals**	metatars/o
less	de-	**middle**	medi/o
	mi/o		medull/o
less than normal	hypo-		meso-
life	bi/o	**middle ear**	tympan/o
	vit/o	**midwife**	obstetr/o
	viv/o	**milk**	galact/o
ligament	ligament/o		lact/o
	syndesm/o	**mimic**	-mimetic
like	phil/o	**mind**	ment/o
lip	cheil/o		phren/o
	labi/o		psych/o
lipid	lip/o		-thymia
little	-ole		-thymic
	-ule	**mixture**	cras/o
liver	hepat/o	**monster**	terat/o
lobe	lob/o	**more**	ple/o
location	top/o	**mouth**	or/o (use with -al)
loin	lumb/o		stomat/o (use with -itis)
loosening	-lysis		-stomia
love	phil/o		
luminous	fluor/o		

Meaning	Combining Form, Suffix, or Prefix	Meaning	Combining Form, Suffix, or Prefix
movement	cine/o	nourishment	troph/o
	kines/o		-trophy
	kinesi/o	nucleus	kary/o
	-kinesia		nucle/o
	-kinesis	nucleus (collection	kern-
	-motor	of nerve cells in	
much	poly-	the brain)	
mucous membrane	mucos/o	numbness	narc/o
mucus	muc/o	obscure	-opaque
	myx/o	obsessive	-mania
muscle	muscul/o (use with -ar, -skeletal)	preoccupation	
	my/o (use with -algia, -ectomy,	off	apo-
	-oma, -neural, -pathy, -rrhaphy,	old age	ger/o, geront/o
	-therapy)		presby/o
	myos/o (use with -in, -itis)	olecranon (elbow)	olecran/o
muscle, heart	myocardi/o	on	epi-
muscle, smooth	leiomy/o	one	mon/o
(visceral)			mono-
muscle, striated	rhabdomy/o		uni-
(skeletal)		one's own	aut/o
muscle tumor	myom/o		auto-
muzzle	phim/o	one who	-er
nail	onych/o		-or
	ungu/o	opening	-tresia
narrowing	-constriction	opening, new	-stomy
	-stenosis	opposite	contra-
nature	physi/o	optic disc (disk)	papill/o
navel	omphal/o	orange-yellow	cirrh/o
	umbilic/o	order	norm/o
-stenosis	para-		tax/o
	proxim/o	organs, internal	viscer/o
neck	cervic/o	ossicle	ossicul/o
neither	neutr/o	other	all/o
nerve	neur/o	other than	par-
nerve root	radicul/o	out, outside	ec-
nest	nid/o		ex-
new	neo-		exo-
network	reticul/o		extra-
network of nerves	plex/o	outer region	cortic/o
neutral	neutr/o	ovary	oophor/o (use with -itis, -ectomy,
neutrophil	neutr/o		-pexy)
night	nocti/i		ovari/o (use with -an)
	nyct/o	own	aut-
nipple	thel/o	oxygen	ox/o
nipple-like	papill/o		-oxia
nitrogen	azot/o	pain	-algia (use with arthr/o, cephal/o,
nitrogen compound	-amine		gastr/o, mast/o, my/o, neur/o,
no, not	a-		ot/o)
	an-		-dynia (use with coccyg/o,
none	nulli-		pleur/o)
normal	eu-		odyn/o
nose	nas/o (use with -al)	pain, excessive	-agra
	rhin/o (use with -itis, -rrhea,	pain, sensitivity to	-algesia
	-plasty)		algesi/o

Meaning	Combining Form, Suffix, or Prefix	Meaning	Combining Form, Suffix, or Prefix
painful	dys-	**pons**	pont/o
palate	palat/o	**pores, condition of**	-porosis
palsy	-plegia	**position**	top/o
	-plegic	**potassium**	kal/i
pancreas	pancreat/o	**pour**	chym/o
paralysis	-plegia		-fusion
	-plegic	**pregnancy**	-cyesis
paralysis, slight	-paresis		gest/o
patella	patell/a (use with -pexy)		gester/o
	patell/o (use with -ar, -ectomy,		gravid/o
	-femoral)		-gravida
			obstetr/o
pelvis	pelv/i		
	pelv/o	**pressure**	bar/o
penis	balan/o		-tension
	phall/o	**process**	-ation
people	dem/o		-ion
perineum	perine/o		-ism
peritoneum	peritone/o		-y
pertaining to	-ac (cardiac)	**produced by** *or* **in**	-genic
	-al (inguinal)	**producing**	-gen
	-an (ovarian)		-genesis
	-ar (palmar)	**prolapse**	-ptosis
	-ary (papillary)	**prostate gland**	prostat/o
	-eal (pharyngeal)	**protection**	immun/o
	-iac (hypochondriac)		-phylaxis
	-ic (nucleic)	**protein**	albumin/o
	-ical (neurologic)		-globin
	-ine (equine)		-globulin
	-ior (superior)		prote/o
	-ose (adipose)	**pubis**	pub/o
	-ous (mucous)	**pulse**	sphygm/o
	-tic (necrotic)		-sphyxia
phalanges	phalang/o	**puncture to remove**	-centesis
pharynx (throat)	pharyng/o	**fluid**	
phrase	-lexia	**pupil**	cor/o
physician	iatr/o		core/o
pineal gland	pineal/o		pupill/o
pituitary gland	hypophys/o	**pus**	py/o, purul/o
	pituit/o	**put**	the/o
	pituitar/o	**put in place**	-pexy
place	-stasis	**pyloric sphincter,**	pylor/o
	the/o	**pylorus**	
	top/o	**radioactivity**	radi/o
plant	phyt/o	**radius** (lower arm	radi/o
	-phyte	bone)	
plaque	ather/o	**rapid**	oxy-
	-plakia	**rash**	exanthemat/o
pleura	pleur/o	**rays**	radi/o
pleural cavity	-thorax	**record**	-gram
plexus	plex/o	**recording, process of**	-graphy
poison	tox/o	**rectum**	rect/o
	toxic/o	**recurring**	cycl/o
pole	styl/o	**red**	eosin/o
polyp	polyp/o		erythr/o

Meaning	Combining Form, Suffix, or Prefix	Meaning	Combining Form, Suffix, or Prefix
redness	erythem/o	severe	acu/o
	erythemat/o	sex glands	gonad/o
reduce	-lytic	sexual intercourse	-pareunia
relaxation	-chalasia, -chalasis	shape	-form
removal	-apheresis		morph/o
	-ectomy	sharp	acu/o
	-pheresis		oxy-
renal pelvis	pyel/o	sheath	thec/o
repair	-plasty	shield	thyr/o
resembling	-form	shin bone	tibi/o
	-oid	shine	-lucent
retina	retin/o	short	brachy-
rib	cost/o	shoulder	om/o
roll, to	vol/o	side	later/o
rosy	eosin/o	sieve	ethm/o
round	spher/o	sigmoid colon	sigmoid/o
rule	norm/o	single	mon/o
run	-drome	sinus	sinus/o
rupture	-rrhexis	skin	cutane/o (use with -ous)
sac, small	alveol/o		derm/o (use with -al)
	follicul/o		-derma (use with erythr/o, leuk/o)
sac of fluid	cyst/o		dermat/o (use with -itis, -logist, -logy, -osis)
sacrum	sacr/o		
safe	immun/o		epitheli/o (use with -al, -lysis, -oid, -oma, -um)
sag, to	-ptosis		
saliva	sial/o	skull	crani/o
salivary gland	sialaden/o	sleep	hypn/o
same	ipsi-		somn/o
	is/o		-somnia
sameness	home/o	sleep, deep	comat/o
scaly	ichthy/o	slender	lept/o
scanty	olig/o	slide, to	lux/o
sclera	scler/o	sliding, condition of	-lapse
scrotum	scrot/o	slipping	-listhesis
sea	thalass/o	slow	brady-
sebum	seb/o	small	-icle
	sebace/o		micro-
	steat/o		-ole
secrete	crin/o		-ule
	-crine	small intestine	enter/o
seed	gon/o	smaller	mi/o
	semin/i	smell	-osmia
seizure	-lepsy	sodium	natr/o
seize, to (take hold of)	-leptic	soft	medull/o
		softening	-malacia
self	aut/o	sole (of the foot)	plant/o
	auto-	solution	-sol
semen	semin/i	sound	echo-
seminal vesicle	vesicul/o		phon/o
send, to	-mission		-phonia
sensation (nervous)	-esthesia		son/o
separate	-crine	spark	scint/i
	-lytic	specialist	-ist
separation	-lysis	speech	phas/o
set, to	-stitial		-phasia

Meaning	Combining Form, Suffix, or Prefix	Meaning	Combining Form, Suffix, or Prefix
sperm cells	sperm/o	**swallowing**	-phagia
(spermatozoa)	spermat/o	**swayback**	lord/o
spinal column	spin/o	**sweat**	diaphor/o (use with -esis)
(spine)	rachi/o		hidr/o (use with -osis)
	vertebr/o	**swift**	oxy-
spinal cord	myel/o	**sword**	xiph/o
spiny	acanth/o	**synovia** (fluid)	synov/o
spitting	-ptysis	**synovial membrane**	synov/o
spleen	splen/o	**tail**	caud/o
split	-fida	**tailbone**	coccyg/o
	schiz/o	**tear**	dacry/o (use with -genic, -rrhea)
split	-schisis		lacrim/o (use with -al, -ation)
stake (pole)	styl/o	**tear** (to cut)	-spadia
stapes	staped/o	**tear gland**	dacryoaden/o
starch	amyl/o	**tear sac**	dacryocyst/o
state of	-sis	**temperament**	cras/o
steal	klept/o	**tendon**	ten/o
sternum	stern/o		tend/o
steroid	ster/o		tendin/o
sticking together	agglutin/o	**tension**	ton/o
stiff	ankyl/o	**testis**	orch/o (use with -itis)
stimulate	-tropin		orchi/o (use with -algia, -dynia,
stomach	gastr/o		-ectomy, -pathy, -pexy, -tomy)
stone	lith/o		orchid/o (use with -ectomy, -pexy,
stop	-suppression		-plasty, -ptosis, -tomy)
stopping	-stasis		test/o (use with -sterone)
	-static	**thick**	pachy-
straight	orth/o	**thigh bone**	femor/o
stranger	xen/o	**thin**	lept/o
strength	-sthenia	**thing**	-um
stretch	tone/o		-us
stretching	-ectasia	**thing that produces**	-gen
	-ectasis	**thirst**	dips/o
stricture	-stenosis	**thorny**	acanth/o
structure	-ium	**three**	tri-
	-plasm	**throat**	pharyng/o
	-um, -us	**through**	dia-
structure, solid	ster/o		per-
study of	log/o		trans-
	-logy	**throw, to**	bol/o
stupor	narc/o	**thymus gland**	thym/o
substance	-in	**thyroid gland**	thyr/o
	-ine		thyroid/o
substance that	-poietin	**tibia**	tibi/o
forms		**tie**	nect/o
sudden	acu/o	**tie together**	-desis
	oxysm/o	**tightening**	-stenosis
sugar	gluc/o	**time**	chron/o
	glyc/o	**tissue**	hist/o
	glycos/o		histi/o
	-ose		-ium
surgical repair	-plasty		-um
surrounding	peri-	**toes**	dactyl/o
suture	-rrhaphy	**together**	con-
swallow	phag/o		sym-
			syn-

Meaning	Combining Form, Suffix, or Prefix	Meaning	Combining Form, Suffix, or Prefix
tongue	gloss/o (use with -al, -dynia, -plasty, -plegia, -rrhaphy, -spasm, -tomy)	uvea	uve/o
	lingu/o (use with -al)	uvula	uvul/o (use with -ar, -itis, -ptosis)
tonsil	tonsill/o		staphyl/o (use with -ectomy, -plasty, -tomy)
tooth	dent/i	vagina	colp/o (use with -pexy, -plasty, -scope, -scopy, -tomy)
	odont/o		
top	acr/o		vagin/o (use with -al, -itis)
toward	ad-	vagus nerve	vag/o
	af-	valve	valv/o
	-ad		valvul/o
trachea	trache/o	varicose veins	varic/o
transmission	-phoresis	varied	poikil/o
treatment	iatr/o	vas deferens	vas/o
	therapeut/o	vein	phleb/o (use with -ectomy, -itis, -tomy)
	-therapy		
trigone	trigon/o		ven/o (use with -ous, -gram)
tube	syring/o		ven/i (use with -puncture)
tumor	-oma	vein, small	venul/o
	onc/o	venereal	vener/o
turn	-tropia	ventricle	ventricul/o
	-verse	vertebra	rachi/o (use with -itis, -tomy)
	-version		spondyl/o (use with -itis, -listhesis, -osis, -pathy)
turning	-tropic		
twisted chains	strept/o		vertebr/o (use with -al)
two	bi-	vessel	angi/o (use with -ectomy, -genesis, -gram, -graphy, -oma, -plasty, -spasm)
tympanic membrane	myring/o		
	tympan/o		vas/o (use with -constriction, -dilation, -motor)
ulcer	aphth/o		
ulna	uln/o		vascul/o (use with -ar, -itis)
umbilicus, navel	omphal/o (use with -cele, -ectomy, -rrhagia, -rrhexis)	view of	-opsy
		viscera	splanchn/o
	umbilic/o (use with -al)	vision	-opia
unchanging	home/o		-opsia
under	hypo-		opt/o
unequal	anis/o		optic/o
unknown	idi/o	visual examination	-scopy
up	ana-	vitreous body	vitr/o
upon	epi-	voice	phon/o
urea	azot/o		-phonia
ureter	ureter/o	voice box	laryng/o
urethra	urethr/o	vomiting	-emesis
urinary bladder	cyst/o (use with cele, -ectomy, -itis, -pexy, -plasty, -plegia, -scope, -scopy, -stomy, -tomy)	vulva	episi/o (use with -tomy)
			vulv/o (use with -ar)
	vesic/o (use with -al)	wander	ion/o
urinary tract	ur/o	washing	-clysis
urination	-uria	wasting away	-phthisis
urine	ur/o	water	aque/o
	-uria		hydr/o
	urin/o	watery flow	rheumat/o
uterus	hyster/o (use with -ectomy, -graphy, -gram, -tomy)	weakness	-paresis
		wedge	sphen/o
	metr/o (use with -rrhagia, -rrhea, -rrhexis)	weight	bar/o
		white	alb/o
	metri/o (use with -osis)		albin/o
	uter/o (use with -ine)		leuk/o

Meaning	Combining Form, Suffix, or Prefix	Meaning	Combining Form, Suffix, or Prefix
wide	mydr/o	**womb**	hyster/o
widening	-dilation		metr/o
	-ectasia		metri/o
	-ectasis		uter/o
	-eurysm	**word**	-lexia
windpipe	trache/o	**work**	erg/o
with	con-	**wrinkle**	rhytid/o
	sym-	**wrist bone**	carp/o
	syn-	**x-rays**	radi/o
within	en-, end-	**yellow**	lute/o
	endo-		jaund/o
	intra-		xanth/o
woman	gynec/o		

appendix I

Plurals

The rules commonly used to form plurals of medical terms are as follows:

1. For words ending in **a**, retain the **a** and add **e**.
   Examples:

Singular	Plural
vertebra	vertebrae
bursa	bursae
bulla	bullae

2. For words ending in **is**, drop the **is** and add **es**.
   Examples:

Singular	Plural
anastomosis	anastomoses
metastasis	metastases
epiphysis	epiphyses
prosthesis	prostheses
pubis	pubes

3. For words ending in **ix** and **ex**, drop the **ix** or **ex** and add **ices**.
   Examples:

Singular	Plural
apex	apices
varix	varices

4. For words ending in **on**, drop the **on** and add **a**.
   Examples:

Singular	Plural
ganglion	ganglia
spermatozoon	spermatozoa

5. For words ending in **um**, drop the **um** and add **a**.
   Examples:

Singular	Plural
bacterium	bacteria
diverticulum	diverticula
ovum	ova

6. For words ending in **us**, drop the **us** and add **i**.
   Examples:

Singular	Plural
calculus	calculi
bronchus	bronchi
nucleus	nuclei

   Two exceptions to this rule are viru<u>ses</u> and sinu<u>ses</u>.

7. Additional rules are used to form plurals in other word families.
   Examples:

Singular	Plural
fora<u>men</u>	fora<u>mina</u>
iri<u>s</u>	iri<u>des</u>
femu<u>r</u>	fem<u>ora</u>
anomal<u>y</u>	anomal<u>ies</u>
biops<u>y</u>	biops<u>ies</u>
aden<u>oma</u>	aden<u>omata</u>

Pronunciations for plural terms as well as other terms can be found on the enclosed CD.

appendix II

Abbreviations, Acronyms, and Symbols

Many of these abbreviations may appear with or without periods and with either a capital or a lowercase first letter.

@	at
ā	before
A, B, AB, O	blood types; may have subscript numbers
ABCD	asymmetry, border, color, diameter (description of skin cancer lesions)
A2, A$_2$	aortic valve closure (heart sound)
AAA	abdominal aortic aneurysm
AAL	anterior axillary line
AB, ab	abortion
Ab	antibody
abd	abdomen; abduction
ABGs	arterial blood gases
a.c.	before meals *(ante cibum)*
AC joint	acromioclavicular joint
ACE	angiotensin-converting enzyme (ACE inhibitors treat hypertension)
ACh	acetylcholine (a neurotransmitter)
ACL	anterior cruciate ligament (of knee)
ACS	acute coronary syndrome(s)
ACTH	adrenocorticotropic hormone (secreted by the anterior pituitary gland)
AD	Alzheimer disease
A.D.	right ear *(auris dextra)*; often better to specify "right ear" rather than abbreviate
ADD	attention deficit disorder
add	adduction
ADH	antidiuretic hormone; vasopressin (secreted by the posterior pituitary gland)
ADHD	attention-deficit hyperactivity disorder
ADL	activities of daily living
ADT	admission, discharge, transfer
ad lib.	as desired
AF	atrial fibrillation
AFB	acid-fast bacillus (bacilli) (the TB organism)
AFO	ankle-foot orthosis (device for stabilization)
AFP	alpha-fetoprotein
Ag	silver
AHF	antihemophilic factor (coagulation factor XIII)
AIDS	acquired immunodeficiency syndrome
AIHA	autoimmune hemolytic anemia
AKA	above-knee amputation
alb	albumin (protein)
alk phos	alkaline phosphatase (elevated in liver disease)
ALL	acute lymphocytic leukemia
ALS	amyotrophic lateral sclerosis (Lou Gehrig disease)
ALT	alanine aminotransferase (elevated in liver and heart disease); formerly called serum glutamic-pyruvic transaminase (SGPT)
AM, a.m.	in the morning or before noon *(ante meridiem)*
AMA	against medical advice; American Medical Association
Amb	ambulate, ambulatory (walking)
AMD	age-related macular degeneration
AMI	acute myocardial infarction
AML	acute myelocytic (myelogenous) leukemia
ANA	antinuclear antibody
ANC	absolute neutrophil count
AP, A/P	anteroposterior
A&P	auscultation and percussion
APC	acetylsalicylic acid (aspirin), phenacetin, caffeine

aq.	water *(aqua)*; aqueous
ARDS	acute respiratory distress syndrome
AROM	active range of motion
AS	aortic stenosis
A.S.	left ear *(auris sinistra)*; better to specify "left ear" rather than abbreviate
ASA	acetylsalicylic acid (aspirin)
ASD	atrial septal defect
ASHD	arteriosclerotic heart disease
AST	aspartate aminotransferase (elevated in liver and heart disease); formerly called serum glutamic-oxaloacetic transaminase (SGOT)
A.U.	both ears *(auris uterque)*; better to specify "in each ear/for both ears" rather than abbreviate
Au	gold
AV	arteriovenous; atrioventricular
AVM	arteriovenous malformation
AVR	aortic valve replacement
A&W	alive and well
Ba	barium
BAL	bronchoalveolar lavage
bands	banded neutrophils
baso	basophils
BBB	bundle branch block
BC	bone conduction
B cells	lymphocytes produced in the bone marrow
BE	barium enema
b.i.d.	twice a day *(bis in die)*
BKA	below-knee amputation
BM	bowel movement
BMR	basal metabolic rate
BMT	bone marrow transplantation
BP, B/P	blood pressure
BPH	benign prostatic hyperplasia (hypertrophy)
BRBPR	bright red blood per rectum (hematochezia)
bs	blood sugar; breath sound(s)
BSE	breast self-examination
BSO	bilateral salpingo-oophorectomy
BSP	bromsulphalein (dye used in liver function testing; its retention is indicative of liver damage or disease)
BT	bleeding time
BUN	blood urea nitrogen
bw, BW	birth weight
Bx, bx	biopsy
C	carbon; calorie
°C	degrees Celsius ("metric" temperature scale); degrees centigrade
c̄	with *(cum)*

C1, C2	first cervical vertebra, second cervical vertebra
Ca	calcium
CA	cancer; carcinoma; cardiac arrest; chronologic age
CABG	coronary artery bypass graft/grafting (surgery)
CAD	coronary artery disease
CAO	chronic airway obstruction
CAPD	continuous ambulatory peritoneal dialysis
cap	capsule
Cath	catheter; catheterization
CBC	complete blood (cell) count
CBT	cognitive behavior therapy
CC	chief complaint
cc	cubic centimeter (same as mL: 1/1000 of a liter)
CCU	coronary care unit; critical care unit
CDC	Centers for Disease Control and Prevention
CDH	congenital dislocated hip
CEA	carcinoembryonic antigen
cf.	compare *(confer)*
CF	cystic fibrosis; complement fixation (test)
cGy	centigray (1/100 of a gray; a rad)
CHD	coronary heart disease; chronic heart disease
chemo	chemotherapy
CHF	congestive heart failure
chol	cholesterol
chr	chronic
μCi	microcurie
CIN	cervical intraepithelial neoplasia
CIS	carcinoma in situ
CK	creatine kinase
CKD	chronic kidney disease
Cl	chlorine
CLD	chronic liver disease
CLL	chronic lymphocytic leukemia
cm	centimeter (1/100 of a meter)
CMA	certified medical assistant
CMG	cystometrogram
CML	chronic myelogenous leukemia
CMV	cytomegalovirus
CNS	central nervous system
Co	cobalt
c/o	complains of
CO	carbon monoxide; cardiac output
CO₂	carbon dioxide
COD	condition on discharge
COPD	chronic obstructive pulmonary disease
CP	cerebral palsy; chest pain
CPA	costophrenic angle
CPAP	continuous positive airway pressure
CPD	cephalopelvic disproportion
CPR	cardiopulmonary resuscitation

CR	complete response; cardiorespiratory
CRF	chronic renal failure
C-section	cesarean section
C&S	culture and sensitivity (testing)
CSF	cerebrospinal fluid; colony-stimulating factor
C-spine	cervical spine (films)
ct.	count
CTA	clear to auscultation
CTS	carpal tunnel syndrome
CT scan	computed tomography (x-ray imaging in axial plane and other planes)
Cu	copper
CVA	cerebrovascular accident; costovertebral angle
CVP	central venous pressure
CVS	cardiovascular system; chorionic villus sampling
c/w	compare with; consistent with
CX, CXR	chest x-ray
Cx	cervix
cysto	cystoscopy
D/C	discontinue
D&C	dilatation (dilation) and curettage
DCIS	ductal carcinoma in situ
DD	discharge diagnosis; differential diagnosis
Decub.	decubitus (lying down)
Derm.	dermatology
DES	diethylstilbestrol; diffuse esophageal spasm
DI	diabetes insipidus; diagnostic imaging
DIC	disseminated intravascular coagulation
DICOM	digital image communication in medicine
diff.	differential count (white blood cells)
DIG	digoxin; digitalis
dL, dl	deciliter (1/10 of a liter)
DLco	diffusion capacity of the lung for carbon monoxide
DLE	discoid lupus erythematosus
DM	diabetes mellitus
DNA	deoxyribonucleic acid
DNR	do not resuscitate
D.O.	Doctor of Osteopathy
DOA	dead on arrival
DOB	date of birth
DOE	dyspnea on exertion
DPI	dry powder inhaler
DPT	diphtheria, pertussis, tetanus (vaccine)
DRE	digital rectal examination
DRG	diagnosis-related group
DSA	digital subtraction angiography
DSM	*Diagnostic and Statistical Manual of Mental Disorders*
DT	delirium tremens (caused by alcohol withdrawal)

DTR	deep tendon reflex(es)
DUB	dysfunctional uterine bleeding
DVT	deep venous thrombosis
D/W	dextrose in water
Dx	diagnosis
EBV	Epstein-Barr virus
ECC	endocervical curettage; extracorporeal circulation
ECF	extended care facility
ECG	electrocardiogram
ECHO	echocardiography
ECMO	extracorporeal membrane oxygenation
ECT	electroconvulsive therapy
ED	emergency department
EDC	estimated date of confinement
EEG	electroencephalogram
EENT	eyes, ears, nose, throat
EGD	esophagogastroduodenoscopy
EKG	electrocardiogram
ELISA	enzyme-linked immunosorbent assay
EM	electron microscope
EMB	endometrial biopsy
EMG	electromyogram
EMT	emergency medical technician
ENT	ear, nose, throat
EOM	extraocular movement; extraocular muscles
eos.	eosinophils (type of white blood cell)
EPO	erythropoietin
ER	emergency room; estrogen receptor
ERCP	endoscopic retrograde cholangiopancreatography
ERT	estrogen replacement therapy
ESR	erythrocyte sedimentation rate
ESRD	end-stage renal disease
ESWL	extracorporeal shock wave lithotripsy
ETOH	ethyl alcohol
ETT	exercise tolerance test
F, °F	Fahrenheit, degrees Fahrenheit
FACP	Fellow of the American College of Physicians
FACS	Fellow of the American College of Surgeons
FB	fingerbreadth; foreign body
FBS	fasting blood sugar
FDA	Food and Drug Administration
Fe	iron
FEF	forced expiratory flow
FEV$_1$	forced expiratory volume in first second
FH	family history
FHR	fetal heart rate
FROM	full range of movement/motion
FSH	follicle-stimulating hormone
F/U	follow-up

5-FU	5-fluorouracil (chemotherapy drug)
FUO	fever of undetermined origin
Fx	fracture
μg	microgram (one millionth of a gram)
G	gravida (pregnant)
g, gm	gram
g/dL	grams per deciliter
Ga	gallium
GABA	gamma-aminobutyric acid (a neurotransmitter); also spelled γ-aminobutyric acid
GB	gallbladder
GBS	gallbladder series (x-ray studies)
GC	gonococcus
G-CSF	granulocyte colony-stimulating factor
GERD	gastroesophageal reflux disease
GFR	glomerular filtration rate
GH	growth hormone
GI	gastrointestinal
GIST	gastrointestinal stromal tumor
G6PD	glucose-6-phosphate dehydrogenase (enzyme missing in inherited red blood cell disorder)
GP	general practitioner
GM-CSF	granulocyte-macrophage colony-stimulating factor
grav. 1, 2, 3	first, second, third pregnancy
GTT	glucose tolerance test
gt, gtt	drop (gutta), drops (guttae)
GU	genitourinary
Gy	gray (unit of radiation; equal to 100 rad)
GYN, gyn	gynecology
H	hydrogen
h., hr	hour
H₂ blocker	H_2 histamine receptor antagonist (inhibitor of gastric acid secretion)
HAART	highly active antiretroviral therapy (for AIDS)
Hb, hgb	hemoglobin
HbA₁c	glycosylated hemoglobin test (for diabetes)
HBV	hepatitis B virus
hCG, HCG	human chorionic gonadotropin
HCl	hydrochloric acid
HCO₃	bicarbonate
Hct, HCT	hematocrit
HCV	hepatitis C virus
HCVD	hypertensive cardiovascular disease
HD	hemodialysis (performed by artificial kidney machine)
HDL	high-density lipoprotein
He	helium
HEENT	head, eyes, ears, nose, throat
Hg	mercury
H&H	hematocrit and hemoglobin (RBC tests)

HIPAA	Health Insurance Portability and Accountability Act (of 1996)
HIV	human immunodeficiency virus
HLA	histocompatibility locus antigen (identifies cells as "self")
h/o	history of
H₂O	water
H&P	history and physical (examination)
HPF; hpf	high-power field (in microscopy)
HPI	history of present illness
HPV	human papillomavirus
HRT	hormone replacement therapy
hs	half-strength
h.s.	at bedtime (hora somni); write out so not to confuse with hs (half-strength)
HSG	hysterosalpingography
HSV	herpes simplex virus
ht	height
HTN	hypertension (high blood pressure)
Hx	history
I	iodine
¹³¹I	radioactive isotope of iodine
IBD	inflammatory bowel disease
ICD	implantable cardioverter/defibrillator
ICP	intracranial pressure
ICSH	interstitial cell–stimulating hormone
ICU	intensive care unit
I&D	incision and drainage
ID	infectious disease
IgA, IgD, IgE, IgG, IgM	immunoglobulins (type of antibodies)
IHD	ischemic heart disease
IHSS	idiopathic hypertrophic subaortic stenosis
IL-1 to IL-15	interleukins
IM	intramuscular; infectious mononucleosis
inf.	infusion; inferior
INH	isoniazid (drug used to treat tuberculosis)
inj.	injection
I&O	intake and output (measurement of patient's fluids)
IOL	intraocular lens (implant)
IOP	intraocular pressure
IPPB	intermittent positive-pressure breathing
I.Q.	intelligence quotient
ITP	idiopathic thrombocytopenic purpura
IUD	intrauterine device
IUP	intrauterine pregnancy
IV	intravenous
IVP	intravenous pyelogram
K	potassium
kg	kilogram (1000 grams)
KJ	knee jerk
KS	Kaposi sarcoma
KUB	kidneys, ureters, bladder (x-ray study)

μL	microliter (one millionth of a liter)
L, l	liter; left; lower
L1, L2	first lumbar vertebra, second lumbar vertebra
LA	left atrium
LAD	left anterior descending (coronary artery)
lat	lateral
LB	large bowel
LBBB	left bundle branch block (heart block)
LBW	low birth weight
LD	lethal dose
LDH	lactate dehydrogenase
LDL	low-density lipoprotein (high levels associated with heart disease)
L-dopa	levodopa (drug used to treat Parkinson disease)
LE	lupus erythematosus
LEEP	loop electrocautery excision procedure
LES	lower esophageal sphincter
LFT	liver function test
LH	luteinizing hormone
LLL	left lower lobe (of lung)
LLQ	left lower quadrant (of abdomen)
LMP	last menstrual period
LMWH	low-molecular-weight heparin
LOC	loss of consciousness
LOS	length of stay
LP	lumbar puncture
lpf	low-power field (in microscopy)
LPN	licensed practical nurse
LS	lumbosacral spine
LSD	lysergic acid diethylamide (hallucinogen)
LSK	liver, spleen, kidneys
LTB	laryngotracheal bronchitis (croup)
LTC	long-term care
LTH	luteotropic hormone (prolactin)
LUL	left upper lobe (of lung)
LUQ	left upper quadrant (of abdomen)
LV	left ventricle
LVAD	left ventricular assist device
L&W	living and well
lymphs	lymphocytes
lytes	electrolytes
MA	mental age
MAC	monitored anesthesia care; *Mycobacterium avium* complex (cause of opportunistic pneumonia)
MAI	*Mycobacterium avium-intracellulare*
MAOI	monoamine oxidase inhibitor (type of antidepressant)
MBD	minimal brain dysfunction
mcg	microgram (one millionth of a gram); also abbreviated μg
MCH	mean corpuscular hemoglobin (average amount in each red blood cell)
MCHC	mean corpuscular hemoglobin concentration (average concentration in a single red cell)
mCi	millicurie
μCi	microcurie
MCP	metacarpophalangeal (joint)
MCV	mean corpuscular volume (average size of a single red blood cell)
MD	Doctor of Medicine
MDI	metered-dose inhaler
MDR	minimum daily requirement
MED	minimum effective dose
mEq	milliequivalent
mEq/L	milliequivalent per liter (measurement of the concentration of a solution)
mets	metastases
MG	myasthenia gravis
Mg	magnesium
mg	milligram (1/1000 of a gram)
mg/cc	milligram per cubic centimeter
mg/dL, mg/dl	milligram per deciliter
MH	marital history; mental health
MI	myocardial infarction; mitral insufficiency
mL, ml	milliliter (1/1000 of a liter)
mm	millimeter (1/1000 of a meter; 0.039 inch)
mm Hg, mmHg	millimeters of mercury
MMPI	Minnesota Multiphasic Personality Inventory
MMR	measles-mumps-rubella (vaccine)
MMT	manual muscle testing
μm	micrometer (one millionth of a meter, or 1/1000 of a millimeter); sometimes seen in older sources as μ (for "micron," an outdated term)
MoAb	monoclonal antibody
MODS	multiple organ dysfunction syndrome
monos	monocytes (white blood cells)
MR	mitral regurgitation; magnetic resonance
MRA	magnetic resonance angiography
MRI	magnetic resonance imaging
mRNA	messenger RNA
MS	multiple sclerosis; mitral stenosis; morphine sulfate
MSL	midsternal line
MTX	methotrexate
MUGA	multiple-gated acquisition scan (of heart)
multip	multipara; multiparous
MVP	mitral valve prolapse
myop	myopia (nearsightedness)
N	nitrogen
NA, N/A	not applicable; not available
Na	sodium
NB	newborn

NBS	normal bowel or breath sounds
ND	normal delivery; normal development
NED	no evidence of disease
neg.	negative
NG tube	nasogastric tube
NHL	non-Hodgkin lymphoma
NICU	neonatal intensive care unit
NKA	no known allergies
NK cells	natural killer cells
NKDA	no known drug allergies
NPO	nothing by mouth *(nil per os)*
NSAID	nonsteroidal anti-inflammatory drug
NSR	normal sinus rhythm (of heart)
NTP	normal temperature and pressure
O, O_2	oxygen
OA	osteoarthritis
OB/GYN	obstetrics and gynecology
OCPs	oral contraceptive pills
O.D.	Doctor of Optometry; right eye *(oculus dexter)*; better to specify "right eye" rather than abbreviate
OD	overdose
OR	operating room
ORIF	open reduction plus internal fixation
ORTH; Ortho.	orthopedics
O.S.	left eye *(oculus sinister)*; better to specify "left eye" rather than abbreviate
os	opening; bone
O.T.	occupational therapy
O.U.	both eyes *(oculus uterque)*; better to specify "both eyes" rather than abbreviate
oz.	ounce
P	phosphorus; posterior; pressure; pulse; pupil
p̄	after
P2, P_2	pulmonary valve closure (heart sound)
PA	pulmonary artery; posteroanterior
P-A	posteroanterior
P&A	percussion and auscultation
PAC	premature atrial contraction
PACS	picture archival communications system
$Paco_2$	partial pressure of carbon dioxide in arterial blood
palp.	palpable; palpation
PALS	pediatric advanced life support
Pao_2	partial pressure of oxygen in blood
Pap smear	Papanicolaou smear (from cervix and vagina)
para 1, 2, 3	unipara, bipara, tripara (number of viable births)
pc, p.c.	after meals *(post cibum)*
PCA	patient-controlled anesthesia

PCI	percutaneous coronary intervention(s)
Pco_2, pCO_2	partial pressure of carbon dioxide
PCP	*Pneumocystis* pneumonia; phencyclidine (a hallucinogen)
PCR	polymerase chain reaction (process allows making copies of genes)
PD	peritoneal dialysis
PDA	patent ductus arteriosus
PDR	*Physicians' Desk Reference*
PE	physical examination; pulmonary embolus
PEEP	positive end-expiratory pressure
PEG	percutaneous endoscopic gastrostomy (feeding tube placed in stomach)
PEJ	percutaneous endoscopic jejunostomy (feeding tube placed in small intestine)
per os	by mouth
PERRLA	pupils equal, round, reactive to light and accommodation
PET	positron emission tomography
PE tube	ventilating tube for eardrum
PFT	pulmonary function test
PG	prostaglandin
PH	past history
pH	hydrogen ion concentration (alkalinity and acidity measurement)
PI	present illness
PICC	peripherally inserted central catheter
PID	pelvic inflammatory disease
PIP	proximal interphalangeal (joint)
PKU	phenylketonuria
PM, p.m.	afternoon *(post meridiem)*
PMH	past medical history
PMN	polymorphonuclear leukocyte
PMS	premenstrual syndrome
PND	paroxysmal nocturnal dyspnea
p/o	postoperative
p.o.	by mouth *(per os)*
Po_2, pO_2	partial pressure of oxygen
poly	polymorphonuclear leukocyte
postop	postoperative (after surgery)
PPBS	postprandial blood sugar
PPD	purified protein derivative (test for tuberculosis)
preop	preoperative
prep	prepare for
PR	partial response
primip	primipara
PRL	prolactin
p.r.n.	as needed; as necessary *(pro re nata)*
procto	proctoscopy
prot.	protocol
Pro. time	prothrombin time (test of blood clotting)
PSA	prostate-specific antigen
pt.	patient
PT	prothrombin time; physical therapy
PTA	prior to admission (to hospital)

PTC	percutaneous transhepatic cholangiography
PTCA	percutaneous transluminal coronary angioplasty
PTH	parathyroid hormone
PTHC	percutaneous transhepatic cholangiography
PTSD	post-traumatic stress disorder
PTT	partial thromboplastin time (test of blood clotting)
PU	pregnancy urine
PUVA	psoralen ultraviolet A (treatment for psoriasis)
PVC	premature ventricular contraction
PVD	peripheral vascular disease
PVT	paroxysmal ventricular tachycardia
PWB	partial weight bearing
Px	prognosis
Q	blood volume; rate of blood flow (daily)
q	every *(quaque)*
qAM	every morning
q.d.	every day *(quaque die)*; better to specify "each/every day" rather than confuse with q.i.d. or q.o.d.
q.h.	every hour *(quaque hora)*
q.2h.	every 2 hours
q.i.d.	four times daily *(quater in die)*
qns	quantity not sufficient *(quantum non sufficit)*
q.o.d	every other day
qPM	every evening
QRS	a wave complex in an electrocardiographic study
q.s.	sufficient quantity *(quantum sufficit)*
qt	quart
R	respiration; right
RA	rheumatoid arthritis; right atrium
Ra	radium
rad	radiation absorbed dose
RBBB	right bundle branch block
RBC, rbc	red blood count; red blood cell
R.D.D.A.	recommended daily dietary allowance
RDS	respiratory distress syndrome
REM	rapid eye movement
RF	rheumatoid factor
Rh (factor)	rhesus (monkey) factor in blood
RhoGAM	drug to prevent Rh factor reaction in Rh-negative women
RIA	radioimmunoassay (minute quantities are measured)
RLL	right lower lobe (lung)
RLQ	right lower quadrant (abdomen)
RML	right middle lobe (lung)
RNA	ribonucleic acid

R/O	rule out
ROM	range of motion
ROS	review of systems
RRR	regular rate and rhythm (of heart)
RT	right; radiation therapy
RUL	right upper lobe (of lung)
RUQ	right upper quadrant (of abdomen)
RV	right ventricle
Rx	treatment; therapy; prescription
s̄	without *(sine)*
S1, S2	first sacral vertebra, second sacral vertebra
S-A node	sinoatrial node (pacemaker of heart)
SAD	seasonal affective disorder
SARS	severe acute respiratory syndrome
SBE	subacute bacterial endocarditis
SBFT	small bowel follow-through (x-ray study of small intestine function)
sed. rate	sedimentation rate (rate of erythrocyte sedimentation)
segs	segmented neutrophils; polys
SERM	selective estrogen receptor modulator
SGOT	*see* AST
SGPT	*see* ALT
SIADH	syndrome of inappropriate antidiuretic hormone
SIDS	sudden infant death syndrome
Sig.	directions (medication instructions)
SIRS	systemic inflammatory response syndrome (severe bacteriemia)
SL	sublingual
SLE	systemic lupus erythematosus
SMAC	automated analytical device for testing blood
SMA 12	blood chemistry profile including 12 different studies/assays
SOAP	subjective, objective, assessment, plan (used for patient notes)
SOB	shortness of breath
s.o.s.	if necessary *(si opus sit)*
S/P	status post (previous disease condition)
SPECT	single photon emission computed tomography
sp. gr.	specific gravity
SQ	subcutaneous
S/S, Sx	signs and symptoms
SSCP	substernal chest pain
SSRI	selective serotonin reuptake inhibitor (type of antidepressant)
Staph.	staphylococci (berry-shaped bacteria in clusters)
stat., STAT	immediately *(statim)*
STD	sexually transmitted disease
STH	somatotropin (growth hormone)
STI	sexually transmitted infection

Strep.	streptococci (berry-shaped bacteria in twisted chains)
sub-Q	subcutaneously
SVC	superior vena cava
SVD	spontaneous vaginal delivery
Sx	symptoms; signs and symptoms
Sz	seizure
T	temperature; time
T tube	tube placed in biliary tract for drainage
T1, T2	first thoracic vertebra, second thoracic vertebra
T$_3$	triiodothyronine (test)
T$_4$	thyroxine (test)
TA	therapeutic abortion
T&A	tonsillectomy and adenoidectomy
TAB	therapeutic abortion
TAH	total abdominal hysterectomy
TAT	Thematic Apperception Test
TB	tuberculosis
Tc	technetium
T cells	lymphocytes produced in the thymus gland
TEE	transesophageal echocardiogram
TENS	transcutaneous electrical nerve stimulation
TFT	thyroid function test
TIA	transient ischemic attack
t.i.d.	three times daily (ter in die)
TLC	total lung capacity
TM	tympanic membrane
TMJ	temporomandibular joint
TNM	tumor-node-metastases (cancer staging system)
tPA	tissue plasminogen activator
TPN	total parenteral nutrition
TPR	temperature, pulse, respirations
TRUS	transrectal ultrasound (examination)
TSH	thyroid-stimulating hormone
TSS	toxic shock syndrome
TUR, TURP	transurethral resection of the prostate

TVH	total vaginal hysterectomy
Tx	treatment
UA	urinalysis
UAO	upper airway obstruction
UC	uterine contractions
UE	upper extremity
UGI	upper gastrointestinal
umb.	navel (umbilicus)
U/O	urinary output
URI	upper respiratory infection
U/S	ultrasound
UTI	urinary tract infection
UV	ultraviolet
VA	visual acuity
VATS	video-assisted thoracic surgery (thorascopy)
VC	vital capacity (of lungs)
VCUG	voiding cystourethrogram
VDRL	test for syphilis (protocol of Venereal Disease Research Laboratory)
VEGF	vascular endothelial growth factor
VF	visual field; ventricular fibrillation
V/Q scan	ventilation-perfusion scan (of lung)
V/S	vital signs; versus
VSD	ventricular septal defect
VT	ventricular tachycardia (abnormal heart rhythm)
VTE	venous thromboembolism
WAIS	Wechsler Adult Intelligence Scale
WBC, wbc	white blood cell; white blood count
WDWN	well developed and well nourished
WISC	Wechsler Intelligence Scale for Children
WNL	within normal limits
wt	weight
XRT	radiation therapy
y/o, yr	year(s) old

ACRONYMS

An *acronym* is the name for an abbreviation that forms a pronounceable word.

ACE ("ace") angiotensin-converting enzyme
AIDS (aydz) acquired immunodeficiency syndrome
APGAR (ap-gahr) appearance, pulse, grimace, activity, respiration
BUN (bun, or bee-yu-en) blood urea nitrogen
CABG ("cabbage") coronary artery bypass graft
CAT ("cat") computerized axial tomography
CPAP (see-pap) continuous positive airway pressure
ELISA ("eliza") enzyme-linked immunosorbent assay
GERD (gerd) gastroesophageal reflux disease
GIST (jist) gastrointestinal stromal tumor
HAART ("heart") highly active anti-retroviral therapy
HIPAA (hip-ah) Health Insurance Portability and Accountability Act of 1996
LASER (lay-zer) light amplification by stimulated emission of radiation
LASIK (lay-sik) laser in situ keratomileusis
LEEP ("leap") loop electrocautery excision procedure
MAC (mak) monitored anesthesia care; *Mycobacterium avium* complex
MICU (mik-yu) medical intensive care unit
MIS ("miss") minimally invasive surgery
MODS (modz) multiple organ dysfunction syndrome
MUGA (myu-gah) multiple-gated acquisition (scan)
NSAID (en-sayd) nonsteroidal anti-inflammatory drug
NICU (nik-yu) neonatal intensive care unit

PACS (paks) picture archival communications system
PALS (palz) pediatric advanced life support
PEEP ("peep") positive end expiratory pressure
PEG ("peg") percutaneous endoscopic gastrostomy
PERRLA (per-lah) pupils equal, round, reactive to light and accommodation
PET ("pet") positron emission tomography
PICU (pik-yu) pediatric intensive care unit
PIP ("pip") proximal interphalangeal (joint)
PUVA (poo-vah) psoralen ultraviolet A
REM (rem) rapid eye movement
SAD ("sad") seasonal affective disorder
SARS (sahrz) severe acute respiratory syndrome
SERM (serm) selective estrogen receptor modulator
SIDS (sidz) sudden infant death syndrome
SIRS (serz) systemic inflammatory response syndrome
SMAC ("smack") sequential multiple analyzer computer (blood testing)
SOAP ("soap") subjective, objective, assessment, plan
SPECT (spekt) single photon emission computed tomography
TENS (tenz) transcutaneous electrical nerve stimulation
TRUS ("truss") transrectal ultrasound
TURP (turp) transurethral resection of the prostate
VATS (vatz) video-assisted thoracic surgery

SYMBOLS

$=$	equal		%	percent
$\neq$	unequal		°	degree; hour
$+$	positive		:	ratio; "is to"
$-$	negative		$\pm$	plus or minus (either positive or negative)
$\uparrow$	above, increase		′	foot
$\downarrow$	below, decrease		″	inch
♀	female		∴	therefore
♂	male		@	at, each
$\rightarrow$	to (in direction of)		$\bar{c}$	with
$>$	is greater than		$\bar{s}$	without
$<$	is less than		#	pound; number
1°	primary to		$\cong$	approximately, about
2°	secondary to		Δ	change
ℨ	dram		p	short arm of a chromosome
℥	ounce		q	long arm of a chromosome

appendix III

Normal Hematologic Reference Values and Implications of Abnormal Results

The implications of abnormal results are major ones in each category. SI units are those used in the International System of Units, which generally are accepted for all scientific and technical uses. All laboratory values should be interpreted with caution because normal values differ widely among clinical laboratories.

cu mm = cubic millimeter (mm^3)
dL = deciliter (1/10 of a liter or 100 mL)
g = gram
L = liter
mg = milligram (1/1000 of a gram)
mL = milliliter
mEq = milliequivalent

mill = million
mm = millimeter (1/1000 of a meter)
mmol = millimole
thou = thousand
U = unit
µL = microliter
µmol = micromole (one millionth of a mole)

CELL COUNTS

	Conventional Units	SI Units	Implications	
Erythrocytes (RBCs)				
Females	4.0–5.5 million/mm³ *or* μL	$4.0–5.5 \times 10^{12}/L$	*High*	♦ Polycythemia
Males	4.5–6.0 million/mm³ *or* μL	$4.5–6.0 \times 10^{12}/L$		♦ Dehydration
			Low	♦ Iron deficiency anemia
				♦ Blood loss
Leukocytes (WBC)				
Total	5000–10,000/mm³ *or* μL	$5.0–10.0 \times 10^{9}/L$	*High*	♦ Bacterial infection
Differential	%			♦ Leukemia
Neutrophils	54–62			♦ Eosinophils high in allergy
Lymphocytes	20–40		*Low*	♦ Viral infection
Monocytes	3–7			♦ Aplastic anemia
Eosinophils	1–3			♦ Chemotherapy
Basophils	0–1			
Platelets	150,000–350,000/mm³ or μL	$200–400 \times 10^{9}/L$	*High*	♦ Hemorrhage
				♦ Infections
				♦ Malignancy
				♦ Splenectomy
			Low	♦ Aplastic anemia
				♦ Chemotherapy
				♦ Hypersplenism

COAGULATION TESTS

	Conventional Units	SI Units	Implications	
Bleeding time (template method)	2.75–8.0 min	2.7–8.0 min	*Prolonged*	♦ Aspirin ingestion
				♦ Low platelet count
Coagulation time	5–15 min	5–15 min	*Prolonged*	♦ Heparin therapy
Prothrombin time (PT)*	11–12.5 sec	11–12.5 sec	*Prolonged*	♦ Vitamin K deficiency
				♦ Hepatic disease
				♦ Oral anticoagulant therapy (warfarin)
Partial thromboplastin time (PTT)	25–34 sec	25–37 sec	*Prolonged*	♦ IV heparin therapy

---

*The INR (international normalized ratio) is a standard for monitoring the effects of an anticoagulant, warfarin; the normal INR value is <1.5.

RED BLOOD CELL TESTS

	Conventional Units	SI Units	Implications	
Hematocrit (Hct)				
Females	37%–47%	0.37–0.47	*High*	♦ Polycythemia
Males	40%–54%	0.40–0.54		♦ Dehydration
			Low	♦ Loss of blood
				♦ Anemia
Hemoglobin (Hb, Hgb)				
Females	12.0–14.0 g/dL *or* 120–140 g/L	1.86–2.48 mmol/L	*High*	♦ Polycythemia
				♦ Dehydration
Males	14.0–16.0 g/dL	2.17–2.79 mmol/L	*Low*	♦ Anemia
				♦ Blood loss

SERUM TESTS

	Conventional Units	SI Units	Implications	
Alanine aminotransferase (ALT; SGPT)	5–30 U/L	5–30 U/L	*High*	♦ Hepatitis
Albumin	3.5–5.5 g/dL	35–55 g/L	*Low*	♦ Hepatic disease
				♦ Malnutrition
				♦ Nephritis and nephrosis
Alkaline phosphatase (ALP)	20–90 U/L	20–90 U/L	*High*	♦ Bone disease
				♦ Hepatitis or tumor infiltration of liver
				♦ Biliary obstruction
Aspartate aminotransferase (AST; SGOT)	10–30 U/L	10–30 U/L	*High*	♦ Hepatitis
				♦ Cardiac and muscle injury
Bilirubin			*High*	♦ Hemolysis
Total	0.3–1.0 mg/dL	5.1–17 μmol/L		♦ Neonatal hepatic immaturity
Neonates	1–12 mg/dL	17–205 μmol/L		♦ Cirrhosis
				♦ Biliary tract obstruction
Blood urea nitrogen (BUN)	10–20 mg/dL	3.6–7.1 mmol/L	*High*	♦ Renal disease
				♦ Reduced renal blood flow
				♦ Urinary tract obstruction
			Low	♦ Hepatic damage
				♦ Malnutrition
Calcium	9.0–10.5 mg/dL	2.2–2.6 mmol/L	*High*	♦ Hyperparathyroidism
				♦ Multiple myeloma
				♦ Metastatic cancer
			Low	♦ Hypoparathyroidism
				♦ Total parathyroidectomy
Cholesterol (desirable range)				
Total	<200 mg/dL	<5.2 mmol/L	*High*	♦ High-fat diet
LDL cholesterol	<130 mg/dL	<3.36 mmol/L		♦ Inherited hypercholesterolemia
HDL cholesterol	>60 mg/dL	>1.55 mmol/L	*Low*	♦ Starvation
Creatine kinase (CK)				
Females	30–135 U/L	30–135 U/L	*High*	♦ Myocardial infarction
Males	55–170 U/L	55–170 U/L		♦ Muscle disease

	Conventional Units	SI Units	Implications	
Creatinine	<1.5 mg/dL	<133 μmol/L	*High*	♦ Renal disease
Glucose (fasting)	75–115 mg/dL	4.2–6.4 mmol/L	*High*	♦ Diabetes mellitus
			Low	♦ Hyperinsulinism
				♦ Fasting
				♦ Hypothyroidism
				♦ Addison disease
				♦ Pituitary insufficiency
Lactate dehydrogenase (LDH)	100–190 U/L	100–190 U/L	*High*	♦ Tissue necrosis
				♦ Lymphomas
				♦ Muscle disease
Phosphate (PO⁻₄)	3.0–4.5 mg/dL	1.0–1.5 mmol/L	*High*	♦ Renal failure
				♦ Bone metastases
				♦ Hypoparathyroidism
			Low	♦ Malnutrition
				♦ Malabsorption
				♦ Hyperparathyroidism
Potassium (K)	3.5–5.0 mEq/L	3.5–5.0 mmol/L	*High*	♦ Burn victims
				♦ Renal failure
				♦ Diabetic ketoacidosis
			Low	♦ Cushing syndrome
				♦ Loss of body fluids
Sodium (Na)	136–145 mEq/L	136–145 mmol/L	*High*	♦ Inadequate water intake
				♦ Water loss in excess of sodium
			Low	♦ Adrenal insufficiency
				♦ Inadequate sodium intake
				♦ Excessive sodium loss
Thyroxine (T₄)	5–12 μg/dL	64–154 nmol/L	*High*	♦ Graves disease (hyperthyroidism)
			Low	♦ Hypothyroidism
Uric acid				
Females	2.5–8.0 mg/dL	150–480 μmol/L	*High*	♦ Gout
Males	1.5–6.0 mg/dL	90–360 μmol/L		♦ Leukemia

appendix IV

Drugs

This is an alphabetized list of the drugs referred to in Chapter 21 (tables), with brand name(s) in parentheses and explanation of use, including category and/or class.

Generic Name (Brand Name)	Explanation of Use
acarbose (Precose)	Antidiabetic (type 2 diabetes)/alpha-glucosidase inhibitor
acetaminophen (Tylenol)	Analgesic/mild
acyclovir (Zovirax)	Antiviral
albuterol (Proventil)	Bronchodilator
alendronate (Fosamax)	Antiosteoporosis/ bisphosphonate
alprazolam (Xanax)	Tranquilizer/minor/benzodiazepine
aluminum antacid (Rolaids)	GI/antacid
aluminum + magnesium antacid (Gaviscon)	GI/antacid
amiodarone (Cordarone)	Cardiovascular/antiarrhythmic
amlodipine (Norvasc)	Cardiovascular/calcium antagonist
amoxicillin trihydrate (Amoxil, Trimox)	Antibiotic/penicillin
amoxicillin + clavulanate (Augmentin)	Antibiotic/penicillin
anastrozole (Arimidex)	Endocrine/aromatase inhibitor
aspirin	Analgesic/mild antiplatelet
atenolol (Tenormin)	Cardiovascular/beta-blocker
atorvastatin (Lipitor)	Cardiovascular/cholesterol-lowering
azithromycin (Zithromax)	Antibiotic/erythromycin class
beclomethasone (Vanceril)	Respiratory/steroid inhaler
buspirone (BuSpar)	Tranquilizer/minor
butabarbital (Butisol)	Sedative-hypnotic
caffeine	Stimulant
carbamazepine (Tegretol)	Anticonvulsant
cefprozil (Cefzil)	Antibiotic/cephalosporin
ceftazidime (Fortaz)	Antibiotic/cephalosporin
cefuroxime axetil (Ceftin)	Antibiotic/cephalosporin
celecoxib (Celebrex)	Analgesic/NSAID
cephalexin (Keflex)	Antibiotic/cephalosporin
cetirizine (Zyrtec)	Antihistamine
chlorpheniramine maleate (Chlor-Trimeton)	Antihistamine
chlorpromazine (Thorazine)	Tranquilizer/major/phenothiazine
cimetidine (Tagamet)	GI/antiulcer/anti-GERD
ciprofloxacin (Cipro)	Antibiotic/quinolone
clarithromycin (Biaxin)	Antibiotic/erythromycin class

Generic Name (Brand Name)	Explanation of Use
clopidogrel bisulfate (Plavix)	Antiplatelet
codeine	Analgesic/narcotic
dalteparin (Fragmin)	Anticoagulant
dextroamphetamine sulfate (Dexedrine)	Stimulant
diazepam (Valium)	Tranquilizer/minor/benzodiazepine
diclofenac (Voltaren)	Analgesic/NSAID
digoxin (Lanoxin)	Cardiovascular/anti-CHF
diltiazem (Cardizem CD)	Cardiovascular/calcium antagonist
diphenhydramine (Benadryl)	Antihistamine
diphenoxylate + atropine (Lomotil)	GI/antidiarrheal
donepezil (Aricept)	Anti-Alzheimer disease
doxycycline	Antibiotic/tetracycline
efavirenz (Sustiva)	Anti-HIV
enalapril maleate (Vasotec)	Cardiovascular ACE inhibitor
enoxaparin sodium (Lovenox)	Anticoagulant
epinephrine	Bronchodilator
erythromycin (Ery-Tab)	Antibiotic/erythromycin
estrogen (Premarin, Prempro, Estradiol)	Endocrine/estrogen
ether	Anesthetic/general
extended insulin zinc suspension (Ultralente)	Antidiabetic (type 1 diabetes)
famotidine (Pepcid)	GI/antiulcer/anti-GERD
felbamate (Felbatol)	Anticonvulsant
fexofenadine (Allegra)	Antihistamine
fluconazole (Diflucan)	Antifungal
flunisolide (AeroBid)	Respiratory/steroid inhaler
fluoxymesterone (Halotestin)	Endocrine/androgen
flutamide (Eulexin)	Endocrine/antiandrogen
fluticasone propionate (Flovent)	Respiratory/steroid inhaler
fulvestrant (Faslodex)	Endocrine/aromatase inhibitor
furosemide (Lasix)	Cardiovascular/diuretic
gabapentin (Neurontin)	Anticonvulsant
glipizide (Glucotrol XL)	Antidiabetic (type 2 diabetes)/sulfonylurea
glyburide	Antidiabetic (type 2 diabetes)/sulfonylurea
halothane (Fluothane)	Anesthetic/general
human insulin (Humalog)	Antidiabetic (type 1 diabetes)
human insulin NPH (Humulin N)	Antidiabetic (type 1 diabetes)
hydrochlorothiazide (Diuril)	Cardiovascular/diuretic
hydrocodone w/APAP	Analgesic/narcotic
hydromorphone (Dilaudid)	Analgesic/narcotic
ibuprofen (Motrin, Advil)	Analgesic/NSAID
ibutilide (Corvert)	Antiarrhythmic
indinavir (Crixivan)	Antiviral/protease inhibitor/anti-HIV
insulin zinc suspension (Lente)	Antidiabetic (type 1 diabetes)
interferon alfa-n1 (Wellferon)	Antiviral/anti-cancer drug
ipratropium bromide + albuterol (Atrovent)	Bronchodilator
irbesartan (Avapro)	Cardiovascular/angiotensin II receptor antagonist
isoniazid or INH (Nydrazid)	Antitubercular
itraconazole (Sporanox)	Antifungal

Generic Name (Brand Name)	Explanation of Use
lamivudine (Epivir)	Antiviral/reverse transcriptase inhibitor/anti-HIV
lansoprazole (Prevacid)	GI/antiulcer/anti-GERD
letrozole (Femara)	Endocrine/aromatase inhibitor
levofloxacin (Levaquin)	Antibiotic
levothyroxine (Levoxyl, Levothroid, Synthroid)	Endocrine/thyroid hormone
lidocaine (Xylocaine)	Anesthetic/local
lidocaine + prilocaine (EMLA)	Anesthetic/local
liothyronine (Cytomel)	Endocrine/thyroid hormone
liotrix (Thyrolar)	Endocrine/thyroid hormone
lisinopril (Prinivil, Zestril)	Cardiovascular/ACE inhibitor
lithium carbonate (Eskalith)	Tranquilizer/major
loperamide (Imodium)	GI/antidiarrheal
loratadine (Claritin)	Antihistamine
lorazepam (Ativan)	Tranquilizer/minor/benzodiazepine
losartan (Cozaar)	Cardiovascular/angiotensin II receptor antagonist
lovastatin (Mevacor)	Cardiovascular/cholesterol-lowering
magnesium antacid (milk of magnesia)	GI/antacid
meclizine (Antivert)	Antihistamine
medroxyprogesterone acetate (Cycrin, Provera)	Endocrine/progestin
megestrol (Megace)	Endocrine/progestin
memantine (Namenda)	Anti-Alzheimer disease
meperidine (Demerol)	Analgesic/narcotic
metaproterenol (Alupent)	Bronchodilator
metformin (Glucophage)	Antidiabetic (type 2 diabetes)/biguanide
methylphenidate (Ritalin)	Stimulant
methylprednisolone (Medrol)	Respiratory/steroid IV or oral
methyltestosterone (Virilon)	Endocrine/androgen
metoclopramide (Reglan)	GI/antinauseant
metoprolol (Lopressor, Toprol-XL)	Cardiovascular/beta-blocker
miconazole (Monostat)	Antifungal
midazolam (Versed)	Sedative-hypnotic
modafinil (Provigil)	Stimulant/sleep antagonist
montelukast (Singulair)	Respiratory/leukotriene modifier
nafcillin (Unipen)	Antibiotic/penicillin
naproxen (Naprosyn, Aleve)	Analgesic/NSAID
nifedipine (Adalat CC, Procardia)	Cardiovascular/calcium antagonist
nilutamide (Casodex)	Endocrine/antiandrogen
nitroglycerin	Cardiovascular/antianginal
nitrous oxide	Anesthetic/general
nystatin (Nilstat)	Antifungal
ofloxacin (Floxin)	Antibiotic/quinolone
olanzapine (Zyprexa)	Tranquilizer/major/antipsychotic
omeprazole (Prilosec)	GI/antiulcer/anti-GERD
ondansetron (Zofran)	GI/antinauseant
oxacillin (Bactocill)	Antibiotic/penicillin
oxycodone (Oxycontin)	Analgesic/narcotic
pamidronate disodium (Aredia)	Anti-osteoporosis/bisphosphonate
paregoric	GI/antidiarrheal
phenobarbital	Sedative-hypnotic/anticonvulsant
phenytoin sodium (Dilantin)	Anticonvulsant

Generic Name (Brand Name)	Explanation of Use
pioglitazone (Actos)	Antidiabetic (type 2 diabetes)
pravastatin (Pravachol)	Cardiovascular/cholesterol-lowering
prednisone	Respiratory/steroid IV or oral
promethazine (Phenergan)	Antihistamine
protamine zinc suspension (PZI)	Antidiabetic (type 1 diabetes)
procaine (Novocaine)	Anesthetic/local
prochlorperazine maleate (Compazine)	GI/antinauseant
propoxyphene (Darvon)	Analgesic/narcotic
propranolol (Inderal)	Cardiovascular/beta-blocker
quinapril (Accupril)	Cardiovascular/ACE inhibitor
raloxifene (Evista)	Endocrine/SERM/antiosteoporosis
ramipril (Altace)	Cardiovascular/ACE inhibitor
ranitidine (Zantac)	GI/antiulcer/anti-GERD
repaglinide (Prandin)	Antidiabetic (type 2 diabetes)/meglitinide
rifampin (Rifadin)	Antitubercular
rosiglitazone (Avandia)	Antidiabetic (type 2 diabetes)
rosuvastatin calcium (Crestor)	Cholesterol-lowering statin
salmeterol (Serevent)	Bronchodilator
simvastatin (Zocor)	Cardiovascular/cholesterol-lowering
sotalol (Betapace)	Cardiovascular/beta-blocker
spironolactone (Aldactone)	Cardiovascular/diuretic
sulfamethoxazole + trimethoprim (Bactrim)	Antibiotic/sulfonamide
sulfisoxazole (Gantrisin)	Antibiotic/sulfonamide
tamoxifen (Nolvadex)	Endocrine/antiestrogen
temazepam (Restoril)	Sedative-hypnotic/benzodiazepine
terbinafine (Lamisil)	Antifungal
tetracycline	Antibiotic/tetracycline
theophylline (Theo-Dur)	Bronchodilator
thiopental (Pentothal)	Anesthetic/general
thioridazine (Mellaril)	Tranquilizer/major/phenothiazine
tissue plasminogen activator (tPA)	Anticoagulant
tramadol (Ultram)	Analgesic/mild
triamcinolone (Azmacort)	Respiratory/steroid inhaler
triamterene (Dyazide)	Cardiovascular/diuretic
triazolam (Halcion)	Sedative-hypnotic/benzodiazepine
trifluoperazine (Stelazine)	Tranquilizer/major/phenothiazine
valproic acid (Depakote)	Anticonvulsant
warfarin (Coumadin)	Anticoagulant
zafirlukast (Accolate)	Respiratory/leukotriene modifier
zidovudine *or* AZT (Retrovir)	Antiviral/reverse transcriptase inhibitor/anti-HIV
zidovudine + lamivudine (Combivir)	Anti-HIV
zileuton (Zyflo Filmtab)	Respiratory/leukotriene modifier
zoledronic acid (Zometa)	Antiosteoporosis/bisphosphonate
zolpidem tartrate (Ambien)	Sedative-hypnotic

appendix V

Complementary and Alternative Medicine Terms*

Following is a listing of common complementary and alternative medicine (CAM) terms. A comprehensive listing of CAM terms, as well as more detailed information on some of the terms listed here, can be found in *Mosby's Dictionary of Complementary and Alternative Medicine*.

Note: The practice of any complementary or alternative medicine techniques and the use of any herbal remedies should be approached with caution and care, or under the supervision of a CAM professional or your physician.

acupoints	Particular locations on the body that allow the practitioner to balance the client's qi (life force) to effect therapeutic changes using acupuncture or acupressure.
acupressure	A technique used to release blocked qi (life force) by applying finger pressure to points on meridians.
acupuncture	A practice in Chinese medicine (developed more than 2000 years ago) in which the skin, at various points along meridians, is punctured with needles to remove energy blockages and to stimulate the flow of qi (life force).
aloe	This plant's leaves are used to treat minor burns, wound healing, GI disorders, menstrual cramps, premenstrual syndrome, and other ailments.
antioxidants	Substances that may protect cells from damage caused by unstable molecules known as "free radicals." Free radicals' damage may lead to cancer. Examples of antioxidants are beta-carotene and vitamins C, E, and A.
apiotherapy	The use of products produced by honeybees for therapeutic and pharmacologic purposes.
applied kinesiology	A physical therapy model that draws on various therapeutic schools of thought; the goal of this therapy is the recovery of muscles that are functionally inhibited with respect to normal range of motion and strength.
aromatherapy	The use of essential oils (extracts and essences) from flowers, herbs, and trees applied topically or inhaled to promote and maintain overall health.
ayurvedic medicine	Also known as *ayurveda;* means the science (veda) of life (ayu). It is an ancient Indian health system that works to reestablish the balance between the body and the mind (with diet and herbal remedies).

---

*Excerpts from Jonas WB: Mosby's Dictionary of Complementary and Alternative Medicine. St. Louis, Mosby, 2005; and from http://nccam.nih.gov/health/bytreatment.htm#s1, on the website of the National Center for Complementary and Alternative Medicine of the National Institutes of Health.

bilberry	This berry is used to treat myopia, retinal problems, inflammation of the mouth and pharynx, GI disorders, varicose veins, and other ailments.
biofeedback	Process in which equipment sensors provide measurements of body functions (such as heart rate or neural activity) and those signals are displayed to the patient, to permit maneuvers to alter the measured function.
black cohosh	This plant's roots are used to treat menopause, menstrual cramps, diarrhea, and other ailments.
chamomile	This plant's dried buds are used to treat inflammatory disease of the GI and upper respiratory tracts and inflammation of the skin and mucous membranes; to promote healing of wounds, rashes, and ulcers (applied topically); and to relieve motion sickness, GI spasms, and restlessness or insomnia, as well as other ailments.
chelation therapy	Medical treatment in which heavy metals are flushed from the bloodstream by means of a chelator that binds metal ions; used in cases of mercury or lead poisoning.
chi	In Tibetan medicine, awareness, one of the three functions of the mind, providing the direction for actions.
chiropractic therapy	A complementary health discipline focusing on the relationship between body structure (primarily of the spine) and function. Chiropractors use manipulative therapy to the client's back, neck, and limbs.
chondroitin	Naturally occurring substance responsible for elasticity and taken as a dietary supplement. Large-scale clinical trials are ongoing to test the effects of this supplement on knee osteoarthritis.
circadian rhythm	The biological patterns (of a specific person) within a 24-hour cycle, usually the course of a day.
coenzyme Q_{10}	A compound made naturally in the body, used for cell growth and to protect cells from damage that could lead to cancer. Animal studies have shown that coenzyme Q_{10} helps the immune system work better and makes the body better able to resist certain infections and types of cancer. Clinical trials have shown that coenzyme Q_{10} helps protect the heart from the damaging side effects of doxorubicin, a drug used to treat cancer.
complementary and alternative medicine (CAM)	A group of diverse medical and health care systems, practices, and products that at present are not considered part of conventional medicine. Complementary medicine is used together with conventional medicine (e.g., aroma therapy to lessen patient discomfort after surgery). Alternative medicine is used in place of conventional medicine (e.g., patient may choose to follow a special diet to treat cancer instead of undergoing surgery, radiation therapy, or chemotherapy).
dehydro-epiandrosterone (DHEA)	A hormone precursor that exists naturally in yams. Examples of common uses are to slow the effects of aging, to support or improve memory, and to treat erectile dysfunction, depression, osteoporosis, and atherosclerosis.
echinacea	This plant's roots, flowers, and leaves are used to treat upper respiratory and urinary tract infections, allergic rhinitis, and other ailments, and to promote wound healing.
electromagnetic fields (EMFs)	Invisible lines of force that surround all electrical devices. Bioelectromagnetic-based therapies involve unconventional use of electromagnets, such as pulsed fields and magnetic currents, to treat asthma and cancer or manage pain from migraine headaches.
ergonomics	Applied study of psychology, anatomy, and physiology relating to people and work environments.

folate	A water-soluble B vitamin that occurs naturally in food. Folic acid is the synthetic form of folate that is found in supplements and added to fortified foods. Folate helps produce and maintain new cells. This is especially important during periods of rapid cell division and growth, such as infancy and pregnancy.
garlic	This plant's bulbs are used to manage and treat elevated cholesterol levels, atherosclerosis, hypertension, upper respiratory tract infections, and other conditions and ailments.
ginger	This plant's roots are used to manage and treat nausea and vomiting, motion sickness, and other conditions and ailments.
ginkgo *(Ginkgo biloba)*	This plant's leaves are used to manage and treat Alzheimer disease, dementia, depression, asthma, retinal disease, heart disease, peripheral arterial occlusive disease, varicose veins, premenstrual syndrome, tinnitus, and other conditions and ailments.
ginseng	This plant's roots are used to manage and treat fatigue, stress, mild depression, decreased libido, and other conditions and ailments.
glucosamine	Natural substance found in and around the cells of cartilage. Glucosamine is an amino sugar that the body produces and distributes in cartilage and other connective tissue. Glucosamine is used in conjunction with chondroitin sulfate; large-scale clinical trials are ongoing to test the effects on knee osteoarthritis.
guided imagery	Directed relaxation and visualization to support changes in health.
herbalism	Study and practice of using plants to treat illnesses and promote health; also called *phytotherapy.*
homeopathy	System of treating disease based on the administration of minute doses of a drug that in massive amounts produces symptoms in healthy persons similar to those of the disease itself.
hydrotherapy	A therapeutic modality that uses water, such as whirlpools or sitz baths.
integrative medicine	Combines mainstream medical therapies and CAM therapies for which there is some high-quality scientific evidence for safety and effectiveness.
kava	This plant's rhizomes and roots are used to treat anxiety, restlessness, fibromyalgia, tension headaches, insomnia, and other ailments.
kinesiology	Study of the body's structure and processes as they relate to movement.
lymphatic drainage	A specific type of massage that supports and assists circulation in the lymphatic system.
macrobiotic diet	Designed to bring yin/yang energies into balance, the macrobiotic diet, developed by Michio Kushi, is part of a larger lifestyle/philosophy and whole-body regimen.
manipulation	In massage therapy, osteopathic medicine, chiropractic, and traditional Chinese medicine, the use of various manual techniques to adjust the joints and spinal column, improve the range of motion of the joints, relax and stretch connective tissue and muscles, and promote overall relaxation.
massage therapy	The application of diverse manual techniques of touch and stroking to muscles and soft tissue to achieve relaxation and to improve sense of well-being.
meditation	Directing one's attention toward a symbol, sound, thought, or breath to alter the state of consciousness, to attain a state of relaxation and stress relief; used for spiritual growth, healing, deepening concentration, and unlocking creativity.
melatonin	Hormone secreted from the pineal glands thought to regulate circadian rhythms; also used in supplement form as a sleep aid.

meridians	In acupuncture, a system of pathways running through the body that connect vital organs and carry qi; channels.
milk thistle	This plant's seeds are used to make a tea to treat liver and gallbladder disease, hepatitis, and dyspepsia, and to support the liver during transplantation recovery.
mistletoe	Leafy shoots and berries of mistletoe are used to make extracts that can be taken by mouth. Mistletoe has been used for centuries to treat seizures, headaches, and other conditions. Clinical trials are ongoing for possible effects on cancer treatment.
naturopathy	Therapeutic system that relies on using natural agents such as light, natural foods, warmth, massage, and fresh air. Naturopaths believe in the power of the body's natural processes to heal illnesses.
omega-3 fatty acids	A group of polyunsaturated fatty acids that come from food sources such as fish, fish oil, some vegetable oils (primarily canola and soybean), walnuts, wheat germ, and certain dietary supplements. Clinical trials are ongoing to test the effects of omega-3 fatty acids on various conditions and for enhancement of general well-being.
osteopathy	A form of medicine that uses joint manipulation, physical therapy, and postural reeducation to restore the structural balance of the musculoskeletal system.
qi	The body's life force. In Chinese philosophy, qi is the force that flows through channels in the body and enlivens all living beings; an imbalance in qi is believed to cause illness.
qi gong	Cultivation of qi. *Qi gong* (chee-GUNG) is the general term for all Chinese techniques of breathing, visualization, and movement, the purpose of which is the promotion of balanced qi flow (vital energy) for enhanced immune function and blood flow.
reflexology	A natural healing system based on the principle that reflexes in the hands and feet correspond to various organs and organ systems in the body; stimulating such reflexes by applying pressure on hands and feet improves circulation, thereby optimizing body functions.
Reiki	A system of spiritual healing/energy medicine developed by Japanese physician Dr. Mikao Usui. Reiki (RAY-kee) is a Japanese word representing universal life energy. It is based on the belief that when spiritual energy is channeled through a Reiki practitioner, the patient's spirit is healed, which then heals the physical body.
Rolfing	A 10-session manual therapy developed to optimize the body's movement and alignment and coordination with the forces of gravity, for relief of muscular and emotional tension.
selenium	A trace mineral that is essential to good health but required only in small amounts. Selenium is incorporated into proteins to make selenoproteins, which are important antioxidant enzymes. The antioxidant effects of selenoproteins help prevent cellular damage from free radicals. Free radicals are natural byproducts of oxygen metabolism that may contribute to the development of chronic diseases such as cancer and heart disease. Clinical trials are ongoing to test the effects of selenium on the treatment and prevention of cancer.
shiatsu	A type of massage developed in Japan; it consists of the application of pressure with the palms and thumbs.
soy	Soybeans in various forms may support healthy body tissues by neutralizing free radicals. Soy may offer a diversity of antioxidant mechanisms in a variety of circumstances.
St. John's wort	This plant's flowers may be used to treat mild to moderate depression, anxiety, sleep disorders, and other ailments.

tai chi

In traditional Chinese medicine, a family of health-promoting exercises that provide benefits for the body, mind, and soul by maintaining balance between the yin and yang components; these exercises comprise flowing movements that imitate the motions and forms of animals, all of which share fundamental elements rooted in qi gong.

valerian

This plant's rhizomes and roots are used to treat sleeping disorders, nervousness, anxiety, restlessness, irritable bowel syndrome, and other ailments.

yin and yang

Governing theory behind traditional Chinese medicine: the idea that life is filled with opposite yet complementary characteristics and qualities on the spiritual and physical levels and on the macro and micro levels. The concept is that each entity can be essentially itself and its opposite; additionally, yang's "seed" is believed to be contained within yin; a balance of yin and yang is considered essential for good health, whereas an imbalance can manifest as disease.

yoga

A family of mind-body disciplines that share the goals of the integrated body and mind or the union of the self with the divine. All yogic systems are aimed at nurturing the body through breath and posture and cultivating the mind through meditation.

zinc

An essential mineral, found in almost every cell, that stimulates the activity of approximately 100 enzymes, which are substances that promote the body's biochemical reactions. Zinc supports a healthy immune system, is needed for wound healing, helps maintain sense of taste and smell, and is needed for DNA synthesis. Zinc also supports normal growth and development during pregnancy, childhood, and adolescence. Clinical trials are ongoing to test the use of supplemental zinc on the effects of the common cold.

Index

Page numbers in *italics* indicate figures; those followed by t indicate tables.

979